Minimally Invasive Thoracic and Cardiac Surgery

Rolf Gilbert Carl Inderbitzi
Ralph Alexander Schmid
Franca M.A. Melfi
Roberto Pasquale Casula
Editors

Minimally Invasive Thoracic and Cardiac Surgery

Textbook and Atlas

Springer

Editors
Rolf G.C. Inderbitzi, M.D.
Thoraxzentrum Zurich
Zurich
Switzerland

Ralph Alexander Schmid, M.D.
Division of General Thoracic Surgery
University Hospital Berne
Berne
Switzerland

Franca M.A. Melfi, M.D.
Department of Cardio-Thoracic Surgery
University of Pisa
Pisa
Italy

Roberto Pasquale Casula, M.D.
Department of Cardiothoracic Surgery
St. Mary's Hospital, Imperial College
Healthcare NHS Trust
London
UK

ISBN 978-3-642-11860-9 ISBN 978-3-642-11861-6 (eBook)
DOI 10.1007/978-3-642-11861-6
Springer Heidelberg New York Dordrecht London

Library of Congress Control Number: 2012953280

Illustrator: Blankvisual GmbH, Thun, Switzerland. www.blankvisual.ch/medicine

Printed on acid-free paper

Springer is part of Springer Science+Business Media (www.springer.com)

Foreword

Surgery in general is associated with the scalpel as the universal instrument for its practice. The scalpel in turn is best described as a sharp as possible bladed instrument which is usually made from hardened stainless steel. However, other materials like obsidian, diamond and ceramics have emerged over time, and further refinements were achieved with specific coatings. Although almost any incision on the surface of the body can be realised with a scalpel, and this includes the thoraco-phreno-laparotomy reaching from the scapula to the pubis which is standard for open repair of the thoraco-abdominal aorta, this is not necessarily the case inside of the body, especially if the access orifice selected is small or minimal as in minimally invasive surgery. Hence, procedures based on electrocautery or laser have emerged.

Visualisation and instrumentation are the two key technologies which are required in addition to skills for successful minimally invasive surgical practice. Video-endoscopy in two or three dimensions can provide direct vision of remote operative targets, and image-guided procedures can be enhanced with fluoroscopy, computerised tomography, ultrasound, magnetic resonance, etc. in real time. Tele-manipulation is at the basis of so-called robotic surgery which is in most cases surgery controlled by a surgeon who manipulates robotic arms that are programmed to follow his instructions. This technology allows for remote procedures through very-small-access orifices which are difficult to access otherwise.

However, robotic surgery is in competition with endoscopic surgery on one side which benefits from increasing sophistication of instrumentation including visualisation, manipulation, suturing and staplers through a single port with a needlescope or even a single instrument which may allow for NOTES (Natural Orifice Transluminal Endoscopic Surgery) versus endovascular procedures which are catheter based and require wire skills. The latter are evolving to full operations through a single stitch with a hollow needle.

It does not require a lot of wisdom to predict that all the technologies mentioned above will eventually grow together, and therefore it is of utmost importance to understand the advantages and drawbacks of all of the different techniques and to recognise their indications as described and perfectly illustrated in this *Textbook and Atlas of Minimally Invasive Thoracic and Cardiac Surgey*.

Lausanne, Switzerland — Ludwig K. von Segesser

Preface

Thoracoscopic surgery made its entry into everyday hospital practice more than 20 years ago and revolutionised conventional surgery. This atlas combines the development of minimally invasive surgery and the resulting experiences and describes and illustrates current surgical techniques.

We are delighted that so many distinguished surgeons who have made a lengthy commitment to the exploration and development of the field of minimal access thoracic and cardiac surgery have now contributed to the creation of this atlas and thank them all for their masterly presentation of the enclosed topics.

Minimally Invasive Thoracic Surgery

In 1989, abdominal and thoracic surgery broke new ground with the use of video technology. Since then, laparoscopic and thoracoscopic procedures have remained the focus of interest. When Springer Verlag published the first monograph on *Thoracoscopic Surgery* in 1993,[1] the author drew on a total of 211 scientific publications on video-thoracoscopy. Eighty-nine of those publications referred to video-thoracoscopic surgery: 18 were principally concerned with this new development and 71 reported on the first clinical experiences from 1,171 thoracoscopies which had been performed on 1,129 patients.

Since then, thoracoscopic surgery has enjoyed equal value with conventional surgery. An increasing number of procedures have in the meantime become routinely carried out as a minimally invasive procedure and no longer performed as an open procedure. Nevertheless, open surgery has also received direct benefit from the knowledge and experience gained from thoracoscopic surgery: anatomical layers and avascular spaces have become clearly visible endoscopically and become routinely accessible to the surgeon, thanks to optical enlargement; careful consideration of these has also led to preparation being perfected for open surgery, to blood saving during operations and, in oncological surgery, to the maintenance of the main postulate and the level of local radicality.

The equivalent outcomes resulting from thoracoscopic procedures mean that minimally invasive tumour resections are beginning to replace the standard open procedures; examples of this are the c-lobectomy (page xy) and VATS lymphadenectomy in the mediastinum (page xy).

[1]Rolf Inderbitzi: Chirurgische Thorakoskopie, Springer Verlag 1993; Rolf Inderbitzi: Surgical Thoracoscopy, Springer Verlag 1994

Developments in thoracoscopic surgery still have a long way to go. At the beginning of the minimally invasive era, diagnostic and predominantly ablative procedures were used, but today we are using ambitious reconstructive procedures, such as sleeve resection for the lung (P.). And, recently, minimally invasive single-port video-assisted thoracoscopic lobectomy (P.) has been added to the range of endoscopic operations via three to four trocar sleeves with or without utility thoracotomy.

Robotic Surgery

Robotic surgery represents a separate new technology within minimally invasive surgery; it provides a digitalised dimension to surgery. Without doubt, it already has an important role in the surgical armoury, although its use in hospitals is not yet fully resolved and its development is proceeding at breakneck speed. Compared to conventional thoracoscopic surgery, which has become a mature, accessible and economical technology everywhere in the last 20 years, robotic surgery remains so far exclusive and expensive, although it has indisputable benefits: 3D visualisation, definitely improved dexterity thanks to 7° of motion, the elimination of physiological tremors caused by the length of instruments, the ability to scale motions, the possibility of carrying out microsurgical steps in operations (e.g. anastomoses), optimised ergonomic position for surgeons and the possibility of telesurgery.

This great potential continues to motivate the purchase of a surgical robot for hospitals specialising in cardiothoracic surgery, in spite of high initial costs and the necessary specialist staff training. The number and manner of procedures in both fields have therefore increased rapidly in the last few years. Since the robot system is also compatible with any computerised information system, the link between CT, MRI and intra-operative video imaging is leading to more targeted and more precise operative steps.

Minimally Invasive Cardiac Surgery

Since the mid-1990s cardiac surgery has shown a progressive and universally rising interest towards the development of minimal invasion and minimal access techniques. However, the total number of minimal access procedures (MICS) performed annually in each country represents an unfair target measure of the actual progress achieved since the 1990s in cardiac surgery given that MICS adoption remains limited to a small percentage of surgeons. The more 'traditional' cardiac surgical community remains concerned about the need of time-consuming and often technically demanding additional training, the increased intra-operative costs and our current clinical practice which takes place in a more-than-ever litigious society. A better picture of the present status of MICS is surely given by the existence of totally converted 'off pump' surgeons and many others who regularly perform their nearly entire annual case loads of isolated aortic and mitral valve procedures via a minimal access route. In the UK only, the percentage of 'off pump' coronary operation has reached a plateau of about 16% in the years 2001–2008, but in real terms, this represents not part but the entire coronary revascularisation workload for an even smaller group of skilful cardiac surgeons.

Robotic surgical systems represent a further adjunct in the surgical armamentarium of cardiac surgeons and probably offer important advantages when used in minimal access coronary revascularization or mitral valve repair surgery; understandably, their efficacy, precision, complication rate and reliability have all been questioned compared to conventional surgical or percutaneous alternatives.

All these aspects have been evaluated favourably in various clinical trials although more evidence is required to demonstrate the superiority of patient reported and functional outcomes of robotic revascularization procedures to justify the additional cost and extensive training required. The totally endoscopic coronary revascularisation procedure with the da Vinci Si appears to be safe with low complication rate and excellent early and midterm reported graft patency rates which grant its role as a safe and efficacious alternative to a LITA to LAD revascularisation via a median sternotomy when performed by an experienced surgical team.

The accessibility to robotic treatment is increasing as the technology becomes more affordable while offered in a multi-disciplinary setting. Furthermore training and mentoring opportunities are currently available for all robotic surgical techniques. However the adoption of robotic technology to current clinical practice is not as widespread as initially anticipated due to several negative drivers and constraints. The safe adoption of all MICS and robotic techniques by cardiac surgeons requires their significant commitment to embark in further time-consuming training which is often very much dissimilar from the previously successfully acquired traditional cardiac surgical one. Robotic surgeons have to undergo a demanding learning curve to achieve clinical proficiency in these modalities. Cardiac robotics and MICS procedures should be safely performed and reproducible; clinical results should be comparable to current results reported with more conventional techniques and standard practice.

Our effort in redeveloping ourselves by approaching new technological tools and learning new techniques has to be weighted against the reality that referral practices in cardiac surgery are constantly changing and are also influenced by the presence of several different therapeutic approaches such the percutaneous ones offered by interventional cardiologists who are ultimately in competition with us for the treatment of the same patients.

Robotic surgery has been extensively applied to perform the LIMA-LAD anastomosis in the contest of a totally endoscopic or atraumatic coronary artery bypass and mitral valve repair. Despite these clinical achievements, the actual penetration of these techniques in most of the industrialised countries remains negligible even following the 2010 publication of the European myocardial revascularisation guidelines by the European task force of the European Society of Cardiology (ESC) and the European Association for Cardiothoracic Surgery (EACTS).

Zurich, Switzerland — Rolf G.C. Inderbitzi
Berne, Switzerland — Ralph A. Schmid
Pisa, Italy — Franca M.A. Melfi
London, UK — Roberto P. Casula

Contents

Part I

Minimally Invasive Thoracic Surgery: General

History of Minimally Invasive Thoracic and Cardiac Surgery

1

Corrado Lavini, Ciro Ruggiero, and Uliano Morandi

Contents

C. Lavini, M.D. (✉) • C. Ruggiero, M.D.
U. Morandi, M.D.
Division of Thoracic Surgery,
Department of General Surgery and Surgical Specialties,
University of Modena and Reggio Emilia,
Policlinico of Modena, Largo del Pozzo 71,
41100 Modena, Italy
e-mail: corrado.lavini@unimore.it;
ciro.ruggiero@unimore.it; uliano.morandi@unimore.it

1.1 Introduction

Minimally invasive thoracic and cardiac surgery has developed into a sound technique over the past 20 years.

It represents an evolution of the early thoracoscopic techniques which were applied in the past century by pulmonologists and internists, mostly aimed at diagnosis and which greatly contributed to the development of an innovative and successful surgical approach.

1.2 Medical Thoracoscopy

The thoracoscope can be considered as the ancestor of the cystoscope, a tool invented in 1807 by the Italian Philippe Bozzini for bladder examination, which employed as a light source the light deriving from a candle reflected in a mirror. Such a tool, called "Lichtleiter", or light conductor, was tested for the first time in Vienna [1].

In 1853, Antoine Jean Desormeaux introduced the term "endoscopist" and created a tool which employed a light source deriving from a lamp burning a mixture of alcohol and turpentine, as well as a lens concentrating the light beam of the flame.

The first thoracoscopy was performed in 1866 by Sir Francis Richard Cruise, who modified Desormeaux's endoscope for the examination of the pleural cavity and introduced it through a fistula in the chest following a metapneumonic empyema [2, 3].

R.G.C. Inderbitzi et al. (eds.), *Minimally Invasive Thoracic and Cardiac Surgery*,
DOI 10.1007/978-3-642-11861-6_1, © Springer-Verlag Berlin Heidelberg 2012

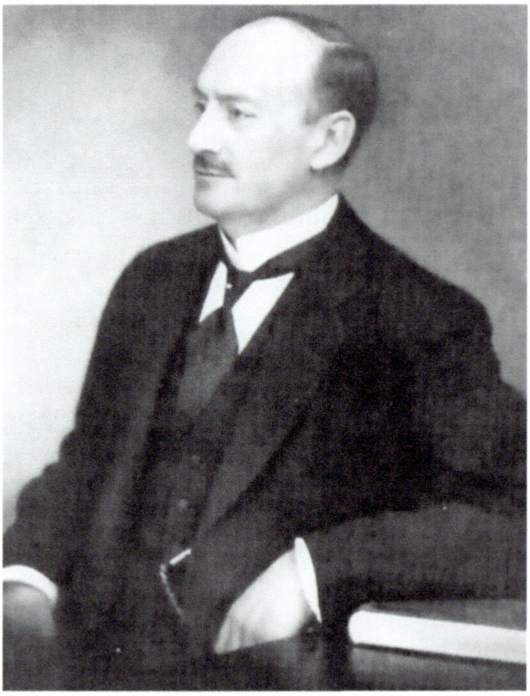

Fig. 1.1 Hans Christian Jacobaeus (1879–1937) (From [4])

In 1886, the thoracoscope was markedly improved when equipped with Thomas Edison's incandescent light bulbs.

However, the technique became steadily performed only at the beginning of the nineteenth century. Its pioneer was the Swedish internist Hans Christian Jacobaeus, who employed a primitive thoracoscope to perform a lysis of pleural adhesions and an effective collapse therapy for cavitary tuberculosis (Fig. 1.1).

In 1882, Forlanini was the first who evidenced how the lobar collapse resulting by pneumothorax or pleural effusion could lead to cavitary tuberculosis remission. He subsequently reproduced the collapse by pneumothorax induction generated injecting air or nitrogen into the pleural cavity [5].

Such technique was then largely performed in the treatment of tuberculosis.

In some patients, the presence of pleural adhesions hindered the ideal goal in the treatment of pneumothorax, i.e. a total lung collapse.

In 1909, Forlanini wrote: "pleural adhesions prevent the occurrence of a complete pneumothorax, and, as a consequence, they prevent the complete rest of the lung treated with pneumothorax".

On these premises, several lung clinicians performed a number of attempts aimed at removing the adhesions from the lung to achieve an effective collapse therapy.

Rowsing was the first to attempt such a procedure by dissecting with the knife two large adhesions through a broad pleurotomy opening. This approach was subsequently applied by other lung clinicians (Jessen, Schottmuller, Sudeck and others), although these attempts were abandoned due to the high frequency of complications such as lung perforations, haemorrhage and pleural cavity infection.

In 1910, H. C. Jacobaeus published on the *Munchener Medizinische Wochenschrift*, a paper with the title "On the Possibility for Performing Cystoscopy in Examinations of Serous Cavities" [4, 6, 7].

In 1911, Jacobaeus published his first experiences on thoracoscopy describing the appearance of the normal pleural cavity and of some pathological alterations, such as exudative pleuritis, pneumothorax and empyema. His first attempt to perform a pleurolysis dates back to 1913 with the technique called "Jacobaeus operation", subsequently described in a paper in 1916.

Such procedure was regarded as extremely relevant in the treatment of tuberculosis and rapidly achieved broad consensus.

Access to the pleural cavity was achieved by positioning bevelled steel cannulae called trocars [8] (Fig. 1.2).

The technique involved patient sedation with bromide or luminal, adhesion identification by fluroroscopy, nearby insertion of a thoracoscope via a first trocar, followed by the insertion of a galvanocautery, a sort of ancestor of the electrical knife, through a second trocar positioned on the anterior axillary line. The galvanocautery was a small metal rod with a platinum loop through which an electrical current could be passed cauterizing and dissecting the adhesion [9]. Pleurolysis usually lasted 1–2 h with constant danger of haemorrhage, especially if the galvanocautery was too strong or if the adhesion was resected too fast.

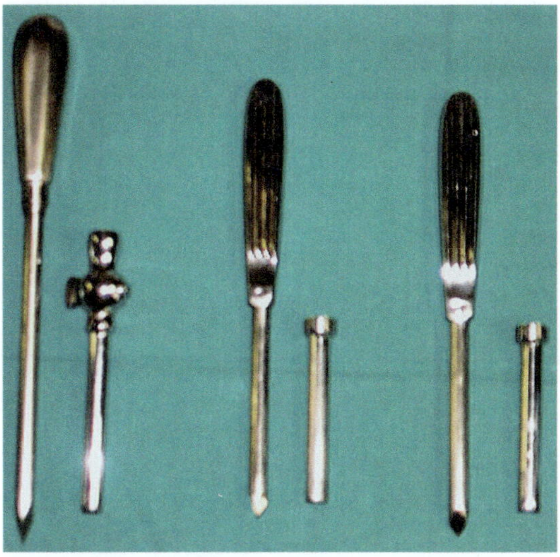

Fig. 1.2 Thoracoscopic trocars (From [8])

Further research by Unverricht [10], Ackermann and Jacobaeus [11] also evidenced that extended adhesions could include areas of alveolar parenchyma up to about 1.5–2 cm from their visceral implant. Therefore, a dissection falling near the adhesion visceral implant could result in a dissection of groups of alveoli, then compressing and eventually leading to early lung perforation (due to direct visceral lesion) or late lung perforation (due to the delayed burn eschar detachment).

The quite high rate of sometimes severe complications secondary to the Jacobaeus operation resulted in a limited number of studies carried on the diagnostic performance of thoracoscopy for many years.

The most commonly used tool was a simple thoracoscope with an optical system, made of a steel tube of 22 cm in length and 0.5 cm in diameter, equipped on the distal tip with a 3-V incandescent light bulb and a 90° side-viewing optic [8] (Fig. 1.3a, b).

Jacobaeus' two-cannula technique was then adopted in Europe and the USA. It was later modified by Davidson and then by Culter, with a single entry port, therefore a single tool. However, the advantage provided by "port-holes" reduction was offset by a limited view of the pleural cavity.

A further but unsuccessful development was the adoption of a bronchoscope to perform thoracoscopy. Such an attempt was soon abandoned due to the high rate of complications, among which fatal haemorrhage. The pulmonologist Felice Cova (1887–1935) played a key role in the development of thoracoscopy in Italy, also writing two books with extensive colour pictures: "*Thoracoscopy – Jacobaeus Operation*" [13], published in 1927 on the experience acquired in diagnostic thoracoscopy and in pleurolysis (Figs. 1.4, 1.5, and 1.6), and *Atlas Thoracoscopicon* [14], published in 1928 with an excellent selection of endoscopic pictures of the pleural cavity.

In the 1930s and 1940s, although indications of thoracoscopy were limited to the treatment of cavitary tuberculosis, some authors started to evidence the diagnosis potential of the procedure.

Sattler played a relevant role in 1937, with pleural endoscopy in the detection and treatment of idiopathic spontaneous pneumothorax [8, 15].

In 1938, Lelong reported a case of *situs viscerum inversus*, and, in another patient, he evidenced an aneurysm of the descending aorta.

In 1939, Sergent diagnosed a case of pleural mesothelioma by biopsy sampling, while Fabbri and co-workers in 1942 applied thoracoscopy to histologically detect a case of pleural neoplasm and nine cases of tuberculosis [8].

Collapse therapy and adhesiolysis by thoracoscopy remained the gold standard in cavitary tuberculosis until 1945, with the introduction of streptomycin antibiotic therapy.

Since then, thoracoscopy was slowly abandoned in the treatment of tuberculosis, while it broadened its scope of application in new diagnostic fields, especially in pleural effusion, also as a result of the increased incidence of mesothelioma in industrialized countries.

Although Jacobaeus technique was gradually discontinued, several European centres continued to perform thoracoscopy providing more precise indications, especially for diagnosis, and broadening the technique by introducing lung biopsy and mediastinal biopsy [8].

In the 1970s, thoracoscopy was revived with a steady diffusion of pleural endoscopy and an increase in the number of scientific papers on the

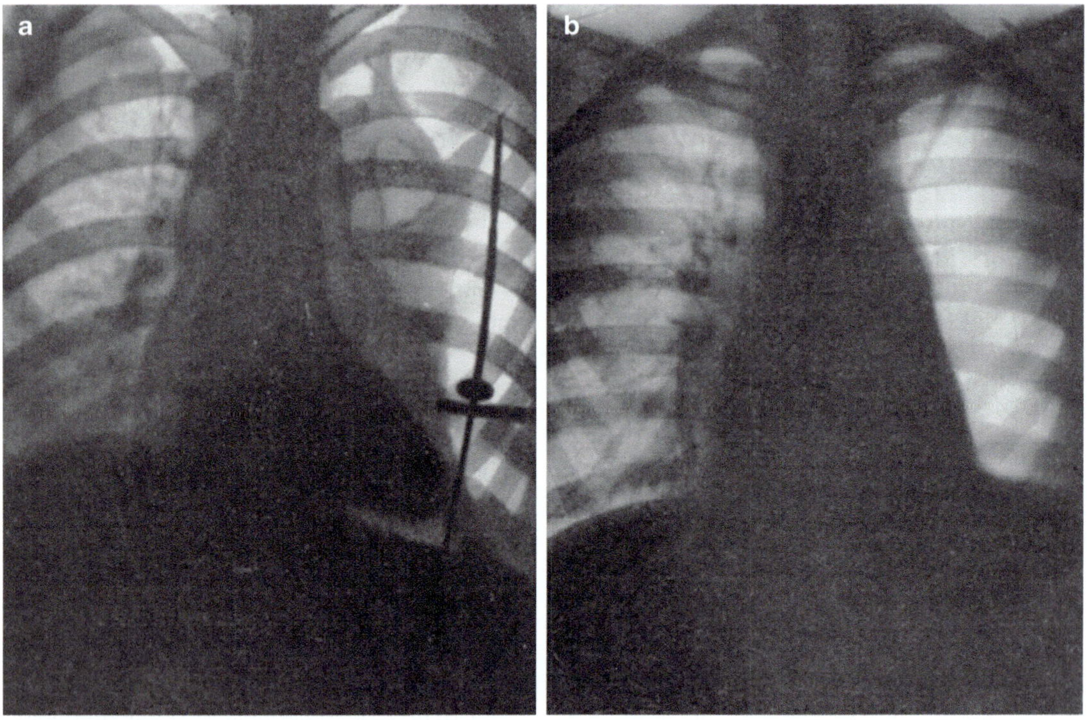

Fig. 1.3 Intrapleural pleurolysis following Jacobaeus. X-rays during and after the intervention. Thoracoscope with galvanocautery applied to a lateral adhesion (**a**). Same case after pleurolysis: total collapse of the left lung (**b**) (From Costantini and Redaelli [12])

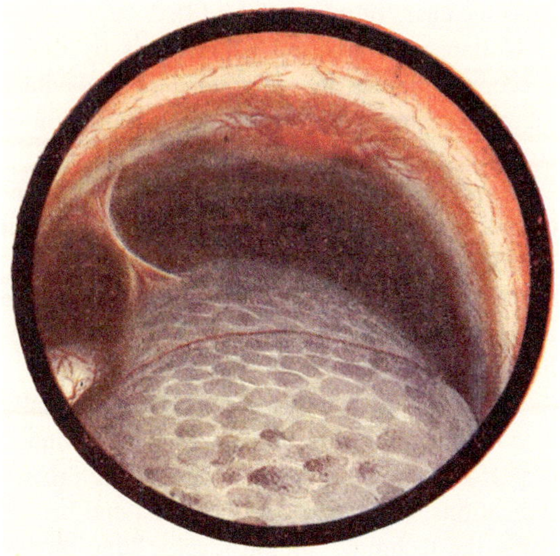

Fig. 1.4 Acute pleuritis with plates. Costal parietal pleura with area of plate hypervascularization. Veiling plate adhesion on the superior lobe (From [14], quoted by kind allowance of B.C.F.)

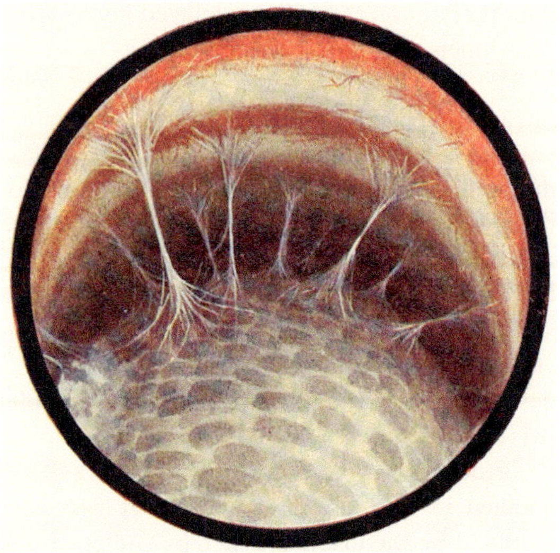

Fig. 1.5 Serofibrinous pleuritis secondary to thoracic trauma. Costal parietal pleura widespread hyperemia with soft fibrinous adhesions on the superior lobe (From [14], quoted by kind allowance of B.C.F.)

subject, leading to an improvement of techniques by the use of cold light sources.

Over that period, a large number of papers reported the higher diagnostic value of thoracoscopy compared with pleural needle biopsy, introduced by De Francis in 1955, and with cytology in cases of chronic pleural effusion [8].

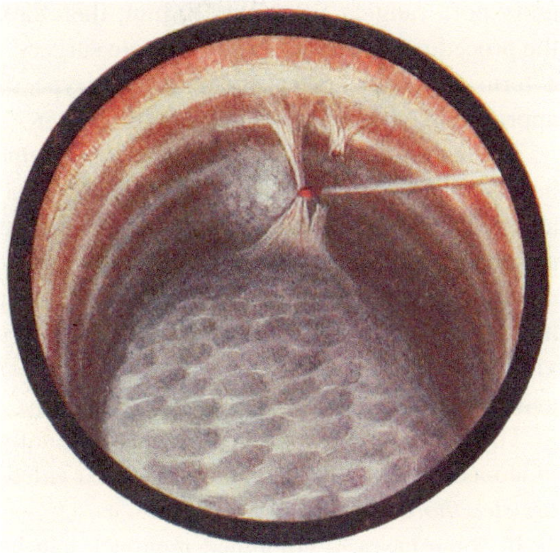

Fig. 1.6 Cavitary tuberculosis. Jacobaeus intervention. Pleurolysis with galvanocautery of cord-like apical adhesion (From [14], quoted by kind allowance of B.C.F.)

In 1978, Bloomberg carried out a comparative study between thoracoscopy and pleural needle biopsy. Analyzing several case loads, needle biopsy proved to achieve diagnostic results in a percentage between 30% and 60%, especially on tuberculosis with widespread pleural involvement. The diagnostic rate was markedly higher with thoracoscopy, also including neoplasms, allowing for etiologic diagnosis in 74% of cases [16].

The first "International Symposium on Thoracoscopy" was held in 1980, aimed at disseminating among pulmonologists and internists the indications and the techniques of thoracoscopy. The event was organized by Boutin in Marseille and received large consensus in the medical community [17].

In the same period, the technique was advanced with the introduction of the operative thoracoscope, in which the optical was separated from the operating channel, making endoscopic biopsies easier and safer (Fig. 1.7).

Different books fully devoted to thoracoscopy date back to that period, among which "*Diagnostic Thoracoscopy*" by G. Alcozer and A. Dorigoni, published in 1984 as the first Italian treaty after the two monographs published by Cova 60 years earlier [8, 17, 18].

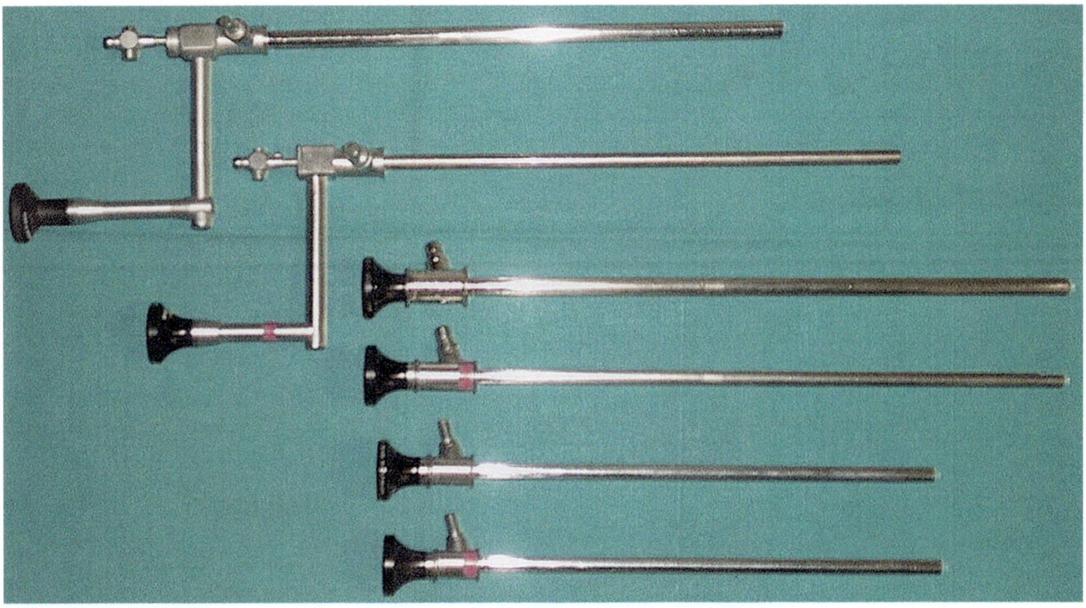

Fig. 1.7 "Bayonet" operative thoracoscopes and thoracoscopic optics (From [8])

In the late 1980s, video-assisted laparoscopy was introduced in general surgery obtaining immediate consensus. Following the success of video-assisted laparoscopy, a new type of thoracoscopic procedure with mainly surgical features started to be gradually performed: video-assisted thoracoscopy.

1.3 Video-Assisted Thoracoscopy

The transition from a mainly diagnostic *medical thoracoscopy* to a fully operative *surgical thoracoscopy* took place in the first 1990s. By connecting the thoracoscope to a video, all the different steps of the procedure could be followed on a screen, allowing the involvement of all the surgical team, while in medical thoracoscopy the endoscopist alone could have the view of the operative field.

With the development of the technological support (miniaturized video cameras, subcentimetre optics, dedicated and innovative equipment, especially endoscopic stapler devices), the methodology further advanced in a few years, allowing to perform even complex procedures. This was the beginning of *video-assisted thoracoscopy*. It requires, as basic equipment, a screen, a light source, an optical and/or magnetic recording device and a thoracoscopic optical connected to a video camera (Figs. 1.8 and 1.9).

This innovative surgical approach allows to explore the pleural cavity and endothoracic organs with minimal incisions and to perform even complex interventions, otherwise inconceivable with the conventional techniques without video-assisted endoscopy of the previous decades.

It is a new and rapidly advancing methodology, raising an extremely large consensus since its very beginning. The video-assisted endoscope is inserted in the pleural cavity through a variable entry port, ranging from 7 to 20 mm; therefore, the procedure is referred to as "keyhole surgery", a term which clearly depicts the new type of approach [8].

The thoracoscopic approach represents a number of advantages versus the conventional "open" approach, among which its application also to patients at risk for thoracotomy, a shorter post-operative recovery, better aesthetic result, lower hospitalization costs, and, from the surgeon's viewpoint, a broader operative view also with 2D and non-stereoscopic images.

The intervention can be performed by totally video-assisted endoscopy, and it is called *video-assisted thoracic surgery – VATS.*

In some cases, a combined approach can be selected, performing both "open", but limited, and video-assisted endoscopic procedures. Such a technique allows even complex procedures to heart, lung, oesophagus and diaphragm, with a remarkably reduced operative traumatism compared with the conventional "open" approach [8].

Overall, these completely or partially video-assisted endoscopic access techniques are defined as *minimally invasive cardiothoracic surgery*.

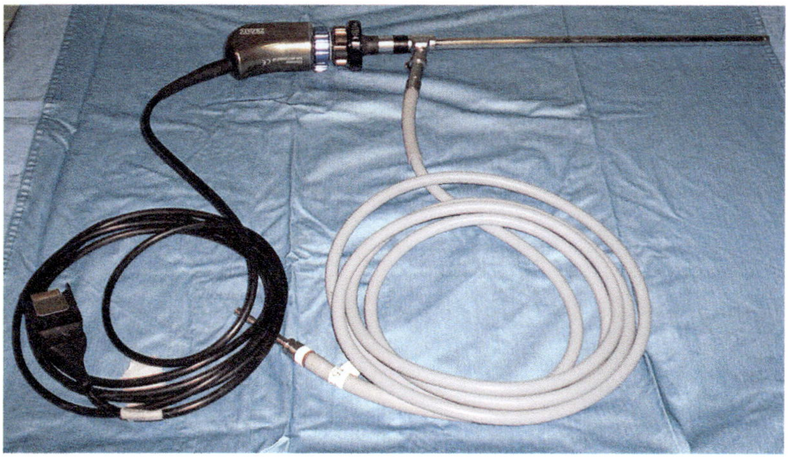

Fig. 1.8 Videothoracoscope

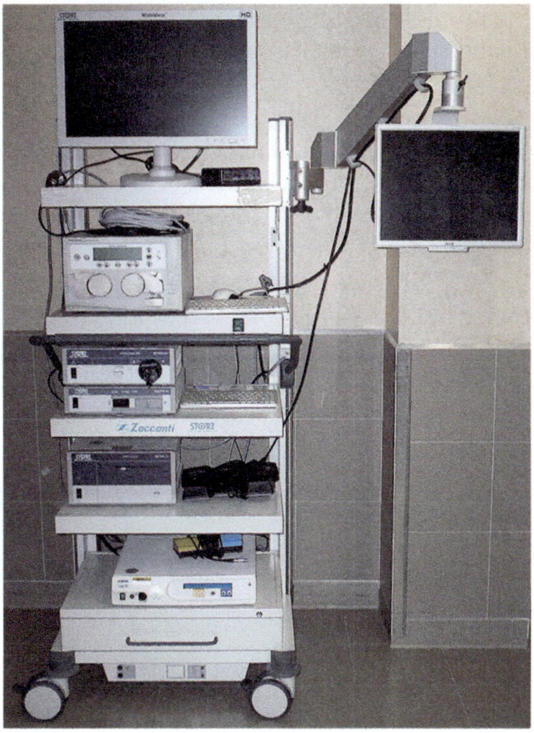

Fig. 1.9 Screen column (Storz)

In 1990, Levi and associates performed the first pleurectomy with video-assisted thoracoscopy to treat pneumothorax [19].

In 1991, Wakabayashi was the first who proposed video-assisted thoracoscopy in the treatment of pleural empyema in adults [20], while Kern and Rogers introduced it in children in 1993 [21].

Landreneau and co-workers, Roviaro and associates (1992) and Kirby and collaborators (1993) published the first caseloads of video-assisted thoracoscopic lung lobectomies [22–24].

In 1994, Inderbitzi and co-workers reported their 3-year experience on video-assisted thoracoscopy for spontaneous pneumothorax [25].

Video-assisted endoscopic examination of thoracic compartments was not just limited to the pleural cavity. Indeed, it was also applied for the mediastinal compartment, with the experiences by Medrano and co-workers, who performed the first thoracoscopic resection of ectopic parathyroid glands in 1992 [26], and of Sugarbaker, who applied the first procedures of thymectomy and of resection of bronchogenic and pleural pericardial cysts in 1993 [27].

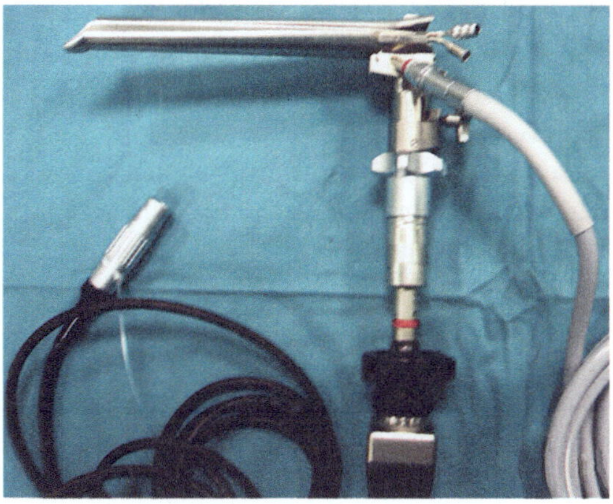

Fig. 1.10 Videomediastinoscope (From [8])

In 1992, Cuschieri and co-workers reported the first video-assisted thoracoscopic esophagectomy [28], while in 1993, Bumm and co-workers performed the first mediastinoscope-assisted transhiatal esophagectomy (MATHE) [29].

In 1993, Kent and Pison proposed the thoracoscopic ligation of the thoracic duct [30], while Cuschieri and co-workers in 1994 reported the first bilateral splanchnicectomy through video-assisted thoracic approach [31].

In 1994, Sortini and co-workers refined mediastinoscopy connecting a video camera to Carlens' speculum (*video-assisted mediastinoscopy – VAM*) [32, 33] (Fig. 1.10).

Technical advances and increased procedure mastering by surgeons lead to a broader application of video-assisted thoracoscopic approaches. The first extensive caseload studies, as well as new indications to video-assisted approaches, were also reported in literature.

In 1996, Kao and co-workers published a caseload review on 9,988 patients treated with video-assisted endoscopic sympathectomy for palmar hyperhidrosis [34].

Mouroux and co-workers in 1996 published an innovative technique for the video-assisted treatment of diaphragmatic eventration, followed in 2005 by a prospective study on 12 patients who underwent the operation [35, 36].

In 1997, Roberts and co-workers reported the first case of descending necrotizing mediastinitis managed through video-assisted thoracoscopic approach [37].

Always in 1997, Jiménez-Merchan carried a comparative retrospective study on the surgical treatment of pneumothorax, comparing 627 patients operated by an "open" conventional technique versus 110 patients by VATS [38].

In 1998, Nuss published a 10-year review of the minimally invasive technique for the correction of pectus excavatum, known as Nuss repair [39].

In 2006, McKenna published his experience of video-assisted thoracic surgery lobectomy with 1,100 cases [40], while Tomulescu and co-workers in the same year conducted a retrospective analysis on 107 patients who underwent thymectomy by thoracoscopic approach for myasthenia gravis [41].

In cardiothoracic surgery, the first video-assisted interventions on congenital pathologies were performed in 1993 by Laborde and co-workers (patent ductus arteriosus) [42] and by Burke and co-workers (vascular ring division) [43].

In the same year, Gersak and co-workers performed the first endoscopic aortic valve replacement [44].

Always in 1993, the pericardial cavity was explored (*pericardioscopy*) on the first contributions by Mack and co-workers [45] as well as Inderbitzi and coworkers (see page 301).

In 1994, Benetti and colleagues described the first beating-heart coronary artery bypass graft surgery performed by video-assisted endoscopic support [46], followed by similar experiences in Europe and the USA [47–49].

After some years from the introduction of video-assisted thoracoscopic techniques, indications to minimally invasive cardiothoracic surgery started to be standardized for diagnosis, staging and therapy. In thoracic surgery, indications involve not only pleural but also mediastinal diseases, lung, oesophageal, diaphragmatic and thoracic malformative diseases and trauma; in cardiac surgery, they comprise pericardial disease, some inborn and valve diseases, and coronary disease.

Consensus on minimally invasive cardiothoracic surgery was supported by a growing scientific literature on the subject, not simply limited to a number of caseload reviews, but also devoting important monographs to the subject.

Of the latter, we list the following: *Thoracoscopic Surgery* by L.R. Kaiser and T.M. Daniel (1993), *Minimally Invasive Surgery* by J.G. Hunter and J.M. Sackier (1993), *Minimally Invasive Surgery* by F.M. Steichen and R. Wetter (1994), *Atlas of Video-Assisted Thoracic Surgery* by W.T. Brown (1994), *Surgical Thoracoscopy* by L. Gossot (1994), *Thoracoscopy for Surgeons. Diagnostic and Therapeutic. Infrequent indications* by R.A. Dieter Jr. (1995), *Laparoscopic and Thoracoscopic Surgery* by T.C. Frantzides (1995), *Surgical Thoracoscopy* by R. Inderbitzi (1994), *Videothoracoscopic Surgery* by J. Krasna (1995), *Video-Assisted Thoracic Surgery* by W.S. Walker (1999), the Italian *Videotoracoscopia* by G. Di Falco (1999), *Thoracoscopic Surgery* by D. Wood and T. Marchioro (2000), the Italian *Chirurgia Toracica Videoassistita* by C. Lavini. C. Ruggiero, U. Morandi (2006).

At present, urgent and elective cardiothoracic surgical procedures are performed by video-assisted thoracoscopic approach with a percentage ranging from 20% to 30%. Such percentage could increase with a further improvement in indications and techniques.

1.4 Robotic Thoracic and Cardiac Surgery

Robotic surgery is the natural evolution of video-assisted surgery.

The term "robot" comes from Czech and means "forced labour" or also "slave".

A robot is but a computer-controlled system that executes a specific set of instructions and that can perform even complex tasks with great precision. It was first used in the second half of the twentieth century for industrial, research (space, interplanetary and deep-sea explorations), transportation and military applications.

Although video-endoscopic techniques opened up new scenarios and rapidly raised broad consensus, they clearly presented with limitations, i.e. the lack of 3D view, the limited degrees of freedom of the tools (just four, as opposed to the

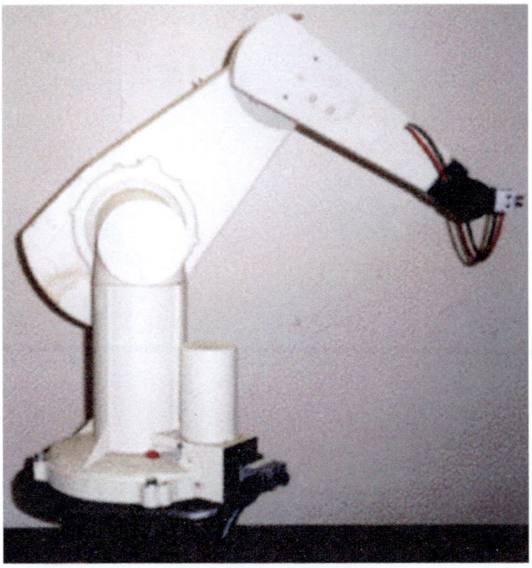

Fig. 1.11 PUMA 560® Surgical System

seven degrees of the human wrist), the transmission to the tools of natural tremors and the lack of tactile feedback. All of these issues could make delicate dissections or complex anastomosis demanding, to the point of hindering them [50].

With a view to overcoming the technical and structural barriers of video-assisted endoscopic surgery, in the mid-1980s, the first attempts were made to apply robotic principles and systems to surgery.

Robotic surgery is defined as a surgical technique that uses a computer-assisted electromechanic system located between the operator and the patient. Thanks to this complex technology, the operator is capable of constantly controlling the entire procedure, though indirectly and remotely from the patient [51, 52].

The first primitive surgical robot to be used was PUMA 560® Surgical System, a modified industrial robot equipped with a mechanical arm which, in 1985, enabled Kwoh and co-workers to perform a CT-guided brain needle biopsy [53] (Fig. 1.11).

In 1988, Davies and co-workers used the same robotic device to perform the first transurethral resection of the prostate [54].

In 1989, Benabid and associates developed a medical robot specially designed for stereotactic neurosurgery, the NEUROMATE® (Renishaw Mayfield SA).

The NEUROMATE® image-guided neurosurgical robot is cleared by European and US regulations and quickly gained an international following. Today, the system is in use at over a dozen top neurosurgical centres and has allowed to perform thousands of interventions [55] (Fig. 1.12).

In 1991, the evolution of the device named PUMA 560® led to the creation of another robot, the PROBOT®, a system specifically conceived to perform urological surgery, and consisting of a computer-driven rotating blade enabling surgeons to safely perform transurethral resections of the prostate [56].

In the same year, Integrated Surgical Supplies Ltd., based in Sacramento, CA, developed ROBODOC®, the first FDA-approved surgical robot to be used specifically for reconstructive and prosthetic surgery of the hip: the robotic arm enables to precisely incise the femur bone to introduce surgical devices therein under the guidance of 3D CT images [57–60] (Fig. 1.13).

In 1993, Computer Motion, based in Goleta, CA, introduced for the first time the AESOP® Surgical System. This system is equipped with a voice- or pedal-controlled robotic arm that is used to hold the video-endoscopic optics, thus allowing the operator to use both hands for surgical manoeuvres. Over 70,000 video-assisted heart, general and urologic procedures were performed with the support of AESOP® [60, 61] (Fig. 1.14).

However, the robotic systems described above did not allow to perform complete robot-assisted surgery procedures. Indeed, they performed quite simple functions and played a substantially limited role in the surgical procedure as a whole. In practice, these were either positioning systems used to assist the surgeon during the procedure, or supporting arms for video-assisted endoscopic techniques which could change their position to meet the needs of the operator.

Only a few years later, a new generation of more complex surgical robots was conceived.

NASA and the US Armed Forces started to develop machines equipped with remote-presence

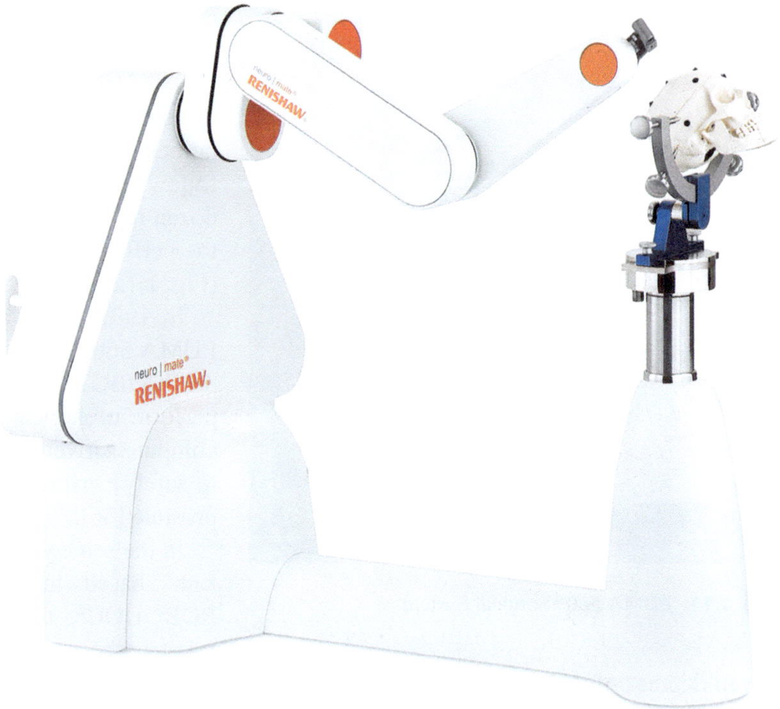

Fig. 1.12 NEUROMATE® Surgical System. ©[2010] *Renishaw Mayfield SA*

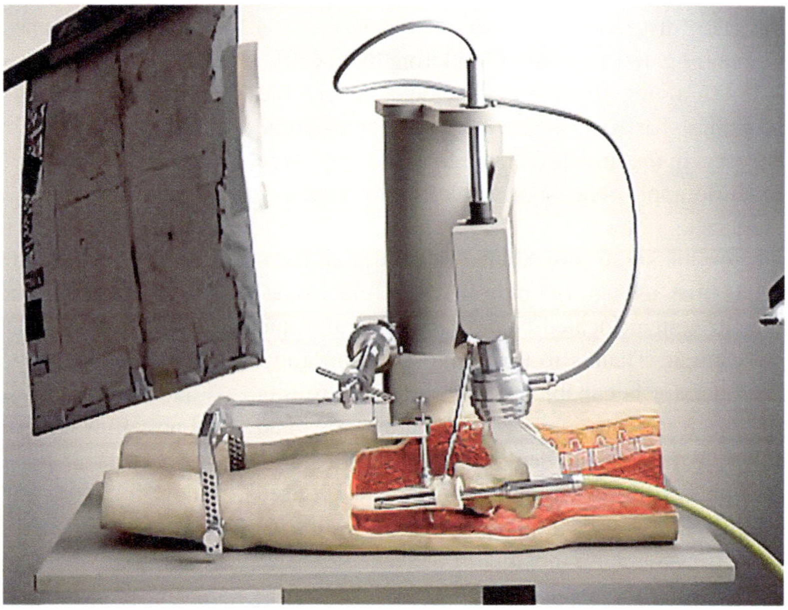

Fig. 1.13 ROBODOC® Surgical System. ©[2010] *Curexo Technology Corporation*

systems, i.e. systems performing actions at a distance through an interface (computer, satellite network, remote systems) and establishing a relationship between the operator and the environment through advanced technological media, sensors and robotic instruments. Remote presence allowed not only to perform actions at a distance but also to have a physical perception of the place.

As a result of the momentum generated by these new technological advances, innovative

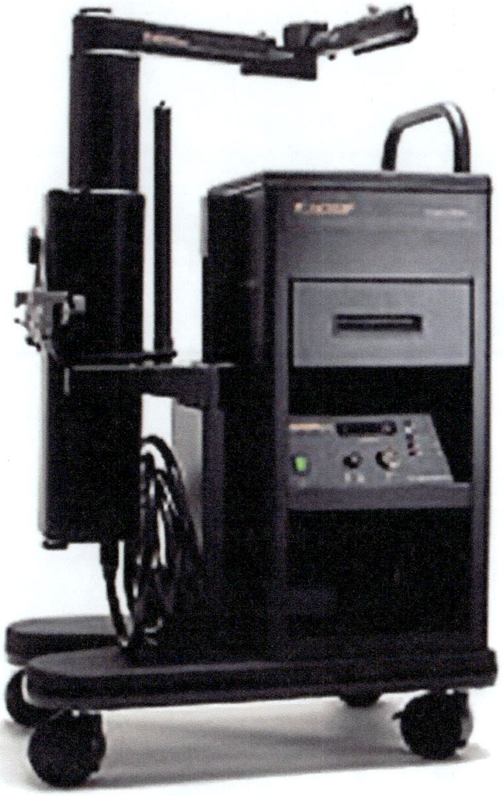

Fig. 1.14 AESOP® Surgical System

surgical robots were designed relying upon a master-slave system of three elements:

- Master, i.e. the control unit, the surgeon's working space, equipped with a screen, a console with knobs, buttons and pedals enabling the operator to move the instruments as part of a sophisticated system that eliminates hand tremors
- Slave, i.e. the executing unit, which actually performs the surgical procedure; it is positioned close to the patient and is composed of the robotic arms and the surgical instruments that can be replaced, including during surgery. This unit is remotely controlled by the movements of the surgeon on the control unit. The instruments are highly mobile, much more than those used in video-assisted endoscopic surgery
- Communication, i.e. the high-tech IT system for information transfer between master and slave and vice versa

The first robot of this generation was ZEUS®, developed in 1998 by Computer Motions, and equipped with a 2D imaging system, a console for the operator and three mechanical arms. The right and left arm corresponded to the operator, while the third arm was provided by a voice-controlled AESOP® robot holding the video endoscope; each arm has four degrees of freedom. In the ZEUS® System, the operator could sit in an ergonomic position in front of an open console, allowing the operator to see the patient and the operating table. The operator could drive the manipulators, which would appropriately filter and transfer the movements to the controlling computer, subsequently moving the robot's arms. A screen was located in front of the surgeon and reproducing 2D images of the operating field. The operator should wear 3D spectacles allowing stereoscopic vision.

ZEUS® was the first system that allowed to perform fully endoscopic robotic heart and general surgery.

In 2001, the ZEUS® robot was used by Jacques Marescaux, based in Strasbourg, to perform the first overseas remote surgery procedure.

Currently, this surgical robot is no longer manufactured because its distributor was taken over by Intuitive Surgery in 2003; however, it continues to be used in many hospitals [50, 52, 62] (Fig. 1.15a, b).

In 1999, Intuitive Surgery, based in Mountain View, CA, further developed the ZEUS® robot into the DA VINCI® Surgical System, FDA-approved in 2001 (Fig. 1.16a, b).

Currently, this is the most widely employed robotic system, with 850 systems installed across the world (2008 data). It is comprised of:

1. A control console. The operator performs the surgical procedure sitting comfortably at the console and looking into a special binocular visor linked to the video endoscope, which, having two parallel chambers that send the images separately to each eye of the surgeon, result in a 3D vision (Fig. 1.17). The operator, plunged in the console's binocular visor, can no longer see the patient and the operating table as he/she used to do with the ZEUS® robot, unless he/she moves away from the workstation with the visor.

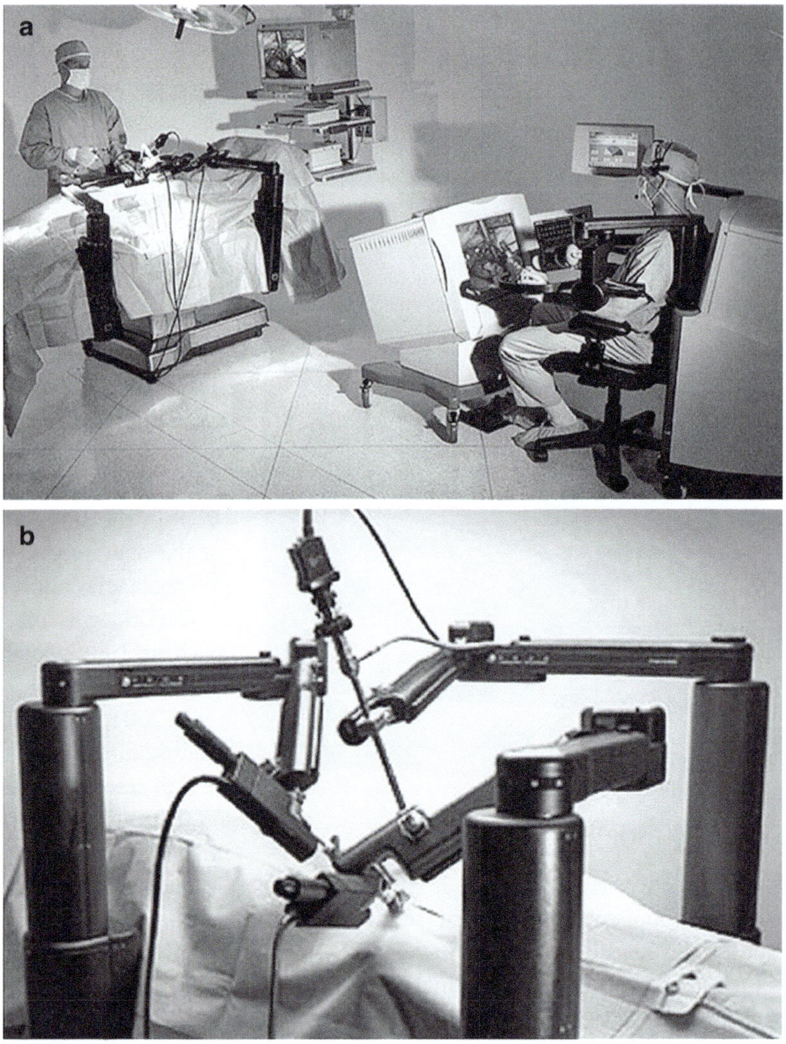

Fig. 1.15 (**a**, **b**) ZEUS® Surgical System

The manipulators are beneath the console level. These are devices equipped with digital sensors used to transmit the movements of the surgeon to the robotic arms; a pedal assembly sits on the floor to control the focus of the visor and the harmonic scalpel and to drive robotic arms (clutch) (Figs. 1.18, 1.19, and 1.20).

2. The surgical robot. Located alongside the operating table on which the patient lies, it is equipped with four arms, of which three are dedicated to the instruments linked to ad hoc trocars, and one to the video endoscope. Each arm has seven degrees of freedom (*EndoWrist*®), allowing all movements in the space without limitations to the operator. The natural human tremor is appropriately filtered and is therefore not transmitted to the instruments (Figs. 1.21 and 1.22).
3. The video trolley. It contains the 3D video camera, one screen allowing the other team members located at the patient's bedside to monitor the timing of the surgical procedure, a light source for the endoscope, an image recording system, a laparoscopic insufflator [50, 52, 62–64].

As compared to ZEUS®, the DA VINCI® System undoubtedly encompasses a number of advantages allowing its broader and more successful application (stereoscopic vision, seven degrees of freedom of movement, filtering of natural

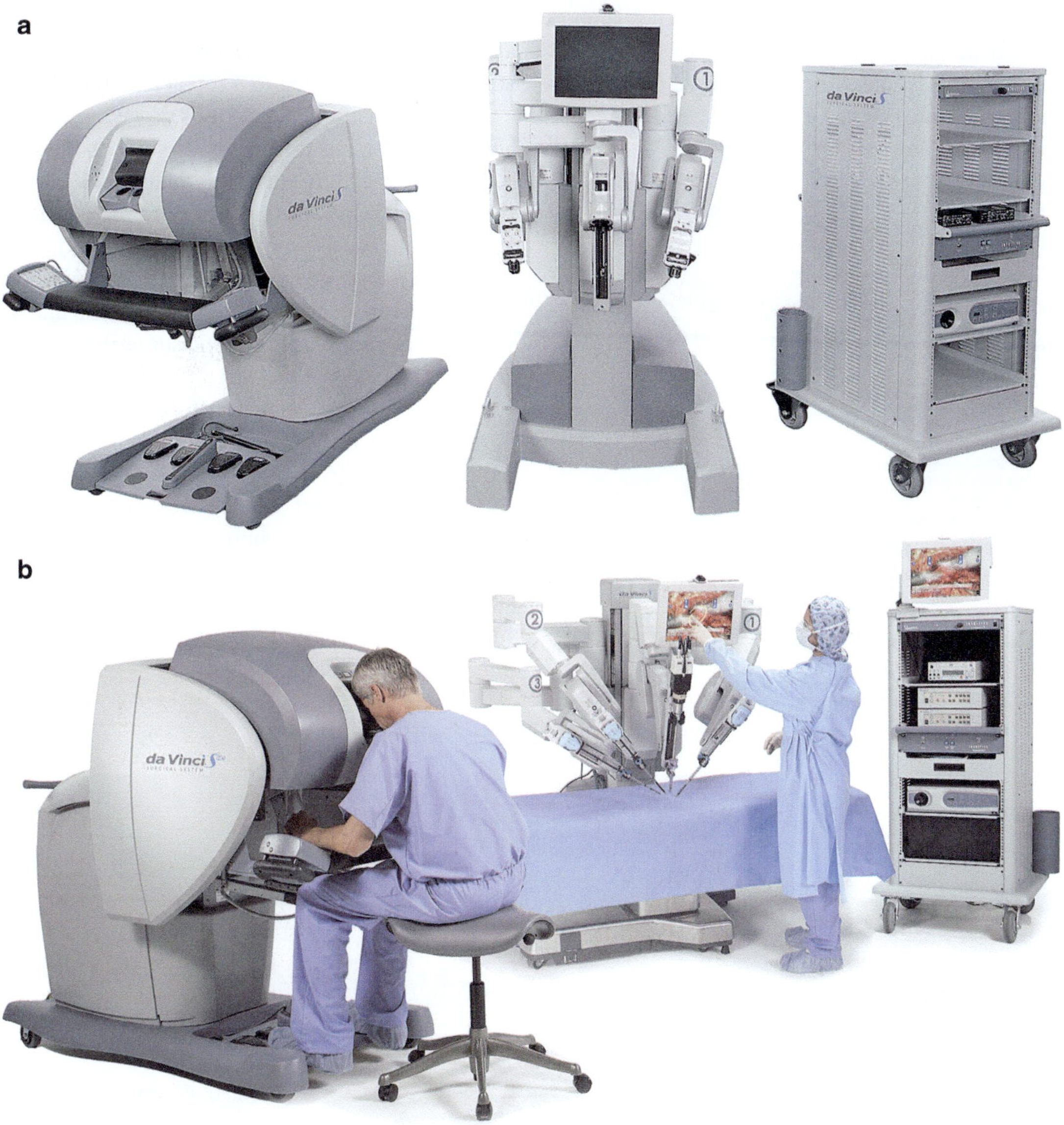

Fig. 1.16 (**a**, **b**) DA VINCI® Surgical System. Full view. ©[2010] *Intuitive Surgical Inc.*

tremor). Its latest evolution provides for the use of two separate consoles occupied by two operators who perform the procedure as a tandem, using all four arms or the robot. The twin console also plays an essential role for surgeon training (Fig. 1.23).

Heart surgery was one of the first branches to apply latest-generation surgical robots.

The benefits derived from ZEUS®, and especially from the DA VINCI® System, in performing complex surgical procedures requiring great accuracy as compared to video-assisted endoscopic techniques, contributed to the immediate application and success of robots in heart surgery, whereas thoracic surgery only adopted robots some years later.

The first robotic surgery procedure ever done was a cholecystectomy, performed in 1997 by the team of the Belgian surgeon Cadiere [65]; just a few months later, the first robotic heart surgical procedures started to be performed, in which, using open-surgery ports, the robot was given a support role to minimize the invasiveness of the "open" approach. Only later, fully endoscopic robotic surgical procedures started to be performed.

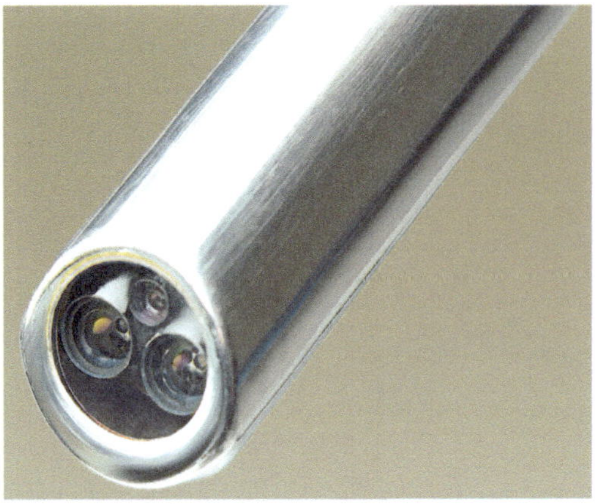

Fig. 1.17 DA VINCI® Surgical System: video-assisted endoscope with parallel chambers allowing 3D vision. ©[2010] *Intuitive Surgical Inc.*

In 1998, Carpentier and co-workers performed a robot-assisted open-heart repair of a broad interatrial defect associated to a septal aneurism [66].

One month after Carpentier's procedure, Mohr and co-workers performed the first robot-assisted repair of the left internal mammary artery (LIMA), which was anastomized to the coronary artery through a left mini-thoracotomy [67].

In that same year, Loulmet and co-workers reported the first cases of two patients who underwent a fully endoscopic robotic surgery for aorto-coronary bypass with LIMA (TECAB) [68].

In 2002, Lange's team performed, with 1-cm ports, the first fully endoscopic robotic repair of the mitral valve [69].

In 2000, Le Bret and co-workers started to perform a robotic interruption of a patent arterial duct [70], and Torracca and co-workers in 2001 and Wimmer-Greinecker and co-workers in 2003 successfully performed the first robotic repairs of interatrial septal defects [71, 72].

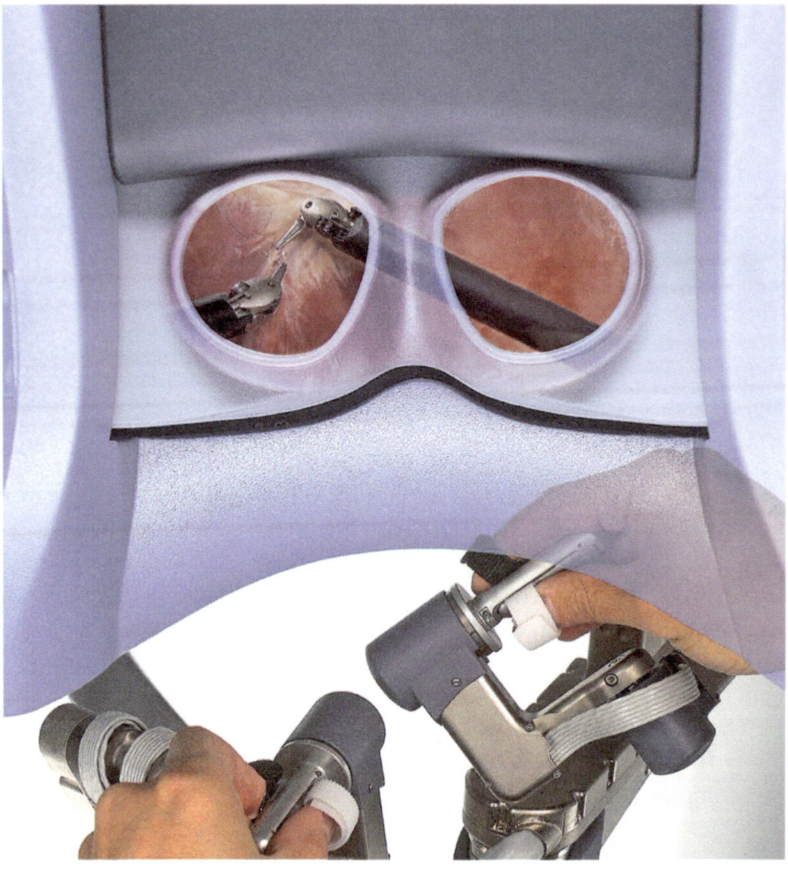

Fig. 1.18 DA VINCI® Surgical System. Control console: binocular visor and manipulators. ©[2010] *Intuitive Surgical Inc.*

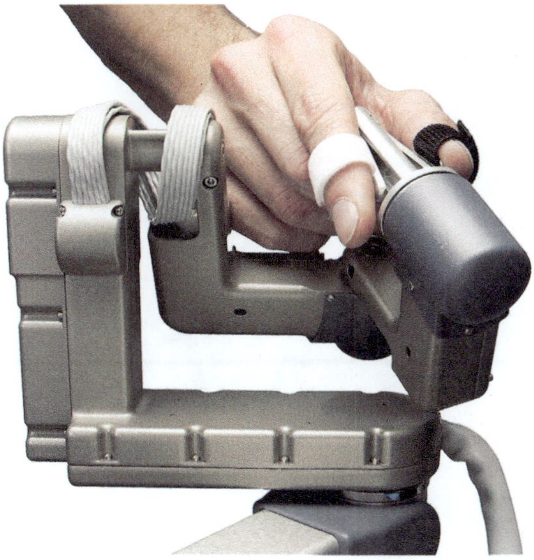

Fig. 1.19 DA VINCI® Surgical System. Manipulator with digital sensors. ©[2010] *Intuitive Surgical Inc.*

In 2004, Folliguet and co-workers performed the first robot-assisted aortic valve replacement using a right anterior mini-thoracotomy [73].

In 2005, Murphy and co-workers reported their experience in treating three atrial myxomas with a robotic approach [74], while almost at the same time, Woo and co-workers removed with a robotic approach an aortic valve papillary fibroelastoma [75].

The first to pioneer atrial fibrillation robotic surgery were Gerosa and co-workers: the electrothermal ablation of the right upper pulmonary vein was smoothly performed with a fully endoscopic approach in 2005 [76].

In the same year, Derose and co-workers reported the first cases of robotic positioning of a left ventricular lead [77].

Among the most significant case reports, mention should be made of the following: the Chitwood

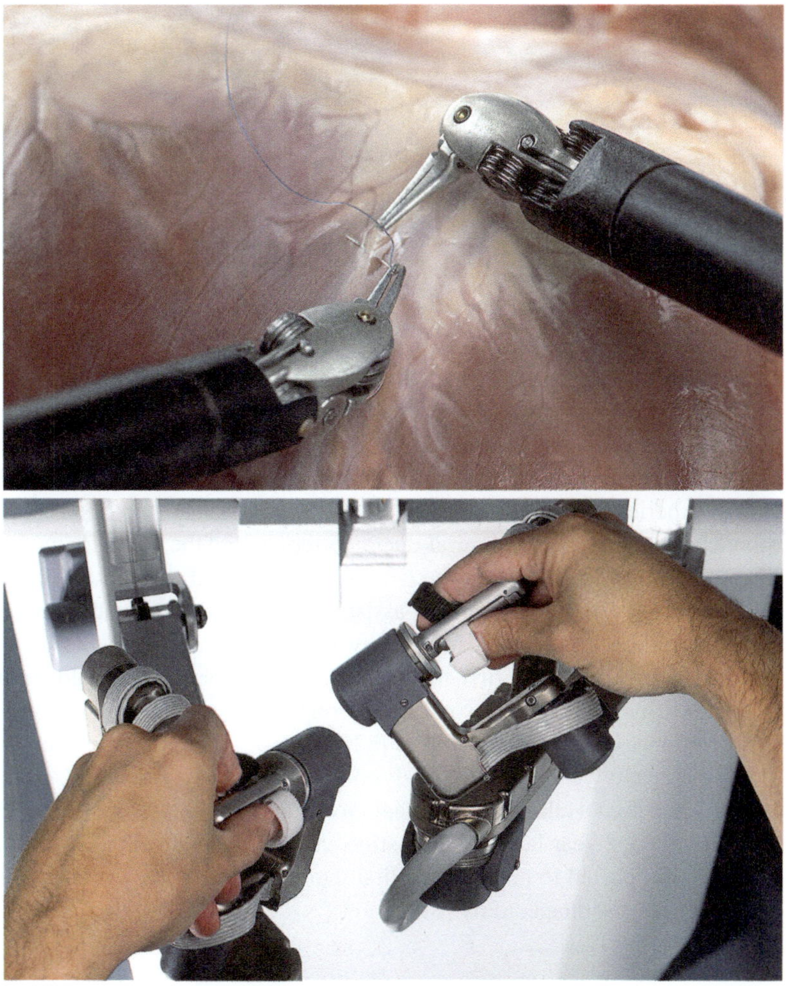

Fig. 1.20 DA VINCI® Surgical System. Movement transmission from manipulators to robotic arms. ©[2010] *Intuitive Surgical Inc.*

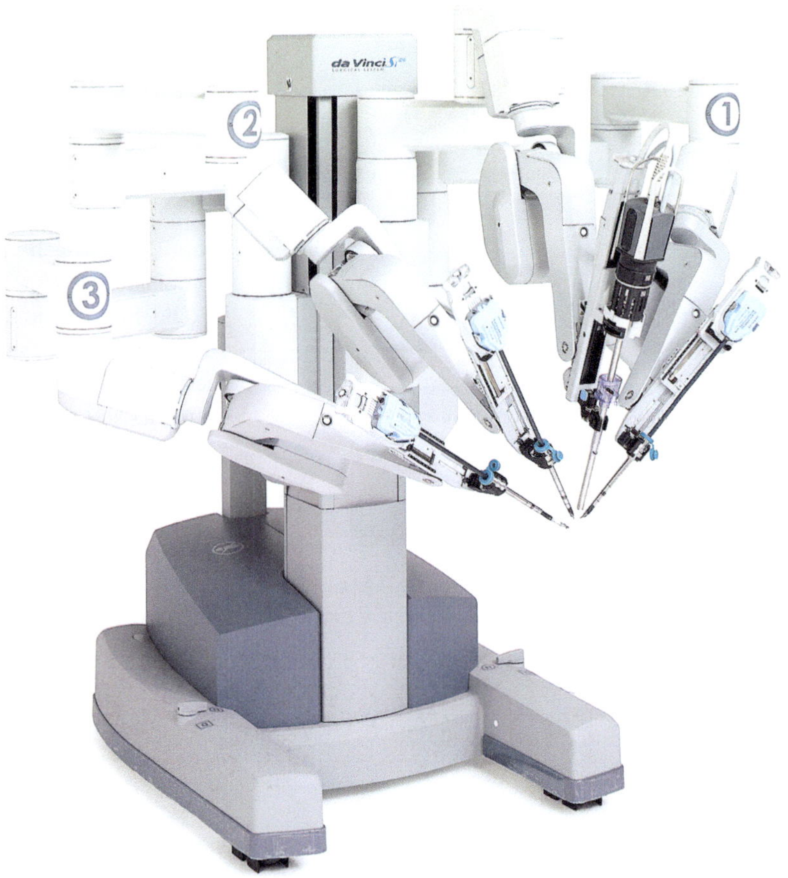

Fig. 1.21 DA VINCI® Surgical System. The four robotic arms. ©[2010] *Intuitive Surgical Inc.*

group, reporting a total of 150 mitral valves operated with robotic surgery in 2005 [78]; de Cannière and co-workers publishing a multicentric review of 228 patients who underwent TECAB in 2007 [79]; and the Del Nido group reporting their 2-year experience with 15 patients treated with robotic surgery for patent arterial duct and repair of vascular rings in 2008 [80].

In thoracic surgery, the first robot-assisted surgical procedures were performed in 2000, by Yoshino and co-workers, with the first thymectomy [81], and in 2001 by Melfi and co-workers reporting the first experiences with lobar resections [82].

In the same year, Melvin and co-workers reported the first Heller oesophageal myotomy [83], followed, 1 year later, by Kernstine and co-workers who started to perform the first thoracoscopic robotic esophagectomy [84].

In 2003, the Argenziano group performed the first robotic implant of a diaphragmatic pacemaker [85], and Elli and co-workers presented the first two oesophageal leiomyoma resections [86].

In the same year, Ruurda and co-workers published the first resection of a neurogenic tumour of the posterior mediastinum [87], while Profanter and co-workers reported in 2004 the first removal of a mediastinal parathyroid adenoma [88].

Among the most significant case reports, mention should be made of the following: Rea and co-workers reporting 33 cases of robotic thymectomies in 2006 [89], Gharagozloo and co-workers presenting their experience with 100 robot-assisted lobectomies in 2009 [90], and Boone and co-workers publishing their 47 thoracoscopic robot-assisted oesophagectomies in 2009 [91].

Undoubtedly, robotic surgery is just at the beginning, and it is gradually gaining consensus throughout the world. However, in order to stand the test of time and pay the price of apprenticeship, it will have to solve the issues relating to high operating costs, operators' training methods and especially some inherent limitations to the system, namely, the lack of tactile feedback.

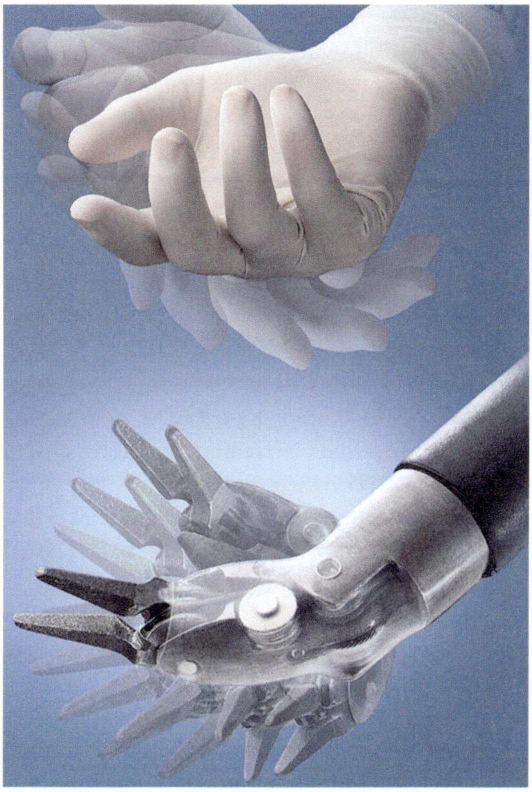

Fig. 1.22 DA VINCI® Surgical System seven degrees of freedom of movement (*Endowrist*). ©[2010] *Intuitive Surgical Inc.*

On this front, studies are underway to achieve intra-operative tactile feedback: the introduction of devices referred to as aptic interfaces, which are capable of reproducing the force feedback, could undoubtedly enable the performance of even more complex, precise and safe surgical procedures.

At the same time, in order to provide more information to the operator, quite interesting research is being carried out on the use of techniques for intra-operative diagnosis and detection that rely upon the principle of "augmented reality", i.e. equipment that displays such anatomical areas that are not visible intraoperatively (CT or MRI images), via a 3D computer reconstruction of the same, and which are also integrated to real images. These techniques result in a "virtual" reconstruction of the previously obtained morphologic data of the patient overlapping real-time intra-operative images, thus allowing the surgeon to locate deep lesions, to choose the proper dissection plane, to spare the vascular structures adjacent to the diseased area, and to perform oncologically radical resections with only minimal sacrifice of the parenchyma. The extremely high intra-operative resolution attained with this technique could drive the surgeon's hand during robotic surgery, thus making the procedure much faster and more effective [92–94].

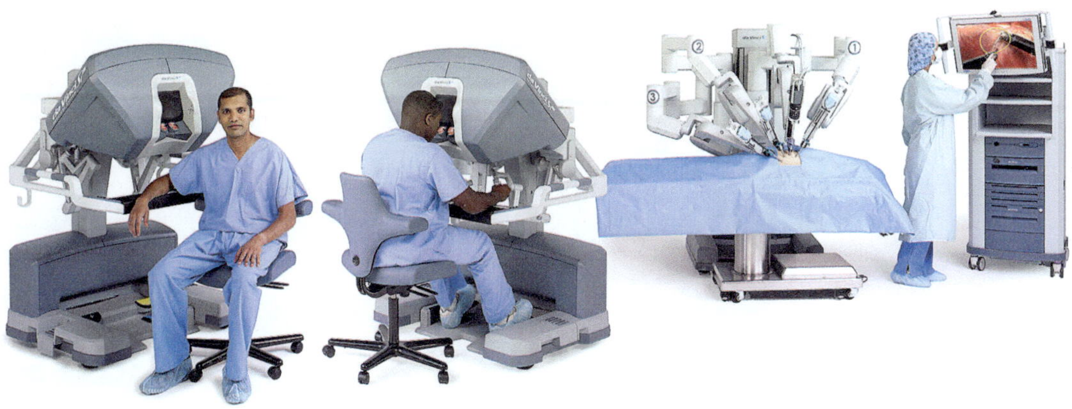

Fig. 1.23 DA VINCI® Surgical System Dual surgeon console. ©[2010] *Intuitive Surgical Inc.*

1.5 Telesurgery

Telesurgery certainly constitutes the extreme application of robotic surgery.

It provides the opportunity to perform remote surgical procedures, even with the surgeon thousands of miles from the patient, by using IT equipment that allows image transmission and control of the robotic arms.

Telesurgery resulted as the development in the following fields:

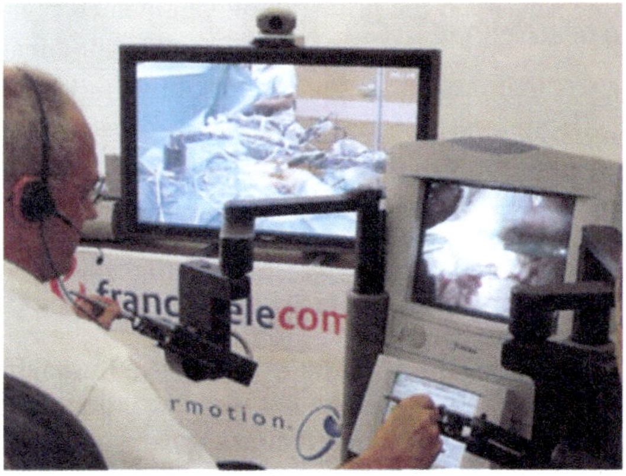

Fig. 1.24 *Lindbergh operation*: operator location on the robotic console in New York (From: Marescaux and co-workers [95], for kind allowance by IRCAD-EITS of Strasbourg)

- IT, allowing to convert images and operating procedures into digital electronic signals
- Telecommunications, allowing to send and receive signals in a very short time
- Digital imaging, allowing to acquire high-resolution 3D images into a digital format
- Robotics, allowing to use sophisticated and extremely precise robotics systems

Robot distance communication of information, images and digital controls travels by optical fibres, as well as on ISDN and ATM networks, allowing very fast data sequence transmission.

The first transatlantic remote surgical procedure (*Lindbergh operation*) consisted in a robotic cholecystectomy, performed in 2001 on a 68-year-old woman by the surgeons of IRCAD-EITS in Strasburg and of the Mount Sinai Medical Center of New York by employing a ZEUS® robot and a complex-integrated telecommunication system called SOCRATES.

The intervention, performed in 2001 at a distance of 7,000 km, was fully successful and lasted only 45 min [63, 95, 96] (Figs. 1.24 and 1.25).

Telesurgery allows:

1. To operate in disadvantaged areas lacking qualified surgeons
2. To make available the professional expertise of a surgeon, providing remote support to the colleagues, but without travelling (*teleconsulting*)

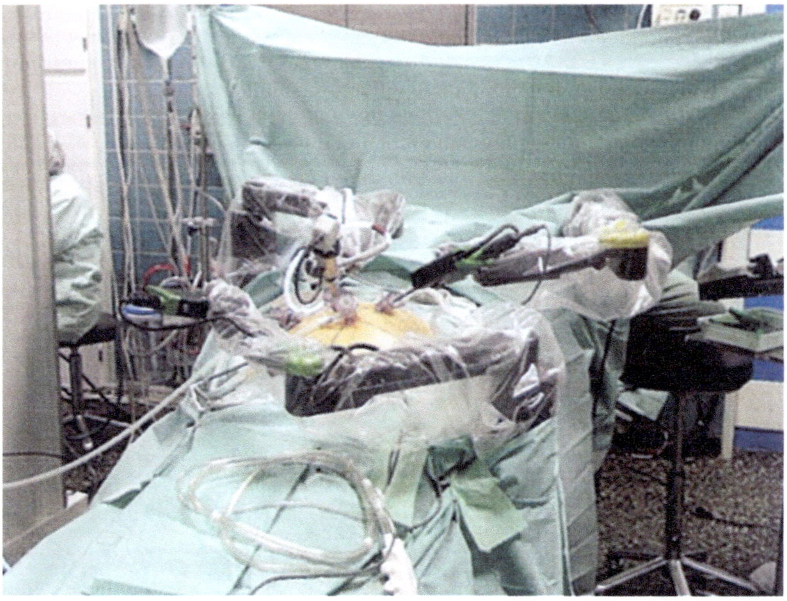

Fig. 1.25 *Lindbergh operation*: ZEUS robot in the remote location in Strasbourg (From: Marescaux and co-workers [95], for kind allowance by IRCAD-EITS of Strasbourg)

3. To have a valuable didactic and training tool addressed to surgeons (*telementoring*) [97]

The technique presents downsides and limitations related to high costs, current lack of ATM network cabling in every hospital [98], but especially due to the difficulty to guarantee a stable signal speed time delay below 300 ms, identified as safety threshold.

In thoracic and cardiac surgery, telesurgery interventions have not yet been performed. However, the resolution of technical problems as well as economic issues related to the procedure will certainly allow it. This will probably happen shortly as a result of the current extremely rapid technological development. After all, only 4 years had elapsed from the first robotic cholecystectomy by Cadiere to the Lindbergh operation.

References

1. Bozzini P (1806) Lichtleiter, eine Erfindung zur Anschauung innerer Theile und Krankheiten nebst der Abbildung (Neues Journal der practischen Heilkunde 17.Band) J den Pract. Arzneykunde und Wundarzneykunst Berlin: CW Hufeland 24 Bd. 1. Stuck:107–124 (mit 2 Abb. pp 177–178)
2. Gordon S (1866) Clinical reports of rare cases, occurring in the Whitworth and Hardwicke Hospitals: most extensive pleuritic effusion rapidly becoming purulent, paracentesis, introduction of a drainage tube, recovery, examination of interior of pleura by the endoscope. Dublin Q J Med Sci 41:83–90
3. Hoksch B, Birken-Bertsch H, Muller JM (2002) Thoracoscopy before Jacobaeus. Ann Thorac Surg 74:1288–1290
4. Ingvar S (1937) Hans Christian Jacobaeus. Acta Med Scand XCIII(6):500–504
5. Forlanini CA (1882) Contribuzioni della terapia chirurgica della tisi – Ablazione del polmone? Pneumotorace artificiale? Gazz Osp 3:537–707
6. Jacobaeus HC (1910) Ueber die Moglichkeit die Zystoskopie bei Untersuchung seroser Hohlungen anzuwenden. Muench Med Woch 57:2090
7. Jacobaeus HC (1921) The cauterization of adhesion in pneumothorax treatment of tuberculosis. Surg Gynaecol Obstet 32:493–500
8. Marchioni A, Lavini C, Morandi U (2006) Storia della Videotoracoscopia. In: Lavini C, Ruggiero C, Morandi U (eds) Chirurgia Toracica Videoassistita. Springer, Milan
9. Jacobaeus HC (1922) The cauterization of adhesion in artificial pneumothorax treatment of pulmonary tuberculosis under thoracoscopic control. Proc R Soc Med 16:45–60
10. Unverricht W (1925) Technik und Methode der Thorakoskopie. Vogel, Leipzig
11. Jacobaeus HC (1925) Die Thorakoskopie und ihre praktische Bedeutung. Ergeb Ges Med 7:122–166
12. Costantini G, Redaelli M (1932) Atlante clinico-radiologico della tubercolosi polmonare. Ed. Stabilimenti Poligrafici Riuniti, Bologna
13. Cova F (1927) Toracoscopia. Operazione di Jacobaeus. Sperling & Kupfer, Milano
14. Cova F (1928) Atlas thoracoscopicon. Sperling & Kupfer, Milano
15. Sattler A (1937) Zur Behandlung des Spontanpneumothorax mit besonderer Berucksich in Thorakoskopie. Beitr Klein Tuberk 89:395–408
16. Bloomberg AE (1978) Thoracoscopy in perspective. Surg Gynaecol Obstet 147:433–443
17. Tassi GF, Marchetti GP (1999) Storia della toracoscopia. In: Di Falco G (ed) Videotoracoscopia. Indicazioni e tecniche chirurgiche. Masson, Milano, pp 1–10
18. Alcozer G, Dorigoni A (1984) La toracoscopia diagnostica. Nardini Editore, Firenze
19. Levi JF, Kleinmann P, Riquet M et al (1990) Percutaneous parietal pleurectomy for recurrent spontaneous pneumothorax. Lancet 336:1577–1579
20. Wakabayashi A (1991) Expanded applications of diagnostic and therapeutic thoracoscopy. J Thorac Cardiovasc Surg 102:721
21. Kern JA, Rodgers BM (1993) Thoracoscopy in the management of empyema in children. J Pediatr Surg 28:1128–1132
22. Landreneau RJ, Hazelrigg SR, Fresón PF (1992) Thoracoscopic resections of 85 pulmonary lesions. Ann Thorac Surg 54:415–419
23. Roviaro G, Rebuffat C, Varoli FC et al (2002) Videoendoscopic pulmonary lobectomy for cancer. Surg Laparosc Endosc Percutan Tech 2:244–247
24. Kirby TJ, Mack MJ, Landreneau RJ et al (1993) Initial experience with video-assisted thoracoscopic lobectomy. Ann Thorac Surg 56:1248–1253
25. Inderbitzi RGC, Leiser A, Furrer M et al (1994) Three years experience in video-assisted thoracic surgery (VATS) for spontaneous pneumothorax. J Thorac Cardiovasc Surg 107:1410–1415
26. Medrano C, Hazelrigg SR, Landreneau RJ et al (2000) Thoracoscopic resection of ectopic parathyroid glands. Ann Thorac Surg 69:221–223
27. Sugarbaker DJ (1993) Thoracoscopy in the management of anterior mediastinal masses. Ann Thorac Surg 56(3):653–656
28. Cuschieri A, Shimi SM, Banting S (1992) Endoscopic esophagectomy through a right thoracoscopic approach. J R Coll Surg Edinb 37:7–11
29. Bumm R, Holscher AH, Feussner H et al (1993) Endodissection of the thoracic esophagus. Technique and clinical results in transhiatal esophagectomy. Ann Surg 218:97–104
30. Kent RB, Pison TW (1993) Thoracoscopic ligation of the thoracic duct. Surg Endosc 7:52–53
31. Cuschieri A, Shimi SM, Crothwaite G et al (1994) Bilateral endoscopic splanchnicectomy through a

posterior thoracoscopic approach. J R Coll Surg Edinb 39:44–47
32. Sortini A, Navarra G, Santini M et al (1994) Video-assisted mediastinoscopy. A new video application in minimally invasive surgery. Minerva Chir 49:803–805
33. Venissac N, Alifano M, Mouroux J (2003) Video-assisted mediastinoscopy: experience from 240 consecutive cases. Ann Thorac Surg 76:208–212
34. Kao MC, Lin JY, Chen YL et al (1996) Minimally invasive surgery: video-endoscopic thoracic sympathectomy for palmar hyperhidrosis. Ann Acad Med Singapore 25:673–678
35. Mouroux J, Padovani B, Poirier NC (1996) Technique for the repair of diaphragmatic eventration. Ann Thorac Surg 62:905–907
36. Mouroux J, Venissac N, Leo F et al (2005) Surgical treatment of diaphragmatic eventration using video-assisted thoracic surgery: a Prospective Study. Ann Thorac Surg 79:308–312
37. Roberts JR, Roy Smythe W, Weber RW et al (1997) Thoracoscopic management of descending necrotizing mediastinitis. Chest 112:850–854
38. Jiménez-Merchán R, Garcia-Diaz F, Arenas-Linares G et al (1997) Comparative retrospective study of surgical treatment of spontaneous pneumothorax. Thoracotomy vs thoracoscopy. Surg Endosc 11(9):919–922
39. Nuss D, Kelly RE, Croitoru DP et al (1998) 10-year review of a minimally invasive technique for the correction of pectus excavatum. J Pediatr Surg 53:545–552
40. McKenna RJ, Houck W, Fuller CB (2006) Video-assisted thoracic surgery lobectomy: experience with 1100 cases. Ann Thorac Surg 81(2):421–426
41. Tomulescu V, Ion V, Kosa A et al (2006) Thoracoscopic thymectomy mid-term results. Ann Thorac Surg 82(3):1003–1007
42. Laborde F, Noirhomme P, Karam J et al (1993) A new video-assisted thoracoscopic surgical technique for interruption of patent ductus arteriosus in infants and children. J Thorac Cardiovasc Surg 105:278–280
43. Burke RP, Rosenfeld HM, Wernovsky G et al (1995) Video-assisted thoracoscopic vascular rings division in infants and children. J Am Coll Cardiol 25:943–947
44. Gersak B, Sostaric M, Kalisnic J (2003) Endoscopic aortic valve replacement. Heart Surg Forum 6(6): E197–E199
45. Mack MJ, Landreneau RJ, Hazelrigg SR et al (1993) Video thoracoscopic management of benign and malignant pericardial effusions. Chest 103:390S–393S
46. Benetti FC, Ballester C (1994) Use of thoracoscopy and a minimal thoracotomy in mammary-coronary bypass to left anterior descending artery, without extracorporeal circulation. Experience in 2 cases. J Cardiovasc Surg 36:159–160
47. Nataf P, Lima L, Regan M et al (1996) Minimally invasive coronary surgery with thoracoscopic internal mammary artery dissection: surgical technique. J Card Surg 11(4):288–292
48. Mack M, Acuff T, Yong P et al (1997) Minimally invasive thoracoscopically assisted coronary artery bypass surgery. Eur J Cardiothorac Surg 12:20–24
49. Duhaylongsod FG, Mayfield WR, Wolf RK (1998) Thoracoscopic harvest of the internal thoracic artery: a multicenter experience in 218 cases. Ann Thorac Surg 66(3):1012–1017
50. Lanfranco R, Castellanos AE, Desai JP et al (2004) Robotic surgery. A current perspective. Ann Surg 239(1):14–21
51. Herron DM, Marohn M (2008) A consensus document on robotic surgery. Surg Endosc 22:313–325
52. Murphy D, Challacombe B, Khan MS et al (2006) Robotic technology in urology. Postgrad Med 82(973):743–747
53. Kwoh YS, Hou J, Jonckheere EA et al (1988) A robot with improved absolute positioning accuracy for CT guided stereotactic brain surgery. IEEE Trans Biomed Eng 35:153–161
54. Davies B (2000) A review of robotics in surgery. Proc Inst Mech Eng H 214:129–140
55. Benabid AL, Hoffmann D, Ashraf A et al (1997) The robotization of neurosurgery: state of the art and future outlook. Bull Acad Natl Med 181(8):1625–1635
56. Harris SJ, Arambula-Cosio F, Mei Q et al (1997) The Probot – an active robot for prostate resection. Proc Inst Mech Eng H 211:317–335
57. Bann S, Khan M, Hernandez J et al (2003) Robotics in surgery. J Am Coll Surg 196:784–795
58. Bargar WL, Bauer A, Börner M (1998) Primary and revision total hip replacement using the RoboDoc system. Clin Orthop 354:82–91
59. Cain P, Kazanzides P, Zuhars J et al (1993) Safety considerations in a surgical robot. Biomed Sci Instrum 29:291–294
60. Satava RM (2002) Surgical robotics: the early chronicles: a personal historical perspective. Surg Laparosc Endosc Percutan Tech 12:6–16
61. Kavoussi LR, Moore RG, Adams JB et al (1995) Comparison of robotic versus laparoscopic camera control. J Urol 154:2134–2136
62. Jung YW, Kim SW, Kim YT (2009) Recent advances of robotic surgery and single port laparoscopy in gynaecologic oncology. J Gynecol Oncol 20(3):137–144
63. Faust A (2007) Robotics in surgery. History, current and future applications. Nova Science Publishers, New York
64. Sung GT, Gill IS (2001) Robotic laparoscopic surgery: a comparison of the da Vinci and Zeus systems. J Urol 58:893–898
65. Himpens J, Lehman G, Cadiere GB (1998) Telesurgical laparoscopic cholecystectomy. Surg Endosc 12(8): 1091
66. Carpentier A, Loulmet D, Aupecle B et al (1998) Computer assisted open heart surgery. First case operated on with success. C R Acad Sci III 321:437–442
67. Mohr FW, Falk W, Diegeler A et al (1999) Computer-enhanced coronary artery bypass surgery. J Thorac Cardiovasc Surg 117:1212–1214
68. Loulmet D, Carpentier A, d'Attellis N et al (1999) Endoscopic coronary artery bypass grafting with the aid of robotic assisted instruments. J Thorac Cardiovasc Surg 118:4–10
69. Mehmanesh H, Henze R, Lange R (2002) Totally endoscopic mitral valve repair. J Thorac Cardiovasc Surg 123:96–97

70. Le Bret E, Papadatos S, Folliguet T et al (2002) Interruption of patent ductus arteriosus in children: robotically assisted versus videothoracoscopic surgery. J Thorac Cardiovasc Surg 123:973–976
71. Torracca L, Ismeno G, Alfieri O (2001) Totally endoscopic computer-enhanced atrial septal defect closure in six patients. Ann Thorac Surg 72:1354–1357
72. Wimmer-Greinecker G, Dogan S, Aybek T et al (2003) Totally endoscopic atrial septal repair in adults with computer-enhanced telemanipulation. J Thorac Cardiovasc Surg 126:465–468
73. Folliguet TA, Vanhuyse F, Magnano D et al (2004) Robotic aortic valve replacement: case report. Heart Surg Forum 7(6):E551–E553
74. Murphy DA, Miller JS, Langford DA (2005) Robot-assisted endoscopic excision of left atrial myxomas. J Thorac Cardiovasc Surg 130:596–597
75. Woo YJ, Grand TJ, Weiss SJ (2005) Robotic resection of an aortic valve papillary fibroelastoma. Ann Thorac Surg 80:110–112
76. Gerosa G, Bianco R, Buja G et al (2004) Totally endoscopic robotic-guided pulmonary veins ablation: an alternative method for the treatment of atrial fibrillation. Eur J Cardiothorac Surg 26:450–452
77. Derose JJ Jr, Belsey S, Swistel DG et al (2004) Robotically assisted left ventricular epicardial lead implantation for biventricular pacing: the posterior approach. Ann Thorac Surg 77:1472–1474
78. Kypson AP, Chitwood WR Jr (2005) The use of robotics in cardiovascular surgery. Future Cardiol 1(1):61–67
79. de Cannière D, Wimmer-Greinecker G, Cichon R et al (2007) Feasibility, safety and efficacy of totally endoscopic coronary artery bypass grafting: multicenter European experience. J Thorac Cardiovasc Surg 134: 710–716
80. Suematsu Y, Mora BN, Mihaljevich T et al (2005) Totally endoscopic robotic-assisted Repair of patent ductus arteriosus and vascular ring in children. Ann Thorac Surg 80:2309–2313
81. Yoshino I, Hashizume M, Shimata M et al (2001) Thoracoscopic thymectomy with the da Vinci computer-enhanced surgical system. J Thorac Cardiovasc Surg 122:783–785
82. Melfi FMA, Menconi GF, Mariani AM et al (2002) Early experience with robotic technology for thoracoscopic surgery. Eur J Cardiothorac Surg 21:864–868
83. Melvin WS, Needleman BJ, Krause KR et al (2002) Computer-enhanced robotic telesurgery: initial experience in foregut surgery. Surg Endosc 16:1790–1792
84. Kernstine KH, DeArmond DT, Shamoun DM et al (2007) The first series of completely robotic esophagectomies with three-field lymphadenectomy: initial experience. Surg Endosc 21(12):2285–2292
85. Morgan JA, Morales DL, John R et al (2003) Endoscopic, robotically assisted Implantation of phrenic pacemakers. J Thorac Cardiovasc Surg 126(2):582–583
86. Elli E, Espat NJ, Berger R et al (2004) Robotic-assisted thoracoscopic resection of esophageal leiomyoma. Surg Endosc 18(4):713–716
87. Ruurda JP, Hanlo PW, Hennipman A et al (2003) Robot-assisted thoracoscopic resection of a benign mediastinal neurogenic tumor: technical note. Neurosurgery 52(2):462–464
88. Profanter C, Schmid T, Prommegger R et al (2004) Robot-assisted mediastinal parathyroidectomy. Surg Endosc 18(5):868–870
89. Rea F, Marulli G, Bortolotti L et al (2006) Experience with the "da Vinci" robotic system for thymectomy in patients with myasthenia gravis: report of 33 cases. Ann Thorac Surg 81:455–459
90. Gharagozloo F, Margolis M, Tempesta B et al (2009) Robot-assisted lobectomy for early-stage lung cancer: report of 100 consecutive cases. Ann Thorac Surg 88(2):380–384
91. Boone J, Schipper MEI, Moojen WA et al (2009) Robot-assisted thoracoscopic Esophagectomy for cancer. Br J Surg 96(8):878–886
92. Kant AJ, Klein MD, Langenburg SE (2004) Robotics in pediatric surgery: perspectives for imaging. Pediatr Radiol 34(6):454–461
93. Marescaux J, Rubino F, Arenas L et al (2004) Augmented-reality-assisted laparoscopic Adrenalectomy. JAMA 292: 2214–2215
94. Shuhaiber JH (2004) Augmented reality in surgery. Arch Surg 139:170–174
95. Marescaux J, Leroy J, Rubino F et al (2002) Transcontinental robot-assisted remote telesurgery: feasibility and potential applications. Ann Surg 235: 487–492
96. Cheah WK, Lee B, Lenzi IE et al (2000) Telesurgical laparoscopic cholecystectomy between two countries. Surg Endosc 14:1085
97. Ballantyne GH (2002) Robotic surgery, telerobotic surgery, telepresence and telementoring. Review of early clinical results. Surg Endosc 16:1389–1402
98. Marescaux J, Rubino F (2004) Robot-assisted remote surgery: technological advances, potential complications, and solutions. Surg Technol Int 12:23–26

General Aspects of Thoracoscopic Surgery

2

Dominique Gossot

Contents

D. Gossot, M.D.
Thoracic Department, Institut Mutualiste Montsouris, 42 Bd Jourdan, 75014 Paris, France
e-mail: dominique.gossot@imm.fr

Thoracoscopic surgical interventions are considered as challenging. Because of the endoscopic vision with its magnification and unusual viewpoints, the anatomical landmarks are changed. In addition, restricted tissue manipulation and use of endoscopic instruments are disturbing. Eventually, as mentioned by T. L. Demmy, performing endoscopic major pulmonary resection means relearning the procedures.

The aim of this chapter is to stress several technical details that we have found helpful. Most of these tips and tricks can be modified according to the surgeon's preferences and will anyway evolve with upcoming technologies.

The key points are:

- Taking time. In most series, these procedures are long lasting because one has to proceed meticulously and step by step. It is thus important to cope with ergonomic issues and adequate positioning of trocars.
- Controlling any oozing or bleeding so that the operative field remains clear and does not deteriorate the quality of vision.
- Achieving a perfect exposure.
- Operating with an outstanding imaging system and preferably with a high-definition camera that gives a sharp image and allows one to operate "as during microscopic surgery."
- Having the right tool for the right task. This means these procedures cannot be performed with just a limited number of instruments. Not only good-quality hand instruments are needed but also hemostatic devices such as ultrasonic shears or bipolar sealing instrument.

R.G.C. Inderbitzi et al. (eds.), *Minimally Invasive Thoracic and Cardiac Surgery*,
DOI 10.1007/978-3-642-11861-6_2, © Springer-Verlag Berlin Heidelberg 2012

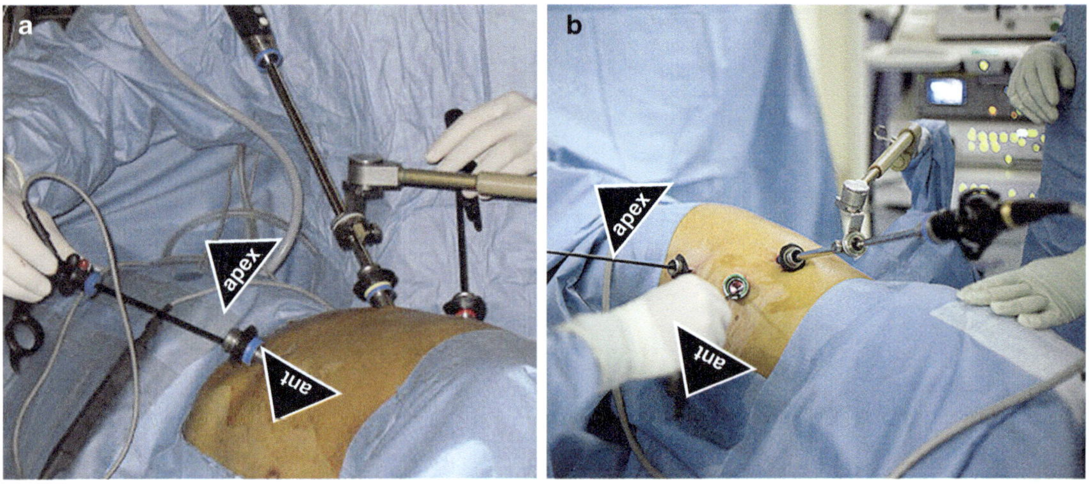

Fig. 2.1 Trocar positioning: (**a**) triangulation with both working instruments opposite one another is uncomfortable; (**b**) example of a left lower lobectomy carried out with both working instruments coming from the front. This position is more ergonomic and less straining

2.1 Ergonomics and Operating Room Setting

It is usually admitted that video-assisted surgery should be done with triangulation of the endoscope and instruments that are positioned opposite one another (Fig. 2.1). This rule is almost impossible to follow during endoscopic major pulmonary resections for the following reasons:

- These procedures last 2–4 h. Maintaining an awkward position with both arms spread apart is exhausting and can provoke shoulder pain and stiffness.
- In these complex operations, there is not just one but several targets (pulmonary hilum, mediastinum, diaphragm…) so that there is not a single ideal position of the scope and instruments. Therefore, whenever possible, we have found it more comfortable manipulating the two working instruments from the back or from the front, depending on the resection to be performed. The opposite side is used for insertion of a lung retractor or a suction device.

The scope is held by a robotic or mechanical scope holder, according to the surgeon preference. Its position should be shrewdly chosen so that the endoscope does not conflict with instruments (Fig. 2.2). Endoscopic instruments and trocars are placed on a dedicated rack, and the conventional thoracic instruments are prepared on a separate table (Fig. 2.3). The list of instruments is given in Table 2.1.

2.2 Trocars

What is the position of trocars is a frequently asked question. Unfortunately, there is no fixed and definite position. It depends not only on the type of resection but also on the patient's morphological type and on the surgeon's habits and preferences. For instance, we prefer performing left resections with the instruments coming from the front (Fig. 2.1), while we do not succeed using this approach for right-sided resections for which we use a combination of dissection from the back and from the front. Other surgeons may feel more comfortable with another approach and different positioning. The only rule we would recommend is inserting the scope in the midaxillary line, in the sixth or seventh intercostal space, depending on the patient's morphological type, because of the need to have an overall view on the whole pleural cavity.

Many tasks can be done with micro-instruments. This avoids large ports and, consequently, large scars.

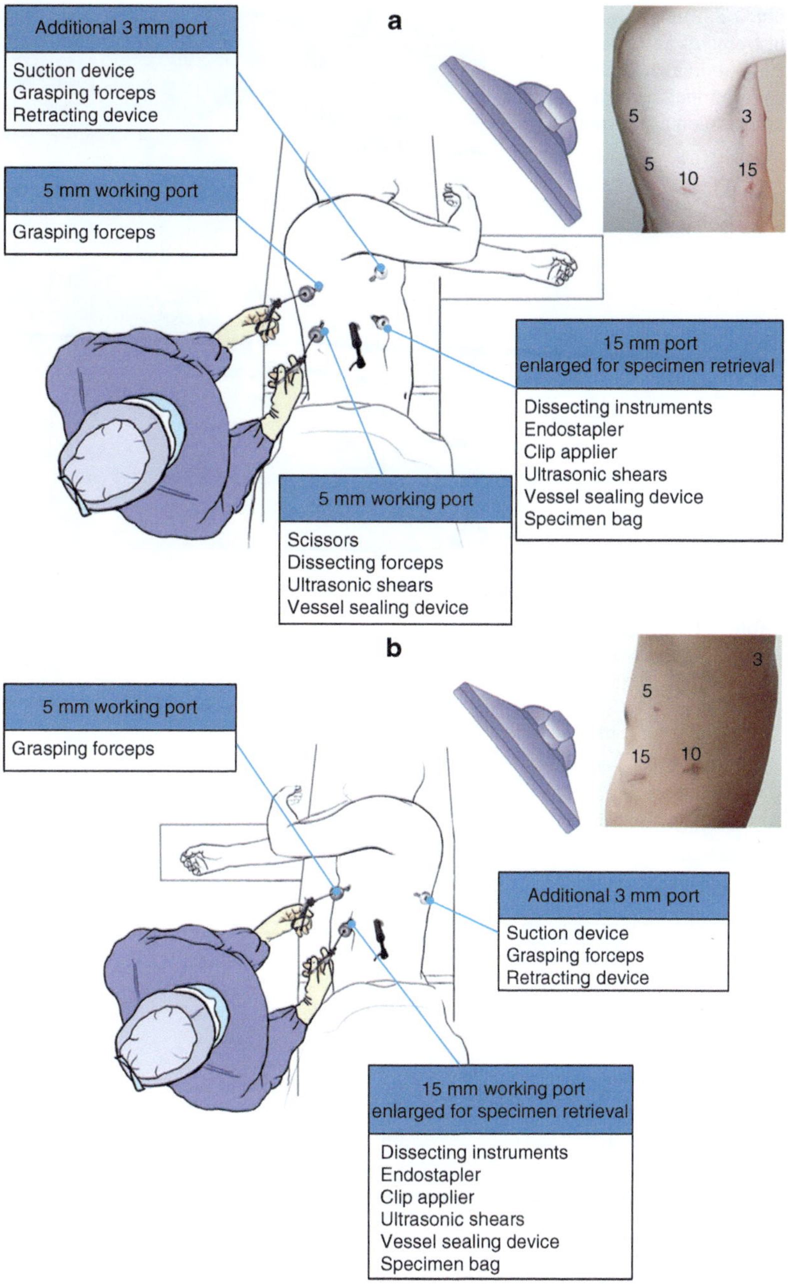

Fig. 2.2 (**a**) Example of ports for a right lobectomy (in this case, a middle lobectomy), with the surgeon standing in the patient's back. Schematic illustration and final aspect on the patient. (**b**) Example of ports for a left lobectomy (in this case, a lower lobectomy), with the surgeon standing in the patient's front. Schematic illustration and final aspect on the patient

2.3 Enhancing Vision and Video Imaging

During open surgery or VATS, the surgeon usually stands at the patient's back because the anatomical landmarks are more familiar to him/her that way. It is sometimes preferable to stand at the patient's front, or to switch from behind to the front, according to the operation steps. This means that at least two monitors should be used. The light in the operating room should be reduced as much as possible to enhance the monitor's contrast. As working many hours in the dark is tiresome for the staff, the best compromise is to have a blue background lighting which offers a nice contrast and does not oblige working in the dark (Fig. 2.4).

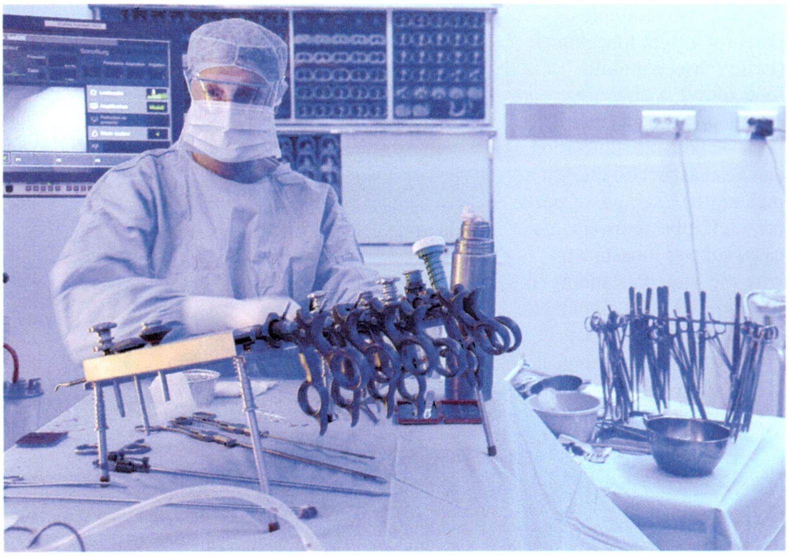

Fig. 2.3 Endoscopic instruments and trocars are laid out on a rack while conventional instruments are available on a separate table

Table 2.1 Standard equipment required for endoscopic major pulmonary resections

Equipment	Type	Remarks
Image		
High-definition camera system	Exera II, Olympus	
High-definition monitors (×2)	Olympus	
Deflectable endoscope	LTF, Olympus	
Scope warmer	Applied Medical	
Scope holder	SH-1, Olympus	
Recording	Sony XDCAM HD PDW-70PM	
Hemostatic tools		
Multifunctional bipolar scissors, 5 mm	Aesculap	Disposable
Vessel sealing device, 5 mm	LigaSure™, Valleylab	Disposable
Vascular endostapler, 12 mm	Endo-GIA 30 V, Covidien	Disposable
Clip applier	Ligaclip 10, Ethicon	Disposable
Hand instruments		
3-mm trocars (×2)	Storz	Reusable
5-mm trocars (×2)	Olympus	Reusable
10-mm trocar (×1)	Olympus	Reusable
12-mm trocar (×1)	Olympus	Reusable
15-mm trocar (×1)	Thoracoport, Covidien	Reusable
Maryland dissecting forceps, 5 mm	Olympus	Reusable
Maryland dissecting forceps, 10 mm	Olympus	Reusable
Metzenbaum scissor, 5 mm	Olympus	Reusable
Hook, 5 mm	Olympus	Reusable
Suction device, 5 mm (with coagulating tip)	Olympus	Reusable
Fenestrated grasping forceps, 5 mm	Olympus	Reusable
Atraumatic grasping forceps, 3 mm	Olympus	Reusable
Pulmonary clamp, 5 mm	Storz	Reusable
Vascular clamp, 5 mm	Storz	Reusable
Bulldog clamps (×3)	Aesculap	Reusable

Table 2.1 (continued)

Equipment	Type	Remarks
Endostaplers	Endo-GIA 45+60 (agrafes 3.5 mm+4.8 mm), Covidien	Disposable
Specimen bag, 15 mm	EndoCatch II, Covidien	Disposable
Deflectable retractor, 5 mm	Goldfinger™, Ethicon or Endo MiniRetract, Covidien	Disposable
Blunt tip dissectors, 5 mm	Endopath®, Ethicon	Disposable
Backup		
Biopsy needle	Bard Monopty® 16 g	Disposable
		For biopsy of nodule for frozen section when no preoperative diagnosis is available
Suction catheter as stapler guide	Gentle-Flow™, 16Ch, Kendlall	Disposable
		For use as a guide for the endostapler tip
Curved instruments, 5 mm	Aesculap	Reusable
		For freeing of some pleural adhesions that are difficult to reach with straight instruments
Needle holder, 5 mm	Olympus	Reusable
		Pulmonary tears, bronchial suture
Conventional instruments	Miscellaneous	Ready on a separate table

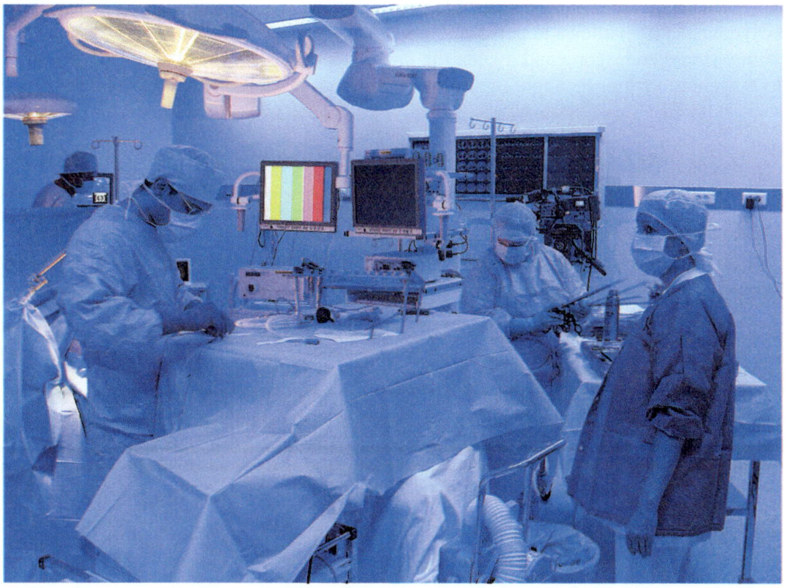

Fig. 2.4 Use of a blue backlight enhances image contrast and does not necessitate reducing light of the operating theater

Since the procedure is long lasting, the endoscope tip may be soiled by blood drops sliding down along the trocar sheath. This annoying issue can be partly overcome by using a 12-mm trocar instead of a 10-mm one. The port is cleaned with a cotton-tipped applicator. Smoke aspiration can be achieved via a 3-mm suction device that is left in place throughout the procedure. The EndoClear™ (Virtual Ports) device is very helpful in efficient cleaning of the optic tip without a need for retrieving the scope.

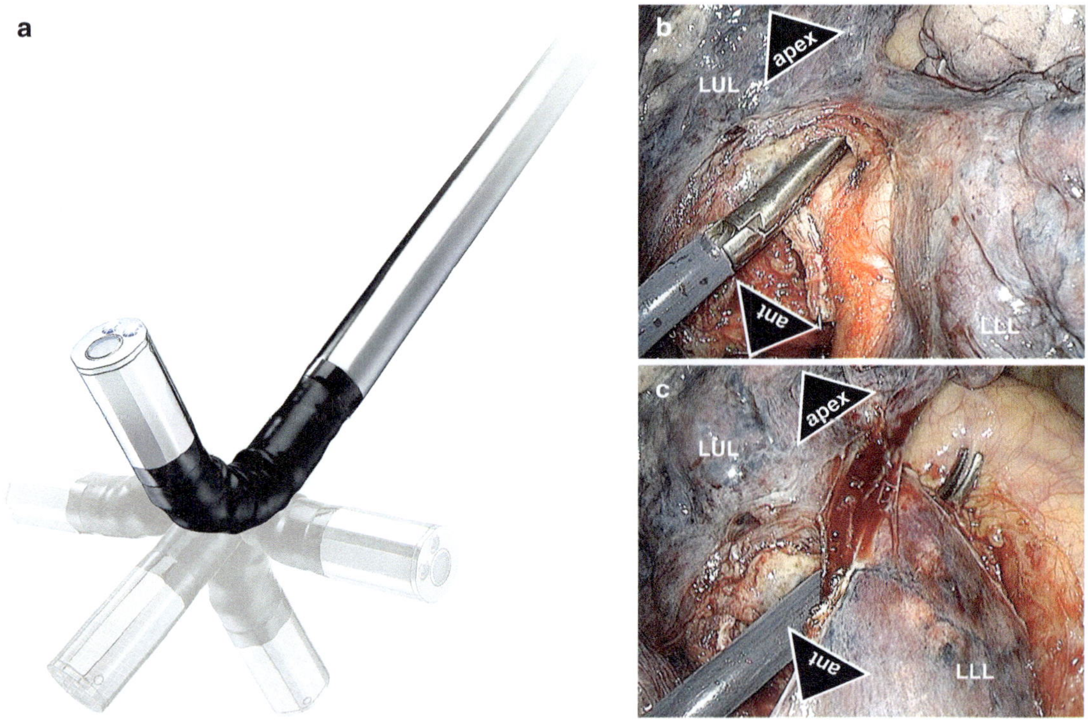

Fig. 2.5 High-definition deflectable tip thoracoscope (Olympus LTF™) allows to perform the whole procedure with a single endoscope and avoids the problems related to tangential vision. Its angle of vision varies from 0° to 100°. (**a**) Example: during the dissection of the posterior part of the left fissure, a 0° vision does not allow to control the instrument tip (**b**) while it becomes clearly visible with a 90° angle of vision (**c**)

Maintaining optimal vision of the whole operative field with a single 0° optic is almost impossible. One of the main concerns with a direct-viewing scope (0°) is the difficulty in controlling the instrument tip, which may be out of the field of vision. Formerly, to overcome this problem, we switched from a direct- (0°) to an oblique-viewing endoscope (30°) as vision became too tangential. However, these maneuvers were time consuming and tedious. The rigid scope with a deflectable tip (Olympus LTF™, Tokyo, Japan) has an angle of vision that varies from 0° to 100° (Fig. 2.5). The flexibility is controlled by a lever located on the handle. Once chosen, the angulation can be locked. This allows the surgeon to have a bird's-eye view, making dissection more natural and safer. The endoscope tip houses a distal CCD connected to a high-definition television (HDTV) camera (Exera II™, Olympus), which provides dramatically sharp viewing, thus allowing for close-up vascular dissections.

2.4 Obtaining Pathological Diagnosis

Patients who are selected for a totally endoscopic major pulmonary resection usually present with a clinical stage I tumor. This means the tumor or nodule is often small and not accessible to a preoperative CT-guided biopsy. Thus, many patients are operated on without confirmed pathological diagnosis. When the nodule is small and subpleural, the easiest way is to perform a wedge resection with frozen section. In other cases, we use a biopsy needle (Bard Monopty®, Covington, GA), which provides a pathological diagnosis in most cases (Fig. 2.6)

2.5 Exposure and Lung Retraction

The most efficient and most natural way to retract the lung is by mean of a 5-mm or 10-mm forceps. However, although it is sometimes necessary, the use of a forceps has two drawbacks: (1) it requires an additional port and (2) it frequently tears the parenchyma, causing oozing or even hemorrhage. Although these minor bleedings are seldom serious, these may be very troublesome. Some have proposed to retract the lung with an endoloop. When there is no need to retract the lung with force, pushing it back with a simple endoscopic peanut is as effective while being less traumatic.

For long-lasting steps where the lung needs to remain retracted, we use either a 3-mm grasping forceps (Fig. 2.7a) or a miniaturized lung forceps that can be released inside the chest cavity (Aesculap©) (Fig. 2.7b). It has a triangular tip, like most lung forceps. A 30-cm-long thread is passed and secured at its ring-shaped basis. Once

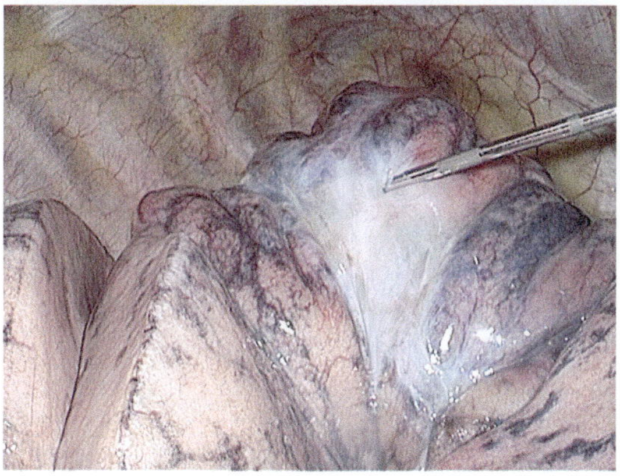

Fig. 2.6 Intraoperative view of a needle biopsy

applied on the portion of the lung to be retracted, the thread is loaded through a 2-mm fascial closure device – whose primary use is port site closure during laparoscopy – and simply passed through the skin. Tension is then adapted by pulling the thread more or less. If needed, two retractors can be used.

2.6 Fissures

The access to the branches of the pulmonary artery is easy or difficult depending on whether the fissure is separated or fused (Fig. 2.8). Opening a largely fused fissure may be a tedious step of the procedure. The main concern is that opening and dissecting the fissure can cause some minor oozing that is troublesome during a thoracoscopic operation where the operative field must remain as dry as possible to maintain optimal vision. One of the keys to a bloodless dissection is to progress step by step, from the periphery to the hilum. We have found thin instruments such as ultrasonic (SonoSurg™, Olympus) or electrothermal bipolar shears (LigaSure™, Valleylab) to be less cumbersome and as effective as stapler for the division of the external part of the fissure. For the inner thick part of the fissure, stapling is however required. A guide is usually necessary to drive the stapler jaws without excessive friction and force on the tissue. We use a small-diameter

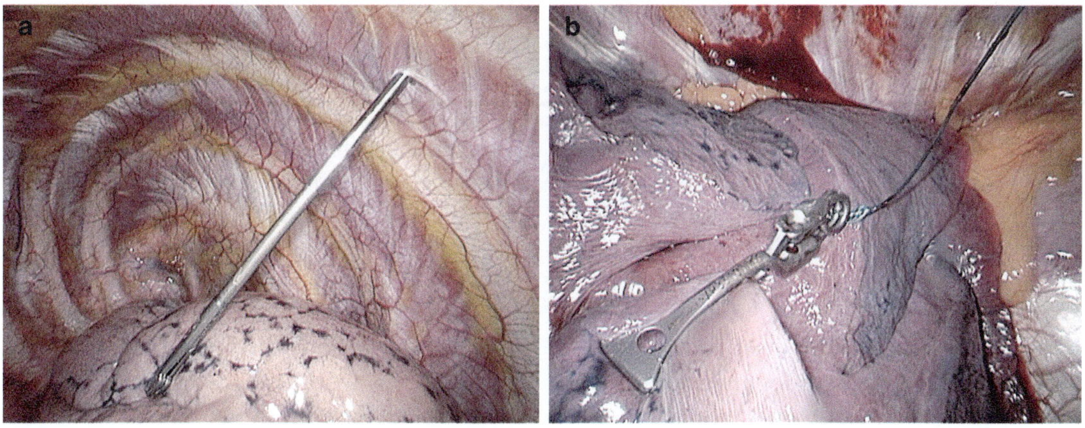

Fig. 2.7 Lung retraction. To avoid using large lung retractors, several solutions are available: (**a**) use of 3-mm grasping forceps; (**b**) use of miniretractors that can be released inside the chest cavity and pulled through the chest wall by a thread

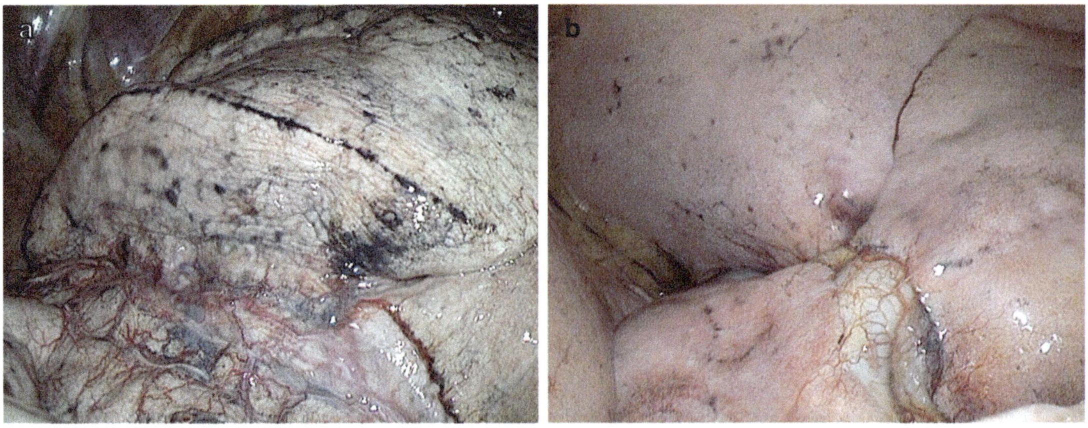

Fig. 2.8 Example of fused (**a**) and separate (**b**) fissure that gives direct access to the pulmonary artery

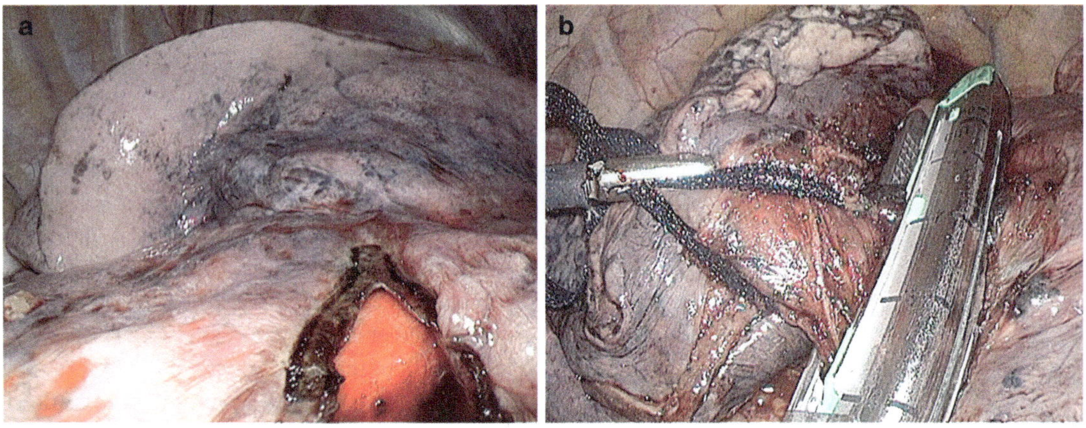

Fig. 2.9 Fissure division: (**a**) division of a thin peripheral part of the left fissure using bipolar sealing, (**b**) stapling of a thick central part of the left fissure

silicone suction tube whose base is connected to the stapler tip, or we retract the fissure with a tape (Fig. 2.9).

With a direct-viewing telescope, the division of the fissure can be difficult because its length may make sharp vision on both of its extremities almost impossible. A deflectable tip thoracoscope is of great help during this step because it allows a bird's-eye view of the whole fissure throughout the dissection.

In case of fused fissures, identifying some branches of the pulmonary artery (PA) is tedious. This is usually not an issue for lower lobectomies but can be a real concern for upper lobectomies, since the branching pattern exhibits many variations, especially on the left side. Therefore, preoperative knowledge of vascular anatomy can be helpful. Three-dimensional reconstruction with volume rendering technique provides an accurate vascular mapping of the lobe or segment to be dissected. This preoperative investigation is time consuming but does not have additional cost or invasiveness, since a preoperative CT with injecting contrast medium is needed anyway.

2.7 Exposure of Bronchial and Vascular Elements

Exposing and retracting a bronchus or a vessel is frequently necessary when it needs to be loaded within the jaws of a clip applier or an endostapler.

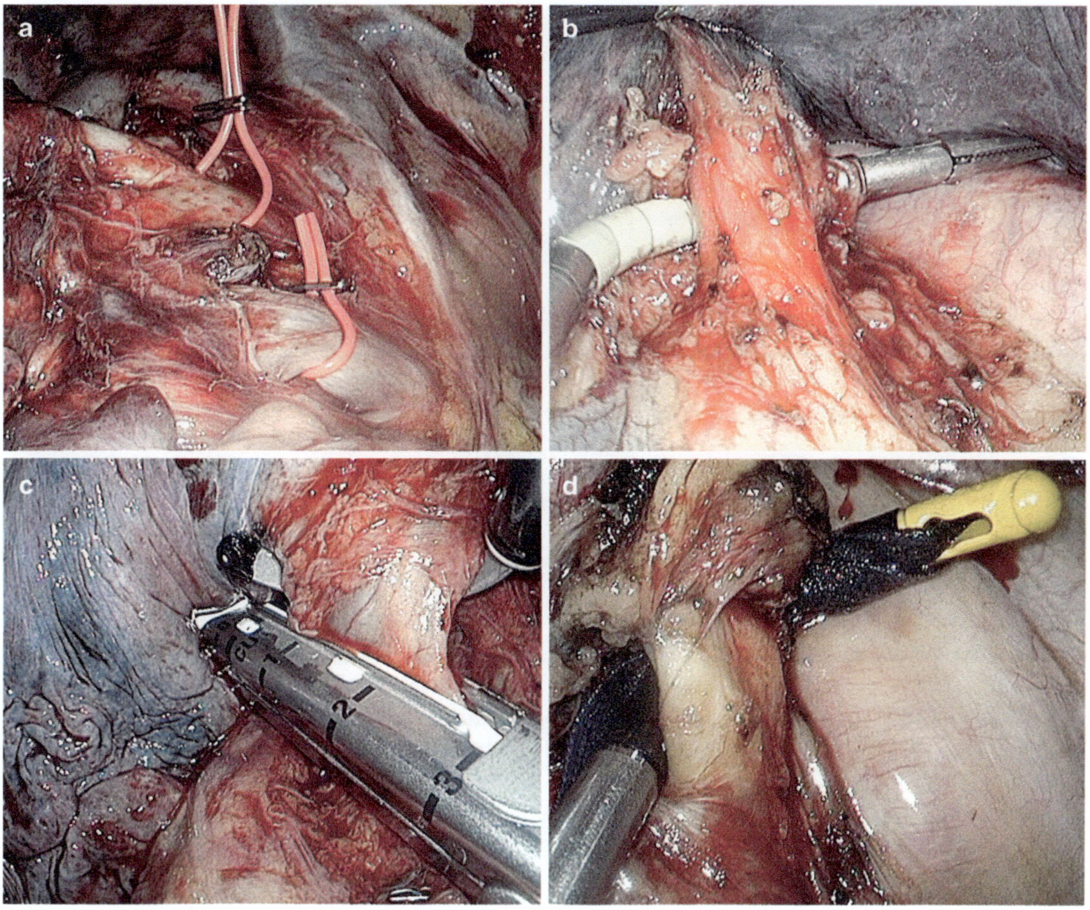

Fig. 2.10 Technical tricks to facilitate retraction of vessels and their exposure: (**a**) use of tapes or slings, (**b**) use of a 5-mm deflectable forceps, (**c**) use of a memory-shape 5-mm retractor, and (**d**) use of a 5-mm deflectable retractor whose tip has a keyhole for a sling

The latter must be passed as smoothly as possible. One can use some deflectable devices (Endo MiniRetract™, Covidien or Goldfinger™, Ethicon whose tip has the advantage of being atraumatic and has a keyhole for a sling) (Fig. 2.10). These instruments can be used both for retraction and for some blunt dissection to create space around the element to be stapled. If this is not sufficient, a guide can be used. We use a chest tube or a 16 Fr suction tube (Gentle-Flow™, Kendall©) (Fig. 2.11). Its base is secured to the anvil by simple pressure. This can be done inside or outside the chest. Its distal end is passed around the structure to be divided and pulled out through the trocar tube. The stapler tip is thus guided around the tissue to be stapled.

2.8 Vascular Control

Whenever possible, clips should be avoided because they may slip or conflict with staples. However, medium-diameter vessels such as some segmental pulmonary branches are too small for an endostapler and too large to be coagulated with electrocautery or ultrasounds. When clips are used, they are doubled or even tripled. Another solution is to apply a clip at the origin of the vessel and complete division with bipolar sealing so that only one clip is present in the operative field. For all other minor vessels, we use ultrasonic shears (US) (EndoSurg™, Olympus) or a bipolar vessel sealing device (VSD) (Ligasure™, Covidien) (Fig. 2.12). Large vessels are stapled.

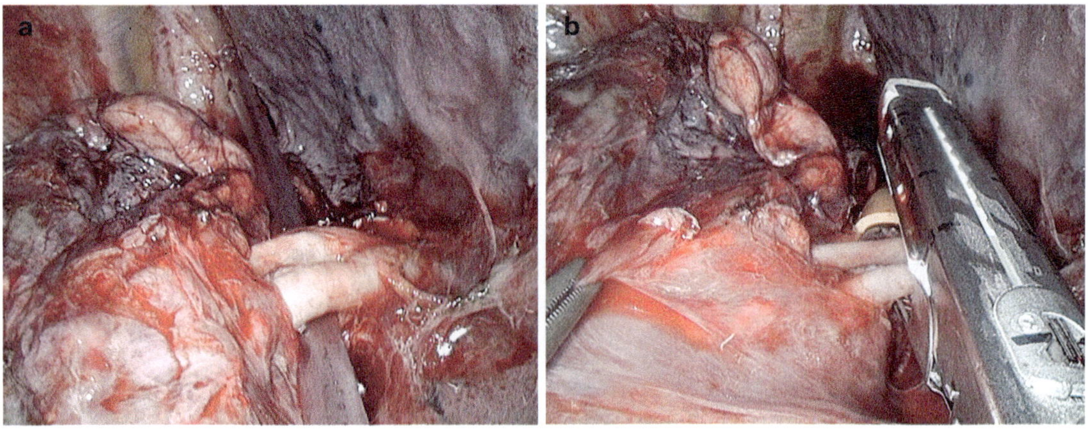

Fig. 2.11 Facilitating the passage of the endostapler for arterial division during a thoracoscopic right basilar segmentectomy using a thin suction catheter as a guide. The tip is first passed behind the vessel (**a**) and then pulled out to attract its basis connected to the stapler jaw (**b**)

Complications related to stapling of bronchus or parenchyma are rare but have been reported, while accidents with vascular stapling are extremely rare. However, the stapler must load the vessel without any force or friction, which implies a perfect vascular dissection. Lymphadenectomy is done only with VSD, and clips are almost never used. A suction device can be activated all over the dissection time for immediate evacuation of smoke and mist.

2.9 Vascular Injuries

Avoiding bleeding and massive vascular injury is a constant concern throughout the procedure. Some authors have advocated clamping the main pulmonary artery using a silk suture in order to control any bleeding. This maneuver can be easily achieved during conventional open procedure or even during some VATS procedures through a utility mini-thoracotomy. But it seems at risk to be done via a totally endoscopic approach because a tear of the main pulmonary artery cannot be controlled. This is one limitation of the endoscopic approach. However, in patients presenting with a regular anatomy, the risk of major vascular injury is minimal due to the close-up dissection and camera magnification. Dissection becomes more risky when neoplastic or inflammatory lymph nodes are present and prevent opening of the vascular sheath that is adherent to the underlying vessel. These situations should lead to convert to an open procedure.

Massive hemorrhage: Although it has never occurred in our experience, a massive bleeding that is not controllable by thoracoscopy should lead to introduce gauzes through the larger port and temporary control bleeding by pressure, while the surgeon convert to thoracotomy. This outlines the importance of having the conventional thoracic instruments ready on a separate operative table.

Minor hemorrhage: A 5-mm clamp must be available (Fig. 2.13a). An alternate solution is the use of throw-off vascular bulldog clips (Aesculap©) (Fig. 2.13b). They are used for controlling a hemorrhage or during the temporary occlusion of a vessel. They are inserted through a 12-mm trocar using a dedicated applier that is withdrawn after the device has been applied. The same instrument is used for retrieving the device.

2.10 Intersegmental Plane and Division of the Parenchyma

Once bronchovascular elements have been controlled and divided, the division of the parenchyma, i.e., intersegmental plane or fused

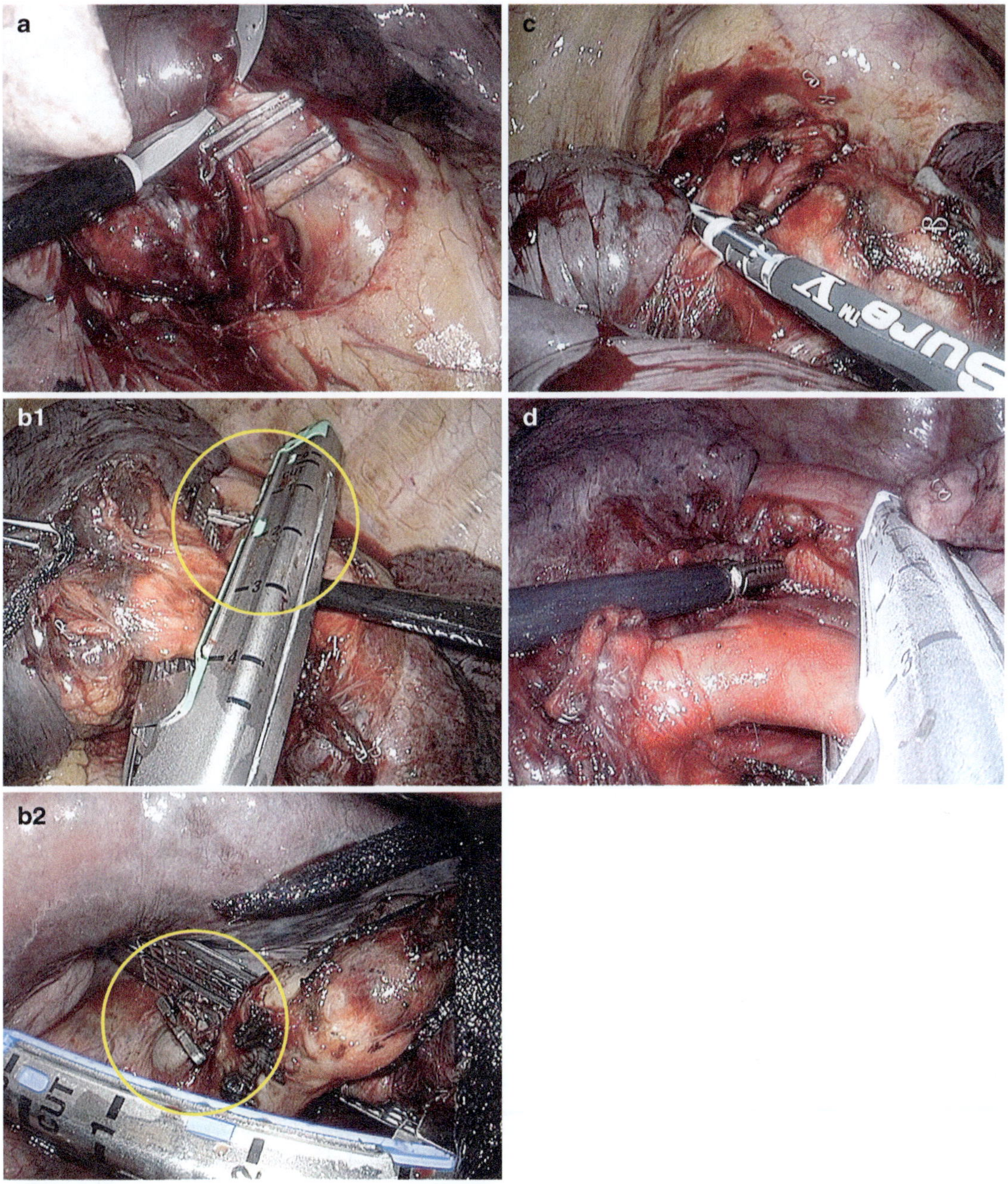

Fig. 2.12 Vessel control. (**a**) Multiple clips. (**b**) Vascular clips can get stuck within stapler anvil (*circle*). (**c**) Combination of clips and bipolar vessel sealing, (**d**) stapling

transverse fissure, can actually be one of the most difficult steps. This is a part of the procedure where one does regret not having the assistance of hand in order to feel and compress the parenchyma and precisely place the stapler. The main concern is that the surgeon usually needs reventilation – after bronchial clamping – to detect the limit between the ventilated and the non-ventilated segments. But reventilation reduces the space and hampers vision. Ventilation must be done with low volumes while a long 5-mm clamp compresses the

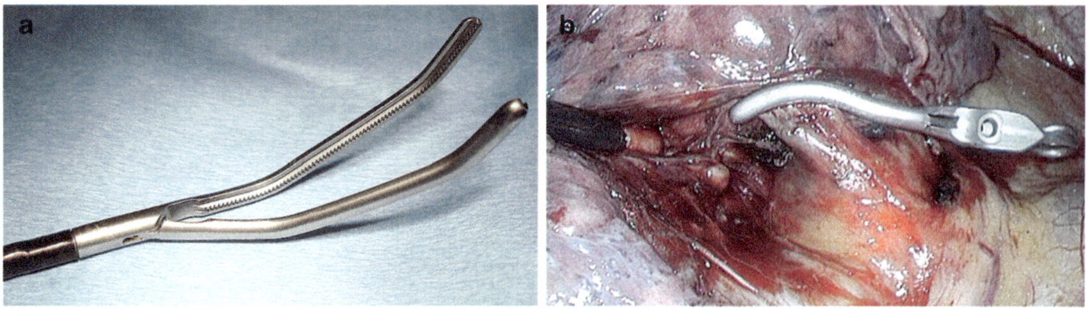

Fig. 2.13 Vascular clamps. (**a**) Conventional thoracoscopic clamp to be inserted through a flexible trocar, (**b**) throw-off bulldog clamp

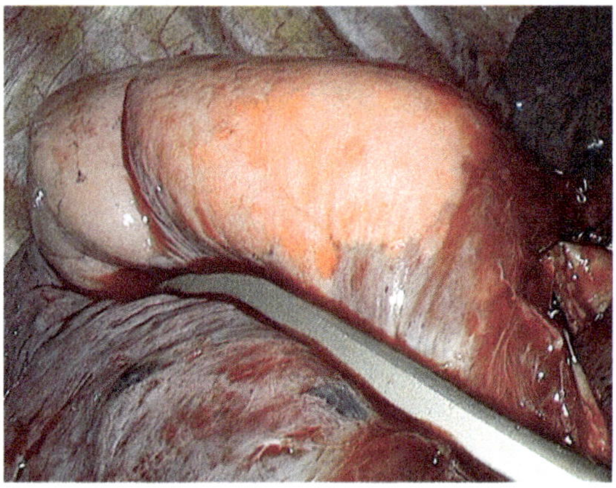

Fig. 2.14 Clamping the parenchyma to determine the intersegmental plane (in this case, a right superior segmentectomy) is achieved with a dedicated endoscopic 5-mm clamp

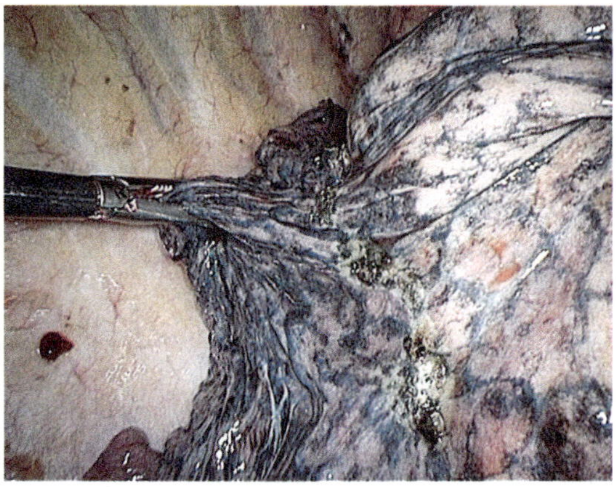

Fig. 2.15 Marking the intersegmental line with dots during a right superior segmentectomy

lung (Fig. 2.14). Once the intersegmental plane has been found and if the stapler cannot be immediately applied, it is sometimes helpful to mark the line between the inflated and the deflated lung parenchyma with small dots using diathermy (Fig. 2.15). Another technique is to reventilate only the lobe or the segment to be resected, using jet ventilation. In this technique, the bronchus to be divided is first intubated with a bronchoscope and selectively reventilated so that the rest of the parenchyma is devoid of air (Fig. 2.16).

2.11 Specimen Retrieval

It would not be recommended to morcellate the specimen as done in other fields of surgery, since it is of outmost importance to analyze the bronchus and the peribronchial lymph nodes and to check that all margins are free. The lobe or segment must be retrieved en bloc. For a segmentectomy, enlarging a port on a 2–3 cm length is sufficient. For a lobectomy, the port must be enlarged on a 35 cm length, depending on the specimen and patient's size. The use of a retractor is never necessary. A solid and large specimen bag must be used (Fig. 2.17). The incision should be done at a site where the intercostal space is soft, preferably in the lower part of the chest on the anterior axillary line or in the axilla (Fig. 2.18).

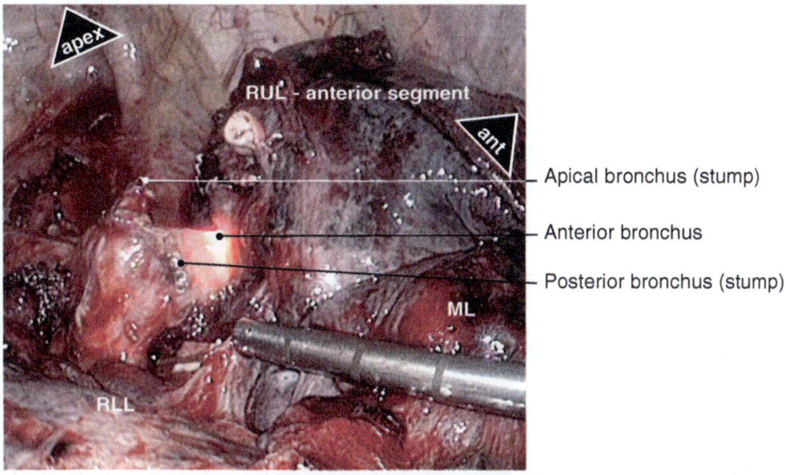

Fig. 2.16 Example of selective endoscopy of a segmental bronchus during a right apico-posterior segmentectomy

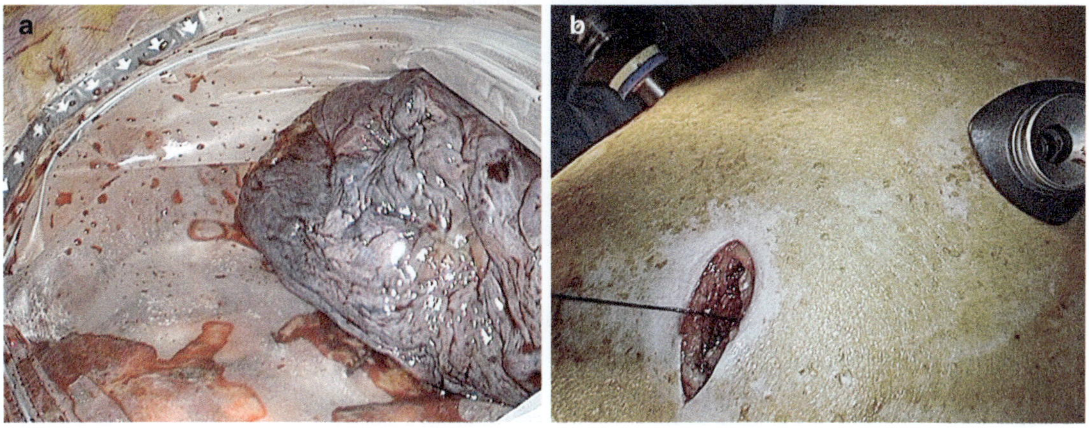

Fig. 2.17 Specimen retrieval. (**a**) Placement of the specimen into a retrieval bag, (**b**) enlargement of one of the ports on a 3–4 cm length

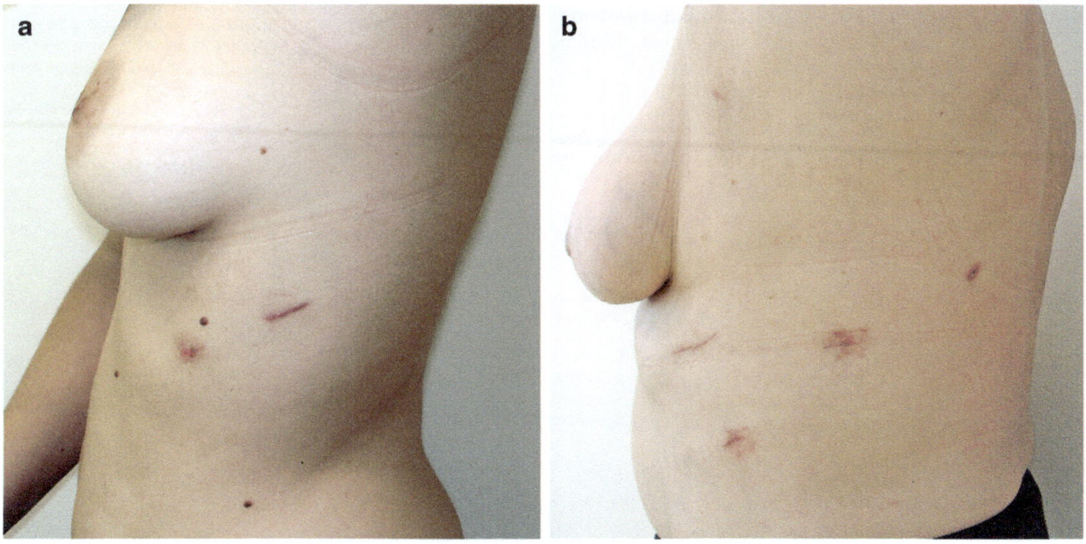

Fig. 2.18 Extraction incisions (*arrows*). Results at 1 month after a segmentectomy (**a**) and a lobectomy (**b**)

Further Reading

General Aspects

Demmy T, James T, Swanson S et al (2005) Troubleshooting video-assisted thoracic surgery lobectomy. Ann Thorac Surg 79:1744–1753

Gossot D (2008) Technical tricks to facilitate totally endoscopic major pulmonary resections. Ann Thorac Surg 86:323–326

Park B, Flores R, Rusch V (2006) Robotic assistance for video-assisted thoracic surgical lobectomy: technique and initial results. J Thorac Cardiovasc Surg 131:54–59

Shiraishi T, Shirakusa T, Miyoshi T et al (2006) A completely thoracoscopic lobectomy/segmentectomy for primary lung cancer: technique, feasibility and advantages. Thorac Cardiovasc Surg 54:202–207

Instruments

Gossot D, Merlusca G, Tudor A et al (2009) Pitfalls related to the use of endostaplers during video-assisted thoracic surgery. Surg Endosc 23:189–192

Ikeda Y, Tamura M, Umezu H et al (2003) Usefulness of mini loop retractor in video-assisted thoracic surgery. Kyobu Geka 56:199–202

Ito N, Suda T, Inoue T et al (2005) Use of a soft silicone tube guide for an automatic suture device in video-assisted lung lobectomy. J Thorac Cardiovasc Surg 130:931–932

Kondo K, Adachi H (2006) Minimally invasive surgery for lung cancer using thoracoscope as a 'microscopic surgery' for the safety endoscopic surgery. Kyobu Geka 59:703–709

Sato Y, Tezuka Y, Kanai Y et al (2008) Novel retractor for lymph node dissection by video-assisted thoracic surgery. Ann Thorac Surg 86:1036–1037

Schoofs J, Gossot D (2004) A neglected but frustrating ergonomic issue: the thoracoscopic trocar. Minim Invasive Ther Allied Technol 13(3):133–137

Hemostatic Devices

Molnar T, Benko I, Szanto Z et al (2006) Lung biopsy using harmonic scalpel: a randomised single institute study. Eur J Cardiothorac Surg 28:604–606

Sakuragi T, Okazaki Y, Mitsuoka M et al (2008) The utility of a reusable bipolar sealing instrument, BiClamp, for pulmonary resection. Eur J Cardiothorac Surg 34:505–509

Santini M, Vicidomini G, Baldi A et al (2006) Use of an electrothermal bipolar tissue sealing system in lung surgery. Eur J Cardiothorac Surg 29:226–230

Tanaka K, Hagiwara M, Kondo Y et al (2006) Usefulness of ultrasonically activated scalpel for pulmonary resection in video-assisted thoracoscopic surgery. Kyobu Geka 59:1171–1175

Technical Tricks

Fukuhara K, Akashi A, Nakane S, Tomita E (2008) Preoperative assessment of the pulmonary artery by three-dimensional computed tomography before video-assisted thoracic surgery lobectomy. Eur J Cardiothorac Surg 34:875–877

Nomori H, Ohtsuka T, Horio H et al (2003) Thoracoscopic lobectomy for lung cancer with a largely fused fissure. Chest 123:619–622

Oda M, Ishikawa N, Tsunezuka Y et al (2007) Closed three-port anatomic lobectomy with systematic nodal dissection for lung cancer. Surg Endosc 21:1464–1465

Okada M, Mimura T, Ikegaki J et al (2007) A novel video assisted anatomic segmentectomy technique: selective segmental inflation via bronchofiberoptic jet followed by cautery cutting. J Thorac Cardiovasc Surg 133:753–758

Watanabe A, Koyanagi T, Nakashima S, Higami T (2007) How to clamp the main pulmonary artery during video-assisted thoracoscopic surgery lobectomy. Eur J Cardiothorac Surg 31:129–131

Wauben L, van Veelen M, Gossot D, Goossens R (2006) Application of ergonomic guidelines during minimally invasive surgery: a questionnaire survey of 284 surgeons. Surg Endosc 20:1268–1274

General Aspects in Robotic Surgery

3

Franca M.A. Melfi, Federico Davini, Andrea Viti, Ralph Alexander Schmid, and Alfredo Mussi

Contents

F.M.A. Melfi, M.D. (✉) • F. Davini, M.D. • A. Mussi
Department of Cardio-Thoracic and Vascular Surgery,
University of Pisa, Via Paradisa 2,
Pisa 56124, Italy
e-mail: f.melfi@med.unipi.it; davinifederico@gmail.com

A. Viti, M.D.
Department of Cardio-Thoracic Surgery,
University of Pisa, Via Paradisa 2,
Pisa 56124, Italy
e-mail: vitimassa@hotmail.it

R.A. Schmid, M.D.
Division of General Thoracic Surgery,
University Hospital Berne,
Freiburgstrasse, Berne CH-3010, Switzerland
e-mail: ralph.schmid@insel.ch

3.1 Introduction

The past two decades have witnessed a revolutionary transition in surgical technique and technology with minimal invasive approaches. Many advantages were obtained by using video thoracoscopic surgery (VTS): less trauma and pain, short hospital stay, cosmetic results [12, 15]. However, limitations still remain due to impaired vision, restricted instrument maneuverability, unstable camera platform, and poor ergonomics for the surgeon. Some of the more prominent limitations involve the technical and mechanical nature of the equipment such as two-dimensional imaging (2D), unsteady camera platform, and limited instrument's maneuverability due to the rigid shaft axis fixed to the thorax by the entry trocar. This implies an unnatural operative feel with hands and the instruments misaligned, fixed instrument tips inside patient and sometimes, inverted surgical movements. The advanced engineering technology on minimally invasive surgery makes it possible to overcome these difficulties. Robotic-assisted minimally invasive surgery represents an extraordinary technological advance for a broad range of procedures

R.G.C. Inderbitzi et al. (eds.), *Minimally Invasive Thoracic and Cardiac Surgery*,
DOI 10.1007/978-3-642-11861-6_3, © Springer-Verlag Berlin Heidelberg 2012

traditionally requiring open surgery. By enabling surgeons to perform complex operations through small incisions, the surgeon's hand movements are scaled and filtered to eliminate hand tremor then translated into micro-movements of the proprietary instruments. These improved ergonomic conditions and instrument mobility at distal articulations seem beneficial in thoracic procedures [11].

3.2 Definitions

"Robotic surgery" is an imprecise accepted term, used by both the medical and lay press. A more scientifically accurate term for current devices would be "remote tele-presence manipulators" since available technology does not generally function without the explicit and direct control of a human operator. In this chapter, we define robotic surgery *as a surgical procedure that adds a computer technology-enhanced device to the interaction between surgeon and patient during a surgical operation and assumes some degree of control heretofore completely reserved for the surgeon.*

3.3 Robot Technical Features

3.3.1 Room Environment

The surgical robot system is a complex device, both electrically and mechanically. It involves direct contact with the patient, both externally and internally. These features differentiate surgical robots from other traditional operating room. In addition, all personnel involved must be appropriately trained to handle this equipment. There are currently standard criteria for nurses, technicians, or surgeons with respect to appropriate training for managing these instruments in the operating room. It is mandatory that teams using such instruments – surgeons, technicians, nurses – meet on a periodic basis to stay current in their training and to learn of updates or changes to the hardware or software. In this way, emerging problems may be quickly identified and addressed.

3.3.2 Surgical Robot System

There are different types of robotic devices, some as simple as the voice control of the camera. Today, the da Vinci™ Robotic System (Surgical Intuitive, Inc., Sunnyvale, CA) is the only complete surgical robot system applied in the surgical practice *which can* overcome some limitations of conventional minimally invasive surgery. The *da Vinci* System is a sophisticated robotic platform designed to expand the surgeon's capabilities, and for the first time offers a minimally invasive option for major surgery.

3.3.3 The *da Vinci*® S™ Surgical System

With *da Vinci,* small incisions are used to introduce miniaturized wristed instruments and a high-definition 3D camera. Seated comfortably at the *da Vinci* console, your surgeon views a magnified, high-resolution 3D image of the surgical site. At the same time, state-of-the-art robotic and computer technologies scale, filter, and seamlessly translate your surgeon's hand movements into precise micro-movements of the *da Vinci* instruments. The system cannot be programmed nor can it make decisions on its own. Rather, the *da Vinci* System requires that every surgical maneuver be performed with direct input from the surgeon.

This system comprehends three different main parts:

- *The Surgeon's Console* (Fig. 3.1):
  It is connected to a surgical manipulator with – three instrument – arms and a central arm to guide the endoscope. Two master handles at the surgeon's console are manipulated by the user. The position and the orientation of the surgeon's hands on the handles trigger highly sensitive motion sensors which transfer the surgeon's movements to the tip of the instrument at a remote location.
- *The Surgical Cart* (Fig. 3.2)
  It provides three degrees of freedom (pitch, yaw, insertion). Attached to the robot arm is the surgical instrument, the tip of which is provided by a mechanical cable-driven wrist

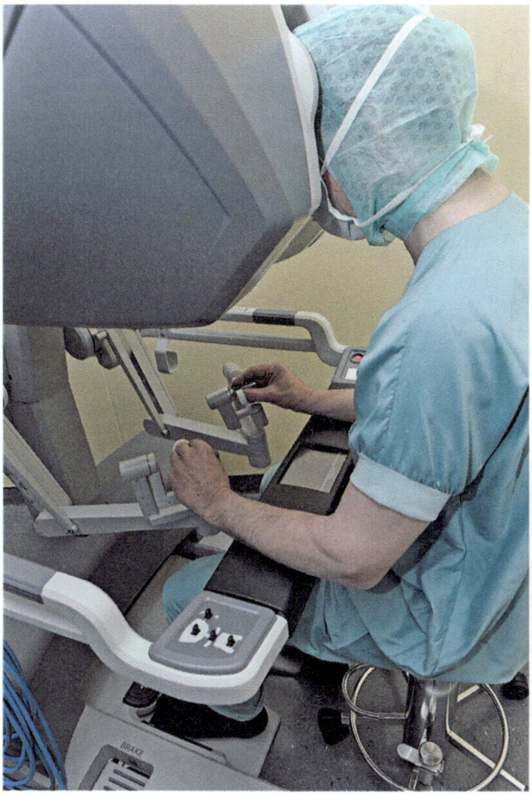

Fig. 3.1 The console (Courtesy of Surgical Intuitive, Inc., Sunnyvale, CA)

(EndoWrist®). This adds four more degrees of freedom (internal pitch, internal yaw, rotation, and grip).

- *The Vision System*
  The computer system which controls the whole system resides in the surgeon's console [6, 8].

The notable features of the da Vinci Surgical System are the surgical instruments with the EndoWrist® move like human hand motion by artificial articulation and the visualization through a high-quality 3D endoscope, which is optimal. This system provides surgeons with an intuitive translation of the instrument handle to the tip movement, thus eliminating the mirror-image effect, scaling, tremor filtering, coaxial alignment of the eyes, hand and tool tip image, and an internal articulated endoscopic wrist providing an additional three degrees of freedom.

3.3.4 Instruments

The *EndoWrist* (Fig. 3.3) Instruments are designed to provide surgeons with natural dexterity and full range of motion for precise operation through tiny incisions. *EndoWrist* Instruments provide enhanced dexterity, thanks to the great range of motion that allows precision and control.

The features instruments:

- Seven degrees of freedom
- 90° of articulation
- *Intuitive* motion and finger tip control
- Motion scaling and tremor reduction

The wrist-like movement, responsiveness, and robotic control afforded by the *da Vinci* System and its exclusive *EndoWrist* Instruments provide surgeons fluid ambidexterity and unparalleled precision.

3.3.5 Dual Console Surgical System

The newly refined *da Vinci* Si Surgical System includes a dual console used for both training and collaboration. During a dual console operation, each surgeon sits at his individual console and can see the same high-definition images of the anatomy from the 3D endoscope (flexible tube with a camera and light at the tip). When the dual console is used for training, control over instruments can be easily and quickly exchanged during surgery – meaning the teaching surgeon can hand over control of the instruments to the resident at any time. This enables a see-and-repeat model of instruction designed to accelerate the learning curve.

For collaborative surgery with the dual console, two surgeons can operate in concert. While one surgeon performs the primary tasks of the operation, the second surgeon can assist with another task, such as retraction.

3.4 Advantages and Disadvantages

This system overcomes many of the obstacles of thoracoscopic surgery. It increases dexterity, restores proper hand-eye coordination and

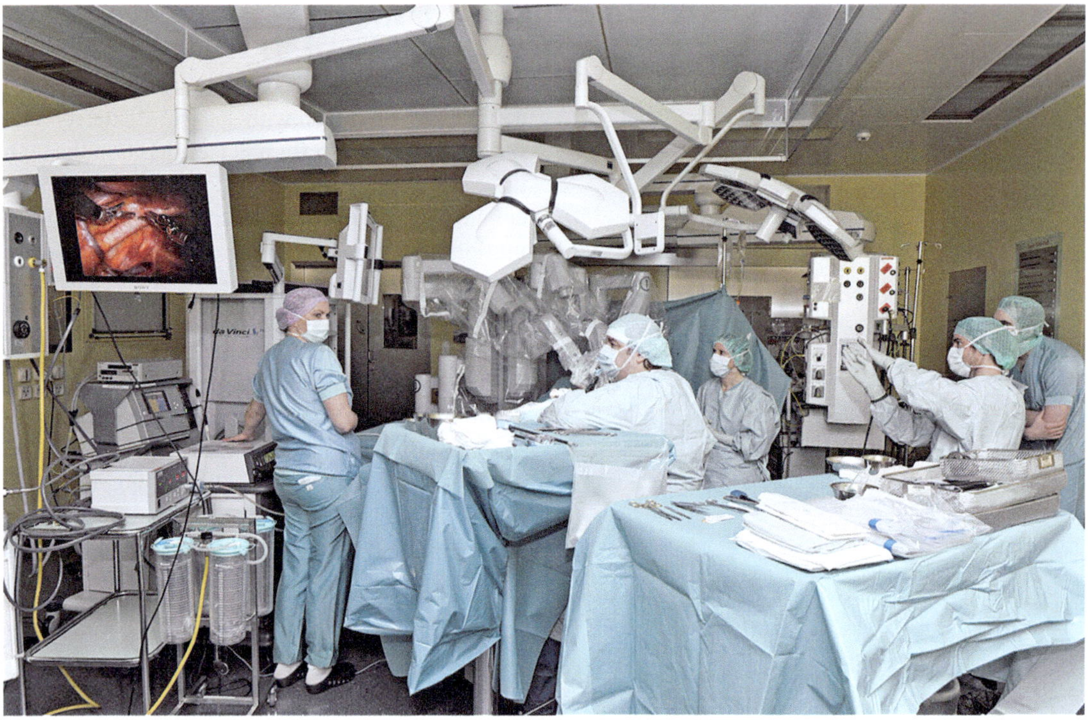

Fig. 3.2 Surgical cart

ergonomic position, and improves visualization. In addition, it makes surgeries that were technically difficult or previously unfeasible, now possible. Instruments with increased degrees of freedom greatly enhance the surgeon's ability to manipulate the tissues. The system is designed so that the surgeons' tremor can be compensated on the end-effector motion through appropriate hardware and software filters. Moreover, this robotic system eliminates the fulcrum effect, making instrument manipulation more intuitive. By most accounts, the enhanced vision afforded by these systems is remarkable. The three-dimensional view with depth perception is a marked improvement over the conventional thoracoscopic camera views. A further advantage is the surgeon's ability to directly control a stable visual field with increased magnification and maneuverability. All of this creates images with increased resolution that, combined with the increased degrees of freedom and enhanced dexterity, greatly enhances the surgeon's ability to identify and dissect anatomic structures as well as to construct microanastomoses.

Nevertheless, there are several disadvantages to the da Vinci Systems. First of all, robotic surgery is a new technology, and its uses and efficacy have not yet been well established. Another disadvantage is the size of this system. This is an important limitation in today's already crowded operating rooms. Moreover, one of the potential disadvantages identified is a lack of compatible instruments and equipment. Lack of certain instruments increases reliance on tableside assistants to perform part of the surgery. This, however, is a transient disadvantage because new technologies have been and will continue to be developed to address these shortcomings. Therefore, most of these disadvantages will be remedied with time and improvements in technology.

3.5 Learning Curve

So far, 1,032 da Vinci Systems have been installed worldwide. Many kinds of surgical operations, such as general surgery, urology, cardiothoracic

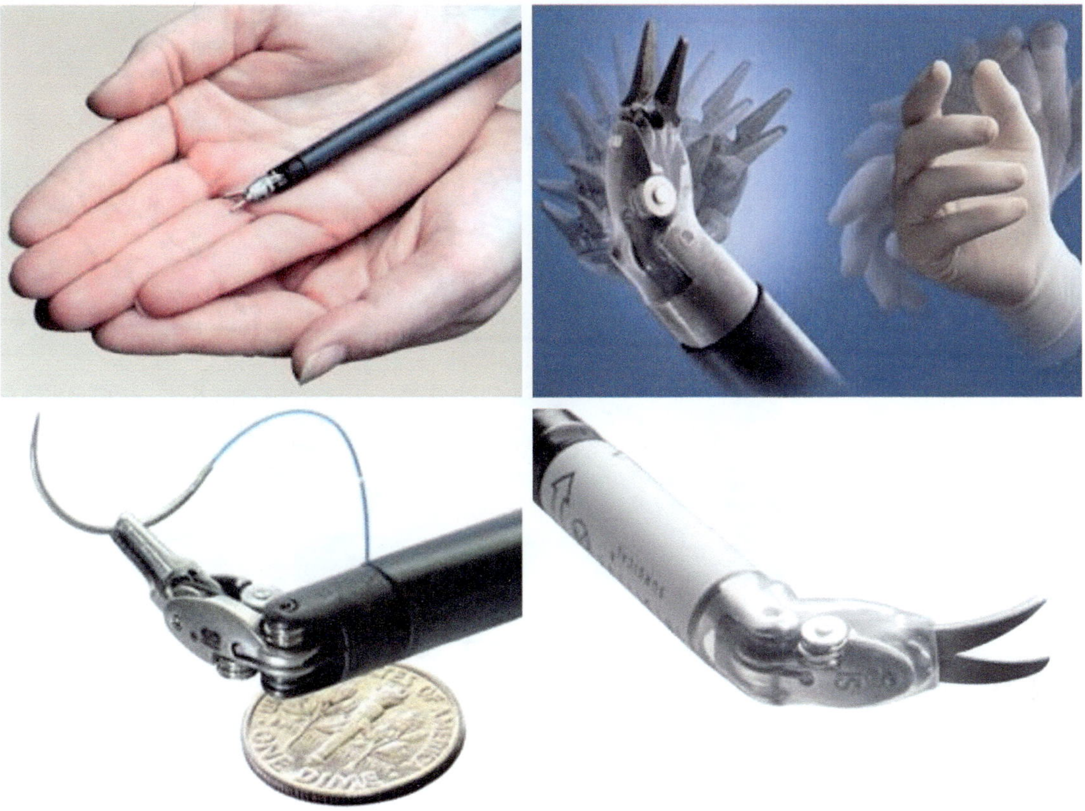

Fig. 3.3 EndoWrist instrumentation (Courtesy of Surgical Intuitive, Inc., Sunnyvale, CA)

surgery, and pediatric surgery, have already been performed using the da Vinci System.

In regard to thoracic surgery, the most frequent procedure recommendable in the initial phase of the learning curve is the treatment of mediastinum lesions (neurinoma, pericardial cysts). These procedures represent an ideal training model, since they provide the means for learning basic procedures combined with a relatively simple technique. Minimum 20 procedures are necessary for the learning curve for both teams to be considered such. In addition, the active cooperation with anesthesiologists is auspicable, mostly with regard to patient and system positioning so as not to hamper patient monitoring.

3.6 Surgical Team

In order to perform robotic surgery in a safe and straightforward manner, it is necessary to standardize procedures and establish operative schemes. This robotic device requires meticulous preparation in terms of setup of the system and its placement at the operating table (Fig. 3.4).

The main body of the machine (surgical cart) must be placed perpendicularly to the camera port. This is mandatory in order to avoid arms impingement. Only when the robotic cart has been positioned appropriately and the patient placed in the chosen position, the robotic arms can be brought into the operative field.

The transition from traditional surgery to advanced totally robotic surgery is not immediate. Just as was necessary in passing from open surgery to minimally invasive technique, here too certain precise organizational and didactic routes must be followed. Advanced training on robotic systems provides surgeon and scrub nurses (surgical team) confidence when operating in tiny intracavitary spaces. This allows the surgical team to activate and maintain the entire

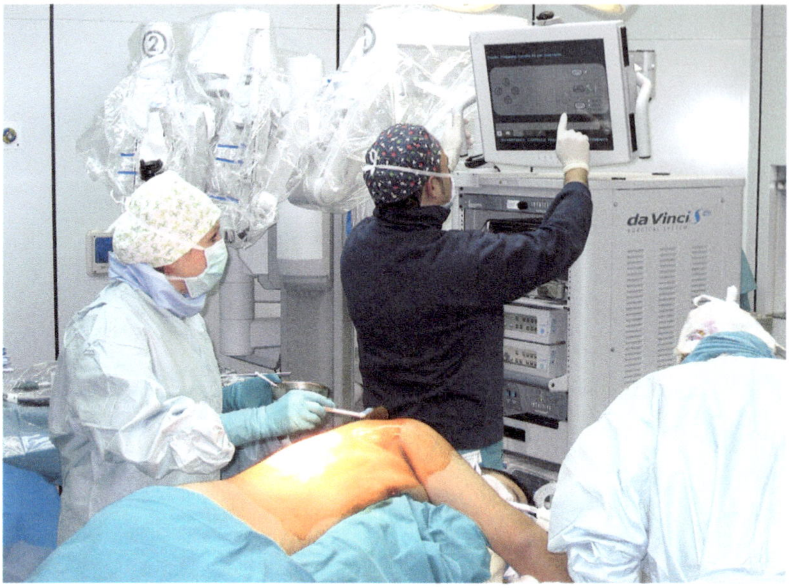

Fig. 3.4 Preparation and setup

operative system, recognize and correct errors, and take charge of handling all materials and instruments. To expand these new capabilities, robotic surgical procedures are developed, and objective-based curriculum levels are designed to optimize surgeon and team training, which is necessary to obtain the best early clinical results.

3.6.1 Indications

Many kinds of surgical operations, such as general surgery, urology, cardiothoracic surgery, and pediatric surgery, have already been performed using the da Vinci System. The most frequent procedure recommendable in the initial phase of the learning curve is the treatment of mediastinum lesions (neurinoma, pericardial cysts) [1]. These procedures represent an ideal training model, since they provide the means for learning basic procedures combined with a relatively simple technique. Minimum 20 procedures are necessary for the learning curve for both teams to be considered such. In addition, the active cooperation with anesthesiologists is auspicable, mostly with regard to patient and system positioning so as not to hamper patient monitoring.

3.6.2 Clinical Applications

Across multiple surgical specialties, robotic surgery was felt to offer the greatest advantage in complex reconstructive processes [2–5]. In thoracic surgery, this new technology offers clear benefits in the treatment of mediastinum lesions, particularly to perform thymectomy [14, 16], and in the treatment of lung cancer, particularly lobectomy in stage I NSCLC patients [9, 10, 13]. Limitations of current robotic technology include, among other technical constraints, lack of haptics (force feedback), instrumentation limitations (both size and variety), lack of flexibility of certain energy devices, and problems with multi-quadrant surgery (current devices are deployed typically for single quadrant application). Overall, the technically exceptional laparoscopic surgeon may derive little benefit from robotic surgery. However, surgical robots may serve as an "enabling technology" for many surgeons, allowing them to provide complex minimally invasive procedures to a broad range of patients.

3.6.3 Technical Considerations: Risks of Robotic Surgery

Current surgical robots are continuously controlled by the surgeon and do not move autonomously.

They possess neither artificial intelligence nor independent functioning. The robot remains a high-level, sophisticated tool used by the surgeon in the conduct of an operative procedure. Risks of robotic surgery can be categorized into those pertaining directly to the use of the robotic system and the general risks of the operative procedure. Theoretically, the lack of haptic feedback in current robotic systems could lead to an increased risk of inadvertent tissue injury [7]. However, to date, robotically performed operations have not been associated with higher clinical complication rates than their standard laparoscopic or open counterparts in experienced hands. In certain instances, evidence exists that robotically performed procedures may be associated with a lower complication rate. Robotic telesurgery, in which the surgeon may be located at some distance from the patient, poses unique risks. For example, precise control of the robot will be dependent upon the quality of the data connection between the surgeon's console and the operating room robot. Issues pertaining to the quality and maintenance of such data connections may be beyond the control of the surgical team but still represent a risk management challenge.

3.6.4 Mechanical Risks

All mechanical and electronic devices are subject to failure. Surgical robots – complex systems relying on a delicate interplay of hardware and software – are no exception. Current systems are designed with features intended to minimize the potentially deleterious effect of such failures on patients. Such features include system redundancy, so-called graceful performance degradation or failure, fault tolerance, just-in-time maintenance, and system alerting. These are standards to which all high-level systems should be held.

References

1. Bodner J, Wykypiel H, Greiner A et al (2004) Early experience with robot-assisted surgery for mediastinal masses. Ann Thorac Surg 78(1):259–265; discussion 265–266
2. Bonatti J, Schachner T, Bernecker O et al (2004) Robotic totally endoscopic coronary artery bypass. Program development and learning curve issues. J Thorac Cardiovasc Surg 127:504–510
3. Chitwood WR Jr (2005) Current status of endoscopic and robotic mitral valve surgery. Ann Thorac Surg 79(Suppl):S2248–S2253
4. Elliott DS, Chow GK, Gettman M (2006) Current status of robotics in female urology and gynecology. World J Urol 24(2):188–192
5. Hanly EJ, Talamini MA (2004) Robotic abdominal surgery. Am J Surg 188(4A Suppl):19S–26S
6. Hashizume M, Shimada M, Tomikawa M, Ikeda Y, Takahashi I, Abe R et al (2002) Early experiences of endoscopic procedures in general surgery assisted by a computer-enhanced surgical system. Surg Endosc 16:1187–1191
7. Lee JW, Yoon YE, Kim DK, Park SY et al (2010) Renal artery injury during robot-assisted renal surgery. J Endourol 24(7):1101–1104
8. Lobontiu A (2001) The da Vinci surgical system performing computer-enhanced surgery. Osp Ital Chir 7:367–372
9. Melfi FM, Menconi GF, Mariani AM et al (2002) Early experience with robotic technology for thoracoscopic surgery. Eur J Cardiothorac Surg 21(5): 864–868
10. Melfi FMA, Ambrogi MC, Lucchi M, Mussi A . Video robotic lobectomy. Video robotic lobectomy. Accessed 2011. Available online: http://mmcts.ctsnetjounals.org/cgi/content/full/2005/0628/mmcts.2004.000448
11. Melfi FM, Mussi A (2008) Robotically assisted lobectomy: learning curve and complications. Thorac Surg Clin 18:289–295
12. Miller DL, Allen MS (1993) Set-up and present indications: video-assisted thoracic surgery. Semin Thorac Cardiovasc Surg 5(4):280–283
13. Park BJ, Flores RM, Rusch VW (2006) Robotic assistance for video-assisted thoracic surgical lobectomy: technique and initial results. J Thorac Cardiovasc Surg 131(1):54–59
14. Rea F, Marulli G, Bortolotti L et al (2006) Experience with the "da Vinci" robotic system for thymectomy in patients with myasthenia gravis: report of 33 cases. Ann Thorac Surg 81(2):455–459
15. Tsuboi M, Sakai H, Magata S et al (1999) The development of a new setup for video-assisted Thoracic Surgery. Diagn Ther Endosc 6(1):43–46
16. Yoshino I, Hashizume M, Shimada M et al (2001) Thoracoscopic thymomectomy with the da Vinci computer-enhanced surgical system. J Thorac Cardiovasc Surg 122(4):783–785

Drainages in Thoracoscopic Surgery

4

Franco Gambazzi

Contents

4.1 Introduction

Because of smaller incisions, thoracoscopic operations are known to be less painful and may therefore lead to a shorter length of hospital stay [1]. However, the variety of surgical procedures have developed to be almost the same for minimally invasive as for conventional open thoracic surgery. In particular, thoracoscopic lobectomy is being conducted in increasing numbers. The reasons to drain the pleural space remain thus the same:

- To evacuate fluid and air
- To re-expand the lung

4.2 Videothoracoscopic Incisions and Position of Chest Tubes

Whereas in open surgery chest tubes should be positioned through separate small incisions, often tunneled, for thoracoscopic procedures, this is not the case. In very tall patients, the use of this on a direct way to applied port incisions may lead to a leakage along the way of the tube trough the chest wall. To avoid subcutaneous emphysema, it is important to close the port incisions around the tube using a deep subcutaneous suture. The other incisions were closed by using the same technique as well.

To fix the tube on the chest wall, a strong non-absorbable filament is applied in a fashion that helps to confine the incision. One or two port incisions can be used to place the tubes. Finally, a

F. Gambazzi, M.D.
Department of Thoracic Surgery, Kantonsspital Aarau, Tellstrasse, 5001 Aarau, Switzerland
e-mail: franco.gambazzi@ksa.ch

R.G.C. Inderbitzi et al. (eds.), *Minimally Invasive Thoracic and Cardiac Surgery*,
DOI 10.1007/978-3-642-11861-6_4, © Springer-Verlag Berlin Heidelberg 2012

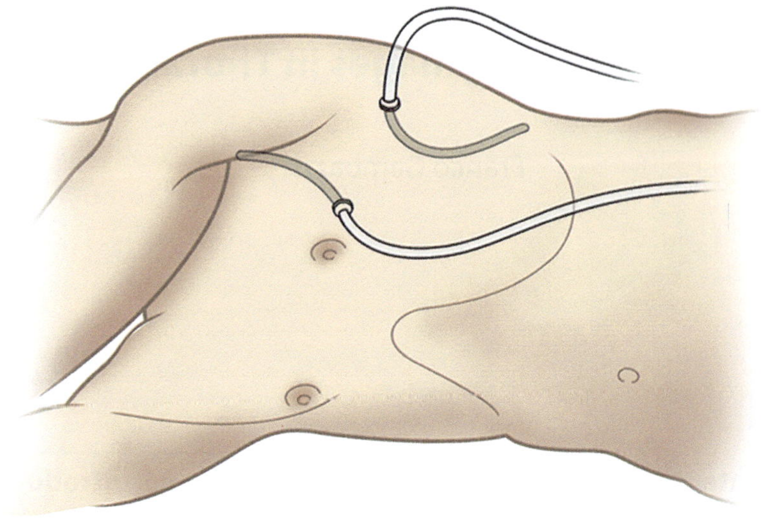

Fig. 4.1 Thoracoscopic-guided positioning of the chest tubes using two tubes

skin suture is prepositioned to close the incision after removal of the drain. Recent studies could show that one tube instead of two is sufficient to drain both air and liquids, even for thoracoscopic lobectomies [2, 3].

If two tubes are used, the following procedure is recommendable:

Before removal of the optic, the tubes are positioned under visual control and guidance of a trocar (Fig. 4.1) through the mini-incisions. The tips of both tubes are located ventroapical and dorsobasal in the phrenicocostal sinus. Finally, the evacuation of the pneumothorax should be done slowly and under visual control, thus avoiding an interstitial edema. Remaining incisions are closed by single sutures.

4.3 Air Leakage, Liquid Amounts, and Chest Tube Removal

Many institutions prefer to have strict guidelines on how to manage chest tubes. Often such guidelines are generated under historical aspects. Air leakage is the main reason to leave the tube in place, whereas for the drainage volume, there are many different recommendations and just a small number of reports in the literature. To assess the air leak, two systems are nowadays common: the standard water seal system and the continuous digital airflow measuring system. With the standard system, air leakage can be evaluated only semiquantitatively by observing air bubbles in the water seal chamber. Often it is difficult to distinguish a real air leak from large swings because of a residual air space. More effective seems to be the digital airflow system allowing a better assessment of air leakage [4].

For the drainage volume, a value of 200 mL/24 h seems to be appropriate for a majority of internal guidelines. Nakanishi and colleagues [5] reported recently on 100 prospective patients with tube removal on the day after thoracoscopic lobectomy independent of the drainage volume. They found no differences among three drainage groups (range from 60 to 1,030 mL/24 h) and concluded that an early removal of chest tube seems to be safe. Even less than 1 day seems to be possible for thoracoscopic diagnostic wedge resections, as published in 2005 by Sienel and colleagues [6]. In absence of a pleural air leakage, they removed the chest tube 2 h postoperatively and found a better pain relief, less x-rays, and a shorter hospital stay. So limits for drainage volumes are no longer indicated, and after cessation of air leak, an early chest tube removal can be recommended [7].

References

1. Hazelrigg SR et al (1993) cost analysis for thovacoscopy: thoracoscopic ledge resection. Ann Thorac Surg 56:633–635
2. Göttgens KWA et al (2011) Early removal of the chest tube after complete video-assisted thoracoscopic lobectomies. Eur J Cardiothorac Surg 39(4):575–578
3. Alex J et al (2003) Comparison of the immediate postoperative outcome of using the conventional two drains versus a single drain after lobectomy. Ann Thorac Surg 76:1046–1049
4. Varela G et al (2009) Postoperative chest tube management: measuring air leak using an electronic device decreases variability in the clinical practice. Eur J Cardiothorac Surg 35:28–31
5. Nakanishi R et al (2009) A prospective study of the association between drainage volume within 24 hours after thoracoscopic lobectomy and postoperative morbidity. J Thorac Cardiovasc Surg 137:1394–1399
6. Sienel W et al (2005) Early chest tube removal after video-assisted thoracoscopic surgery. Results of a prospective randomized study. Chirurg 76:1155–1160
7. Cerfolio RJ et al (2008) Results of a prospective algorithm to remove chest tubes after pulmonary resection with high output. J Thorac Cardiovasc Surg 135: 269–273

Anesthesia

5

Andreas Vogt

Contents

A. Vogt, M.D.
Division of General and Thoracic Surgery, University Department of Anaesthesiology and Pain Therapy, Berne University Hospital/Inselspital, and University of Bern, Berne 3010, Switzerland
e-mail: andreas.vogt@insel.ch

5.1 Introduction

The last two decades have shown a trend toward "minimal invasive surgery" in many surgical subspecialties, and thoracic procedures are increasingly performed as video-assisted thoracoscopic surgery (VATS) or robotic-assisted surgery (RATS) [18]. VATS generated less pain and cytokine production and preserved the early pulmonary function better compared to standard posterolateral thoracotomy [29]. The concept of fast-track thoracic surgery was evaluated only with very few studies showing that VATS can be performed with minimal complications and reduced costs [6]. A prerequisite for a successful surgical performance during a closed chest approach is the optimal deflation of the operated lung with the need of lung separation and one-lung ventilation. Pre-VATS indications for one-lung ventilation were divided into absolute and relative groups (Table 5.1). The expectations that are imposed today upon thoracic anesthesiologists may be better defined by lung isolation and lung separation [18]. The goal of lung isolation is to protect the nondiseased contralateral lung from massive bleeding, pus, or alveolar proteinosis and avoid complications of positive pressure ventilation in the case of bronchopleural fistula. In contrast lung separation is used and mandatory to optimize lung deflation and to improve surgical exposure especially required in closed chest approaches like VATS. Thus thoracic anesthesiologists have to become familiar with minimal invasive surgical techniques and the pathophysiological impact of

R.G.C. Inderbitzi et al. (eds.), *Minimally Invasive Thoracic and Cardiac Surgery*,
DOI 10.1007/978-3-642-11861-6_5, © Springer-Verlag Berlin Heidelberg 2012

Table 5.1 Absolute and relative indications for one-lung ventilation, subdivided in lung isolation (to protect the non-diseased lung) and lung separation (to improve surgical exposure) [3, 18]

Absolute indications		Relative indications
Lung isolation	Lung separation	Lung separation
Lung abscess	Video-assisted thoracoscopy	Open, middle, and lower lobectomy
Lung bleeding	Pneumonectomy	Esophageal resection
Large bronchopleural fistula	Upper lobe resection	
Bronchopleural cutaneous fistula	Repair of thoracic aortic aneurysm	
Giant unilateral lung cyst	Unilateral bronchopulmonary lavage for alveolar proteinosis	

lung separation and one-lung ventilation. Slinger [37] has proposed the following "ABC" for lung isolation:

- A = Anatomy. Lack of familiarity with distal airway anatomy is one of the major problems in achieving successful lung isolation.
- B = Bronchoscopy. Is highly recommended for the positioning of bronchial blockers and double-lumen tubes.
- C = Chest imaging for the detection of airway abnormalities and size to chose the optimal method for lung isolation.

This chapter aims to summarize the key features of (i) monitoring, (ii) airway and ventilation strategy, and (iii) anesthetic implications and perioperative analgesia for minimal invasive thoracic surgery.

5.2 Monitoring

The incidence of hypoxemia during one-lung ventilation in pulmonary surgery may be up to 10% [26]. During VATS, vital intrathoracic organs may be injured which needs rapid identification and treatment. An increase in inspired oxygen fraction or hypoxic pulmonary vasoconstriction cannot always compensate the effects of the obligatory right-to-left shunt. Limitations of noninvasive pulse oximetry to provide information about patient oxygenation include inadequate readings, i.e., in the setting of poor peripheral perfusion. In patients with good overall clinical condition [(American Society of Anesthesiologists (ASA) I–II)] undergoing short lasting procedures (<30 min of OLV), an indwelling arterial catheter may be omitted. The majority of VATS patients, however, are at higher risk for intraoperative hypoxemia requiring rapid and intermittent arterial blood gas sampling to confirm noninvasive pulse oximetry readings for a safe management of oxygenation during one-lung ventilation [18]. Large bore venous access is recommended to control hemorrhage due to large vessel bleeding. In case of massive hemorrhage during VATS, the surgeon may change to an open approach. It may be rather challenging to maintain stable hemodynamics in these situations, and large bore venous access prior to start of the procedure may be highly supportive [18]. Central venous access provides reliable and effective administration of vasoactive medications in case of cardiovascular comorbidities or rapid volume restoration if peripheral venous access is difficult.

5.3 Airway Management and Ventilation Strategy

5.3.1 Double-Lumen Tube

The currently single-use double-lumen tubes are manufactured in several sizes (26, 28, 32, 35, 37, 39, 41 Charrière or French) from different producers (Rusch-Teleflex, Mallinckrodt-Tyco, Portex-Smiths, Hudson-Teleflex) [28]. The outer diameter in millimeters is converted according the formula Charrière/3.14 or French/3.

Many authors prefer left-shaped double-lumen tubes due to the higher length and margin of safety (16–19 mm) of the left main stem bronchus compared with the right main stem bronchus (<9 mm) [28]. In 1,170 patients, left double-lumen tubes were chosen for 1,166 patients, and successful lung separation was achieved in 1,145 procedures (98.2%) [5]. Right-shaped double-lumen tubes have a murphy eye at the endobronchial end to avoid obstruction of the right superior lobar bronchus. However, correct positioning remains difficult (i) due to anatomical abnormalities (origin next to the carina) and (ii) small intraoperative displacements may lead to obstruction and atelectasis of the right upper lobe [28]. Contraindications for the placement of double-lumen tubes are obstructions by tumors or compression by aortic aneurysms, lacerations, or near carina surgery of the main bronchus (sleeve resections). The correct size of a double-lumen tube is highly dependent on the inner diameter of the corresponding main bronchus. The tube has to pass atraumatically through the glottis, advance easily along the trachea till a slight resistance is felt. Several methods for the evaluation of the correct size of a double-lumen tube have been reported:

1. The assessment of the tracheal diameter by chest X-ray. The diameter of the left main bronchus is calculated as follows: 0.75 × inner diameter of the trachea (males) and 0.77 × inner diameter of the trachea (females) [28].
2. Main stem bronchus diameter can be measured by computer tomography, and in addition, morphology and patency of the airway can be evaluated [10, 16].
3. Anthropometric parameters like age, sex, height, and weight correlated weak but significant with left bronchial width, however, multivariate statistical analysis showed that left bronchial diameter was best predicted by tracheal width.

There is compelling evidence that correct position of the double-lumen tube after placement has to be confirmed [4, 12]. It is a matter of debate whether clinical signs (auscultation, observation of chest wall movement, peak inspiratory pressures) are reliable enough, or if fiber-optic bronchoscopy should be used per routine [12]. In previous work, fiber-optic bronchoscopy found 20–40% of clinically verified double-lumen tubes malpositioned [38]. Typical examples are shown in Fig. 5.1. At the author's institution, fiber-optic bronchoscopy is routinely used for this purpose. Left-sided tubes are "blindly" positioned but controlled by fiber-optic bronchoscopy immediately after placement and after each change of patients' position. If fiber-optic bronchoscopy is performed via the tracheal lumen of a left-sided double-lumen tube, the right main stem bronchus can be identified by the typical orifice of the right upper lobe. In case of any doubt concerning the anatomy, fiber-optic bronchoscopy will be performed via the bronchial lumen, and the double-lumen tube will be withdrawn above the carina. Both main stem bronchi will be evaluated, and afterward, the left-sided double-lumen tube advanced under fiber-optic guidance into the left main stem bronchus. This maneuver is illustrated in Fig. 5.2. Right-sided tubes are only advanced into the trachea, and the anatomy of the right main stem bronchus especially with regard to the anatomy of the right upper bronchus will be evaluated by bronchoscopy via the bronchial lumen. Afterward, the tube will be advanced under fiber-optic guidance to the correct place. With this approach, one should be able to eliminate malpositioning of left- or right-shaped double-lumen tubes. This is a key feature of successful lung separation and one-lung ventilation keeping in mind that correction of a malpositioned double-lumen tube after the start of surgery in the lateral decubitus position may be very difficult or impossible [12]. Turning the patient from supine to the lateral decubitus position will displace the double-lumen tube, and correct position has always to be verified after final positioning of the patient. During thoracic surgery, up to 12% of all double-lumen tubes may be dislodged or malpositioned requiring immediate fiber-optic monitoring [23].

5.3.2 Bronchial Blocker and Difficult Airway

Bronchial blockers are alternative tools to achieve lung separation and one-lung ventilation. In case of a difficult airway insertion of a double-lumen tube may be very challenging or impossible due to its rigidity and increased outer diameter compared with single-lumen tubes [31]. Bronchial

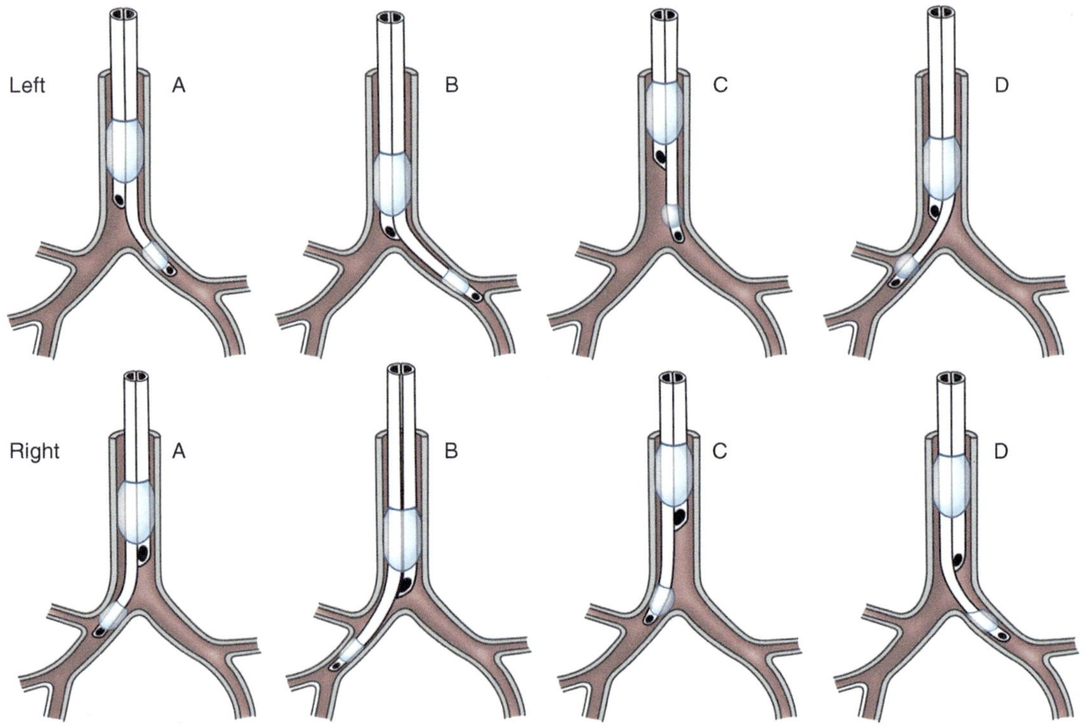

Fig. 5.1 Tube misplacement during one lung ventilation may lead to hypoxemia. The correct position (*Left A*) and possible misplacements (*Left B–D*) of the left-sided double-lumen tube are shown. In the lower four figures, correct position (*Right A*) and possible misplacements (*Right B–D*) of the right sided double-lumen tube are shown (modified from Karzai and Schwarzkopf [23]).

blockers require a single-lumen tube for placement with the following advantages: (i) to evaluate the bronchial stump at the end of surgery, an adult bronchoscope not fitting through a DLT may be needed; (ii) there will be no need to change from a double-lumen tube to a single-lumen tube at the conclusion of surgery if the patient cannot be extubated; the bronchial blocker has only to be removed from the single-lumen tube.

In the past, Fogarty catheters were used for bronchial blockade [31]. However, they were not designed for thoracic surgery (low-volume, high-pressure balloons), and more suitable devices have been invented for providing one-lung ventilation. Key features of the currently used bronchial blockers are a wire loop at tip to snare fiber-optic scope (5F, 7F, 9F, Arndt®), tip deflecting (9F, Cohen®), tip with prefixed bend (5F, 9F, Uniblocker®), preshaped tip for guidance (5F, 9F Fuji®), and single-lumen tube with incorporated channel containing the bronchial blocker (3.5- to 9-mm ID, Univent Tube®). In a prospective, randomized, controlled trial with 48 patients, no difference was found for positioning time of the Cohen bronchial blocker or the Arndt blocker with a trend to a longer positioning time compared with the double-lumen tube [15]. The Cohen device had more difficulty to block the left main bronchus compared with the right one. The least satisfactory lung collapse was achieved with the Arndt blocker. For patients requiring one-lung ventilation with potentially difficult airway, the placement of an orally or nasotracheally single-lumen tube with the aid of flexible fiber-optic bronchoscopy is recommended. Lung isolation can then be achieved by the use of an independent bronchial blocker which can also be used through a tracheostomy [8]. A flexible fiber-optic bronchoscope is needed to verify optimal position

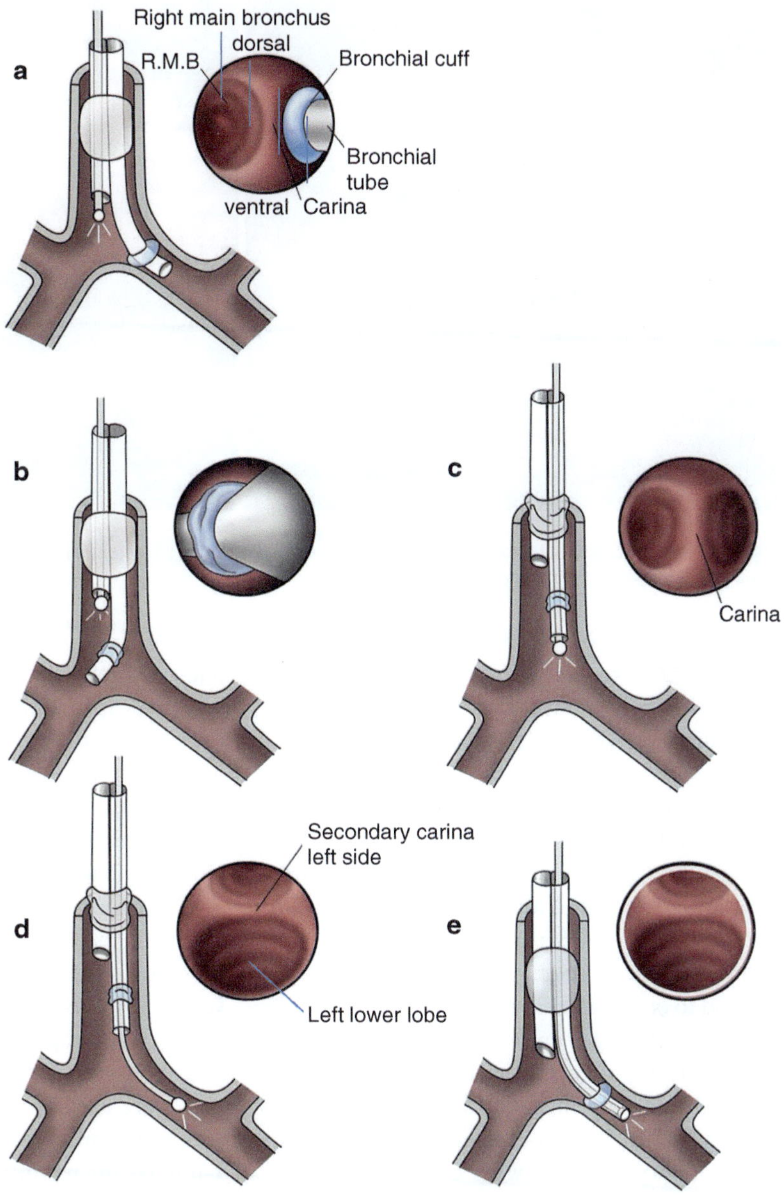

Fig. 5.2 Fiberoptic controlled positioning of a left sided double-lumen tube. Correct position (*panel a*); misplacement in the right main stem bronchus, fiberoptic in the tracheal lumen (*panel b*); withdrawal of double-lumen tube above carina, fiberoptic in bronchial lumen; advancement of fiberoptic in the left main bronchus (*panel d*); correct placement of double-lumen tube proximal the secondary carina left side (modified from Cohen. [12])

of the bronchial blocker at least 10 mm below the tracheal carina after inflation of the high-volume, low-pressure balloon with 5–8 mL of air (Fig. 5.3). Disadvantages of bronchial blockers consist in (i) difficult right lung isolation because of right upper lobe anatomy and (ii) bronchoscopy of the isolated lung impossible and suction very limited [37].

5.3.3 Ventilatory Mode and Settings

Hypoxemia during one-lung ventilation with arterial oxygen saturation lower than 90% has been reported in up to 4% of patients receiving an inspiratory oxygen fraction greater than 50% [23]. First of all, correct position of the double-lumen tube or bronchus blocker has to be checked

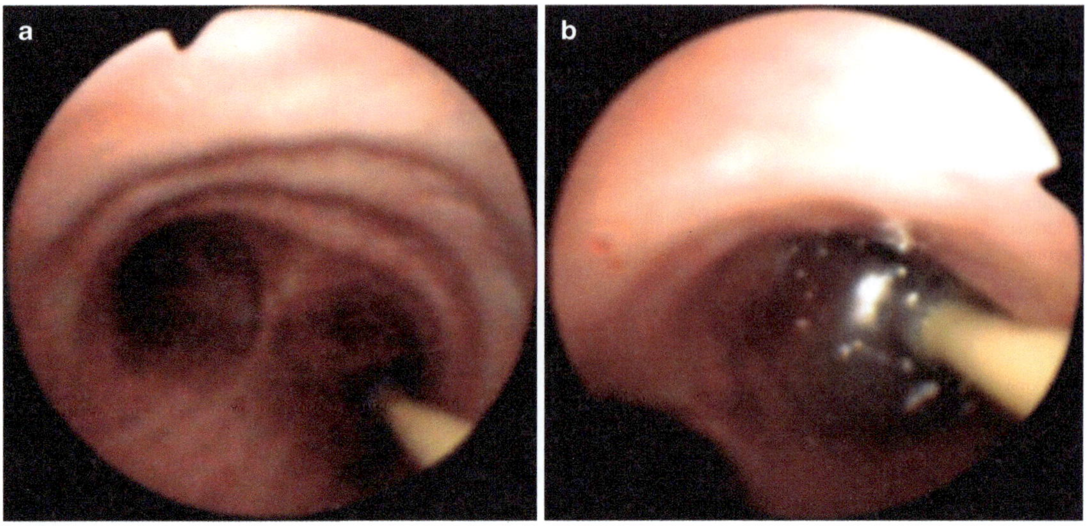

Fig. 5.3 Arndt bronchial blocker with deflated (*panel* **a**) and inflated (*panel* **b**) spherical balloon in the right main stem bronchus. To be checked concerning resolution

by fiber-optic bronchoscopy. Right-sided thoracic surgery has been identified as an important factor in predicting hypoxemia (when the smaller left lung is the ventilated lung). As a paradoxical effect, obstructive airway disease reduced hypoxemia which may be explained by auto-positive end-expiratory pressure (PEEP) due to air trapping in the ventilated lung [23]. In the literature, the application of 5 cm H_2O PEEP after lung recruitment maneuvers was reported the best method to employ PEEP during one-lung ventilation [20]. A larger intraoperative tidal volume (8–12 mL/kg) may be associated with ventilatory-induced lung injury (VILI) and respiratory failure; however, data of the effect on pulmonary inflammatory response were contradictory [27]. At the authors' institution, smaller tidal volumes (6 mL/kg predicted body weight [1]) are used during OLV from the following reasons: (i) some evidence for a lung-protective effect [36, 42] and (ii) to maximize surgical exposure and to minimize mediastinal shift as an important prerequisite for successful VATS [27]. Continuous positive airway pressure (CPAP) may be useful in open thoracic surgery to treat hypoxemia but will prevent an optimal deflation of the nondependent lung reducing visualization and identification of pathological lung processes during VATS [20]. In one case report, oxygenation was improved by selective ipsilateral segmental insufflation of oxygen via the bronchoscope [26]. In patients with previous lobectomy or contralateral pneumonectomy not tolerating complete lung collapse, selective lobar blockade has been reported to maintain arterial oxygenation [7].

Two randomized clinical trials in 58 [40] and 110 patients [34] found no effect of the ventilatory mode [pressure-controlled ventilation (PCV) versus volume-controlled ventilation (VCV)] on intra- and postoperative gas exchange. In both trials, an FIO_2 of 1.0 and zero end-expiratory pressure were used; however, tidal volumes were set to 9 and 8 mL/kg, respectively. In 13 patients, a 1-min lasting recruitment maneuver of the dependent lung during one-lung ventilation followed by 5 cm H_2O PEEP improved the PaO_2/FIO_2 ratio from 235 ± 113 to 351 ± 120 mmHg; cardiac index decreased from 3.04 ± 0.7 to 2.4 ± 0.6 L/m^2, returning to baseline postrecruitment maneuver [11].

As previously mentioned, optimal lung deflation is crucial for successful minimal invasive thoracoscopic surgery. In 100 patients, the use of air (AIR, $N = 33$) during two-lung ventilation resulted after 10 and 20 min of OLV in the lowest lung deflation score (0 = no collapse, 10 = fully collapsed) compared with 100% oxygen (O_2, $N = 33$) or nitrous

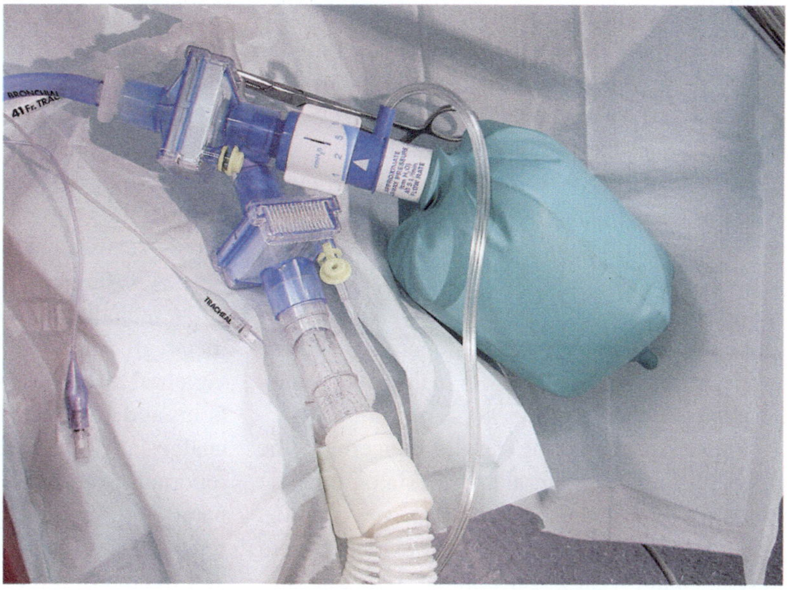

Fig. 5.4 Mallinckrodt CPAP system delivering oxygen 3 L/min to the nondependent lung

oxide (N_2O, $N=34$; best lung deflation score) [24]. The oxygen group had the highest PaO_2 values in the first 10 min after initiation of one-lung ventilation. The very low incidence of clinically important desaturation ($SpO_2 < 90\%$) was similar in each group (group AIR = 2, group $O_2 = 1$, group $N_2O = 2$). At our institution, one-lung ventilation is initiated immediately after fiber-optic verification of the correct double-lumen tube position with oxygen 3 L/min delivered by a Mallinckrodt CPAP system to the nondependent lung (Fig. 5.4).

5.4 Anesthetic Implications and Perioperative Analgesia

A major concern of one-lung ventilation is transpulmonary right-to-left shunt resulting in arterial deoxygenation and hypoxemia [3]. From surgical reasons, especially during VATS, the nondependent lung has to be fully collapsed and non-ventilated; however, it remains under perfusion. Most commonly, this type of surgery is performed in the lateral decubitus position. Gravity is one factor that diverts blood from the nondependent to the dependent and ventilated lung. Hypoxic pulmonary vasoconstriction (HPV) resulting from airway hypoxia is an intrinsic feature of the pulmonary circulation increasing pulmonary vascular resistance in atelectatic areas, pneumonia, asthma, or the adult respiratory distress syndrome [30]. Thereby, the resulting ventilation-perfusion mismatch or shunt is decreased by a reduction of blood flow in non-ventilated and hypoxic areas. Hypoxic pulmonary vasoconstriction causes a large difference on arterial oxygenation in intermediate hypoxic lungs (30–70%) reducing the shunt fraction from the expected 40–50% to 20–25% [3].

Numerous anesthesiological interventions modify hypoxic pulmonary vasoconstriction [30]; decrease by dextran volume replacement, halothane, verapamil, alkalosis, nitroprusside and pregnancy; increase by lateral decubitus positioning, thoracic epidural anaesthesia, lidocaine and high-frequency positive pressure ventilation; and propofol, enflurane, isoflurane and fentanyl without impact on hypoxic pulmonary vasoconstriction. However, a systematic Cochrane review of Bassi et al. [2] (9 trials that enrolled 291 patients) evaluating safety and effectiveness of intravenous versus inhalational anesthesia for one-lung ventilation found no important differences in outcomes. The authors highlighted the need for further clinical trials with standardized outcomes such as death, adverse postoperative events, and intraoperative awareness. Two clinical trials in 80 and 36 patients undergoing one-lung ventilation comparing bispectral index-guided administration of propofol and sevoflurane found similar effects of intravenous and inhalational anesthesia on intraoperative oxygenation [19, 35]. However, one trial in 54 patients undergoing thoracic surgery found that TNF-α, interleukin 6, interleukin 8, and monocyte chemoattractant protein 1, representing the inflammatory response to one-lung ventilation, increased less in the sevoflurane group compared with propofol [14]. Also important clinical endpoints like postoperative adverse events were significantly lower in the sevoflurane-treated patients (18 versus 40; $P<0.05$).

There are conflicting results concerning the effect of thoracic epidural anesthesia on hypoxic pulmonary vasoconstriction and oxygenation [30, 33]. However, there is some evidence from several smaller and larger clinical trials that thoracic epidural anesthesia has no clinically relevant effect on pulmonary shunt and intraoperative oxygenation (regardless whether inhalational or intravenous technique was used) [9, 22, 33, 43]. Some authors concluded that thoracic epidural anesthesia can be used safely with both anesthesia techniques.

One of the advantages of a thoracoscopic procedure compared with thoracotomy is reduced postoperative pain. In 153 patients undergoing thoracoscopic lobectomy, mean pain score (on a scale of 0–3; 0 = no pain; 1 = mild pain; 2 = moderate pain, and 3 = severe pain) was 0.6 (median 0; range 0–3) [32]. Local anesthetics for intercostal nerve block or by intrapleural route, nonsteroidal anti-inflammatory drugs or opioids have been reported to be effective [39]. Decortication with pleurodesis, however, may cause significant postoperative pain requiring paravertebral block or epidural analgesia. In a clinical trial of 46 patients undergoing VATS, epidural analgesia resulted in significantly lower pain scores compared with diclofenac and pentazocine but a higher incidence of nausea and vomiting (29% vs. 5%, $P<0.05$) [44]. Single-dose paravertebral nerve block has been shown to be effective. Vogt et al. found significantly lower pain scores during the first 24 h postoperatively compared with morphine patient-controlled analgesia [41]. In another trial, multilevel paravertebral nerve block reduced pain only during the 6 h after nerve blockade [21]. Because of time-limited effect, the authors concluded that this technique is not indicated for thoracoscopic pain treatment. There is some evidence that single-shot paravertebral block might be suited for pain treatment in simple VATS procedures; however, for longer and more complex surgery, catheter techniques should be considered [13]. A systematic review of Kotze published in 2009 including 25 trials with 763 patients for metaregression concluded that continuous paravertebral techniques were superior to intermittent bolus and higher dose local anesthetics improved analgesia [25]. Paravertebral block has been reported to provide similar pain relief compared with epidural analgesia but with less side effects like urinary retention, nausea, vomiting, and hypotension [13]. In a series of 18 patients undergoing video-assisted thoracic surgery, sympathectomy preemptive local infiltration with lidocaine before surgical incision reduced pain significantly with the clinical impact of early discharge and return to work [17].

5.5 Summary of Evidence and Authors Recommendations

Minimally invasive thoracic procedures will be increasingly performed generating less pain and inflammatory response with a better preservation of early pulmonary function. Thoracic anesthesiologists have to become familiar with all aspects of lung separation and one-lung ventilation including detailed knowledge of distal airway anatomy, skills in fiber-optic bronchoscopy, and correct interpretation of radiological chest imaging.

Optimal surgical conditions for thoracoscopic surgery require a fully collapsed nondependent, non-ventilated lung. Lung separation and one-lung ventilation can be achieved either by the insertion of double-lumen tubes or the placement of a bronchial blocker via a single-lumen tube. Beside clinical signs, fiber-optic bronchoscopy is highly recommended for the correct placement and control during surgery. In case of doubt concerning the correct position of a "blindly" introduced double-lumen tube, it should be withdrawn above the carina and both main stem bronchi visualized by fiber-optic bronchoscopy in order to place the double-lumen under vision into the corresponding main stem bronchus.

There is some evidence that lung-protective ventilation with a tidal volume up to 6 mL/kg predicted body weight may be beneficial for one-lung ventilation. No difference could be found for volume-controlled versus pressure-controlled ventilatory mode. Adequate oxygenation maintaining peripheral oxygenation saturation >90% can be achieved (i) with 5 mbar PEEP on the dependent, ventilated lung; (ii) application of continuous positive airway pressure with 100% oxygen on the nondependent lung at the start of one-lung ventilation; (iii) recruitment maneuvers of the ventilated lung followed by PEEP; and (iv) increase of inspired oxygen fraction from 80% to 100%.

Hypoxic pulmonary vasoconstriction is one of the most powerful intrapulmonary mechanisms to reduce the inevitable right-to-left shunt during one-lung ventilation. It is influenced by many anesthesiological interventions. There is no clear evidence that intravenous or inhalational anesthesia might be beneficial in terms of intraoperative oxygenation. However, sevoflurane might reduce inflammatory response and postoperative adverse events.

For thoracoscopic procedures, single-shot and continuous thoracic paravertebral block provide effective perioperative pain treatment with fewer incidences of side effects like urinary retention, nausea, vomiting, and hypotension compared with epidural analgesia. Less invasive strategies like surgical infiltration of side ports with short-acting local anesthetics, intercostal block, systemic opoids, or anti-inflammatory agents can be considered in appropriate procedures as well.

References

1. The Acute Respiratory Distress Syndrome Network (2000) Ventilation with lower tidal volumes as compared with traditional tidal volumes for acute lung injury and the acute respiratory distress syndrome. N Engl J Med 342:1301–8
2. Bassi A, Milani WR, El Dib R et al (2008) Intravenous versus inhalation anaesthesia for one-lung ventilation. Cochrane Database Syst Rev: CD006313
3. Benumof JL (1985) One-lung ventilation and hypoxic pulmonary vasoconstriction: implications for anesthetic management. Anesth Analg 64:821–833
4. Brodsky JB (2004) Fiberoptic bronchoscopy need not be a routine part of double-lumen tube placement. Curr Opin Anaesthesiol 17:7–11
5. Brodsky JB, Lemmens HJ (2003) Left double-lumen tubes: clinical experience with 1,170 patients. J Cardiothorac Vasc Anesth 17:289–298
6. Campos JH (2009) Fast track in thoracic anesthesia and surgery. Curr Opin Anaesthesiol 22:1–3
7. Campos JH (2009) Update on selective lobar blockade during pulmonary resections. Curr Opin Anaesthesiol 22:18–22
8. Campos JH (2010) Lung isolation techniques for patients with difficult airway. Curr Opin Anaesthesiol 23:12–17
9. Casati A, Mascotto G, Iemi K et al (2005) Epidural block does not worsen oxygenation during one-lung ventilation for lung resections under isoflurane/nitrous oxide anaesthesia. Eur J Anaesthesiol 22:363–368
10. Chow MY, Liam BL, Thng CH et al (1999) Predicting the size of a double-lumen endobronchial tube using computed tomographic scan measurements of the left main bronchus diameter. Anesth Analg 88:302–305
11. Cinnella G, Grasso S, Natale C et al (2008) Physiological effects of a lung-recruiting strategy applied during one-lung ventilation. Acta Anaesthesiol Scand 52:766–775
12. Cohen E (2004) Double-lumen tube position should be confirmed by fiberoptic bronchoscopy. Curr Opin Anaesthesiol 17:1–6
13. Daly DJ, Myles PS (2009) Update on the role of paravertebral blocks for thoracic surgery: are they worth it? Curr Opin Anaesthesiol 22:38–43
14. De Conno E, Steurer MP, Wittlinger M et al (2009) Anesthetic-induced improvement of the inflammatory response to one-lung ventilation. Anesthesiology 110:1316–1326
15. Dumans-Nizard V, Liu N, Laloe PA et al (2009) A comparison of the deflecting-tip bronchial blocker with a wire-guided blocker or left-sided double-lumen tube. J Cardiothorac Vasc Anesth 23:501–505
16. Eberle B, Weiler N, Vogel N et al (1999) Computed tomography-based tracheobronchial image reconstruction allows selection of the individually appropriate double-lumen tube size. J Cardiothorac Vasc Anesth 13:532–537
17. Fiorelli A, Vicidomini G, Laperuta P et al (2010) Pre-emptive local analgesia in video-assisted thoracic surgery sympathectomy. Eur J Cardiothorac Surg 37: 588–593
18. Fischer GW, Cohen E (2010) An update on anesthesia for thoracoscopic surgery. Curr Opin Anaesthesiol 23:7–11
19. Fukuoka N, Iida H, Akamatsu S et al (2009) The association between the initial end-tidal carbon

dioxide difference and the lowest arterial oxygen tension value obtained during one-lung anesthesia with propofol or sevoflurane. J Cardiothorac Vasc Anesth 23:775–779
20. Grichnik KP, Shaw A (2009) Update on one-lung ventilation: the use of continuous positive airway pressure ventilation and positive end-expiratory pressure ventilation – clinical application. Curr Opin Anaesthesiol 22:23–30
21. Hill SE, Keller RA, Stafford-Smith M et al (2006) Efficacy of single-dose, multilevel paravertebral nerve blockade for analgesia after thoracoscopic procedures. Anesthesiology 104:1047–1053
22. Jung SM, Cho CK, Kim YJ et al (2010) The effect of thoracic epidural anesthesia on pulmonary shunt fraction and arterial oxygenation during one-lung ventilation. J Cardiothorac Vasc Anesth 24:456–462
23. Karzai W, Schwarzkopf K (2009) Hypoxemia during one-lung ventilation: prediction, prevention, and treatment. Anesthesiology 110:1402–1411
24. Ko R, McRae K, Darling G et al (2009) The use of air in the inspired gas mixture during two-lung ventilation delays lung collapse during one-lung ventilation. Anesth Analg 108:1092–1096
25. Kotze A, Scally A, Howell S (2009) Efficacy and safety of different techniques of paravertebral block for analgesia after thoracotomy: a systematic review and metaregression. Br J Anaesth 103:626–636
26. Ku CM, Slinger P, Waddell TK (2009) A novel method of treating hypoxemia during one-lung ventilation for thoracoscopic surgery. J Cardiothorac Vasc Anesth 23:850–852
27. Lytle FT, Brown DR (2008) Appropriate ventilatory settings for thoracic surgery: intraoperative and postoperative. Semin Cardiothorac Vasc Anesth 12:97–108
28. Merli G, Guarino A, Della Rocca G et al (2009) Recommendations for airway control and difficult airway management in thoracic anesthesia and lung separation procedures. Minerva Anestesiol 75:59–78; 79–96
29. Nagahiro I, Andou A, Aoe M et al (2001) Pulmonary function, postoperative pain, and serum cytokine level after lobectomy: a comparison of VATS and conventional procedure. Ann Thorac Surg 72:362–365
30. Nagendran J, Stewart K, Hoskinson M et al (2006) An anesthesiologist's guide to hypoxic pulmonary vasoconstriction: implications for managing single-lung anesthesia and atelectasis. Curr Opin Anaesthesiol 19:34–43
31. Neustein SM (2009) The use of bronchial blockers for providing one-lung ventilation. J Cardiothorac Vasc Anesth 23:860–868
32. Nicastri DG, Wisnivesky JP, Litle VR et al (2008) Thoracoscopic lobectomy: report on safety, discharge independence, pain, and chemotherapy tolerance. J Thorac Cardiovasc Surg 135:642–647
33. Ozcan PE, Senturk M, Sungur Ulke Z et al (2007) Effects of thoracic epidural anaesthesia on pulmonary venous admixture and oxygenation during one-lung ventilation. Acta Anaesthesiol Scand 51:1117–1122
34. Pardos PC, Garutti I, Pineiro P et al (2009) Effects of ventilatory mode during one-lung ventilation on intraoperative and postoperative arterial oxygenation in thoracic surgery. J Cardiothorac Vasc Anesth 23:770–774
35. Pruszkowski O, Dalibon N, Moutafis M et al (2007) Effects of propofol vs. sevoflurane on arterial oxygenation during one-lung ventilation. Br J Anaesth 98: 539–544
36. Schultz MJ (2008) Lung-protective mechanical ventilation with lower tidal volumes in patients not suffering from acute lung injury: a review of clinical studies. Med Sci Monit 14:RA22–RA26
37. Slinger P (2008) Con: the new bronchial blockers are not preferable to double-lumen tubes for lung isolation. J Cardiothorac Vasc Anesth 22:925–929
38. Smith GB, Hirsch NP, Ehrenwerth J (1986) Placement of double-lumen endobronchial tubes. Correlation between clinical impressions and bronchoscopic findings. Br J Anaesth 58:1317–1320
39. Thomsen RW (2008) Mediastinoscopy and video-assisted thoracoscopic surgery: anesthetic pitfalls and complications. Semin Cardiothorac Vasc Anesth 12: 128–132
40. Unzueta MC, Casas JI, Moral MV (2007) Pressure-controlled versus volume-controlled ventilation during one-lung ventilation for thoracic surgery. Anesth Analg 104:1029–1033, tables of contents
41. Vogt A, Stieger DS, Theurillat C et al (2005) Single-injection thoracic paravertebral block for postoperative pain treatment after thoracoscopic surgery. Br J Anaesth 95:816–821
42. Wolthuis EK, Choi G, Dessing MC et al (2008) Mechanical ventilation with lower tidal volumes and positive end-expiratory pressure prevents pulmonary inflammation in patients without preexisting lung injury. Anesthesiology 108:46–54
43. Xu Y, Tan Z, Wang S et al (2010) Effect of thoracic epidural anesthesia with different concentrations of ropivacaine on arterial oxygenation during one-lung ventilation. Anesthesiology 112:1146–1154
44. Yoshioka M, Mori T, Kobayashi H et al (2006) The efficacy of epidural analgesia after video-assisted thoracoscopic surgery: a randomized control study. Ann Thorac Cardiovasc Surg 12:313–318

Imaging

6

Bernd Kläeser and Jakub Wiskirchen

Contents

6.1 Conventional Radiographs

For a period of approximately 80 years, conventional chest X-ray was the only available non-invasive modality for imaging of the chest. Although planar chest X-ray is generally limited by poor soft tissue contrast and superposition of anatomic structures, it offers the possibility to get an impression of infectious and/or tumourous pathologies of the lung and chest wall such as pneumonia, effusion or pulmonary nodules (Fig. 6.1). With further developments such as fluoroscopy, conventional tomography and bronchography, hilar pathologies also became visible, possible nodules disappeared and potential bronchial occlusions or bronchiectases were detected. Furthermore, planar chest X-ray offered the opportunity to estimate preoperatively whether or not a surgical approach would be helpful (e.g. in case of a peripheral solitary nodule), or futile with regard to the expected overall patient outcome (e.g. documentation of multiple pulmonary nodules or bone metastases). Even with the widespread availability of cross-sectional imaging, conventional planar radiographs remain a cost-effective diagnostic tool and first choice for a number of applications, e.g. for preoperative screening, and documentation and monitoring of infectious lung pathologies. The chest X-ray is especially helpful in the postoperative management, e.g. to verify the position of tubes, drains and catheters and to document acute pathologies, e.g. pneumothorax or pleural effusion. Also treatment-associated complications such as pulmonary

B. Kläeser, M.D. (✉)
Department of Nuclear Medicine,
University Hospital Berne, CH-3010, Berne, Switzerland
e-mail: bernd.klaeser@insel.ch

J. Wiskirchen, M.D.
Klinik für Radiologie und Nuklearmedizin,
Franziskus Hospital gem. GmbH,
Kiskerstraße 26, 33615 Bielefeld, Deutschland
e-mail: jakub.wiskirchen@franziskus.de

R.G.C. Inderbitzi et al. (eds.), *Minimally Invasive Thoracic and Cardiac Surgery*,
DOI 10.1007/978-3-642-11861-6_6, © Springer-Verlag Berlin Heidelberg 2012

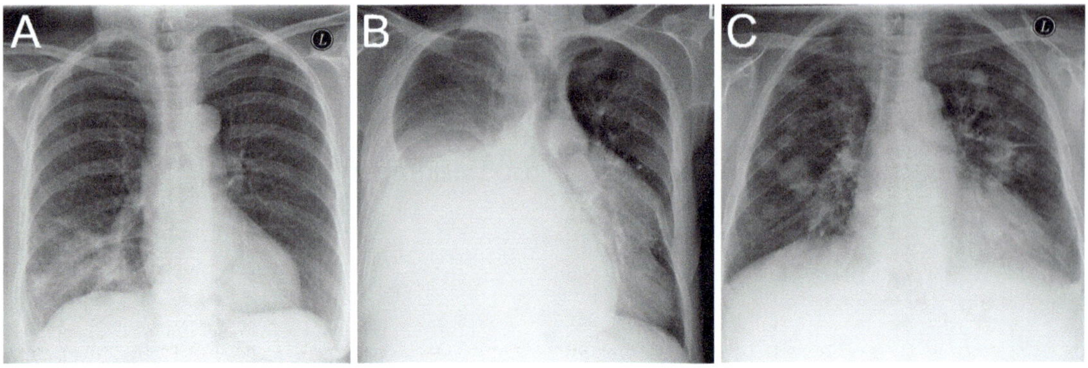

Fig. 6.1 Chest X-ray examinations of a patient with diffuse pulmonary infiltration in the right lower lobe of the lung indicating pneumonia (**a**), a patient presenting with a large pleural effusion on the right side of the chest leading to a shift of the heart and the mediastinum to the left (**b**), and a patient with a history of bladder cancer 2 years before presenting with bilateral pulmonary metastases and a subtle pleural effusion in the left lateral recessus (**c**)

abscess, pneumothorax or fluid lung due to an aggressive peri- and postoperative management can be detected reliably.

6.2 Computed Tomography

With the introduction of computed tomography (CT) at the beginning of the 1970s, the era of modern chest imaging started. At the beginning, examination times were long and image resolution was limited. However, the introduction of spiral CT in 1988 and of multi-slice spiral CT (MSCT) in 1998 boosted CT-based chest imaging. Today, using a modern MSCT examination time of a chest ranges between 4 and 6 s so that even dyspnoeic patients can be examined with good image resolution. Submillimetre slices allow reconstruction of images in all planes and volume data sets for 3D reconstruction and for precise treatment planning, e.g. for tumour surgery, paediatric cardiac surgery and reconstructive surgery. Using modern computer technology, it is possible to simulate surgery in a virtual reality setup before treating the patient (e.g. when using robotics for surgery).

Contrast-enhanced CT helps to differentiate benign (e.g. pneumonic infiltrations, hamartomas, granulomas, vessel malformation) from malignant processes (e.g. primary lung tumours like lung cancer, secondary lung tumours like metastases) and in case of underlying malignancy can be used for effective T staging. Due to the contrast between solid processes and ventilated lung, the T staging of peripheral lesions can be done appropriately. However, lesions close to the mediastinum, the chest wall or the large vessels may be over- or understaged as tissue of the same or equal density cannot be differentiated appropriately [60]. Lymph node (LN) staging of the mediastinum is more accurate with CT and especially with MSCT than with conventional imaging (Fig. 6.2). The bases for the evaluation of LNs with CT are morphological criteria like node size, shape and contrast agent enhancement. While the size of LNs is generally associated with a certain probability of metastatic involvement, a reliable prediction of metastases in a single LN is not possible with CT [9]. CT of the trunk may also be used for M staging. However, PET/CT detects distant metastases in a significant proportion of patients without suspicious findings in CT and is the modality of choice for whole-body staging of NSCLC (see Chap. 4).

6.3 Magnetic Resonance Imaging

Magnetic resonance imaging (MRI) – although feasible – did not find its way into routine chest imaging. It is equivalent to CT in differentiating between benign and malignant lesions and may

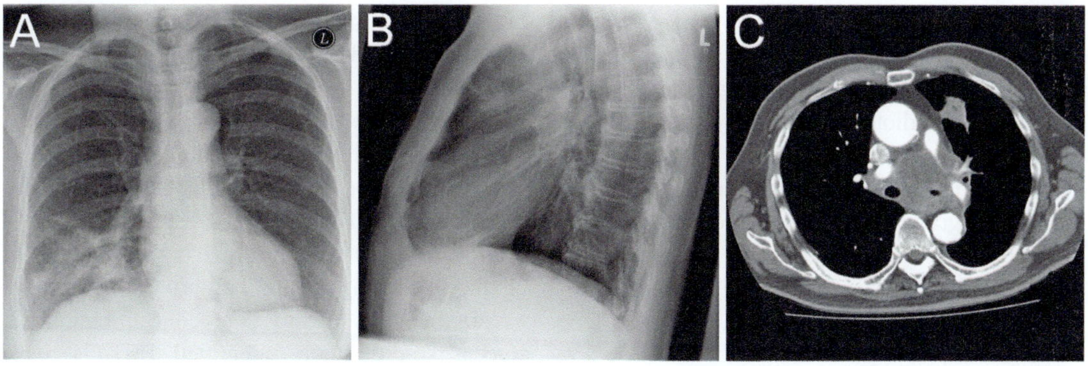

Fig. 6.2 53-year-old male patient presenting with dyspnoea. Chest X-ray in the p.a. projection (**a**) shows only subtle changes in the hilar region on the left and a compression of the left main bronchus. The lateral projection (**b**) shows a prominent left hilar region and an additional pulmonary nodule. The CT scan shows a large central tumour (**c**) encasing the main left bronchus with infiltration of the mediastinum. Note the additional pulmonary lesion on the left

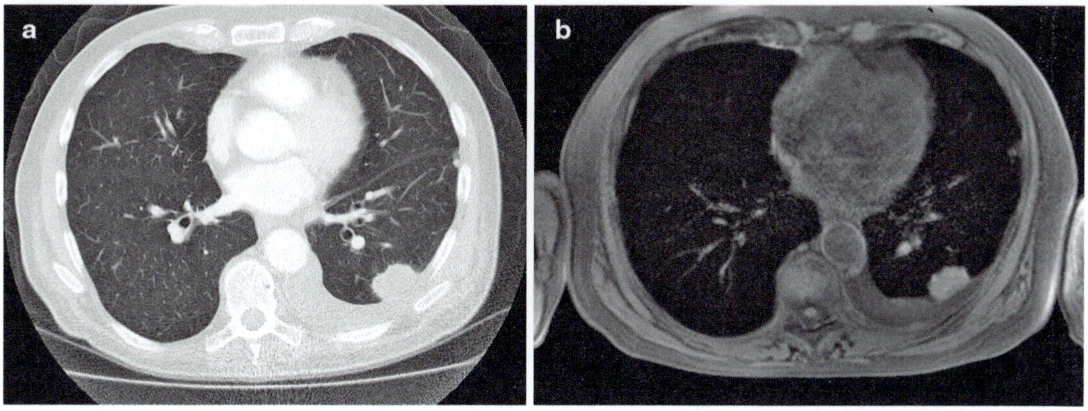

Fig. 6.3 89-year-old patient with shortness of breath. Due to being afraid of X-ray exposure, the patient insisted on MR tomography of the chest. The MR (**a**) revealed a spiculated lesion in the left lower lobe with a diameter of 3 cm. Note the pleural effusion and the subtle pleural droplets. The CT scan (**b**) – acquired before image-guided puncture – showed the same picture. However, the pleural droplets were invisible even in the soft tissue window (not shown). The soft tissue contrast of the MR examination – although the examination was performed without IV contrast agent – is much better than the contrast of CT

be more accurate than CT and PET/CT for diagnosing chest wall infiltration and T stage when breath-hold techniques are applied (Fig. 6.3). MRI is superior to CT in defining the nodal status, but again PET/CT is more sensitive and specific for N staging than MRI [55]. For M staging of lung cancer, the overall performance of whole-body MRI seems to be comparable to PET/CT with advantages to detect hepatic and brain metastases [52, 55, 69], but overall also with a higher number of false-positive lesions with MRI [28].

6.4 Positron Emission Tomography

Since the 1990s, positron emission tomography (PET) with the glucose derivate F-18-fluorodeoxyglucose (FDG) has become the standard of care imaging modality for the pre-surgical staging of thoracic malignancies. With the introduction and widespread availability of combined PET/CT systems since 2000, PET imaging alone has been widely replaced by hybrid PET/CT imaging that provides fused images of PET metabolism and CT morphology. Hybrid imaging further improved the diagnostic accuracy of PET and established the basis for planning and performing minimally invasive surgery, image-guided interventions and radiotherapy directly based on the metabolic information of PET. The development of systems for instrument guidance and video-assisted surgery integrating PET/CT data for planning and navigation will further facilitate the effective use of PET/CT information in the clinical setting.

6.4.1 Patient Preparation

A careful patient preparation is essential to maintain high-quality FDG-PET examinations. All patients must have a carbohydrate-free diet for at least 6 h before the examination. Fasting time may be prolonged to 12 h in patients with impaired glucose tolerance or adult-onset diabetes to assure normal blood glucose and insulin levels at the time of FDG injection. Patients rest comfortably in a well-tempered environment between injection of the radiopharmaceutical and PET acquisition to avoid increased FDG uptake in muscles and brown fat [15, 24].

Relevant details of patient history must be provided by the referring physician and are necessary for the correct interpretation of PET/CT findings, i.e. results of other diagnostic tests, previous biopsies, previous or concurrent bacterial or fungal infections, tuberculosis and other conditions potentially associated with increased FDG uptake (e.g. silicosis, sarcoidosis).

6.4.2 Non-small Cell Lung Cancer

6.4.2.1 Primary Staging

Surgery with curative intent represents the treatment of choice in patients with non-small cell lung cancer (NSCLC) but is only an option in patients with stages I, II, and selected cases of stage III. As only 30% of NSCLC cases present at early stages [11], an accurate preoperative stage grouping is required to identify patients in a palliative situation that are not candidates for surgery. PET/CT is a robust imaging modality for staging NSCLC in clinical routine, with a very high level of interobserver agreement for both staging LNs and distant metastases [30].

6.4.2.2 T Staging

The T staging of NSCLC is mainly based on morphological criteria and aims at the preoperative differentiation of T1–3 from T4 stages. In clinical routine, contrast-enhanced CT is the modality of choice for T staging and has proven to be more accurate in this regard than conventional PET. Recent studies with integrated PET/CT have shown an advantage for T staging based on integrated PET/contrast-enhanced CT compared to separate PET and CT examinations, e.g. to differentiate tumour and atelectasis [12, 27, 44].

6.4.2.3 N Staging

Preoperative N staging has to discriminate patients with no or only ipsilateral hilar LN metastases (N1), which are candidates for direct surgery, from patients with ipsilateral (N2) and contralateral or supraclavicular LN metastases (N3). Patients with N2 stage typically undergo neo-adjuvant chemotherapy before surgery; N3 stage would preclude surgery and determine treatment in palliative intent. While the diagnosis of LN metastases with CT is based on morphological criteria, mainly the short axis nodal diameter with an upper limit defining abnormal nodes of 1 cm, FDG-PET relies on the detection of the increased glucose metabolism. The additional value of PET is given by the fact that the size of a LN alone is not reliable as a parameter to define the nodal status. As about three-fourths of enlarged mediastinal LNs are not metastatic, and nearly half of all LN metastases of NSCLC are found in non-enlarged LNs (diameter less than 10 mm) [57], the accuracy of CT for LN staging is limited (pooled sensitivity 57%, specificity 82% [71]). By detecting increased tumour metabolism, PET can also detect metastases in non-enlarged LNs and is more accurate than CT. Combined PET/CT has proven significantly better staging accuracy for LNs than PET and CT alone [12, 44], with a sensitivity and specificity for second-generation PET/CT machines (reconstructed resolution 5 mm or less) in the range of 72–82% and 93–94%, respectively [70, 73].

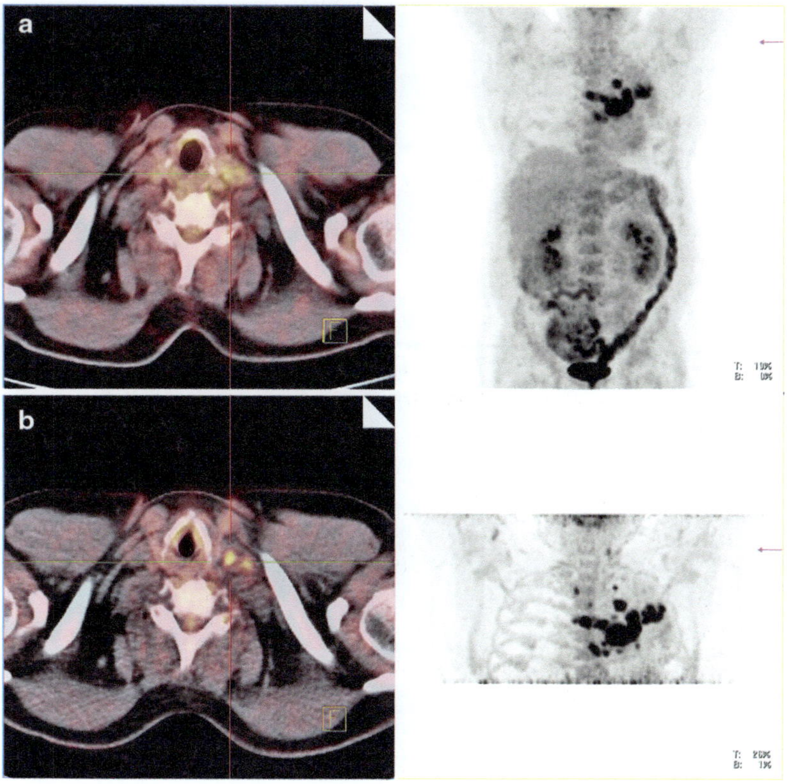

Fig. 6.4 54-year-old patient with left hilar NSCLC. Whole-body PET/CT (image resolution <5 mm) shows ipsilateral mediastinal LN metastases but is negative in the left supraclavicular region (**a**). In contrast, the regional high-resolution PET/CT acquisition (image resolution 2 mm) shows additional FDG avid LNs in the contralateral mediastinum as well as supraclavicular on the left (**b**). The left supraclavicular LN was histologically proven to represent a LN metastasis (pN3)

Last-generation PET/CT machines again offer a markedly improved image resolution and may further improve the sensitivity and NPV of LN staging with PET/CT (Fig. 6.4).

6.4.2.4 M Staging

PET and PET/CT examinations usually comprise the whole trunk from the base of the orbit to the legs and allow for a reliable screening for distant metastases, e.g. in the liver, in the adrenal glands, in bones and soft tissue and in the lung (Figs. 6.5 and 6.6). In this context, PET may detect distant metastases before morphological abnormalities of metastases become visible in CT [38]. Depending on the patient collective, PET/CT identifies distant metastases previously unrecognized after conventional staging in 6–24% of patients [21, 51]. LN and distant metastases exclusively detected by PET lead to a modified stage grouping and major changes of planned treatment in up to 30% of patients [21, 51, 58, 67]. In a prospectively randomized trial, Fischer et al. found that PET spared futile thoracotomies in nearly 50% of patients in a palliative situation but did not negatively affect overall survival [21]. Stage grouping by PET but not discordant findings of conventional staging correlates with patient outcome [78]. Several studies in different health care systems have shown that the use of PET/CT for the primary staging of NSCLC is cost-effective, i.e. does not increase overall health care costs or even reduces costs as it minimizes the number of futile therapies [4, 23, 36, 39, 49, 51, 66, 75].

6.4.2.5 Recurrence

FDG PET/CT is useful in selected cases in the follow-up of NSCLC, e.g. for patients with suspected recurrence and inconclusive findings in conventional imaging, or when distant metastases should be excluded in patients with localized recurrence before treatment (Fig. 6.7). The diagnostic accuracy of PET and PET/CT for restaging is comparable to what was reported for primary staging. PET defines the extent of disease significantly more accurate than CT and changes treatment in a high proportion of patients [29, 34].

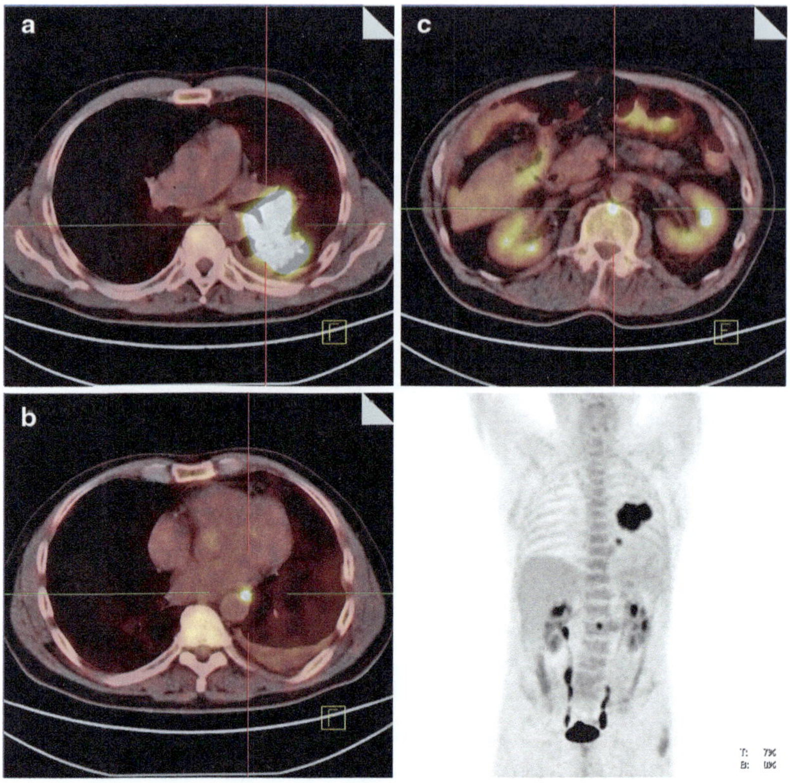

Fig. 6.5 72-year-old patient with NSCLC in the left lower lobe and hilar LN metastases (**a**). An additional mediastinal LN metastasis was found in a non-enlarged LN adjacent to the aorta/pulmonary ligament (**b**, cN2). Solitary bone metastasis in the lumbar spine (**c**, cM1)

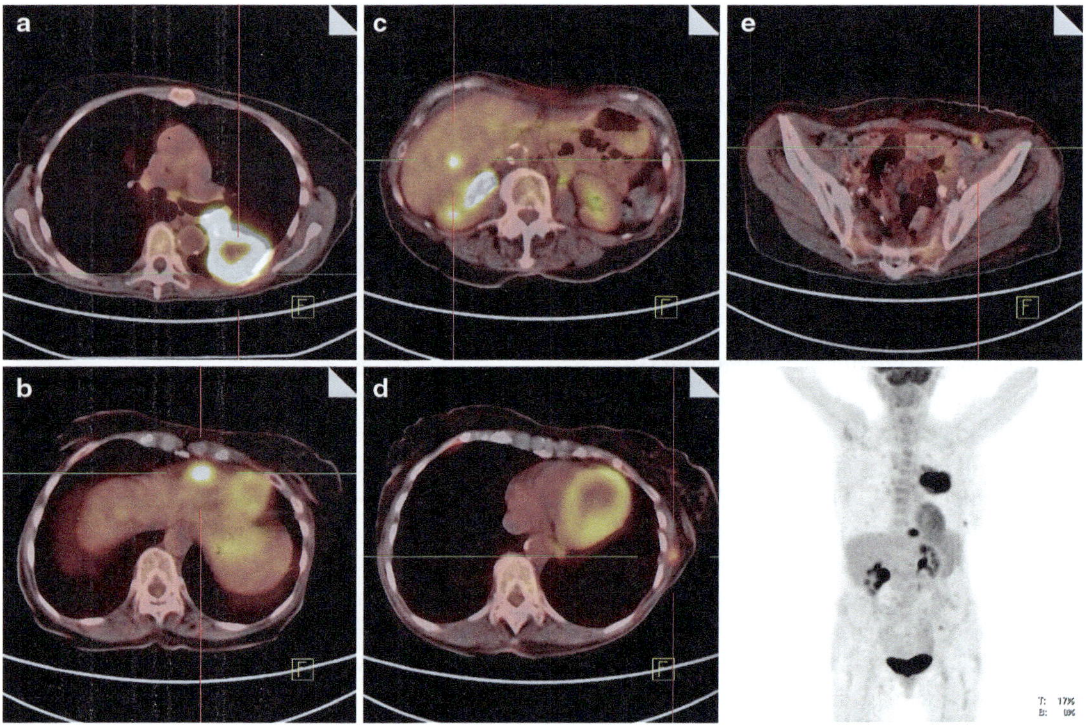

Fig. 6.6 77-year-old patient with NSCLC in left lower lobe infiltrating the chest wall (cT3) and hilar LN metastases (**a**, cN1). Atypical distant metastatic spread with LN metastases in the right cardiophrenic angle (**b**), a solitary liver metastasis (**c**) and small soft tissue metastases in the left anterior serratus muscle (**d**) and in the abdomen adjacent to the abdominal wall (**e**)

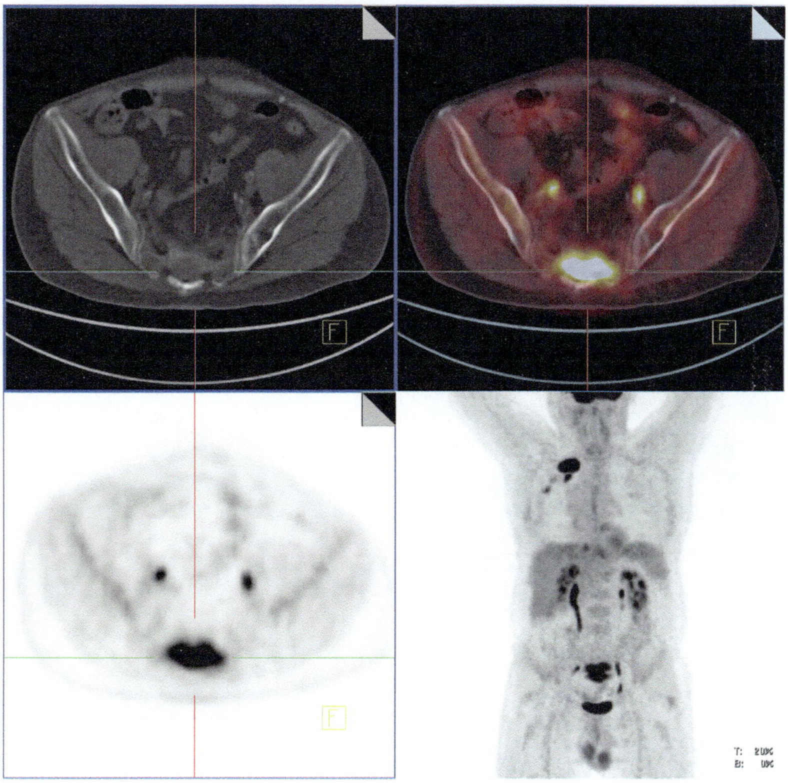

Fig. 6.7 65-year-old patient with tumour recurrence in the right lower lobe 12 months after resection of a NSCLC pT2 pN2 cM0 in the right upper lobe. PET/CT shows a LN metastasis in the ipsilateral anterior mediastinum. In addition, PET/CT detected a distant metastasis in the sacrum that is not evident in CT

6.4.3 Neuroendocrine Tumours of the Lung

Typical and atypical carcinoid tumours of the lung have variable FDG uptake that is often lower than expected from malignant tumours. Given a lower sensitivity than for other thoracic malignancies, FDG-PET might only be indicated as a staging test for atypical carcinoids [14, 17, 40, 65]. Based on somatostatin receptor expression of neuroendocrine tumours, well-differentiated carcinoids are suited for specific imaging with somatostatin analogues labelled with 111-In for SPECT imaging (octreotide) or Ga-68 for PET/CT (e.g. DOTA-TOC) [26, 35, 41].

High-grade neuroendocrine malignancies such as small cell lung cancer (SCLC) usually have an intense FDG uptake. Available data suggest that PET/CT may be more accurate than conventional imaging including CT in the staging of SCLC [10, 63]. PET was reported useful to identify unknown LN and distant metastases in patients with SCLC and to change planned treatment in about 20%, predominantly concerning radiotherapy in patients with limited vs. extended disease [6, 33, 50, 76]. Corresponding to a better stage grouping, PET predicts the outcome of patients with SCLC better than CT [6].

6.4.4 Solitary Pulmonary Nodules

The detection of solitary pulmonary nodules (SPN) in chest radiographs or CT requires further clarification, and malignancy has to be ruled out. The recommended diagnostic strategy depends on the pretest probability of malignancy and comprises resection and histopathology for SPN judged at high risk for malignancy, the use of FDG-PET(/CT) to characterize nodules at low or and intermediate risk and "wait-and-see" with repeated imaging follow-up for SPN at very low risk [2]. Overall, already conventional PET has proven excellent diagnostic accuracy for SPN with a sensitivity and specificity of 91–96% and 78%, respectively [22, 25]. However, the sensitivity of PET to detect malignant pulmonary lesions correlates with the size of the SPN and the resolution of the PET or PET/CT machine used and was shown

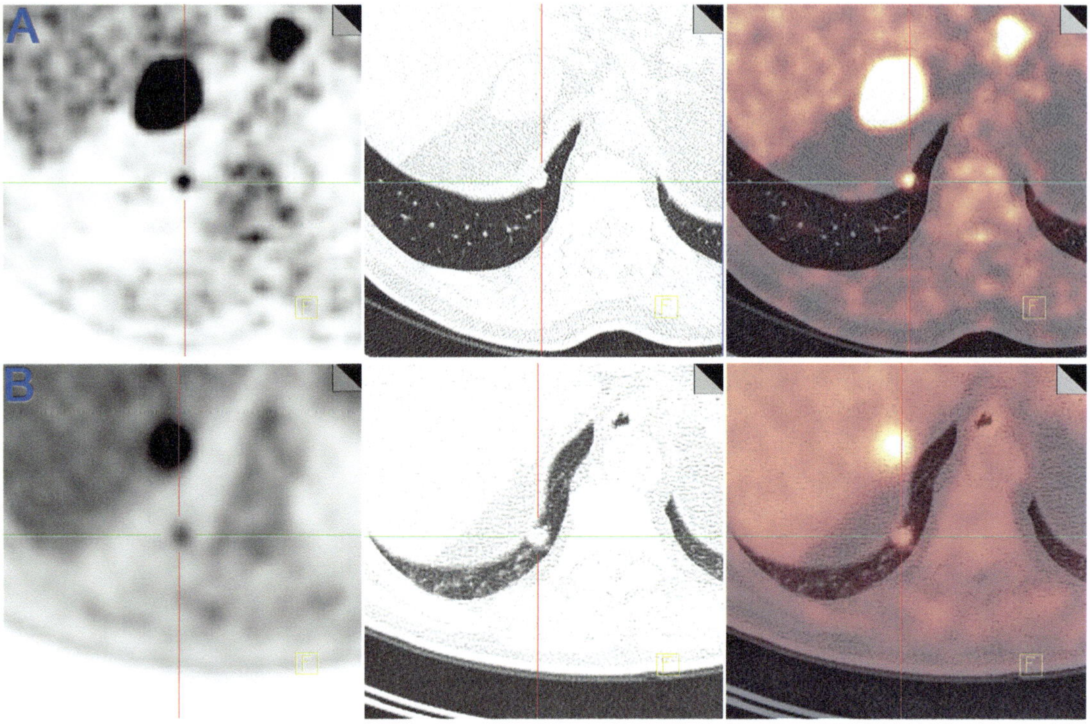

Fig. 6.8 68-year-old patient with malignant melanoma referred for whole-body staging before resection of a suprarenal metastasis and a retroperitoneal LN metastasis. Whole-body PET showed a lesion with apparently low FDG uptake in the right lower lobe (**a**). An additional breath-hold acquisition of that area (20 s acquisition time) characterized the lesion as highly FDG avid, compatible with a further metastasis of malignant melanoma (**b**)

to decrease for lesions less than 8–10 mm in diameter [74, 77]. Recently introduced deep inspiration breath-hold (DIBH) acquisition techniques reduce the partial volume effect caused by the motion of lung lesions during the breathing cycle and were shown to significantly improve the probability of detection of hypermetabolic lung lesions either small or situated in the basal parts of the lungs. [3, 16, 47, 72]. With modern PET/CT systems, such additional DIBH acquisitions comprising a deep inspiration CT and a breath-hold PET can be performed as one exam in less than 1 min (Fig. 6.8).

6.4.5 Pleural Mesothelioma

FDG-PET/CT can differentiate malignant pleural mesothelioma (MPM) from benign lesions of the pleura, such as pleural plaques, diffuse pleural thickening and benign asbestos-related pleural effusion (sensitivity 94–100%; specificity 95–100% [53, 81]). Similar to CT, PET/CT has limitations for T staging but offers better accuracy for N and M staging [54, 80]. In a direct comparison of CT, PET, MRI and PET/CT, Plathow and colleagues found PET/CT to have the best diagnostic accuracy, not only being significantly more accurate than all other techniques in stages II and III but also having the best interobserver agreement [56].

FDG-PET/CT can also be used in the follow-up of MPM. However, the interpretation of PET may be complicated after talc pleurodesis, as the foreign material causes an inflammatory reaction that can persist for years. To avoid unnecessary false-positive PET results, pleural FDG uptake has to be interpreted with caution together with the morphological appearance in CT: Increased FDG uptake in areas with increased density in CT usually represents talc-induced granulomatous lesions, and malignancy is unlikely [1, 42, 46, 48, 79]. A careful correlation with previous CT studies is recommended, and further follow-up with CT or PET/CT as well as a biopsy may be necessary to definitely exclude pleural recurrence.

6.4.6 Thymic Carcinoma

Several thymic pathologies, besides thymic carcinoma, including hyperplasia, thymoma, carcinoids and lymphoma, can show increased FDG uptake [20]. Consequently, FDG-PET uptake alone cannot reliably differentiate benign from malign thymic tumours. However, an inhomogeneous pattern of thymic uptake with focal lesions is generally suspicious for malignancy and would guide further examinations. PET may have a role in whole-body staging patients with histologically verified thymic carcinoma and can help to identify recurrence [19, 32].

6.4.7 Metastases

The lung is a common target organ for distant metastases of many extrapulmonary primary tumours. FDG-PET/CT used for whole-body staging of FDG avid malignancies, including gastrointestinal malignancies, breast cancer, gynaecologic malignancies, melanoma, lymphoma and head-and-neck cancer, accurately detects pulmonary metastases. As discussed earlier, even small pulmonary lesions in CT can be characterized with appropriate breath-hold acquisition techniques. However, a negative nodule in PET/CT finally does not preclude a metastasis, as several factors such as FDG avidity and partial necrosis may be responsible for the negative appearance of a lesion in PET. Consequently, a further follow-up with CT or PET/CT might be necessary in selected cases even when the PET study is negative.

6.4.8 Limitations and Pitfalls

PET/CT is generally more sensitive to detect lymphatic spread than imaging modalities based on criteria such as CT, and an excellent imaging modality to identify macroscopic metastatic spread to distant sites. PET can detect tumour metabolism in normal-sized LNs and organs, and even lesions with a diameter smaller than the resolution of a PET machine can be detected if the metabolic activity of a lesion is high enough to compensate for partial volume effects. However, the probability to detect metastases decreases with the lesion size and is less than 50% for metastases smaller than the system resolution. Consequently, a negative PET cannot definitely exclude microscopic disease.

False-negative PET results can occur in malignant primary tumours with a low FDG uptake, e.g. carcinoid tumours or mucin-producing NSCLC [64]. Tumours with a diffuse growth pattern such as the bronchioalveolar carcinoma (BAC) can also be false-negative and mistaken for inflammatory changes, especially in early stages. A careful evaluation of areas with low and homogenous lung uptake together with CT is necessary, and ground glass nodules should raise the suspicion of BAC [5, 7, 45, 68]. Non-FDG avid metastases of extrapulmonary tumours, e.g. differentiated thyroid carcinoma, prostate cancer and extrapulmonary neuroendocrine tumours, can also occur.

While a focal FDG uptake in a lesion is often associated with malignancy, this metabolic feature is not tumour specific. A variable increase of glucose metabolism may also be noticed in chronic and acute inflammatory processes of the chest, e.g. bacterial or fungal infections, tuberculosis, sarcoidosis, amyloidosis, vasculitis or chronic unspecific inflammatory changes of hilar and/or mediastinal LNs, and can lead to a false-positive PET interpretation [8, 13, 18, 59, 62]. In complex situations, when discrimination between metastatic and inflammatory changes of mediastinal LNs is difficult, PET/CT may not be perceived as a tool for definite LN staging but for image guidance and targeted histological verification of LNs, e.g. using mediastinoscopy or endoscopical fine needle aspiration.

6.5 Image-Guided Interventions

6.5.1 CT-Guided Interventions

Image-guided tissue sampling with CT is well established in clinical routine. Two possible approaches for punctures exist: the step-by-step technique and the fluoroscopic technique.

The step-by-step technique is the traditional approach. After defining the puncture site, a needle is introduced. Step by step – using several CT

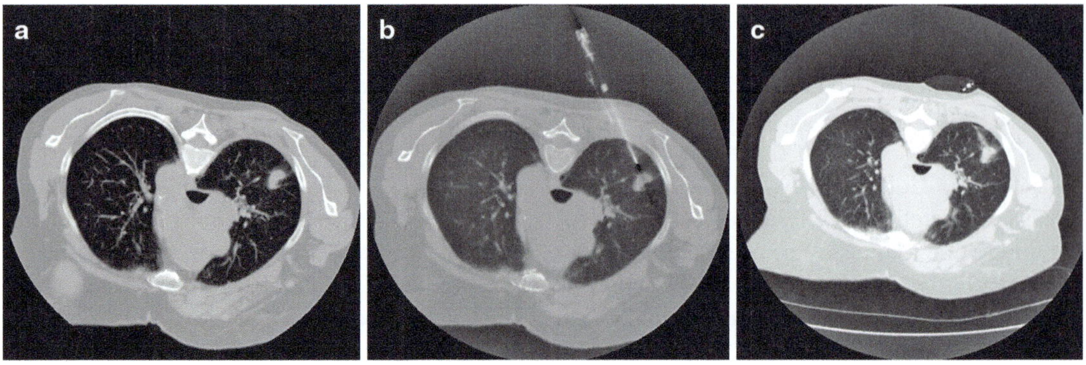

Fig. 6.9 56-year-old patient who presented with a wide mediastinum in a routine preoperative chest X-ray (not shown). CT revealed a lesion in the left upper lobe of the lung (**a**) that was sampled percutaneously in prone position under CT guidance (**b**). Subtle pulmonary haemorrhage was visible after puncture (**c**)

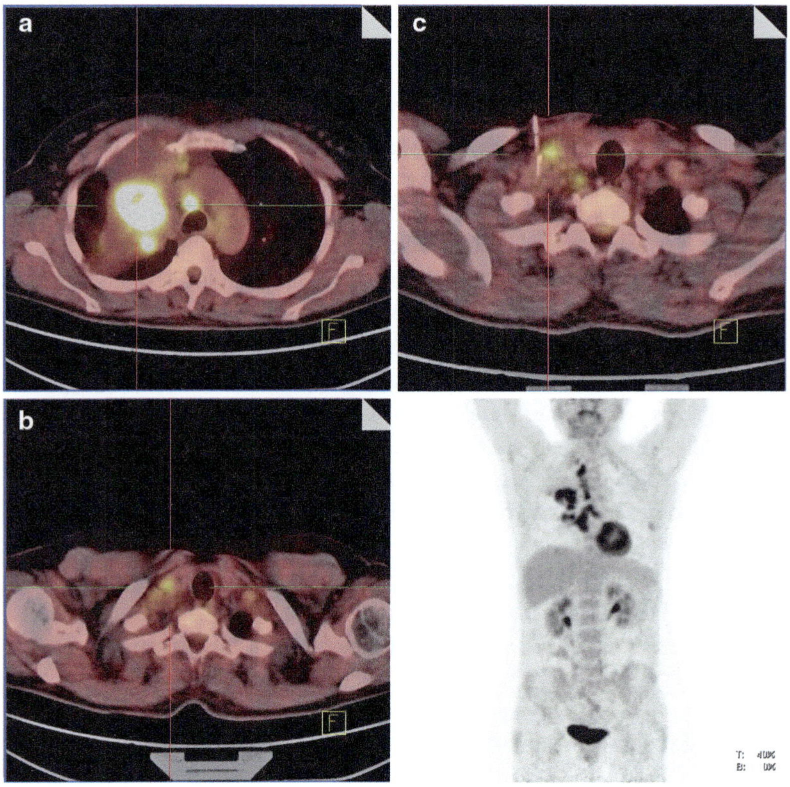

Fig. 6.10 54-year-old patient with NSCLC of the partially atelectatic right upper lobe, a satellite lesion in the same lobe (cT4) and ipsilateral mediastinal LN metastases (**a**). An only moderately FDG avid, non-enlarged right supraclavicular LN (**b**) was wire marked under PET/CT guidance (**c**) and was histologically proven to represent a LN metastasis (pN3)

control scans – the needle is advanced until a tissue sample can be obtained. The advantages of this technique are that it can be done with every CT scanner and that the radiation exposure of both – the patient and the staff – is low (Fig. 6.9). However, it is difficult to obtain a sample from tiny pathologies as well as from structures close to the heart or the great vessels.

The fluoroscopic approach is advantageous when aiming at tiny pathologies or when pathologies are close to the heart. However, continuous radiation is accompanied by a high radiation exposure of patient and staff, and this technique can only be performed with new generation CT machines.

In the last years, CT-guided minimally invasive local therapies such as radiofrequency ablation

(RFA) or cryotherapy gained more attention because these therapeutic modalities can be performed even in patients not qualifying for chest surgery in combination with general anaesthesia.

6.5.2 PET/CT-Guided Interventions

As increased FDG uptake is not tumour specific and can also occur in a number of benign conditions, a histological verification of singular and/or morphologically indeterminate lesions can be necessary in a small proportion of patients. In order to make such lesions reliably accessible, PET/CT is increasingly used for image guidance of percutaneous, transbronchial and surgical biopsies, wire marking (Fig. 6.10) and image-guided treatment, e.g. radiofrequency ablation [31, 37, 38, 43, 61].

References

1. Ahmadzadehfar H, Palmedo H, Strunk H et al (2007) False positive 18F-FDG-PET/CT in a patient after talc pleurodesis. Lung Cancer 58:418–421
2. Alberts WM (2007) Diagnosis and management of lung cancer executive summary: ACCP evidence-based clinical practice guidelines (2nd edition). Chest 132:1S–19S
3. Allen-Auerbach M, Yeom K, Park J et al (2006) Standard PET/CT of the chest during shallow breathing is inadequate for comprehensive staging of lung cancer. J Nucl Med 47:298–301
4. Alzahouri K, Lejeune C, Woronoff-Lemsi MC et al (2005) Cost-effectiveness analysis of strategies introducing FDG-PET into the mediastinal staging of non-small-cell lung cancer from the French healthcare system perspective. Clin Radiol 60:479–492
5. Aquino SL, Halpern EF, Kuester LB et al (2007) FDG-PET and CT features of non-small cell lung cancer based on tumor type. Int J Mol Med 19:495–499
6. Azad A, Chionh F, Scott AM et al (2010) High impact of (18)F-FDG-PET on management and prognostic stratification of newly diagnosed small cell lung cancer. Mol Imaging Biol 12(4):443–451
7. Balogova S, Huchet V, Kerrou K et al (2010) Detection of bronchioloalveolar cancer by means of PET/CT and 18F-fluorocholine, and comparison with 18F-fluorodeoxyglucose. Nucl Med Commun 31: 389–397
8. Beggs AD, Hain SF (2002) F-18 FDG-positron emission tomographic scanning and Wegener's granulomatosis. Clin Nucl Med 27:705–706
9. Beyer F, Buerke B, Gerss J et al (2010) Prediction of lymph node metastases in NSCLC. Three dimensional anatomical parameters do not substitute FDG-PET-CT. Nuklearmedizin 49:41–48; quiz N41
10. Brink I, Schumacher T, Mix M et al (2004) Impact of [18F]FDG-PET on the primary staging of small-cell lung cancer. Eur J Nucl Med Mol Imaging 31: 1614–1620
11. Buccheri G, Ferrigno D (2000) Prognostic value of stage grouping and TNM descriptors in lung cancer. Chest 117:1247–1255
12. Cerfolio RJ, Ojha B, Bryant AS et al (2004) The accuracy of integrated PET-CT compared with dedicated PET alone for the staging of patients with nonsmall cell lung cancer. Ann Thorac Surg 78:1017–1023; discussion 1017–1023
13. Chang JM, Lee HJ, Goo JM et al (2006) False positive and false negative FDG-PET scans in various thoracic diseases. Korean J Radiol 7:57–69
14. Chong S, Lee KS (2007) Spectrum of findings and usefulness of integrated PET/CT in patients with known or suspected neuroendocrine tumors of the lung. Cancer Imaging 7:195–201
15. Cohade C (2010) Altered biodistribution on FDG-PET with emphasis on brown fat and insulin effect. Semin Nucl Med 40:283–293
16. Daisaki H, Shinohara H, Terauchi T et al (2010) Multi-bed-position acquisition technique for deep inspiration breath-hold PET/CT: a preliminary result for pulmonary lesions. Ann Nucl Med 24:179–188
17. Daniels CE, Lowe VJ, Aubry MC et al (2007) The utility of fluorodeoxyglucose positron emission tomography in the evaluation of carcinoid tumors presenting as pulmonary nodules. Chest 131:255–260
18. Divgi CR (2009) Molecular imaging of pulmonary cancer and inflammation. Proc Am Thorac Soc 6:464–468
19. El-Bawab HY, Abouzied MM, Rafay MA et al (2010) Clinical use of combined positron emission tomography and computed tomography in thymoma recurrence. Interact Cardiovasc Thorac Surg 11(4):395–399
20. Ferdinand B, Gupta P, Kramer EL (2004) Spectrum of thymic uptake at 18F-FDG PET. Radiographics 24:1611–1616
21. Fischer B, Lassen U, Mortensen J et al (2009) Preoperative staging of lung cancer with combined PET-CT. N Engl J Med 361:32–39
22. Fischer BM, Mortensen J, Hojgaard L (2001) Positron emission tomography in the diagnosis and staging of lung cancer: a systematic, quantitative review. Lancet Oncol 2:659–666
23. Gambhir SS, Hoh CK, Phelps ME et al (1996) Decision tree sensitivity analysis for cost-effectiveness of FDG-PET in the staging and management of non-small-cell lung carcinoma. J Nucl Med 37:1428–1436
24. Garcia C, Bandaru V, Van Nostrand D et al (2010) Effective reduction of brown fat FDG uptake by controlling environmental temperature prior to PET scan: an expanded case series. Mol Imaging Biol 12(6): 652–656

25. Gould MK, Maclean CC, Kuschner WG et al (2001) Accuracy of positron emission tomography for diagnosis of pulmonary nodules and mass lesions: a meta-analysis. JAMA 285:914–924
26. Halley A, Hugentobler A, Icard P et al (2005) Efficiency of 18F-FDG and 99mTc-depreotide SPECT in the diagnosis of malignancy of solitary pulmonary nodules. Eur J Nucl Med Mol Imaging 32:1026–1032
27. Halpern BS, Schiepers C, Weber WA et al (2005) Presurgical staging of non-small cell lung cancer: positron emission tomography, integrated positron emission tomography/CT, and software image fusion. Chest 128:2289–2297
28. Heusner TA, Kuemmel S, Koeninger A et al (2010) Diagnostic value of diffusion-weighted magnetic resonance imaging (DWI) compared to FDG PET/CT for whole-body breast cancer staging. Eur J Nucl Med Mol Imaging 37:1077–1086
29. Hicks RJ, Kalff V, MacManus MP et al (2001) The utility of (18)F-FDG PET for suspected recurrent non-small cell lung cancer after potentially curative therapy: impact on management and prognostic stratification. J Nucl Med 42:1605–1613
30. Hofman MS, Smeeton NC, Rankin SC et al (2009) Observer variation in FDG PET-CT for staging of non-small-cell lung carcinoma. Eur J Nucl Med Mol Imaging 36:194–199
31. Hsu LH, Ko JS, You DL et al (2007) Transbronchial needle aspiration accurately diagnoses subcentimetre mediastinal and hilar lymph nodes detected by integrated positron emission tomography and computed tomography. Respirology 12:848–855
32. Ito H, Shimada K, Isogami K et al (2006) Recurrent thymoma: radiological (CT and FDG-PET) and histological (WHO criteria) features. Radiat Med 24: 292–296
33. Kamel EM, Zwahlen D, Wyss MT et al (2003) Whole-body (18)F-FDG PET improves the management of patients with small cell lung cancer. J Nucl Med 44: 1911–1917
34. Kanzaki R, Higashiyama M, Maeda J et al (2010) Clinical value of F18-fluorodeoxyglucose positron emission tomography-computed tomography in patients with non-small cell lung cancer after potentially curative surgery: experience with 241 patients. Interact Cardiovasc Thorac Surg 10:1009–1014
35. Kayani I, Bomanji JB, Groves A et al (2008) Functional imaging of neuroendocrine tumors with combined PET/CT using 68 Ga-DOTATATE (DOTA-DPhe1, Tyr3-octreotate) and 18F-FDG. Cancer 112: 2447–2455
36. Kee F, Erridge S, Bradbury I et al (2010) The value of positron emission tomography in patients with non-small cell lung cancer. Eur J Radiol 73(1):50–58
37. Klaeser B, Mueller MD, Schmid RA et al (2009) PET-CT-guided interventions in the management of FDG-positive lesions in patients suffering from solid malignancies: initial experiences. Eur Radiol 19: 1780–1785
38. Klaeser B, Wiskirchen J, Wartenberg J et al (2010) PET/CT-guided biopsies of metabolically active bone lesions: applications and clinical impact. Eur J Nucl Med Mol Imaging 37:2027–2036
39. Kosuda S, Ichihara K, Watanabe M et al (2002) Decision-tree sensitivity analysis for cost-effectiveness of whole-body FDG PET in the management of patients with non-small-cell lung carcinoma in Japan. Ann Nucl Med 16:263–271
40. Kruger S, Buck AK, Blumstein NM et al (2006) Use of integrated FDG PET/CT imaging in pulmonary carcinoid tumours. J Intern Med 260:545–550
41. Kumar A, Jindal T, Dutta R et al (2009) Functional imaging in differentiating bronchial masses: an initial experience with a combination of (18)F-FDG PET-CT scan and (68)Ga DOTA-TOC PET-CT scan. Ann Nucl Med 23:745–751
42. Kwek BH, Aquino SL, Fischman AJ (2004) Fluorodeoxyglucose positron emission tomography and CT after talc pleurodesis. Chest 125:2356–2360
43. Lamprecht B, Porsch P, Pirich C et al (2009) Electromagnetic navigation bronchoscopy in combination with PET-CT and rapid on-site cytopathologic examination for diagnosis of peripheral lung lesions. Lung 187:55–59
44. Lardinois D, Weder W, Hany TF et al (2003) Staging of non-small-cell lung cancer with integrated positron-emission tomography and computed tomography. N Engl J Med 348:2500–2507
45. Liu S, Cheng H, Yao S et al (2010) The clinical application value of PET/CT in adenocarcinoma with bronchioloalveolar carcinoma features. Ann Nucl Med 24:541–547
46. Murray JG, Erasmus JJ, Bahtiarian EA et al (1997) Talc pleurodesis simulating pleural metastases on 18F-fluorodeoxyglucose positron emission tomography. AJR Am J Roentgenol 168:359–360
47. Nagamachi S, Wakamatsu H, Kiyohara S et al (2010) The reproducibility of deep-inspiration breath-hold (18)F-FDG PET/CT technique in diagnosing various cancers affected by respiratory motion. Ann Nucl Med 24:171–178
48. Nguyen NC, Tran I, Hueser CN et al (2009) F-18 FDG PET/CT characterization of talc pleurodesis-induced pleural changes over time: a retrospective study. Clin Nucl Med 34:886–890
49. Nguyen VH, Peloquin S, Lacasse Y (2005) Cost-effectiveness of positron emission tomography for the management of potentially operable non-small cell lung cancer in Quebec. Can Respir J 12:19–25
50. Niho S, Fujii H, Murakami K et al (2007) Detection of unsuspected distant metastases and/or regional nodes by FDG-PET [corrected] scan in apparent limited-disease small-cell lung cancer. Lung Cancer 57:328–333
51. Nosotti M, Castellani M, Longari V et al (2008) Staging non-small lung cancer with positron emission

tomography: diagnostic value, impact on patient management, and cost-effectiveness. Int Surg 93:278–283
52. Ohno Y, Koyama H, Onishi Y et al (2008) Non-small cell lung cancer: whole-body MR examination for M-stage assessment–utility for whole-body diffusion-weighted imaging compared with integrated FDG PET/CT. Radiology 248:643–654
53. Orki A, Akin O, Tasci AE et al (2009) The role of positron emission tomography/computed tomography in the diagnosis of pleural diseases. Thorac Cardiovasc Surg 57:217–221
54. Otsuka H, Terazawa K, Morita N et al (2009) Is FDG-PET/CT useful for managing malignant pleural mesothelioma? J Med Invest 56:16–20
55. Plathow C, Aschoff P, Lichy MP et al (2008) Positron emission tomography/computed tomography and whole-body magnetic resonance imaging in staging of advanced nonsmall cell lung cancer – initial results. Invest Radiol 43:290–297
56. Plathow C, Staab A, Schmaehl A et al (2008) Computed tomography, positron emission tomography, positron emission tomography/computed tomography, and magnetic resonance imaging for staging of limited pleural mesothelioma: initial results. Invest Radiol 43:737–744
57. Prenzel KL, Monig SP, Sinning JM et al (2003) Lymph node size and metastatic infiltration in non-small cell lung cancer. Chest 123:463–467
58. Prevost A, Papathanassiou D, Jovenin N et al (2009) Comparison between PET(–FDG) and computed tomography in the staging of lung cancer. Consequences for operability in 94 patients. Rev Pneumol Clin 65:341–349
59. Reichert M, Bensadoun ES (2009) PET imaging in patients with coal workers pneumoconiosis and suspected malignancy. J Thorac Oncol 4:649–651
60. Schaefer-Prokop C (2010) Conventional and CT diagnostics of bronchial carcinoma. Radiologe 50:675–683
61. Schoellnast H, Larson SM, Nehmeh SA et al (2010) Radiofrequency ablation of non-small-cell carcinoma of the lung under real-time FDG PET CT guidance. Cardiovasc Intervent Radiol 34:S182–S185
62. Seo JH, Lee SW, Ahn BC et al (2010) Pulmonary amyloidosis mimicking multiple metastatic lesions on F-18 FDG PET/CT. Lung Cancer 67:376–379
63. Shen YY, Shiau YC, Wang JJ et al (2002) Whole-body 18F-2-deoxyglucose positron emission tomography in primary staging small cell lung cancer. Anticancer Res 22:1257–1264
64. Shim SS, Han J (2010) FDG-PET/CT imaging in assessing mucin-producing non-small cell lung cancer with pathologic correlation. Ann Nucl Med 24:357–362
65. Shin V, Bhargava P, Brown J et al (2007) Multimodality imaging features in a case of bronchial carcinoid including FDG PET. Med Sci Monit 13:CS4–CS8
66. Sloka JS, Hollett PD, Mathews M (2004) Cost-effectiveness of positron emission tomography for non-small cell lung carcinoma in Canada. Med Sci Monit 10:MT73–MT80
67. Subedi N, Scarsbrook A, Darby M et al (2009) The clinical impact of integrated FDG PET-CT on management decisions in patients with lung cancer. Lung Cancer 64:301–307
68. Sun JS, Park KJ, Sheen SS et al (2009) Clinical usefulness of the fluorodeoxyglucose (FDG)-PET maximal standardized uptake value (SUV) in combination with CT features for the differentiation of adenocarcinoma with a bronchioloalveolar carcinoma from other subtypes of non-small cell lung cancers. Lung Cancer 66:205–210
69. Takenaka D, Ohno Y, Matsumoto K et al (2009) Detection of bone metastases in non-small cell lung cancer patients: comparison of whole-body diffusion-weighted imaging (DWI), whole-body MR imaging without and with DWI, whole-body FDG-PET/CT, and bone scintigraphy. J Magn Reson Imaging 30: 298–308
70. Tasci E, Tezel C, Orki A et al (2010) The role of integrated positron emission tomography and computed tomography in the assessment of nodal spread in cases with non-small cell lung cancer. Interact Cardiovasc Thorac Surg 10:200–203
71. Toloza EM, Harpole L, McCrory DC (2003) Noninvasive staging of non-small cell lung cancer: a review of the current evidence. Chest 123:137S–146S
72. Torizuka T, Tanizaki Y, Kanno T et al (2009) Single 20-second acquisition of deep-inspiration breath-hold PET/CT: clinical feasibility for lung cancer. J Nucl Med 50:1579–1584
73. Tournoy KG, Maddens S, Gosselin R et al (2007) Integrated FDG-PET/CT does not make invasive staging of the intrathoracic lymph nodes in non-small cell lung cancer redundant: a prospective study. Thorax 62:696–701
74. Ung YC, Maziak DE, Vanderveen JA et al (2007) 18Fluorodeoxyglucose positron emission tomography in the diagnosis and staging of lung cancer: a systematic review. J Natl Cancer Inst 99:1753–1767
75. Verboom P, van Tinteren H, Hoekstra OS et al (2003) Cost-effectiveness of FDG-PET in staging non-small cell lung cancer: the PLUS study. Eur J Nucl Med Mol Imaging 30:1444–1449
76. Vinjamuri M, Craig M, Campbell-Fontaine A et al (2008) Can positron emission tomography be used as a staging tool for small-cell lung cancer? Clin Lung Cancer 9:30–34
77. Wahidi MM, Govert JA, Goudar RK et al (2007) Evidence for the treatment of patients with pulmonary nodules: when is it lung cancer?: ACCP evidence-based clinical practice guidelines (2nd edition). Chest 132:94S–107S
78. Wauters I, Stroobants S, De Leyn P et al (2010) Impact of FDG-PET-induced treatment choices on long-term outcome in non-small cell lung cancer. Respiration 79:97–104

79. Weiss N, Solomon SB (2003) Talc pleurodesis mimics pleural metastases: differentiation with positron emission tomography/computed tomography. Clin Nucl Med 28:811–814
80. Wilcox BE, Subramaniam RM, Peller PJ et al (2009) Utility of integrated computed tomography-positron emission tomography for selection of operable malignant pleural mesothelioma. Clin Lung Cancer 10:244–248
81. Yildirim H, Metintas M, Entok E et al (2009) Clinical value of fluorodeoxyglucose-positron emission tomography/computed tomography in differentiation of malignant mesothelioma from asbestos-related benign pleural disease: an observational pilot study. J Thorac Oncol 4:1480–1484

Part II

Minimally Invasive Thoracic Surgery: The Lung

Technique for Complete Video-Assisted Thoracic Lobectomy (c-VATS Lobectomy)

7

Jan Siebenga

Contents

J. Siebenga, M.D.
Division of Thoracic Surgery, Department of General Surgery, Atrium Medical Centre,
Henri Dunantstraat 5, 6401 CX Heerlen,
The Netherlands
e-mail: j.siebenga@atriummc.nl

7.1 Introduction

There is mounting evidence that c-VATS lobectomy is an oncologic adequate procedure and thereby an advantage for our patients [16]. While in the late 1990s and early 2000s, the question was if c-VATS lobectomy is comparable to open lobectomy, the accent has moved to studies which proof that c-VATS lobectomy is better than open lobectomy.

Areas in which c-VATS lobectomy performs better are reduced postoperative pain [8], shorter hospital stay [12, 16], better recovery [6], better pulmonary function [8], lower overall complication rate [9, 16], shorter chest tube drainage [5, 12, 16], and better compliance to adjuvant chemotherapy [10].

One of the causes for the relatively slow introduction of c-VATS lobectomy is the technically difficult procedure with a relatively long learning curve [2, 7]. Furthermore, it is difficult to perform an RCT because of the limited compliance with the approach (for VATS surgeons, a thoracotomy is a more morbid operation) and patients request a less invasive approach.

In this chapter, the technical aspects of the c-VATS lobectomy are described. There are different definitions for the VATS lobectomy [13]. For this chapter, the definition of report CALGB 39802 will be used: "we prefer to standardize the definition of a VATS lobectomy to encompass a true anatomic lobectomy with individual ligation of lobar vessels and bronchus as well as hilar

R.G.C. Inderbitzi et al. (eds.), *Minimally Invasive Thoracic and Cardiac Surgery*,
DOI 10.1007/978-3-642-11861-6_7, © Springer-Verlag Berlin Heidelberg 2012

lymph node dissection or sampling using the video screen for guidance, two or three ports, and no retractor use or rib spreading" [14].

7.2 General Considerations

The techniques described make use of conventional instruments. This has the advantage that it is easier to learn the c-VATS lobectomy because the handling of the instrumentation is the same as in open thorax surgery. Conventional instruments are usually shorter than endoscopic instruments, and therefore, they have a more "direct" feel which gives more confidence. Because no CO_2 insufflation is used, it is necessary to use single-lung ventilation.

The video camera and stapling devices are introduced through a trocar, but instruments can be put into the thorax straight through the incisions. This enhances the handling and reduces pressure on intercostal nerves.

A 45-mm stapler filling is used; for wedge resections, 60-mm fillings are more convenient. Different stapler heights are used for different tissues, the white stapler (open 2.5 mm, closed 1 mm) is used for vascular structures. For lung parenchyma, a blue stapler is used (open 3.5 mm, closed 1.5 mm), and for the bronchus, the green stapler is used (open 4.1 mm, closed 2 mm). There should be no traction on any of the tissues [4]. It is a good habit to check staple formation, because this will give an indication if you use the right stapler height. Furthermore, it is important to remove any unused staples which are lost in the thoracic cavity and especially remove staples which are left in the crotch; they have the potential to create a disaster by striping staples from the next filling [1].

7.2.1 Trocars

A 30° scope is inserted in the midaxillary line, in the seventh intercostal space, so it is possible to have an overview of the entire pleural cavity. This is also the place where the thoracic drain is left. An anterior and posterior port are made according to Fig. 7.1. The ventral port is in line with the fissure. The utility incision is made to remove the lobe after the resection. For right upper and middle lobe and for left upper lobe, it is made directly above the superior pulmonary vein. For right and left lower lobe, it is made directly above the inferior pulmonary vein.

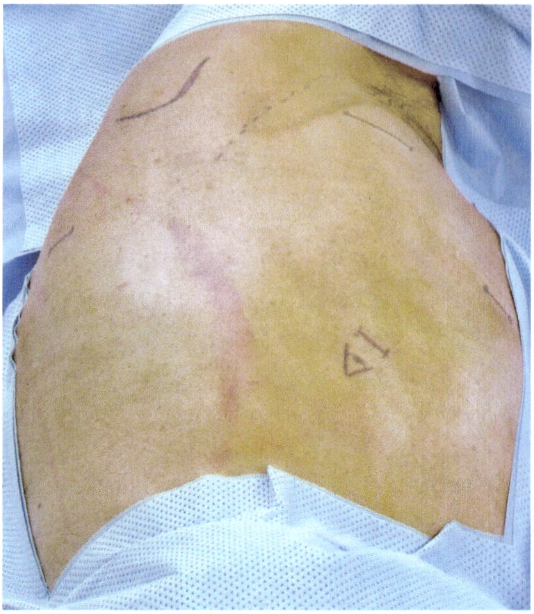

Fig. 7.1 Positions of the trocars and utility incision. The camera port is used for the thoracic drain. Anterior port is in line with the fissure. The utility incision is directly above the superior pulmonary vein for upper and middle lobe, and above the inferior pulmonary vein for lower lobe

7.2.2 Positioning

During c-VATS lobectomy, the surgeon stands at the front of the patient because the dissection is from anterior to posterior. The first assistant is standing opposite the surgeon and can play a very active role during preparation by maneuvering the lung and presenting tissue. Therefore, it is obligatory to use at least two monitors during the procedure. The assistant holding the scope is standing next to the surgeon and the scrub nurse is in the opposite position. See Fig. 7.1. With a 30° scope it is possible to have a good view on

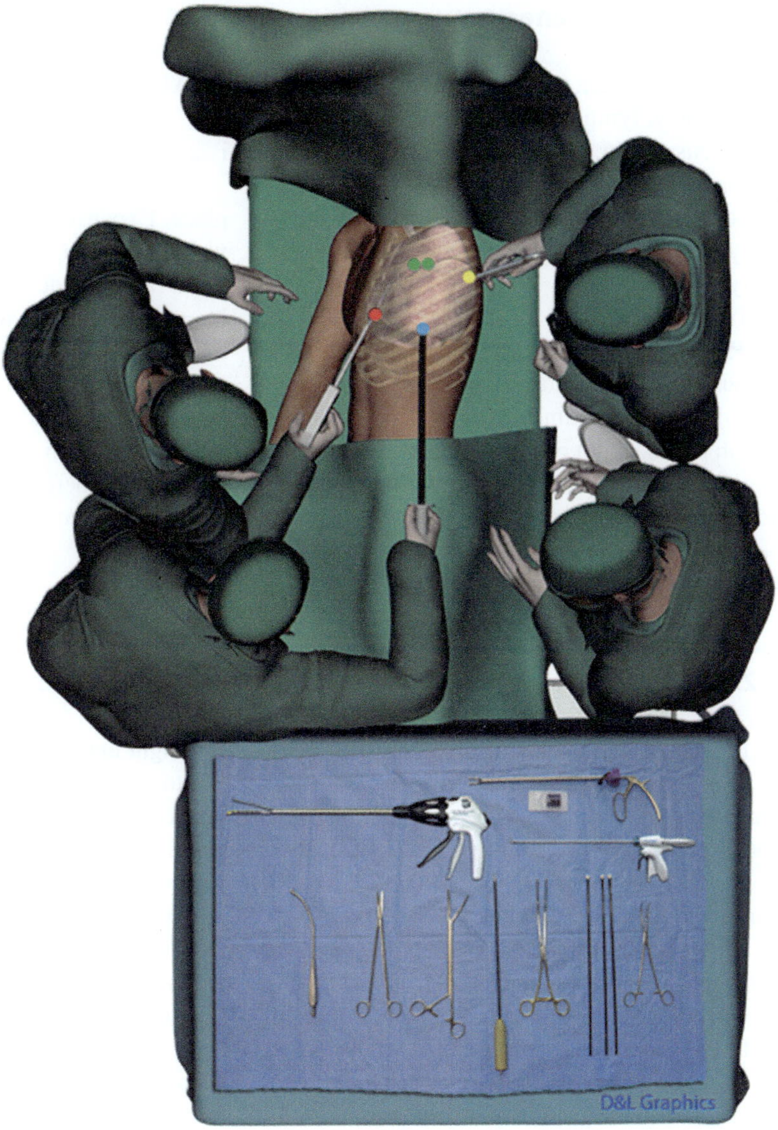

Fig. 7.2 Positioning of the operating team in the OR

every anatomic structure. The surgeon can use a Foerster clamp to give tissue traction and has in his other hand scissors, clamp, cautery, or ultrasonic instruments. The assistant uses a Foerster clamp and Yankauer to retract the lung and present the tissues (Fig. 7.2).

7.2.3 Exposure and Lung Retraction

While in open surgery lung handling is not an issue, in VATS surgery it is an important factor and influencing operation comfort. The lobe which is resected can be retracted with a Foerster clamp. The Foerster clamp is not traumatic and can be used in different ways. In video surgery, it is always handy to use curved instruments, so they are not in direct view. The lobe(s) which are not resected are handled as much as possible indirectly without grasping the lung directly. This lowers the change for parenchymal damage and consequent air leakage. The Yankauer can also be used for indirect and non-traumatic manipulation of the lung.

7.2.4 Lymphadenectomy

In this subchapter, the indications for lymphadenectomy, lymph node picking, etc., will not be discussed [6, 17]. The technique for the lymphadenectomy is important in c-VATS lobectomy. Lymphadenectomy in c-VATS lobectomy can be just as adequate as in open lobectomy [12, 15].

Tissue dissection is performed with the HARMONIC ACE® (Ethicon Endo-Surgery) because this has the advantage of reducing blood loss through sometimes very well-vascularized lymph nodes, and it can also be used for preparation. The c-VATS procedure starts with the lymph node dissection. Hereby, already a significant part of preparation is performed which makes the lobectomy easier.

7.2.5 Vascular Control

To isolate vascular structures, the same principles as in open lobectomy apply. A conventional preparation clamp can be used. For emergencies, an endoscopic vascular clamp is on the set. If there is unexpected bleeding, most bleeders can be controlled with a gauze ball.

Clips should be used very judiciously. They can slip of or they conflict with stapling later in the operation. If an artery is too small for stapling and there is no alternative, a Hem-o-lok® (Weck) can be used. These clips are removable, and they have a very good grip; they are even used on the renal artery [11]. We use two locks on the patient side and one on the specimen side.

Small vessels are coagulated with electrocautery or ultrasounds, e.g., HARMONIC ACE® (Ethicon Endo-Surgery).

Complications related to stapling of vascular structures are extremely rare [3]. The stapler must be used without any force, and it must be very easy to put the stapler in place. There should be no traction on the vessel, and there should be no bunching of the vessel in the crotch [1]. This can give folding of the vessel, and when the stapler is released, the vessel will not be stapled completely.

7.2.6 Thoracic Drainage

c-VATS lobectomy fits very well in fast-track lung surgery. An important factor in this concept is a fast protocol for thoracic drainage. After a c-VATS lobectomy, one 28 Ch drain is left in place. Expansion of the lung is controlled under vision through the video scope. Postoperative X-thorax is made to see if the lung is expanded. No suction is used, and the drain is left on water seal. On the first postoperative day, the drain is checked for air leakage and production. If there is no air leakage and production is not more than 400 cc, the drain is removed [5]. An X-thorax is made when there is clinical suspicion or deterioration of the patient's clinical condition.

7.3 Technique

7.3.1 Right Upper Lobe

The right upper lobe (RUL) is retracted to posterior to get a good view of the hilum. The pleura is opened just superior to the azygos vein. It is easy to create room in this space so that the pleura can be opened to inferior so that the superior pulmonary vein is exposed and the branch to the middle lobe is identified. Care should be taken not to touch the phrenic nerve. The azygos vein is then isolated and can be divided. This gives good exposure of the mediastinum; now a lymphadenectomy can be performed of nodes two and four right. Dissection can be made into the subcarinal space; if a radical lymph node dissection is wanted after dissection, a gauze ball can be left in the subcarinal space. The RUL is now retracted to anterior.

The pulmonary ligament is released up to the inferior pulmonary vein; hereby, lymph node nine can be resected. The pleura is opened posterior up till the azygos vein. The stump of the azygos vein is released from the RUL by opening the pleura completely around the upper part of the RUL. Lymph node eight is removed, and now it is possible to dissect to the subcarinal space from posterior to resect lymph node seven. A complete resection is achieved when the gauze ball you left anterior is seen and the complete subcarinal space is opened. It is important to make sure there is no bleeding because this will have an adverse effect on the rest of the procedure and will hinder the view. Sometimes, it is necessary to leave a low end hemostat (collagen or cellulose) in the subcarinal space. Now the RUL is retracted back to posterior.

Now it is time for the actual lobectomy. First, the branch to the RUL from the superior pulmonary vein is isolated. The branch to the middle lobe is also identified. After dissection, a Vicryl which is wetted with paraffin is pulled through, so it will be easier to pass a stapler. Before dividing the vein, the fissure is first opened.

The right lung is positioned so that a stapler which is introduced from the anterior port can easily staple the horizontal fissure. It is important that the lung tissue goes easily into the stapler and that no force is used. Aim the anvil of the stapler to the division between the upper and middle lobe vein. Most of the time, one or two staplers will open the fissure up to the vein. Now it is easier to move in the stapler from posterior to divide the branches of the vein going up to the RUL. The RUL is retracted to posterior.

The pulmonary artery and the truncus anterior will be in view and can be dissected. The truncus anterior must be isolated. Beware of anatomic anomalies; sometimes, the truncus divides itself directly. With the 30° scoop, it is possible to look behind the truncus to be sure there are no surprises. After dissection, a Vicryl which is wetted with paraffin is pulled through, and the truncus can be divided with a stapler from the posterior port. After division, most of the time, it is possible to take a little bit more of the fissure. Next step will be the dissection of the bronchus, so the RUL is retracted to posterior and inferior.

Because of the lymph node dissection at the start, the main bronchus and the bronchus to the RUL should be in view. The bronchus to the RUL is further dissected by releasing the tissue direct to the left of the bronchus. Beware of the posterior branch of the pulmonary artery. After dissection, a Vicryl which is wetted with paraffin is pulled through, and the bronchus to the RUL can be divided with a stapler which is inserted from the posterior port. The RUL is now retracted to posterior.

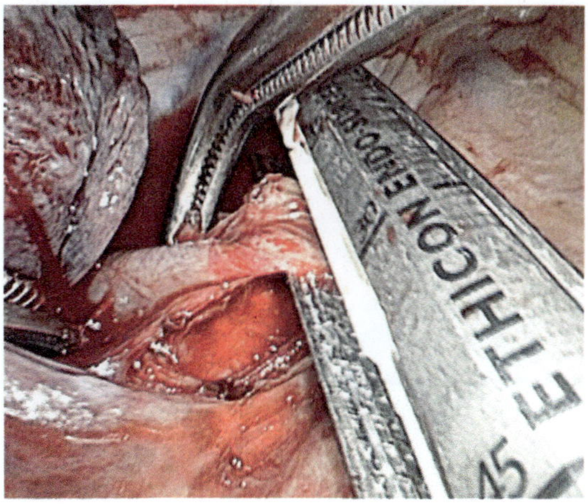

Fig. 7.3 After opening up of the mediastinal pleura, the azygos vein is dissected facilitate the mediastinal lymphadenectomy

If the posterior branch of the pulmonary artery is easily identified, this can be divided separately, but this is not strictly necessary. It should be possible to see the branch of the middle lobe artery. The fissure is now completed with the stapler introduced through the anterior port. Because this port is in the same plane as the fissure, it is possible to complete the fissure in one straight line.

Now the RUL can be retrieved in an endobag through the utility incision. We clean the thoracic cavity with warm water. The procedure is completed with spraying TISSEEL® (Baxter) over all parenchymal staple lines and on the bronchus stump; this is to make sure that even minimal air leakages are prevented and thoracic drainage will be as sort as possible (Figs. 7.3, 7.4, 7.5, 7.6, 7.7, 7.8, 7.9, 7.10, 7.11, 7.12, and 7.13).

Pitfalls:

- Early branching of truncus anterior pulmonary artery
- Creating the dissection plane between posterior branch of the pulmonary artery and bronchus

7.3.2 Right Middle Lobe

The procedure for the right middle lobe (RML) is started like the RUL. The right upper lobe (RUL) is retracted to posterior to get a good view of the

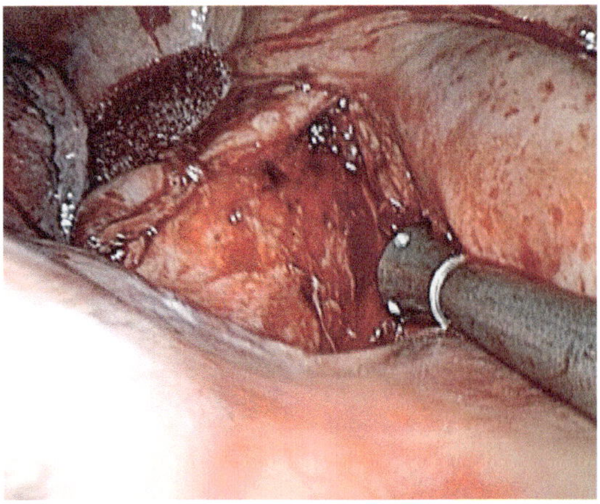

Fig. 7.4 After completion of the lymphadenectomy, the paratracheal space is cleared and the anatomic landmarks are clearly identifiable

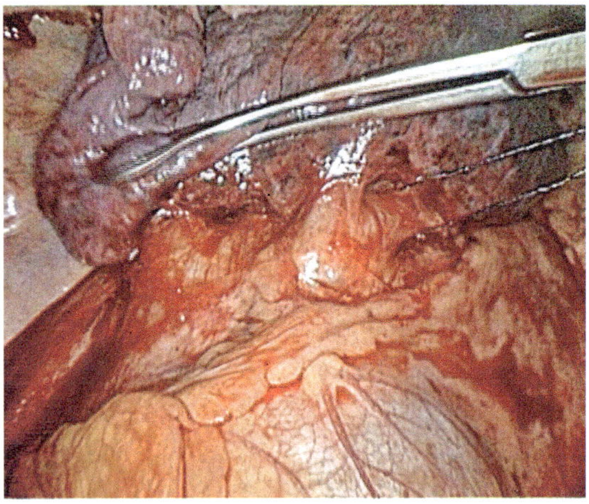

Fig. 7.5 View on the right superior and inferior pulmonary vein. The superior pulmonary vein is made free; the segmental veins for the upper lobe are identified and isolated. The middle lobe vein can be clearly seen in the middle of the screen

hilum. The pleura is opened just superior to the azygos vein. It is easy to create room in this space so that the pleura can be opened to inferior so that the superior pulmonary vein is exposed and the branch to the middle lobe is identified. Care should be taken not to touch the phrenic nerve. The azygos vein is then isolated and can be divided. This gives good exposure of the mediastinum; now a lymphadenectomy can be performed of nodes two and four right. Dissection

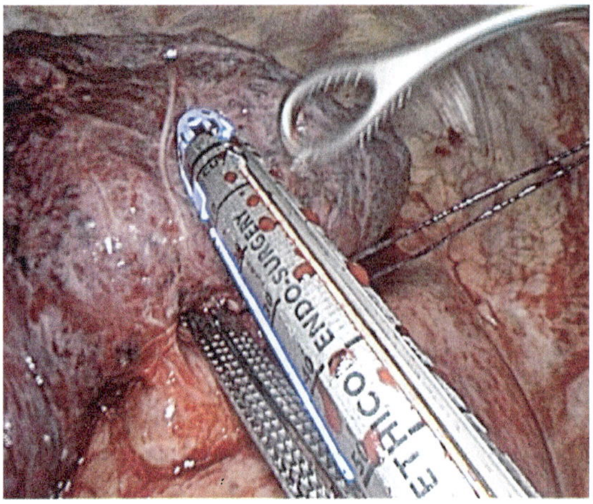

Fig. 7.6 Opening up of the horizontal fissure. The anvil of the stapler is placed in the division of middle and upper lobe vein. Now the lung can be retracted into the stapler and the fissure can be opened

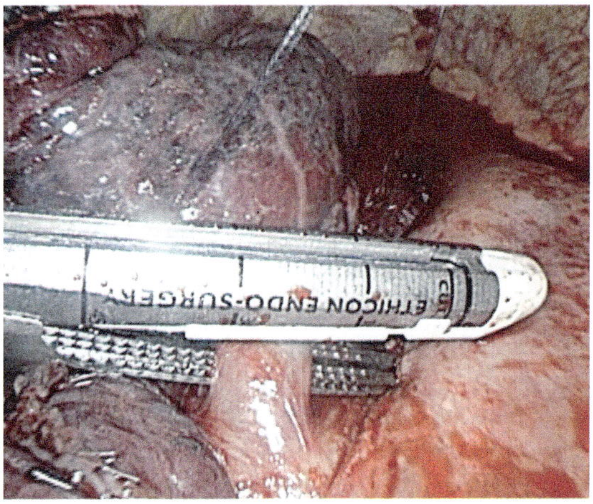

Fig. 7.7 The vein to the upper lobe is dissected. Because of the opening of the fissure, there is enough space to maneuver around the vein

can be made into the subcarinal space; if a radical lymph node dissection is wanted after dissection, a gauze ball can be left in the subcarinal space. The RUL is now retracted to anterior.

The pulmonary ligament is released up to the inferior pulmonary vein, hereby lymph node nine can be resected. The pleura is opened posterior up till the azygos vein. The stump of the azygos vein is

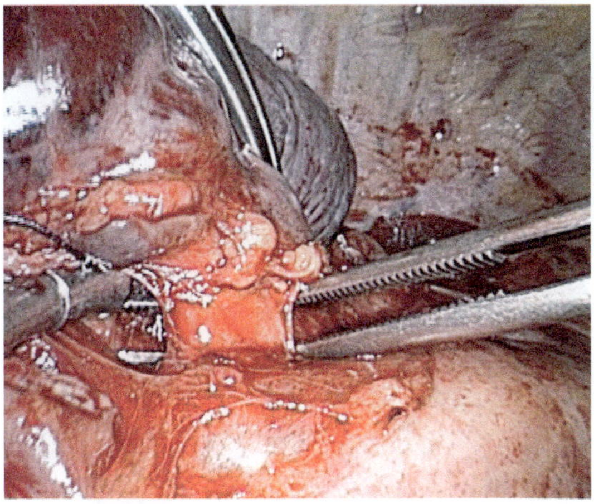

Fig. 7.8 Preparation of the anterior trunk

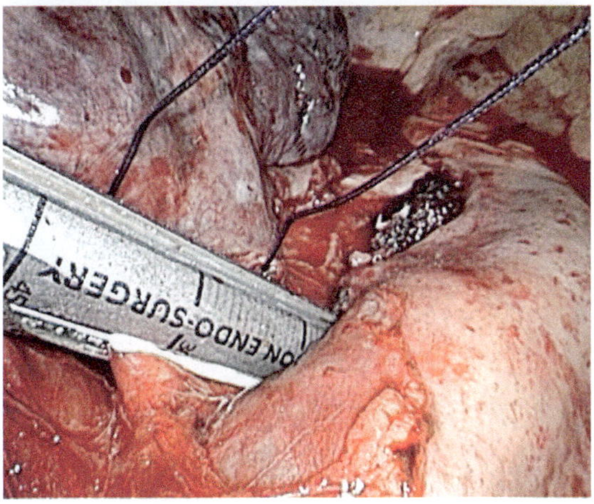

Fig. 7.9 The anterior trunk is stapled. Make sure to immobilize the stapler while firing to make sure there is no traction on the artery

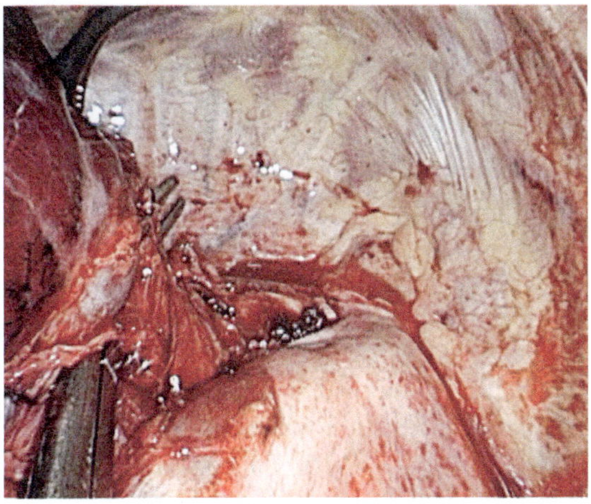

Fig. 7.10 Isolation of the right upper lobe bronchus

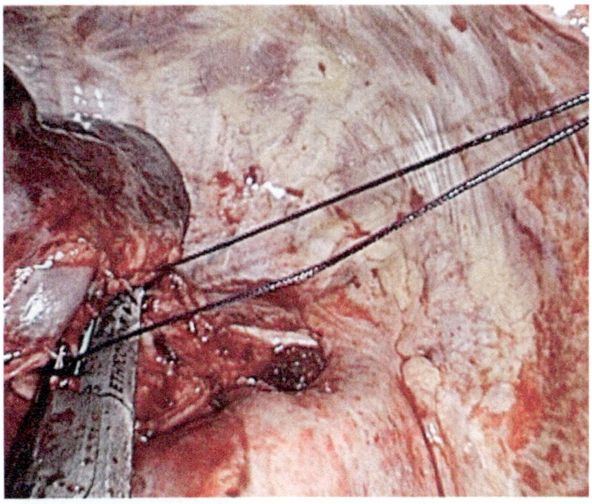

Fig. 7.11 The right upper lobe bronchus is stapled

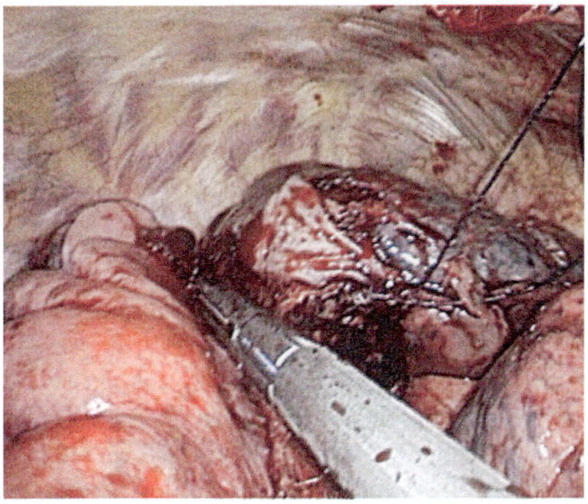

Fig. 7.12 The fissure is completed. The posterior ascending artery is taken together with the fissure. If necessary, it is possible to clip the artery before completing the fissure

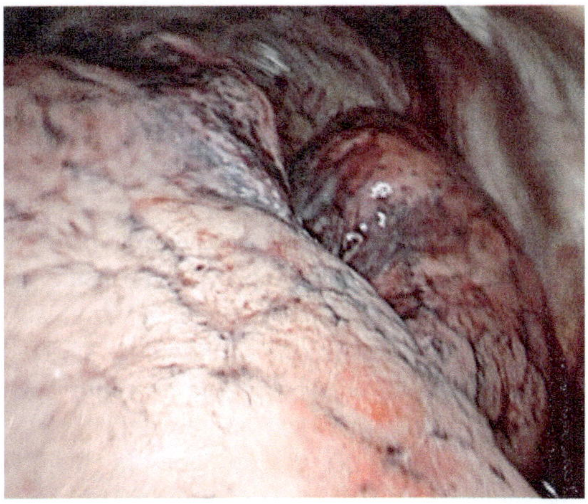

Fig. 7.13 Insufflation of middle and lower lobe. Check that the middle lobe has no rotation

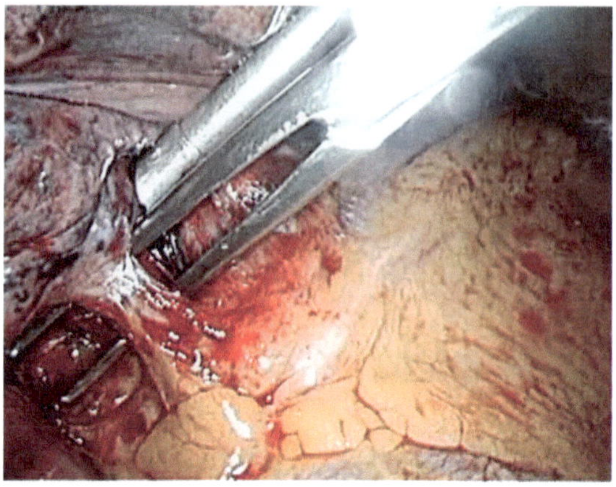

Fig. 7.14 The right middle lobe vein is isolated

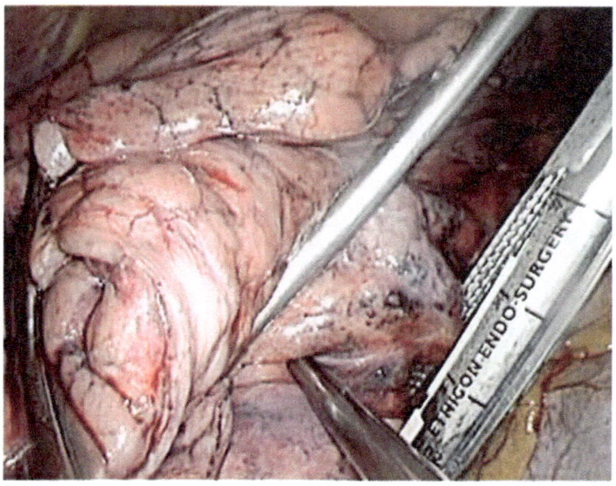

Fig. 7.15 Stapling of the right middle lobe vein

released from the RUL by opening the pleura completely around the upper part of the RUL. Lymph node eight is removed, and now it is possible to dissect to the subcarinal space from posterior to resect lymph node seven. A complete resection is achieved when the gauze ball you left anterior is seen and the complete subcarinal space is opened. It is important to make sure there is no bleeding because this will have an adverse effect on the rest of the procedure and will hinder the view. Sometimes, it is necessary to leave a low end hemostat (collagen or cellulose) in the subcarinal space. Now the RUL is retracted back to posterior.

Now it is time for the actual lobectomy. First, the branch to the RML from the superior pulmonary vein is isolated. After dissection, a Vicryl which is wetted with paraffin is pulled through, so it will be easier to pass a stapler. Before dividing the vein, the fissure is first opened.

The right lung is positioned so that a stapler which is introduced from the anterior port can easily staple the horizontal fissure. It is important that the lung tissue goes easily into the stapler and that no force is used. Aim the anvil of the stapler to the division between the upper and middle lobe vein. Most of the time, one or two staplers will open the fissure up to the vein. Next step is completing the oblique fissure; you can use the stapler, but it is important not to use any force. In this way, the stapler will not divide any anatomical structure. Sometimes, it will be necessary to develop the last part of the fissure with sharp or blunt dissection. Now introduce the stapler from posterior to divide the branch of the vein going up to the RML. The RML is retracted to anterior and superior.

Further dissection into the oblique fissure will reveal the RML bronchus. Directly behind the bronchus is the artery for the RML, so preparation should be cautious. Often, lymph nodes will be in this place; after careful removal of the lymph nodes, the anatomic structures will be clearly seen. Tissue around the bronchus is removed and the bronchus isolated. A Vicryl wetted in paraffin is put around the bronchus, and the stapler is introduced through the posterior port. Be aware of the ML artery and advance the stapler cautiously. After the bronchus is divided, one should have a clear view on the RML artery which is also isolated and a Vicryl wetted in paraffin is pulled around it. The artery is also stapled from the posterior port. Now the middle lobe is only hold by the fissure. Both the fissures are completed through stapling. When the fissures are not developed, this last part can be difficult when there is a lot of parenchyma left. It can be convenient to use a 60-mm stapler. Now the RML can be retrieved in an endobag through the utility incision. We clean the thoracic cavity with warm water. The procedure is completed with spraying TISSEEL® (Baxter) over all parenchymal staple lines and on the bronchus stump; this is to make sure that even minimal air leakages are prevented and thoracic drainage will be as sort as possible (Figs. 7.14, 7.15, 7.16, 7.17, 7.18, 7.19, 7.20, 7.21, 7.22, and 7.23).

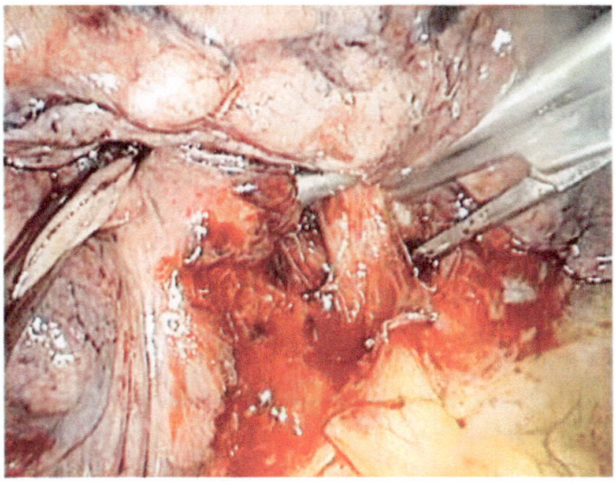

Fig. 7.16 Isolation of the right middle lobe bronchus. Clearing of the lymph nodes makes preparation easier

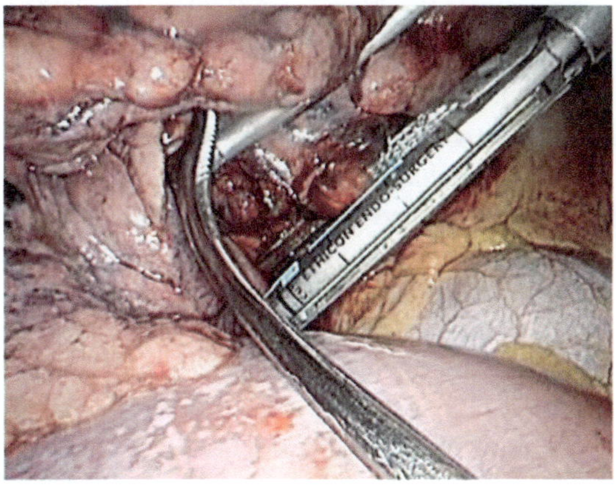

Fig. 7.17 The right middle lobe bronchus is stapled. Before firing, insufflate upper and lower lobe to make sure there is no tenting which compromises the bronchus

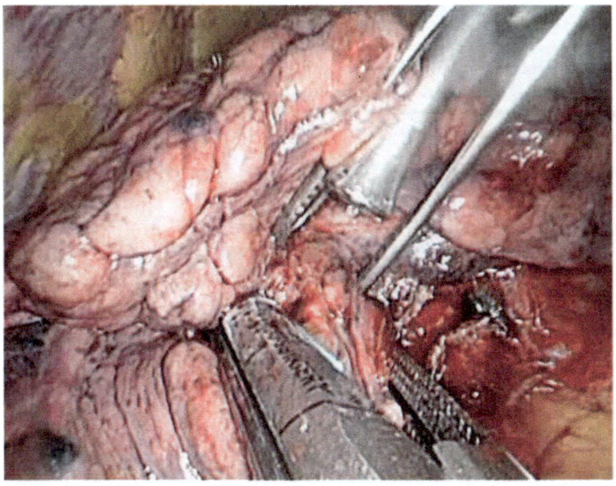

Fig. 7.18 Opening up of the oblique fissure. No force should be used

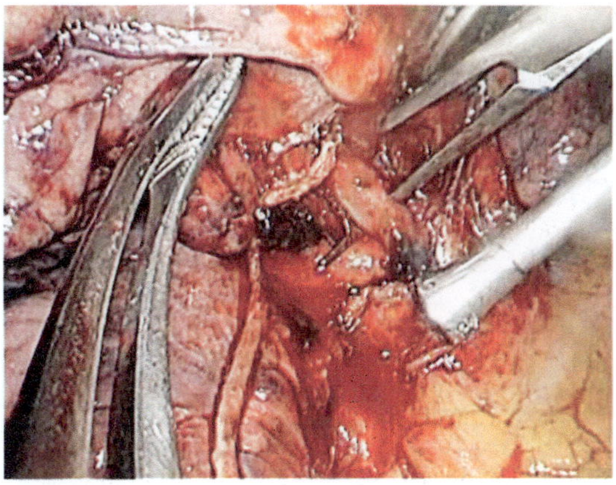

Fig. 7.19 The oblique fissure is opened up, giving access to the artery. The middle lobe artery is isolated

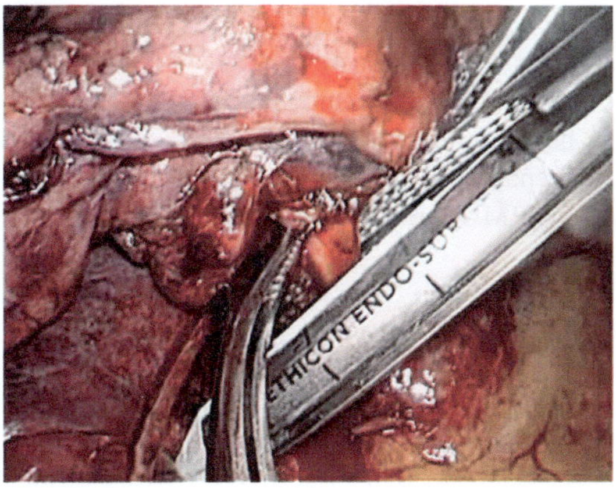

Fig. 7.20 The middle lobe artery is stapled

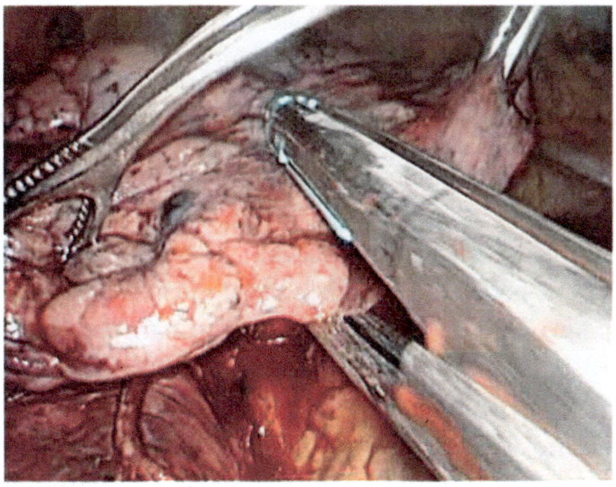

Fig. 7.21 Opening up of the horizontal fissure

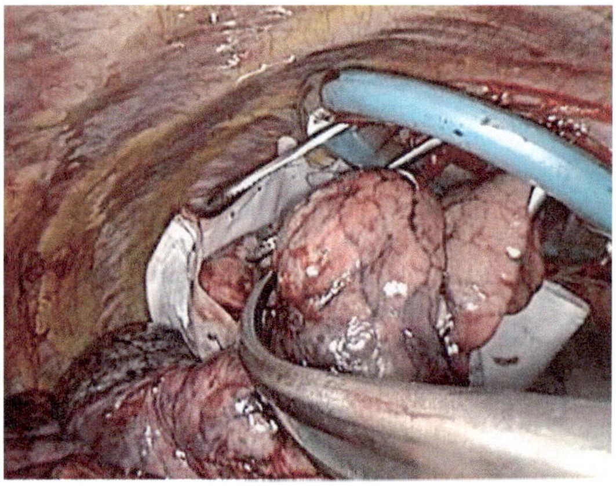

Fig. 7.22 After completion of both fissures, the middle lobe is free. The lobe is put into a specimen bag and removed through the utility incision

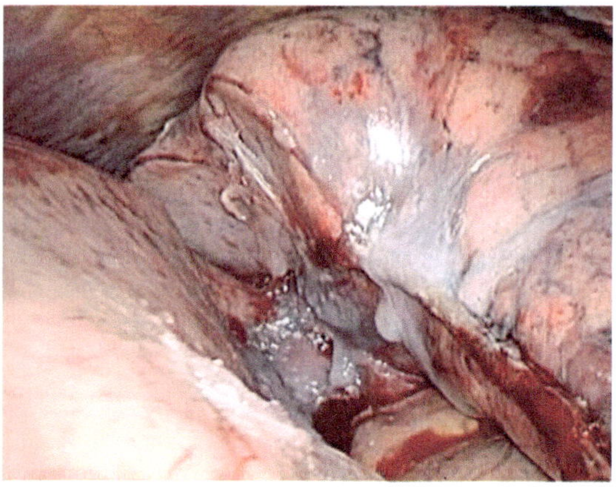

Fig. 7.23 Insufflation of right upper and lower lobe

Pitfalls:

- Developing the fissures and finding the RML bronchus and artery
- Preparation of the bronchus without seeing the RML artery

7.3.3 Right Lower Lobe

Because of the lymph node dissection, the procedure for the right lower lobe (RLL) is started in the same way as the RUL. The RUL is retracted to posterior to get a good view of the hilum. The pleura is opened just superior to the azygos vein. It is easy to create room in this space so that the pleura can be opened to inferior so that the superior pulmonary vein is exposed and the branch to the middle lobe is identified. Care should be taken not to touch the phrenic nerve. The azygos vein is then isolated and can be divided. This gives good exposure of the mediastinum; now a lymphadenectomy can be performed of nodes two and four right. Dissection can be made into the subcarinal space; if a radical lymph node dissection is wanted after dissection, a gauze ball can be left in the subcarinal space. The RUL is now retracted to anterior.

The pulmonary ligament is released up to the inferior pulmonary vein, hereby lymph node nine can be resected. The pleura is opened posterior up till the azygos vein. The stump of the azygos vein is released from the RUL by opening the pleura completely around the upper part of the RUL. Lymph node eight is removed, and now it is possible to dissect to the subcarinal space from posterior to resect lymph node seven. A complete resection is achieved when the gauze ball you left anterior is seen and the complete subcarinal space is opened. It is important to make sure there is no bleeding because this will have an adverse effect on the rest of the procedure and will hinder the view. Sometimes, it is necessary to leave a low end hemostat (collagen or cellulose) in the subcarinal space. Now the RUL is kept retracted to anterior.

The inferior pulmonary vein is freed from its surrounding tissue and most of the time it is easy to isolate this vein. When the inferior pulmonary vein is isolated, a Vicryl wetted in paraffin is put around it. Before the vein is divided, the oblique fissure is developed first. A stapler introduced thorough the anterior port will easily be put in position for the fissure. In most cases, one or two staplers can be used. Opening of the fissure will give more space for the division of the inferior pulmonary vein. This is divided by a stapler introduced through the posterior port. The lobe is now retracted upward.

The oblique fissure is dissected until the bronchus. From posterior is the most convenient way to find the RLL bronchus. If the bronchus is identified, the RLL can be retracted to posterior. The RLL arteries will be superior to the bronchus; also in this place, when carefully removing lymph nodes, the anatomic structures will show

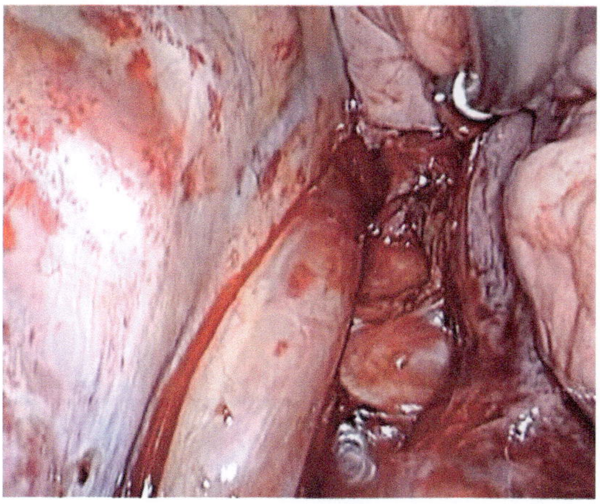

Fig. 7.24 The inferior pulmonary ligament is dissected and the inferior pulmonary vein isolated. The posterior pleura is opened to cranial giving exposure to the subcarinal space. The esophagus is clearly seen. In the subcarinal space, lymph node seven is removed. In this figure, the subcarinal space is cleared, and there is a clear view on the anatomic structures

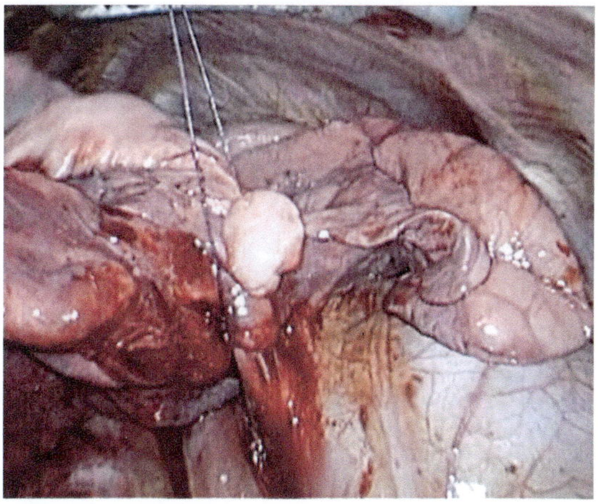

Fig. 7.25 The inferior pulmonary vein is isolated

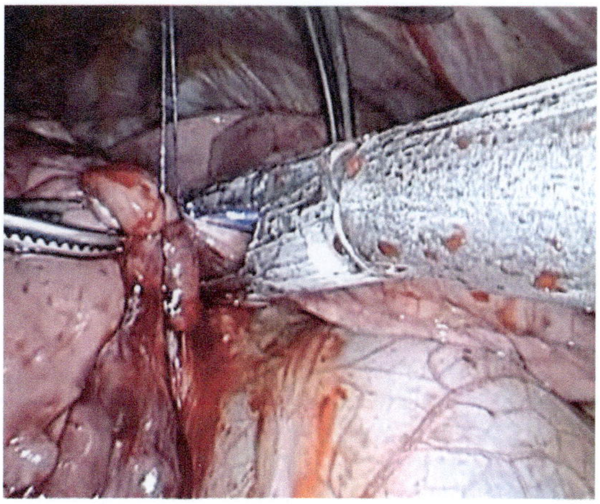

Fig. 7.26 The oblique fissure is opened. The anvil of the stapler is placed between the superior and inferior pulmonary vein

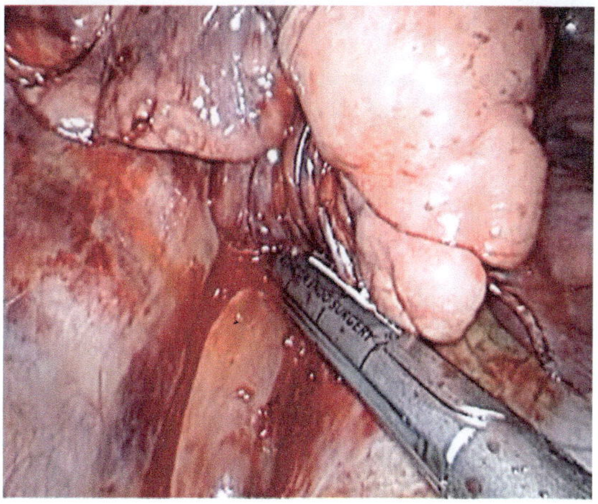

Fig. 7.27 Dissection of the inferior pulmonary vein by stapler

themselves. When a space is made cranial from the arteries, it is possible to staple some of the parenchyma and pleura to get more space. Isolate the arteries by removing surrounding tissue. A wet Vicryl is put around the arteries, and they are divided by a stapler introduced from the anterior port. Now there is enough room to isolate the bronchus to the RLL, and this is divided in the same way. The fissure can now be completed by stapling from the anterior port. In the end, one should have one long straight stapler line.

Now the RLL can be retrieved in an endobag through the utility incision. We clean the thoracic cavity with warm water. The procedure is completed with spraying TISSEEL® (Baxter) over all parenchymal staple lines and on the bronchus stump; this is to make sure that even minimal air leakages are prevented and thoracic drainage will be as sort as possible (Figs. 7.24, 7.25, 7.26, 7.27, 7.28, 7.29, 7.30, 7.31, and 7.32).

Pitfalls:

- Developing the fissures and finding the RLL bronchus and artery

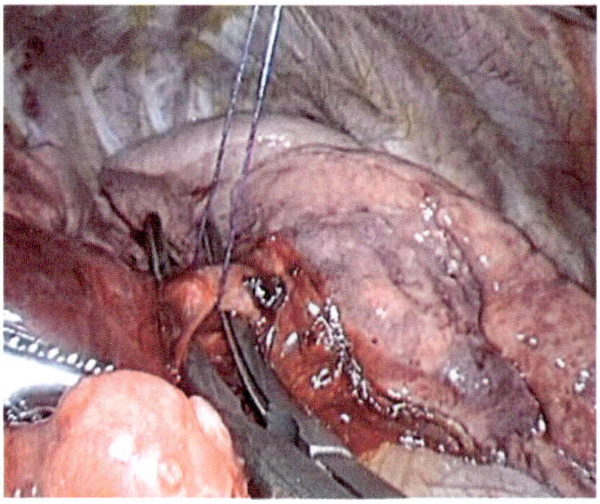

Fig. 7.28 By opening up of the oblique fissure, the segmental arteries to the right lower lobe are isolated

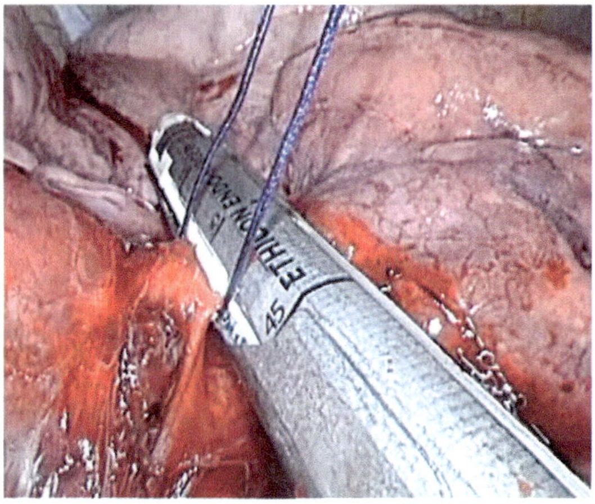

Fig. 7.29 Stapling of the lower lobe artery

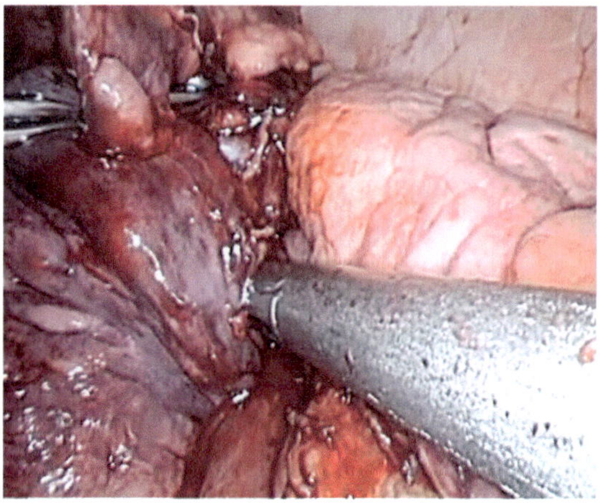

Fig. 7.30 Before firing the stapler to dissect the right lower lobe bronchus, the lung is insufflated. Make sure the middle lobe bronchus is not compromised. In this figure, the insufflation of the middle lobe is shown

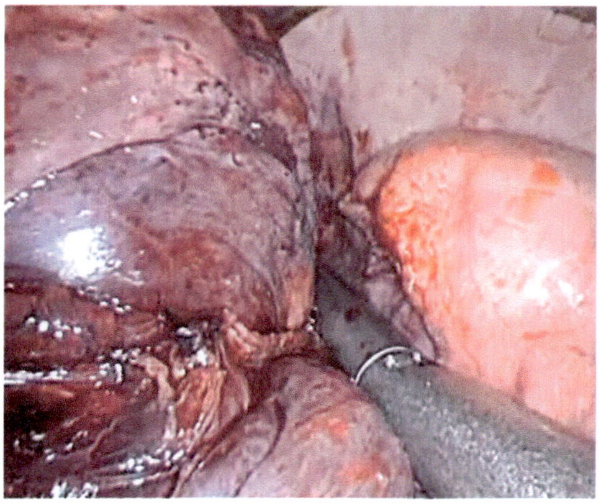

Fig. 7.31 The oblique fissure is completed

7.3.4 Left Upper Lobe

The left upper lobe (LUL) is retracted to posterior so that a clear view on the hilum is achieved. The pleura lying over the aortopulmonary window is widely opened. This gives access to lymph nodes five and six. The lymph nodes are removed; it is important to identify the vagus nerve and to identify the recurrent nerve which lies over the aortic arch. Care should be taken not to touch the phrenic nerve. Now the LUL is retracted to anterior. The pulmonary ligament is dissected, and the pleura dorsal to the LUL is opened to cranial so that the complete pleura around the LUL is opened; this will facilitate the lobectomy. Lymph nodes nine and eight can be dissected. The inferior pulmonary vein is identified. The left main bronchus is identified from posterior; in this way, it is possible to dissect up onto the carina and remove lymph node seven. It is important to make sure there is no bleeding because this will have an adverse effect on the rest of the procedure and will hinder the view. Sometimes, it is necessary to leave a low end hemostat (collagen or cellulose) in the subcarinal space. Now the LUL is retracted to posterior.

The superior pulmonary vein is released from surrounding tissue and is isolated. A Vicryl wetted with paraffin is put around the vein. Before

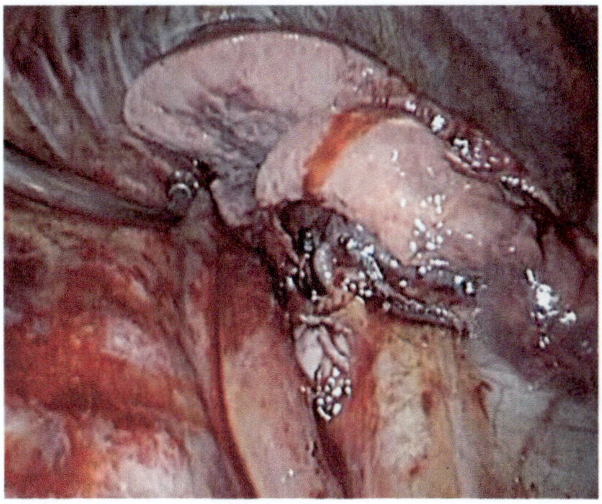

Fig. 7.32 Situation with the right lower lobe removed. Make sure that by insufflation the middle lobe is not rotated

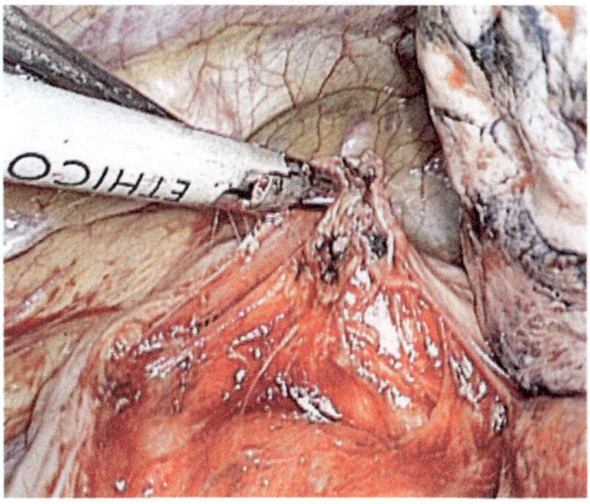

Fig. 7.33 Lymph node dissection of the aortopulmonary window. Lymph nodes and fatty tissue are cleared to give a clear view on the anatomic structures. Care should be taken to keep the recurrent nerve intact

division of the vein, the fissure should be opened. The left lung is put in neutral position; in this way, a stapler introduced into the anterior port will be right into the fissure. The superior pulmonary vein is used as landmark, and the stapler is directed just to the right side of the vein. Mostly one or two staplers will be sufficient to open the fissure. The LUL is now retracted to posterior.

After this, there will be enough space to introduce the stapler from the posterior point and to divide the superior pulmonary vein. After division of the vein, the bronchus to the LUL can be identified. Be aware that it is relatively easy to do the preparation to centrally and to isolate the main left bronchus, so it is important to identify the bronchus to the left lower lobe. If dissection is made to distal, also the bronchus to the lingual can be identified. Careful dissection is necessary around the bronchus because the pulmonary artery is direct beyond the bronchus. After isolating the bronchus, a Vicryl wetted in paraffin is put around it. Sometimes, it can be convenient at this stage to open up the fissure a little more with one stapler. A stapler is introduced from the posterior port, and the bronchus to the LUL is divided. At this stage, the left pulmonary artery will be in view. Tissue surrounding the artery is dissected, and in this way, a good exposure of the artery can be achieved. The LUL is retracted to superior to give exposure to the pulmonary artery.

In this way, the arterial branches, truncus anterior, posterior, and lingual branch can be seen. The truncus anterior is freed from surrounding tissue and isolated. A Vicryl wetted in paraffin is pulled around the truncus. From posterior, a stapler is introduced and the truncus is divided. Because the other branches are in view and there should be a lot of space at this stage of the lobectomy, it often is possible to divide the last branches to lingula and posterior segment with one or two staplers including the fissure and parenchyma. In this way, it is prevented that too much pulling force is put on the little arterial branches which could lead to unnecessary and uncomfortable bleeding.

Now the LUL can be retrieved in an endobag through the utility incision. We clean the thoracic cavity with warm water. The procedure is completed with spraying TISSEEL® (Baxter) over all parenchymal staple lines and on the bronchus stump; this is to make sure that even minimal air leakages are prevented and thoracic drainage will be as sort as possible (Figs. 7.33, 7.34, 7.35, 7.36, 7.37, 7.38, 7.39, 7.40, 7.41, and 7.42).

Pitfalls:

- Preparation of the bronchus and developing the plane between bronchus and pulmonary artery
- Stapling last part of the fissure including arterial branches

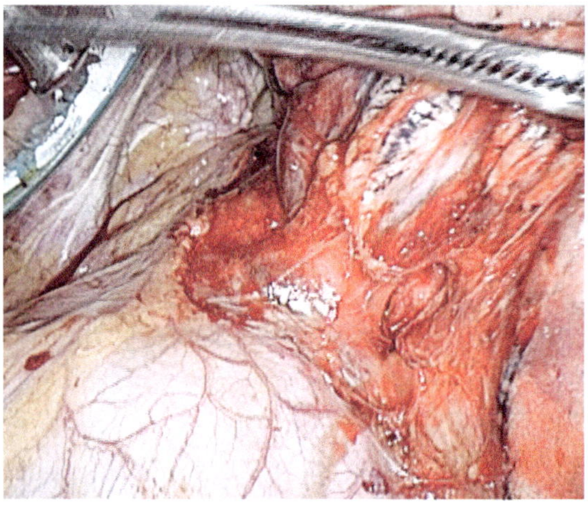

Fig. 7.34 The pleura over the hilum is opened. The superior pulmonary vein is isolated

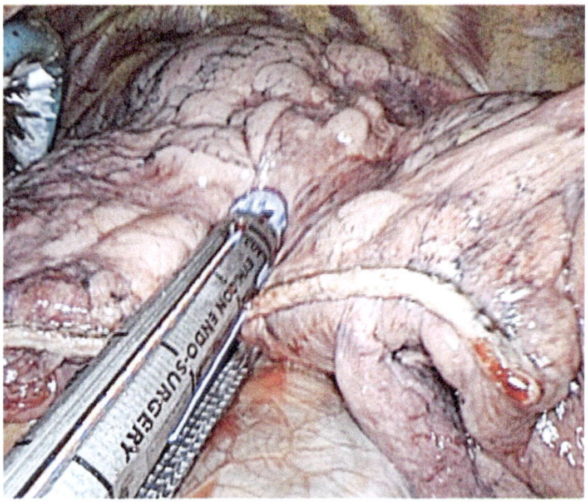

Fig. 7.35 Before dissecting the superior pulmonary vein, the oblique fissure is opened so that space is created. The anvil is directed at the division of superior and inferior pulmonary vein

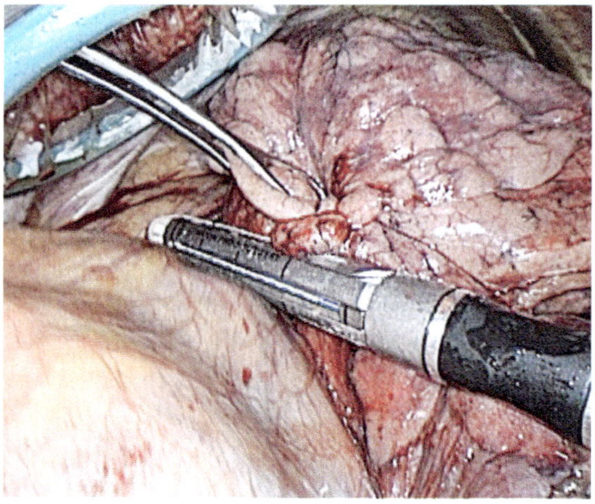

Fig. 7.36 Stapling of the superior pulmonary vein. (Note that the utility incision is direct above the superior pulmonary vein)

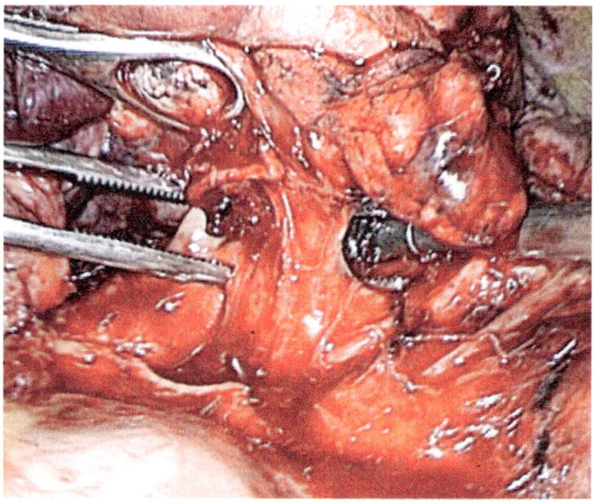

Fig. 7.37 Isolation of the left upper lobe bronchus. To the right, the lower lobe bronchus can be identified. Also the anterior trunk is exposed

7.3.5 Left Lower Lobe

The c-VATS lobectomy of the left lower lobe (LLL) is started in the same way as the LUL. The LLL is retracted to posterior so that a clear view on the hilum is achieved. The pleura lying over the aortopulmonary window is widely opened. This gives access to lymph nodes five and six. The lymph nodes are removed; it is important to identify the vagus nerve and to identify the recurrent nerve which lies over the aortic arch. Care should be taken not to touch the phrenic nerve. Now the LLL is retracted to anterior. The pulmonary ligament is dissected and the pleura dorsal to the LLL is opened to cranial. Lymph nodes nine and eight can be dissected. The inferior pulmonary vein is identified. The left main bronchus is identified from posterior; in this way, it is possible to dissect up onto the carina and remove lymph node seven. It is important to make sure there is no bleeding because this will have an adverse effect on the rest of the procedure and will hinder the view. Sometimes, it is necessary to leave a low end hemostat (collagen or cellulose) in the subcarinal space. Now the LLL is retracted to posterior.

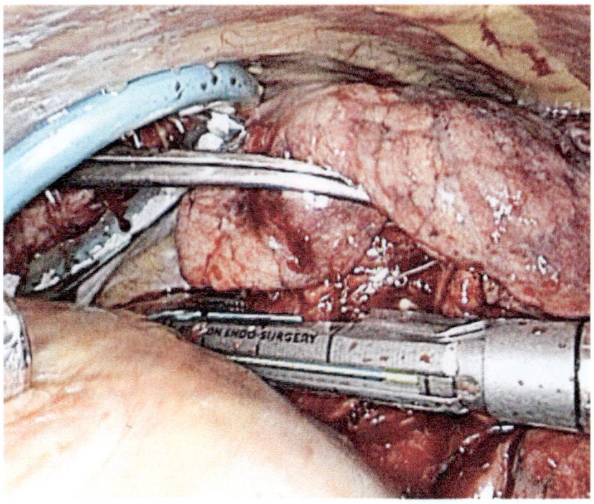

Fig. 7.38 Stapling of the upper lobe bronchus

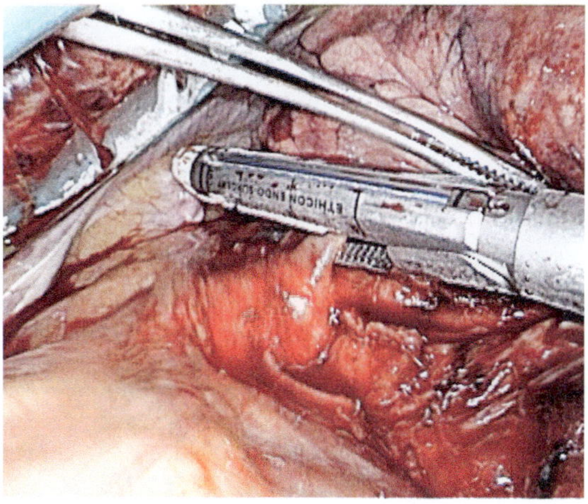

Fig. 7.40 Stapling of the anterior trunk

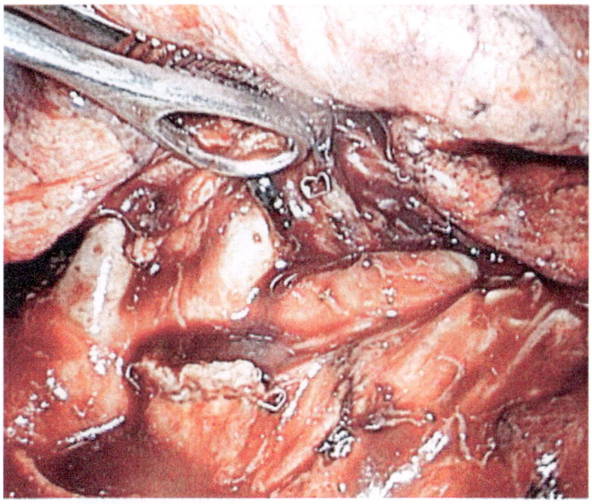

Fig. 7.39 The pulmonary artery and its branches to the upper lobe are exposed. There is a clear view on the lower lobe bronchus

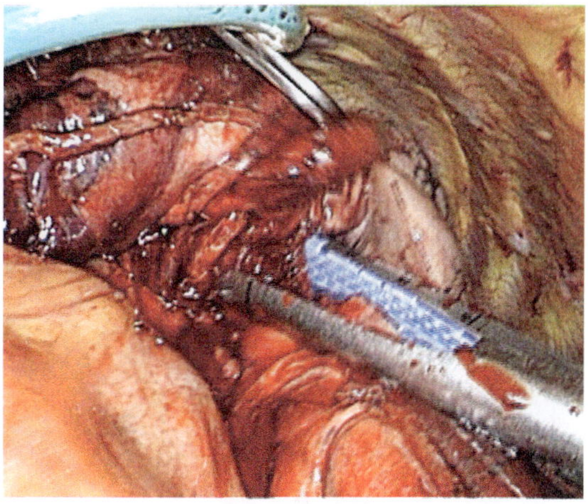

Fig. 7.41 Completion of the oblique fissure. The anvil of the stapler is on top of the pulmonary artery. In this way, posterior ascending arteries are also dissected together with the fissure

The inferior pulmonary vein is already freed from the pulmonary ligament, and most of the time, it is easy to isolate the vein. A Vicryl wetted with paraffin is pulled around the vein. Before division of the vein, the fissure should be opened. The left lung is put in neutral position; in this way, a stapler introduced into the anterior port will be right into the fissure. The inferior pulmonary vein is used as landmark, and the stapler is directed just to the left side of the vein. Mostly, one or two staplers will be sufficient to open the fissure. The LLL is now retracted to posterior. The stapler is introduced from the anterior port, and the inferior pulmonary vein is divided. If necessary, the fissure can be opened using sharp or blunt dissection until the bronchus is in view. It can be difficult to find the bronchus if there is no fissure; another possibility is to retract the LLL to anterior and to approach the bronchus from posterior. Tissue around the bronchus is dissected, and especially lymph nodes are removed to give good exposure. Keep in mind that the artery lies directly behind the bronchus. A Vicryl wetted with paraffin is pulled around the bronchus, and the bronchus is stapled from the posterior port. Now the artery will be in view; if there are lymph nodes, a good access to the

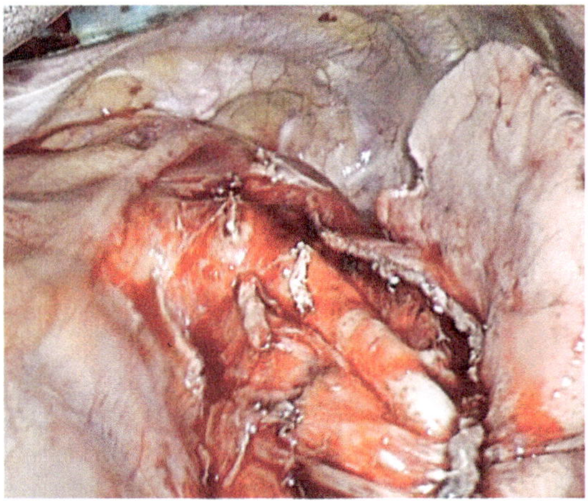

Fig. 7.42 The left upper lobe is removed. The left lower lobe is insufflated. There is a clear view on the pulmonary artery

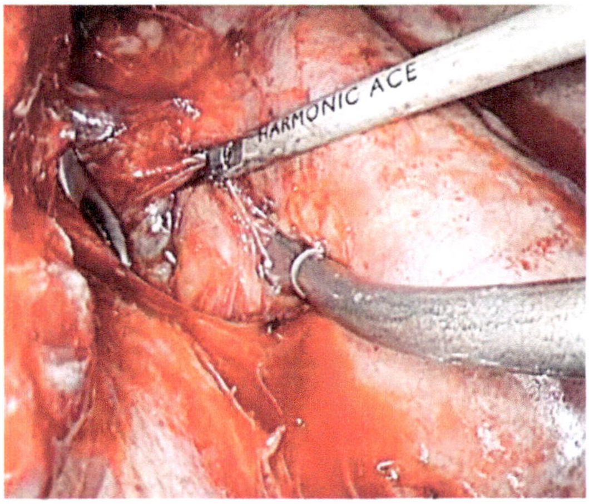

Fig. 7.43 The posterior pleura is opened. The descending aorta and esophagus can be seen. In the subcarinal space, lymph node seven is cleared

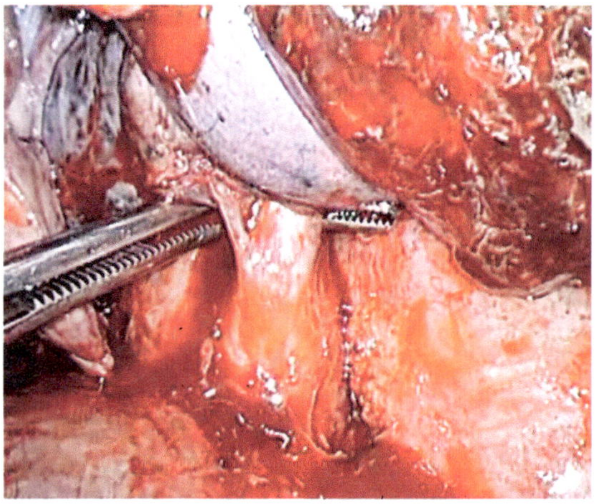

Fig. 7.44 The inferior pulmonary ligament is dissected and the inferior pulmonary vein is isolated

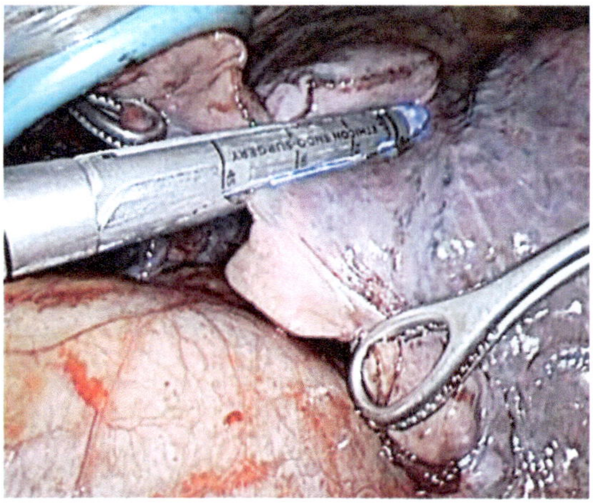

Fig. 7.45 The oblique fissure is opened. The tip of the anvil is directed between the superior and inferior pulmonary vein

artery can be achieved by removing these lymph nodes.

The artery is isolated and a wet Vicryl is put around it. Through the anterior port, the stapler is introduced and the artery is divided. The only thing whereby the LLL is attached to the body is the fissure. The fissure is completed from anterior so that in the end one can see one straight continuous staple line.

Now the LLL can be retrieved in an endobag through the utility incision. We clean the thoracic cavity with warm water. The procedure is completed with spraying TISSEEL® (Baxter) over all parenchymal staple lines and on the bronchus stump; this is to make sure that even minimal air leakages are prevented and thoracic drainage will be as sort as possible (Figs. 7.43, 7.44, 7.45, 7.46, 7.47, 7.48, 7.49, and 7.50).

Pitfalls:

- Preparation of the bronchus and developing the plane between bronchus and pulmonary artery

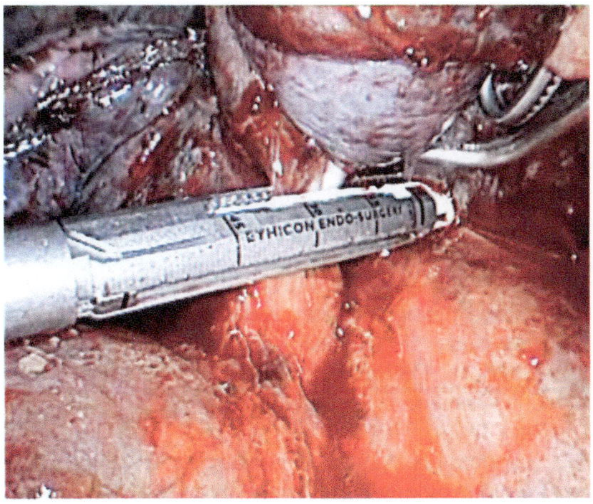

Fig. 7.46 The inferior pulmonary vein is stapled

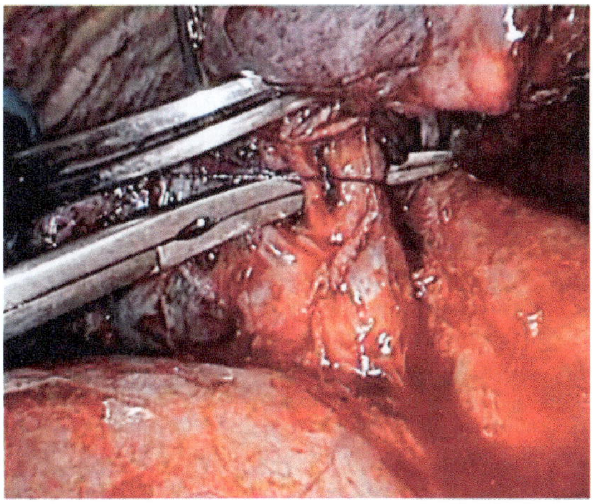

Fig. 7.47 Isolation of the left lower lobe bronchus

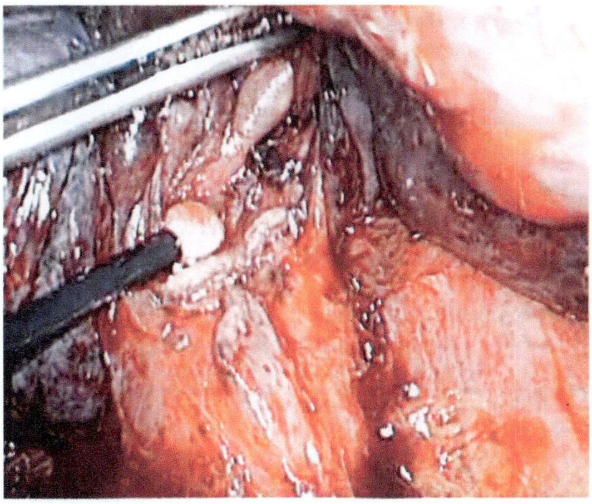

Fig. 7.48 The left lower lobe bronchus is dissected. The lower lobe arteries are in view. Behind the cherry dissector is the lingular artery

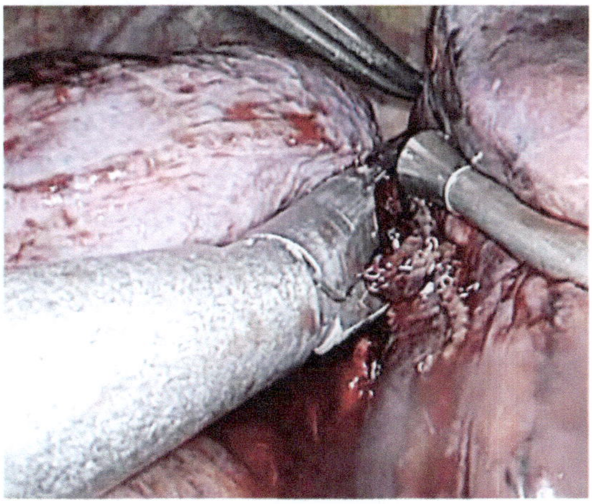

Fig. 7.49 Completion of the oblique fissure. The lower lobe arteries can be stapled independently

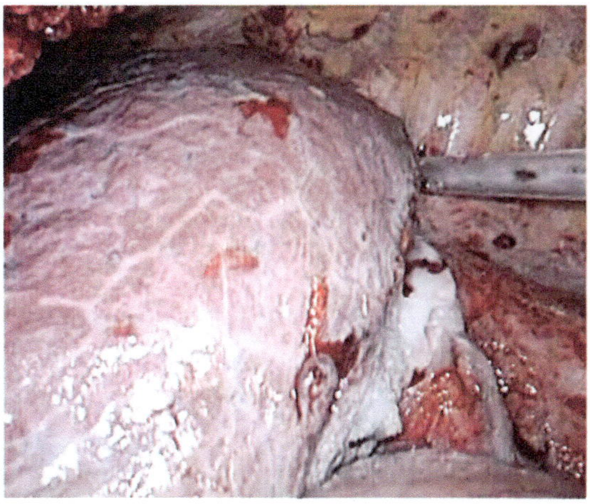

Fig. 7.50 Situation with the lower lobe removed. The left upper lobe is insufflated

Acknowledgement I would like to thank R. McKenna Jr, M.D., for opening my eyes for the c-VATS lobectomy.

References

1. Baker R, Foote J, Kemmeter P et al (2004) The science of stapling and leaks. Obes Surg 14(10):1290–1298
2. Belgers EH, Siebenga J, Bosch AM et al (2010) Complete video-assisted thoracoscopic surgery lobectomy and its learning curve. A single center study introducing the technique in The Netherlands. Interact Cardiovasc Thorac Surg 10(2):176–180
3. Craig SR, Walker WS (1995) Potential complications of vascular stapling in thoracoscopic pulmonary resection. Ann Thorac Surg 59(3):736–738
4. Gossot D, Merlusca G, Tudor A et al (2009) Pitfalls related to the use of endostaplers during video-assisted thoracic surgery. Surg Endosc 23(1):189–192
5. Gottgens KW, Siebenga J, Belgers EH et al (2011) Early removal of the chest tube after complete video-assisted thoracoscopic lobectomies. Eur J Cardiothorac Surg 39(4):575–578
6. Handy J, Asaph JW, Douville EC et al (2010) Does video-assisted thoracoscopic lobectomy for lung cancer provide improved functional outcomes compared with open lobectomy? Eur J Cardiothorac Surg 37(2):451–455
7. McKenna J (2008) Complications and learning curves for video-assisted thoracic surgery lobectomy. Thorac Surg Clin 18(3):275–280
8. Nagahiro I, Andou A, Aoe M et al (2001) Pulmonary function, postoperative pain, and serum cytokine level after lobectomy: a comparison of VATS and conventional procedure. Ann Thorac Surg 72(2):362–365
9. Paul S, Altorki NK, Sheng S et al (2010) Thoracoscopic lobectomy is associated with lower morbidity than open lobectomy: a propensity-matched analysis from the STS database. J Thorac Cardiovasc Surg 139(2):366–378
10. Petersen RP, Pham D, Burfeind WR et al (2007) Thoracoscopic lobectomy facilitates the delivery of chemotherapy after resection for lung cancer. Ann Thorac Surg 83(4):1245–1249
11. Ponsky L, Cherullo E, Moinzadeh A et al (2008) The Hem-o-Lok clip is safe for laparoscopic nephrectomy: a multi-institutional review. Urology 71(4):593–596
12. Scott WJ, Allen MS, Darling G et al (2010) Video-assisted thoracic surgery versus open lobectomy for lung cancer: a secondary analysis of data from the American College of Surgeons Oncology Group Z0030 randomized clinical trial. J Thorac Cardiovasc Surg 139(4):976–983
13. Shigemura N, Akashi A, Funaki S et al (2006) Long-term outcomes after a variety of video-assisted thoracoscopic lobectomy approaches for clinical stage IA lung cancer: a multi-institutional study. J Thorac Cardiovasc Surg 132(3):507–512
14. Swanson SJ, Herndon JE, D'Amico TA et al (2007) Video-assisted thoracic surgery lobectomy: report of CALGB 39802 – a prospective, multi-institution feasibility study. J Clin Oncol 25(31):4993–4997
15. Watanabe A, Koyanagi T, Ohsawa H et al (2005) Systematic node dissection by VATS is not inferior to that through an open thoracotomy: a comparative clinicopathologic retrospective study. Surgery 138(3):510–517
16. Whitson BA, Groth SS, Duval SJ et al (2008) Surgery for early-stage non-small cell lung cancer: a systematic review of the video-assisted thoracoscopic surgery versus thoracotomy approaches to lobectomy. Ann Thorac Surg 86(6):2008–2016
17. Zhong W, Yang X, Bai J et al (2008) Complete mediastinal lymphadenectomy: the core component of the multidisciplinary therapy in resectable non-small cell lung cancer. Eur J Cardiothorac Surg 34(1):187–195

VATS Lobectomy: The Copenhagen Experience

8

Henrik Jessen Hansen and René H. Petersen

Contents

H.J. Hansen, M.D. (✉) • R.H. Petersen
Department of Cardiothoracic Surgery 2.15.2,
The Heart Centre, Rigshospitalet, The National
University Hospital, DK 2100 Copenhagen, Denmark
e-mail: henrik.jessen@rh.regionh.dk

8.1 Introduction

Video-assisted thoracoscopic surgery (VATS) lobectomy is now a well-accepted way to perform a minimally invasive lobectomy and has been done almost in two decades.

The 2007 ACCP (American College of Chest Physicians) guidelines states with a grade of recommendation of 1B: "In patients with stage I NSCLC (non small cell lung cancer) who are considered appropriate candidates for thoracoscopic anatomic lung resection (lobectomy or segmentectomy), the use of video-assisted thoracic surgery by surgeons experienced in these techniques, is an acceptable alternative to open thoracotomy" [1].

Likewise, a consensus statement of the International Society for Minimally Invasive Cardiothoracic Surgery (ISMICS) in 2007 concluded that: "VATS lobectomy can be recommended to reduce overall postoperative complications, acute and chronic pain and loss of pulmonary function." Multiple measures of postoperative function are improved with VATS compared with open lobectomy. The VATS procedure improves delivery of adjuvant chemotherapy, and most importantly, it is concluded that there are no proven differences in stage-specific 5-year survival [2]. Two recently published systematic reviews do even suggest that there might be an improved long-term survival rate [3, 4].

Although there is mounting evidence favouring this minimally invasive procedure, it is only performed routinely in few centres. It seems likely

R.G.C. Inderbitzi et al. (eds.), *Minimally Invasive Thoracic and Cardiac Surgery*,
DOI 10.1007/978-3-642-11861-6_8, © Springer-Verlag Berlin Heidelberg 2012

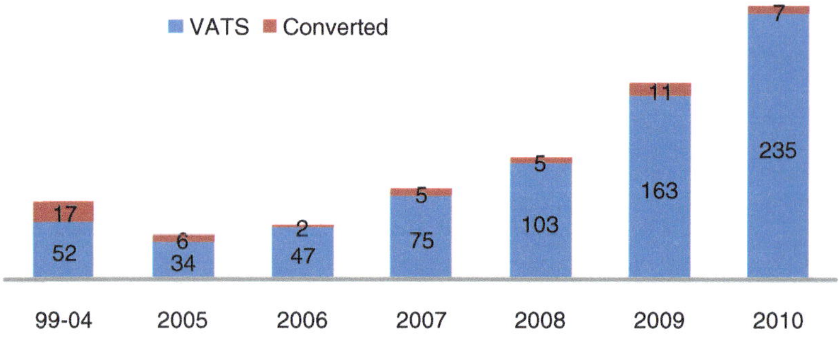

Fig. 8.1 VATS lobectomy numbers in Copenhagen until 1.1.2011

that the lack of success of the procedure is more due to the challenging learning curve than due to the lack of randomized studies. Different approaches have been described including the simultaneously stapled lobectomy, a VATS assisted operation with some rib spreading and, what there now is a general agreement on is a true VATS lobectomy defined by no rib spreading and with anatomical hilar dissection and only monitor based, so the surgeon does not look through the 5-cm utility incision. Different incisions, instruments and camera positions have also been described.

In Copenhagen, we now have a huge experience with over 1000 cases performed by a standardized three-port anterior approach, fulfilling the above-mentioned criteria for a true VATS lobectomy and it allows us to perform VATS lobectomies in the majority of the cases even if they do present co-morbidity [5]. We find that our standardized three-port anterior approach facilitates VATS lobectomy, and it is our experience from visiting surgeons that our technique can easily be adapted by many surgeons, especially those who are used to an open anterior approach.

It has been a yearlong slowly process after the beginning in 1999. The first 51 cases were performed by a four-port posterior technique with a posterior camera position as studied by Mr. W. Walker in Edinburgh, but by the end of 2004, the technique was changed to our standard three-port access. This and the fact that the author was pointed ahead of the thoracic program created focus on VATS lobectomies and the number has raised ever since (Figs. 8.1 and 8.2). This was finally accelerated by January 2009 when the two units in Copenhagen were centralized into one serving 2.4 million people.

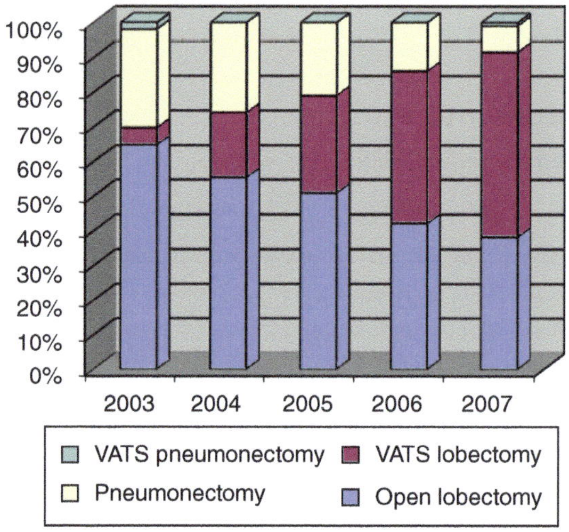

Fig. 8.2 The change in surgical profile by focusing on VATS lobectomies

8.2 Indication for a VATS Lobectomy

VATS lobectomy is commonly performed for selected peripherally located T1 or T2 tumours and usually reserved for patient where complications are not expected. Due to the advantages of a minimally invasive approach, we ask the following question in our daily clinically practice: Is there any contraindication to perform the planned lobectomy as a VATS procedure?

At present, we find the following contraindications:

- T3 or T4 tumours
- Tumours larger than 6 cm
- Tumours visible at bronchoscopy
- Possible sleeve resection
- Centrally placed tumours in the hilum

All our patients have a preoperative examination with lung function testing and PET/CT, bronchoscopy and EBUS/mediastinoscopy for preoperative staging.

With growing experience, we find indication to do a lobectomy by VATS in the majority of the cases in our institution, even if they do present co-morbidity. In 2009, 71% of all cancer lobectomies in our institution were performed by VATS, and alone in 2010, we did perform 235 VATS lobectomies and 10 anatomical VATS segmentectomies with only seven conversions in total.

8.3 The OR Set-up and Basic Principles (Fig. 8.3)

A standard set-up is with one monitor placed on each side of the table in front of the surgeons and the scrub nurse. A screen placed centrally on the wall can allow other persons in the theatre to follow the procedure. We use primarily a dedicated VATS theatre designed by the author together with Olympus Inc. This VATS theatre is only used for thoracoscopic procedures. The basic principle is that the theatre is symmetrical so it is suitable for both right- and left-sided procedures. The light setting is a dynamic and coloured lightning which enhances the surgical ergonometric.

All VATS lobectomies are performed with a 10-mm, 30° angled HD digital video thoracoscope. The 30° angulation allows a superior view within the chest cavity, and in a 10-mm camera, the power of the light source is stronger than the light source in the existing 5-mm cameras, which is easily absorbed by even a minor bleeding.

The surgeon and the assistant are positioned on the anterior (abdominal) side of the patient and with the surgeon cranially. The scrub nurse is opposite to the assistant and follows the operation on a separate screen and still positioned face to face with the surgeon (Fig. 8.3). Initially, a 4- to 5-cm anterior utility incision is made without any tissue retractor or rib spreading. This incision is later used to specimen retraction, and it is positioned between the breast and the lower angel of the scapula in the fourth intercostal space just anterior to the m. latissimus dorsi. The cavity is evaluated with the camera through this incision looking for unexpected pathology, adhesions and the level of the diaphragm. A low anterior 1- to 1.5-cm camera port is positioned at the level of the top of the diaphragm and anterior to the level of the hilum and the phrenic nerve. The final 1.5-cm incision is positioned at the same level but more posterior in a straight line down from the scapula. This results in a triangle with two approximately 10-cm legs and the camera positioned in the middle, with a working channel on each side, which makes the procedure more easy and natural to the surgeon. The camera is in the lower anterior corner of the chest cavity with a good overview, and it is generally not necessary to change port during the procedure (Fig. 8.4).

To palpate, free and prepare the structures, we use a mixture of a peanut or sponge stick and an electrocautery blade hook controlled with a normal surgical handhold. The tip of the hook can be used to lift and divide the tissue. To present vessels and other structures to be divided, we use an elastic vessel loop made of rubber as slings of other materials presents a risk of tearing, especially the fragile arteries to upper lobes. We do not place clamps on the vessels before stapling, but two vessel clamps are ready on the table in case of an emergency bleeding, and furthermore, a set-up for open surgery is present in the theatre.

Vessels, the fissures and the bronchus are divided one by one, with appropriate endostaplers. For the majority of the vessels, staplers with 2.5-mm clips are used; for parenchyma and the fissure, 3.5-mm clips are used, and the bronchus is transected with staplers with 4.8-mm clips. The new generation named Tristaplers (Covidien, USA) are very promising and do now replace the former models. Any specimen with suspicion of malignancy is removed with an endobag.

Energy-based devises can also be used, and we have some experience with an electrothermal bipolar tissue sealing system (Ligasure, Valleylab Inc., USA) and find it useful to transect minor pulmonary arteries up to the size of 3–4 mm, and

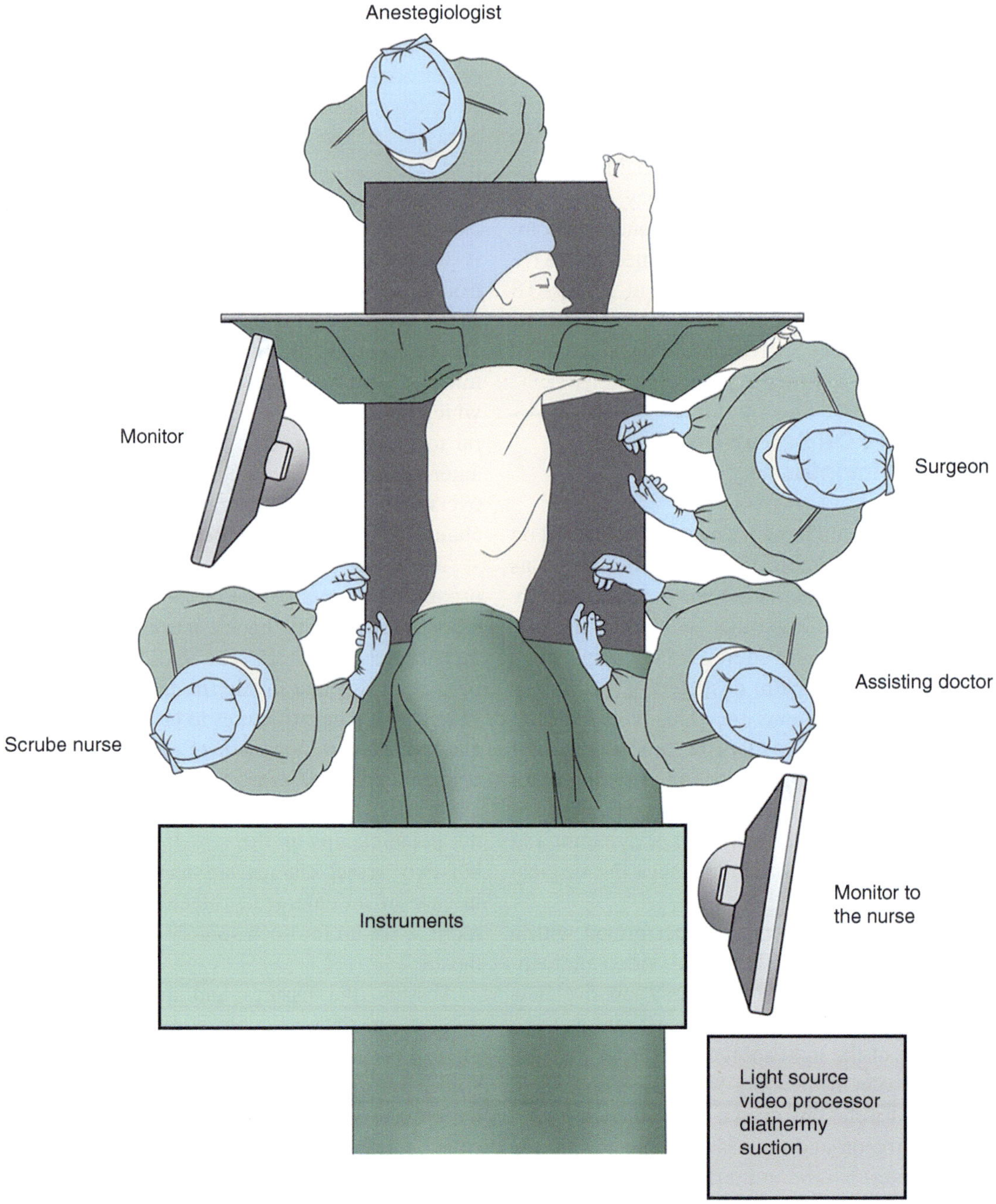

Fig. 8.3 VATS Endosuite

they are very useful for lymphadenectomy where it facilitates a proper "en bloc" dissection.

Due to a high percentage of patients with prolonged air leakage early in our experience, we have changed to a "no touch fissure technique." This means no dissection or use of electrocautery in the fissure. Instead, the fissure is stapled with the visceral pleura intact as a seal above the parenchyma, giving a more tight closure within the stapling line, and no scars in the tissue next to the clips. To facilitate this, the fissure stapling is performed quite late in the procedure when the majority of the hilar structures are divided [5].

At the end, one tube is placed in through the camera incision, and after surgery the patient is transferred to an intermediate ward and next day to the normal ward. The patients are mobilized on the day of surgery, and lung physiotherapy is provided for training. The tube is removed when there is no air leakage and less than 500 cc of fluid in 24 h. Patients are usually discharged 1 day after tube removal and seen 1 week later in the outpatient clinic.

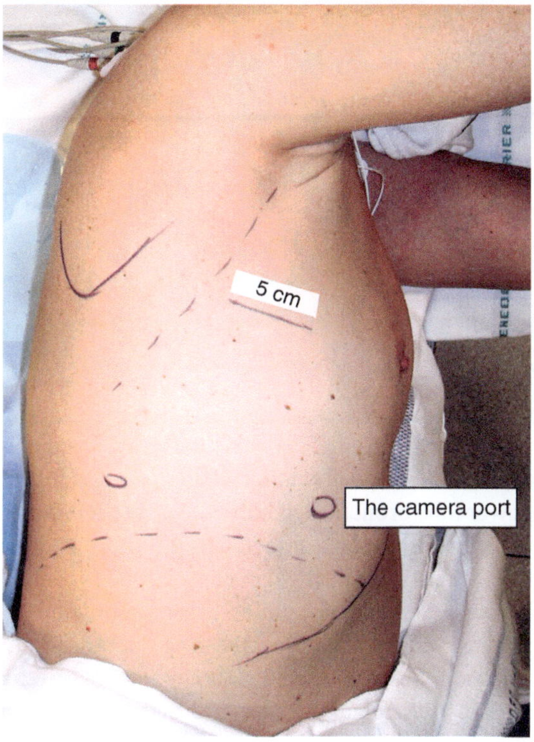

Fig. 8.4 The place of the incisions

8.4 Sequence for Each Lobe

After inspection of the cavity and confirmation of the indication for a lobectomy, the structures are divided as you meet them during the operation going from anterior and posteriorly.

8.4.1 Right Upper Lobe

First, the pleura over the anterior hilum and along the azygos vein is divided, and next a thoracoscopic DeBakey forceps, introduced through the posterior port, is passed behind the superior pulmonary vein after clear identification of the middle lobe vein. The superior pulmonary vein is then encircled with a vascular sling (Fig. 8.5), and enough space to introduce a stapler around the vessel is created. The endovascular stapler is introduced through the posterior port, and the thin blade is passed behind the superior pulmonary vein, which is then divided after removal of the vascular sling.

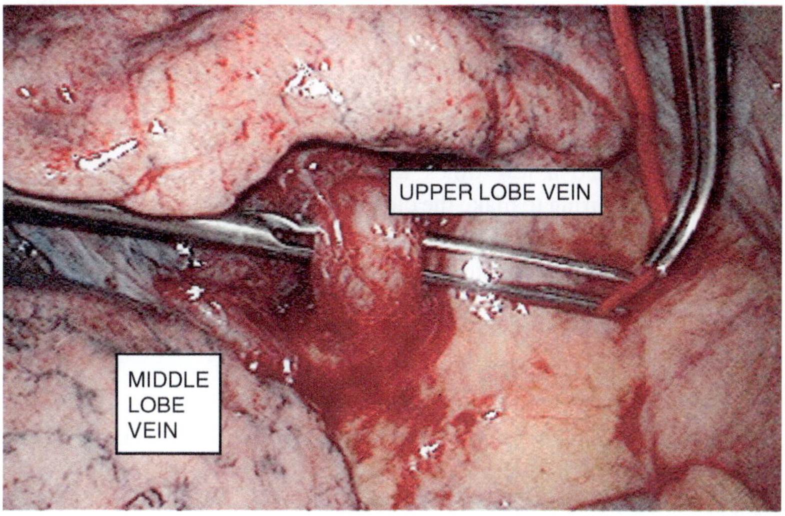

Fig. 8.5 Presentation of the vein to the upper lobe as first step in a lobectomy

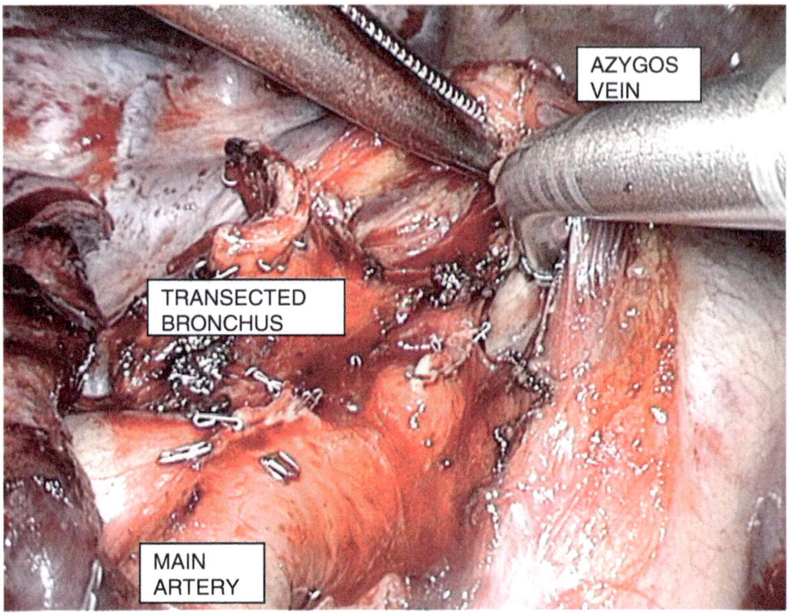

Fig. 8.6 After a right upper lobe lobectomy

When the pulmonary vein is divided, the pulmonary artery and the superior truncus arteriosus are visualized and the superior trunk is transacted in the same way as the vein.

The pulmonary artery can then be visualized down to the branches to the middle lobe and the minor fissure is divided with endostaplers. The centrally landmark is the posterior border of the artery just above the middle lobe and below the divided vein to the upper lobe. After the transection of the fissure past the artery, the middle lobe drops down and exposes the posterior part of the artery and the remaining arterial branches to the upper lobe is transected. Next, the posterior part of the fissure and the bronchus is divided one by one. The bronchus is transacted with a 4.8-mm endostapler, and the device is closed and opened a few times to crunch the bronchus before firing to make the closure tighter. The lobe is then placed in an endobag and removed via the utility incision (Fig. 8.6).

8.4.2 Left Upper Lobe

The plane between the artery and the upper lobe vein is opened so the vein can be slinged and transacted. Next step is the superior branch of the pulmonary artery (Fig. 8.7) where after there can be created a plane between the artery and the bronchus. The bifurcation of the left upper and lower lobe bronchi is identified, and the left upper lobe bronchus is transected from the posterior port by a 4.8-mm endostapler. The lobe is pushed posterior, and the remaining branches on the pulmonary artery including the lingular artery are exposed and transected. The major fissure is finally transected with several endostaplers via the posterior port.

8.4.3 Middle Lobe

The anterior part of the pleura over and between the veins is divided with the hook to expose and allow division of the middle lobe vein. Next is the anterior part of the major fissure and thereafter the middle lobe bronchus (Fig. 8.8). There is now a good view of the artery, and branches to the middle lobe are exposed, encircled and transected. The fissures are then completed beginning with stapling of the central part next to the artery via the posterior port.

8.4.4 Lower Lobes

The lower lobe is retracted superiorly, and the inferior pulmonary ligament is transected. This

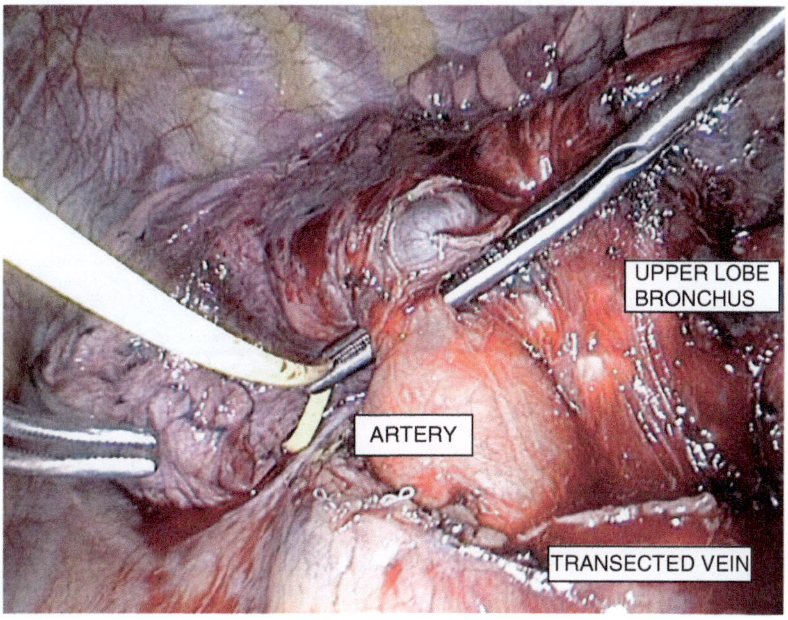

Fig. 8.7 Superior trunk of the artery in a left upper lobe after transaction of the vein

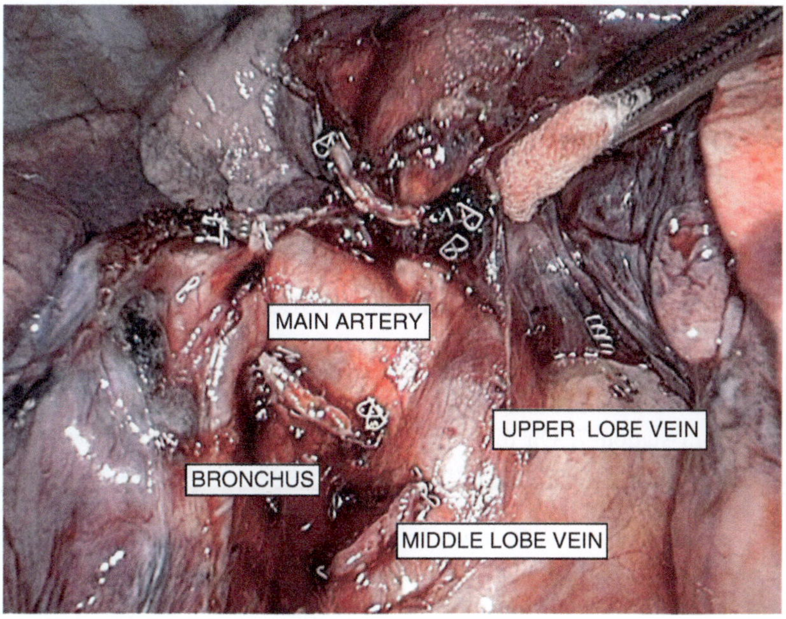

Fig. 8.8 Middle lobe with vein and bronchus divided

exposes the inferior pulmonary vein which can be encircled and transected. Next is the artery where the pleura above are opened to allow the artery to be dissected in the sheet. The artery is lifted away from the parenchyma with a vascular sling and divided. In some cases, the segment 6 artery has to be divided separately. The anterior part of the fissure is divided before or after the artery and the bronchus and the posterior fissure can be transacted step by step.

Take care not to compromise the airflow to the middle lobe on the right side and when in doubt then close the stapler and inflate the lung with one or two ventilations.

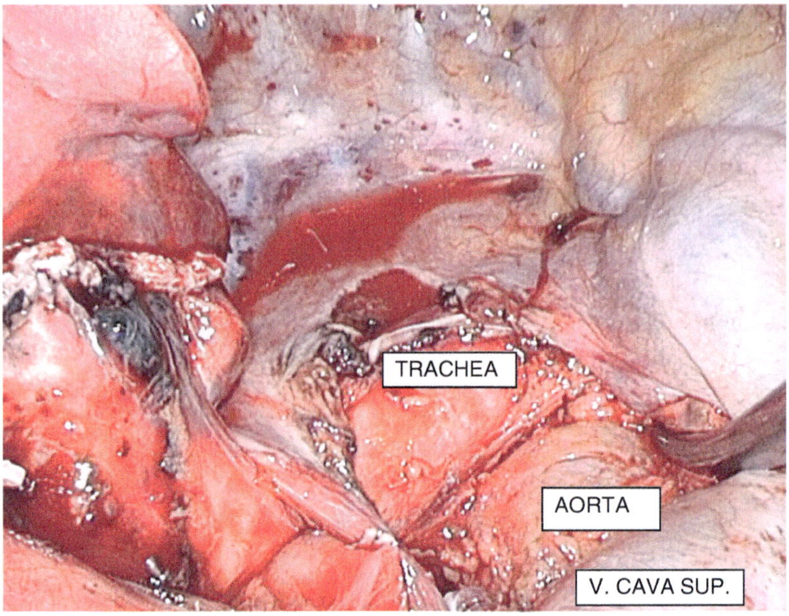

Fig. 8.9 The right upper mediastinum after lymph node removal

8.4.5 Lymph Node Dissection

It remains unclear if a complete mediastinal lymph node dissection has an actual therapeutic benefit, or if lymph node sampling only relates to stage migration by the increased probability of indentifying metastatic lymph nodes. In all our cases, we do a systematic lymph node dissection using the electrothermal system or electrocautery with removal of lymph nodes from at least 3 stations of N2 nodes according to the IASLC/Mountain classification.

In right-sided procedures, the nodes removed are from stations 2R and 4R en bloc (Fig. 8.9) and from station 7. On the left side, nodes are removed from station en bloc from stations 5 and 6, and station 7 is removed after division of the lower pulmonary vein. In lower lobe resections, nodes from stations 8 and 9 on the affected site are removed as well. Station 10 nodes are in upper lobe resections removed during the procedure to expose other structures. N1 nodes along the bronchus to the resected lobe are removed together with the specimen.

8.5 Conversion

Although the center has got a vast experience in dealing with peri-operative surgical problems related to VATS lobectomy, there are still a few cases with unexpected pathology or a bleeding complication that will be necessary to convert to an open procedure. And with growing experience, more difficult cases are also scheduled for a VATS lobectomy, and this will also create a few conversions but now the rate is below 5%.

It is important to keep in mind that conversion is not a failure. If there is a need to convert to a thoracotomy, the utility incision is expanded to 10–12 cm anterior to the latissimus dorsi muscle and along the fibres of the serratus anterior muscle giving an anterolateral muscle sparring approach within 1–2 min.

Conclusions

We have now in Copenhagen a VATS lobectomy program that deals with the majority of the institutions major pulmonary resections. The operations are performed with a standardized three-port anterior approach with a low conversion rate and a low morbidity. There is no need for extra incisions, rib spreading or changing camera position.

The "no touch fissure technique," new stabling devises and digitalized drainage systems reduce the postoperative tube time, the in-hospital stay and the percentage of patents with prolonged air leakage. In 2009, we did have a median postoperative tube time of 4 days and median postoperative in hospital stay of 5 days, and this was further cut in 2010. This is rather low in a public European setting and will be beneficial to the costs and production of the institution.

References

1. Michael Alberts W (2007) Diagnosis and management of lung cancer executive summary. ACCP evidence-based clinical practice guidelines (2nd edition). Chest 132:1S–19S
2. Downey RJ, Cheng D, Kernstine K, Stanbridge R, Shennib H, Wolf R, Ohtsuka T, Schmid R, Waller D, Fernando H, Yim A, Martin J (2007) Video-assisted thoracic surgery for lung cancer resection. A consensus statement of the International Society of Minimally Invasive Cardiothoracic Surgery (ISMICS) 2007. Innovations 2:293–302
3. Whitson BA, Groth SS, Duval SS, Swanson SJ, Maddaus MA (2008) Surgery for early-stage non small cell lung cancer: a systematic review of the video-assisted thoracoscopic surgery versus thoracotomy approaches to lobectomy. Ann Thorac Surg 86:2008–2018
4. Yan TD, Black D, Bannon PG, McCaughan BC (2009) Systematic review and meta-analysis of randomized and nonrandomized trials on safety and efficacy of video-assisted thoracic surgery lobectomy for early-stage non-small-cell lung cancer. J Clin Oncol 27:2553–2562
5. Hansen HJ, Petersen RH, Christensen M (2010) Video-assisted thoracic surgery (VATS) lobectomy using a standardized anterior approach. Surg Endosc. 2011;25:1263–9 doi:10.1007/s00464–010–1355–9, published online 07 October 2010

Single-Port Video-Assisted Thoracoscopic Lobectomy

9

Diego Gonzalez-Rivas

Contents

D. Gonzalez-Rivas, M.D.
Department of Thoracic Surgery, Coruña University Hospital, Xubias 84, 15006 Coruña, Spain
e-mail: diego.gonzalez.rivas@sergas.es

9.1 Material

Although uniportal video-assisted thoracoscopic (VATS) lower lobectomy can be performed with conventional instruments, the use of especially adapted conventional material (such as instrumentation with both proximal and distal articulations) seems to be more fitted for successful single-incision lobectomy.

The *material* recommended is:

- 30° and 10- or 5-mm-long thoracoscope (10 mm high definition recommended)
- High definition monitor screen (recommended)
- Long- and short-curved ring forceps (×2)
- Long scissors
- Curved suction (plastic yankauer recommended)
- Long thoracoscopic dissector
- Endopath 10 mm endoscopic, blunt cherry dissector (×2)
- Ligasure, harmonic scalpel, bipolar scissors, or electrocautery
- Protective bag
- Endostaplers

9.2 General Aspects

Single-incision video-assisted thoracoscopic lobectomy follows the oncological principles of major pulmonary resections by VATS: individual dissection of veins, arteries, and lobar bronchus, likewise complete mediastinal lymphadenectomy

R.G.C. Inderbitzi et al. (eds.), *Minimally Invasive Thoracic and Cardiac Surgery*,
DOI 10.1007/978-3-642-11861-6_9, © Springer-Verlag Berlin Heidelberg 2012

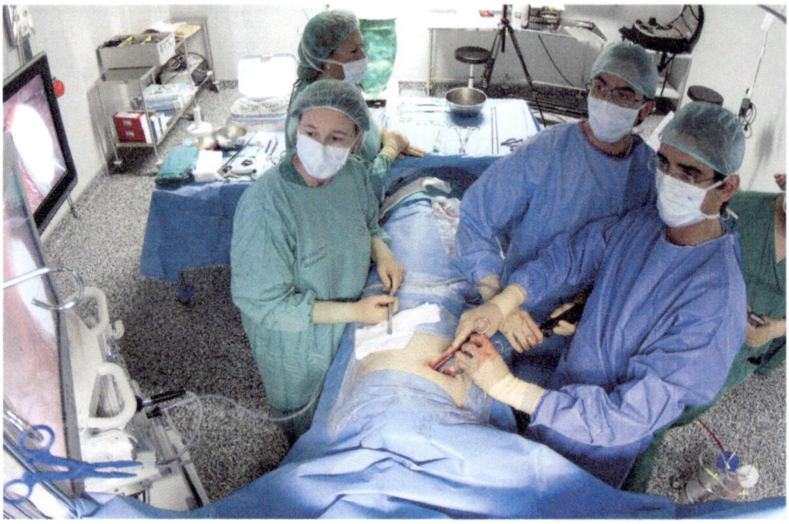

Fig. 9.1 Surgeons position in front of the patient

with a video-assisted thoracoscopic approach, with no rib spreading.

The surgeon and the assistant must to be placed in front of the patient in order to have the some thoracoscopic vision during all steps of the procedure and be more coordinated with the movements (Fig. 9.1).

The camera must be of 30° in order to enable us to achieve a panoramic view (10 mm scope high definition preferred). Instruments must preferably be long and curved to allow the insertion of 3 or 4 instruments simultaneously.

Optimal exposure of the lung is key in order to facilitate the dissection of the structures and to avoid instrument malposition. Even thought the field of vision is only obtained through the anterior access site, the movement of the camera alongside the incision as well as its rotation will create different angles of vision. The advantage of using the camera in coordination with the instruments is that the vision is direct to the target tissue, bringing the instruments to address the target lesion from a vertical perspective.

Lower lobectomies seem to carry less difficulty due to the fact that in the double- and triple-port approach, the whole procedure is performed through the utility incision. On the other hand, single-port upper lobectomy requires a completely different approach than multiport, since the surgeon will have to adapt through the utility incision the staplers in order to access hilar structures, which are usually accessed through posterior and/or inferior incisions in conventional VATS. We consider previous experience in double-port approach a necessary requirement to successfully perform the technique

9.3 Surgical Technique

9.3.1 Lower Lobectomies

Under general anesthesia and double lumen intubation, the patient is placed in a lateral decubitus position as usual for a conventional VATS. A 4-cm incision with no rib spreading is made in the fifth intercostal space in the anterior position just inferior to the breast and pectoralis major. Insertion of the finger helps to detect pleural adhesions. The 10 mm 30° thoracoscope is inserted in the lower part of the incision to explore the chest cavity. If adhesions are found, we detach them with blunt dissection or electrocoagulation with instruments placed in the upper portion of incision. After the lobe is detached, we confirm the location of the lesion by digital palpation and tracking the lower lobe toward the incision. The lobectomy is different whether the fissure is complete or not. If fissure is complete, we try to expose the artery in the fissure by blunt dissection. We insert the instruments through the upper part of the incision. There is no need to use

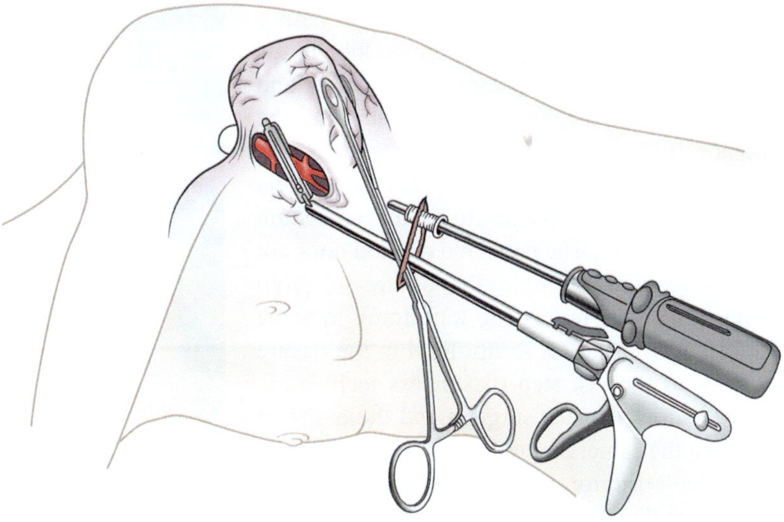

Fig. 9.2 Drawing of the procedure for staple the artery in the fissure

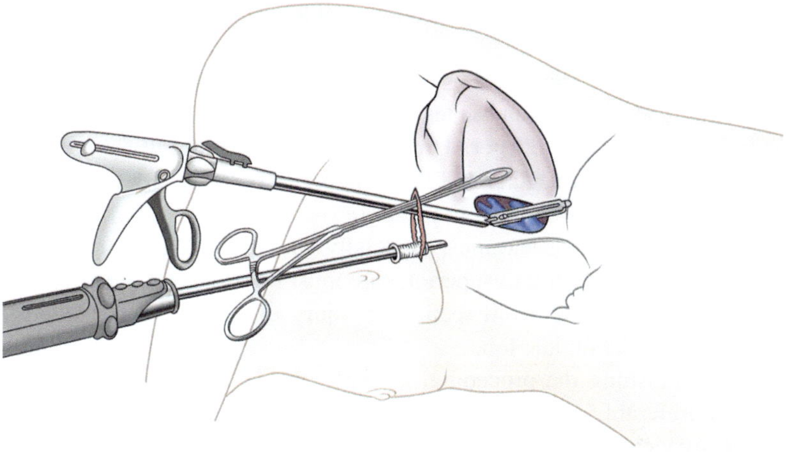

Fig. 9.3 Drawing of the procedure for exposure and staple the inferior pulmonary vein

a trocar for the camera. Avoiding the trocar allowed us to have more mobility of the camera, hence obtaining bigger and better angles of vision. If the patient is obese, a Weitlander retractor may be used to hold the soft tissues of the chest wall open for easier insertion of instruments and to prevent the lung from expanding when suction is used.

The first step is to dissect the artery in the fissure, holding the lower lobe with a ring forceps positioned above the dissector. We can use blunt dissection and suction. To staple the artery, we recommend to move the camera to the upper part of the utility incision and insert the stapler below the camera to be more comfortable (Fig. 9.2).

The next step is to dissect the vein. For inferior pulmonary vein, bronchus, and fissure, the thoracoscope is usually placed in the posterior part of the incision. However, the location of the camera varies depending on the anatomy of each patient. With a long ring forceps, we hold the lower lobe and cut the pulmonary ligament to find the vein for dissect and staple it (Fig. 9.3). We expose the inferior bronchus and with blunt dissection and suction. We dissect and staple it in the same way as mentioned for the vein. The last step is to staple the anterior or posterior fissure and put the lobe into a protective bag. It is helpful to orientate the bag inlet on the left (bag bottom located to the apex) and lower lobe on the right (piece located close to the diaphragm). With a long curve ring forceps, we insert the lobe in the bag and remove the specimen. Irrigation and insufflation of the upper lobe confirms the absence of bronchial air leaks.

Regarding lobectomies with incomplete fissure or with no visible artery, the procedure must be different. The preferred method does not involve dissection within the fissure to avoid postoperative air leaks. The lobectomy must be performed from down to up, leaving the fissure stapling as the last step (fissureless technique). Coordination between surgeon and the assistant handling the camera is crucial. We recommend to open the posterior mediastinal pleura and to expose the division of the bronchus before starting the lobectomy. After cranially retraction of the lobe, the sequence of the dissection should be inferior pulmonary ligament, inferior vein, and inferior bronchus, creating thus a plane between bronchus and artery. Sometimes it is easier to individually divide the arterial branches of the superior and basilar segments. Fissure is the last step performed from anterior to posterior.

For right lower lobectomies, especially when performed from inferior to superior, care must be taken to identify and avoid section or injury of the artery for the middle lobe.

After finishing the procedure, a single chest tube is preferably placed in the posterior part of the utility incision (Fig. 9.4). It is vital to properly close this sort of incision.

9.3.2 Upper Lobectomies

The incision, about 4–5 cm long, is performed preferably in the 5th or 6th intercostal space, more lateral than a conventional VATS. This location of the incision provides better angles for hilar dissection and stapler insertion to the upper lobe. This incision has the same size as we used for double- or triple-port VATS technique.

The sequence for left upper lobectomies is similar as for conventional VATS, but we recommend to first divide the upper lobe truncus anterior when possible in order to facilitate the insertion of the staplers in the upper lobe vein.

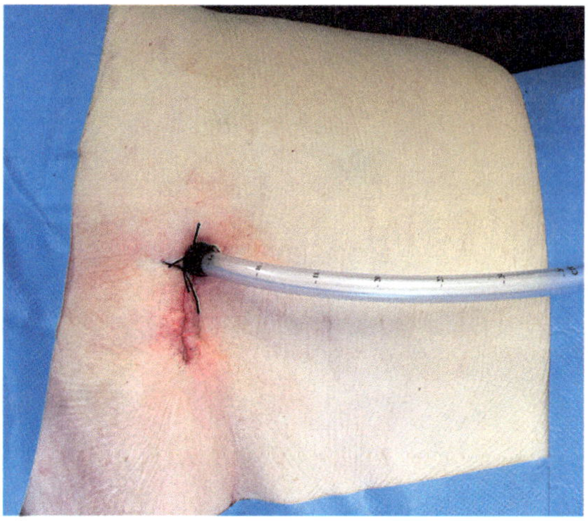

Fig. 9.4 Postoperative result with chest tube placed in the posterior portion of the utility incision

For upper lobes, we try to use staplers for all of these anatomic hilar structures (Fig. 9.5), but when there is no angle for stapler insertion or is difficult from the incision, as occur with lingular vein in left upper lobe, we use clips for vascular control (Click'aV, Grena) (Fig. 9.6).

We recommend the following sequence of dissection when possible: apical-anterior arterial trunk, upper lobe vein, bronchus, lingular artery, posterior ascending artery, and fissure. We must to be careful with bronchus dissection in order to avoid injury of lingular artery, which is usually behind the bronchus. We recommend to staple the fissure as the last step of the procedure, after dividing the hilar structures, from anterior to posterior (fissureless technique). When the fissure is complete, the lingular artery dissection can be done from the fissure. This maneuver facilitates the bronchus dissection.

Right upper lobectomy is probably more difficult than left upper lobectomy, because both the horizontal and oblique fissures must be managed. We recommend first to expose the posterior bifurcation between the upper lobe and intermediate bronchus by dividing the posterior pleural reflection. This maneuver facilitates the following anterior bronchial dissection. We prefer to staple first the arterial truncus anterior when possible to help the insertion of staplers to the upper vein as described in the left upper lobe. The

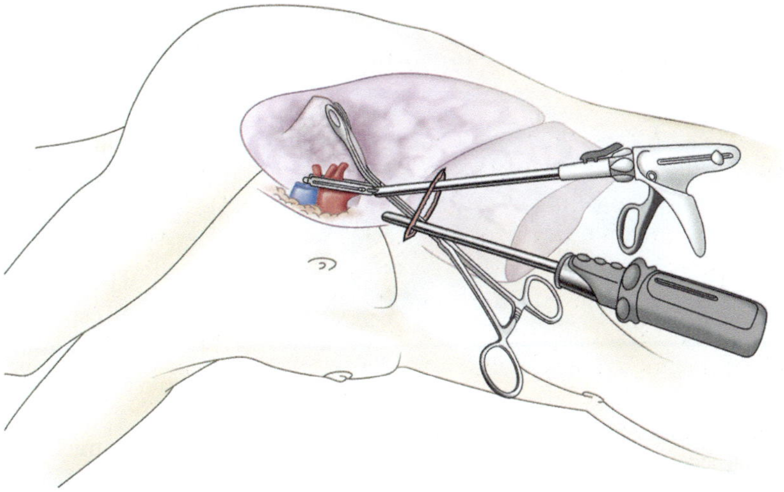

Fig. 9.5 Diagram of the procedure for staple superior pulmonary vein

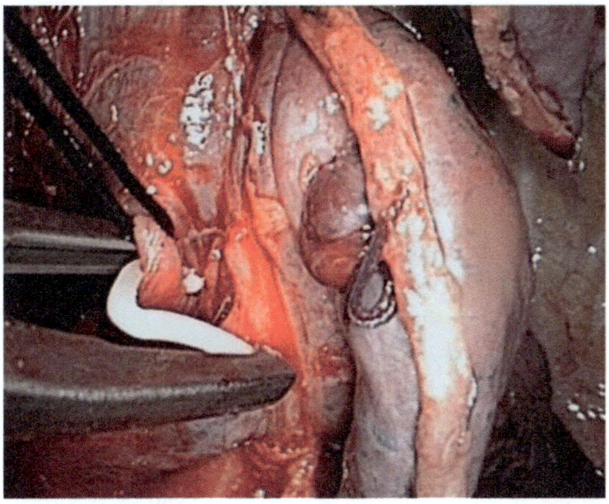

Fig. 9.6 Surgical image of vascular clip placement for lingular vein in left upper lobectomy

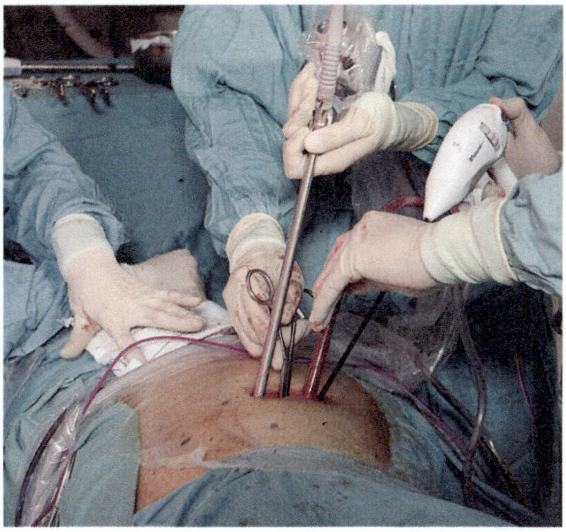

Fig. 9.7 Surgical image of instruments inserted through the incision for lobectomy

sequence of surgical steps is similar to left upper lobectomy: truncus anterior, upper vein, posterior ascending artery, upper bronchus, and fissure.

Sometimes it is helpful to divide the anterior fissure as the first step (stapler placed between the upper and middle lobe vein) in order to get better angle for insertion staplers to the upper vein. Moreover, after carrying out the vein transection and after identifying the artery for the middle lobe, we can continue to divide the fissure by placing the stapler over the intermediate artery, pulling the parenchyma anteriorly making sure that the middle lobe artery is left out to the left side of the stapler. This maneuver will provide us with a much better field of vision in order to dissect and transect the RUL bronchus or the ascending arteries. The last step would be to complete the posterior fissure.

For right upper lobes, the camera placement is usually at the upper part of the utility incision working with the instruments in the lower part. For left upper lobectomies, the camera placement varies depending on the anatomy of each patient, being frequently moved along the incision (Fig. 9.7).

It is helpful to rotate the surgical table backwards in order to place the lung posteriorly (help the hilar dissection). When the lobectomy is completed, the lobe is removed in a protective bag

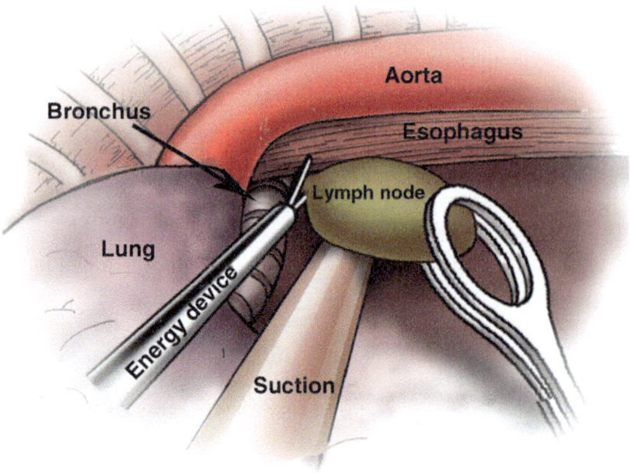

Fig. 9.8 Drawing of the procedure for left subcarinal lymph node dissection

and a systematic lymph node dissection is accomplished.

Once the surgery is finished, we insert a single chest tube in the posterior part of the utility incision. We infiltrate the intercostal spaces with bupivacaine at the end of the surgery under thoracoscopic vision.

9.3.3 Lymphadenectomy

A complete lymph node dissection is probably the most difficult step during the single-incision approach but can be performed with similar results as conventional VATS.

During the lymph node dissection, it is important to rotate the patient anteriorly in order to move the lung to the anterior mediastinum.

The best approach is to place the camera in the posterior part of the incision. The camera placement may vary depending on the anatomy of each thorax. We can insert 3 or 4 instruments below the camera to complete the systematic dissection of the subcarinal space and paratracheal on the right side and subcarinal and aortopulmonary window on the left side.

For subcarinal dissection, it is helpful to insert 2 crossed 10 mm endopath endoscopic dissectors in the lower part of the utility incision to retract the aorta, esophagus, and lung. This operation facilitates the dissection with instruments placed above the peanuts and below the camera. The use of a curved suction device is most useful especially in the single-port approach (Fig. 9.8). Sectioning the pulmonary ligament first gives us a better exposure to the subcarinal space.

For paratracheal lymph node dissection, we recommend to carry out the procedure by opening the pleura inferiorly to the acygos vein, lifting the acygos, and retracting the superior vena cava to the right side with an endopath instrument. This technique will create a plane that will allow us to successfully dissect the paratracheal space from an inferior approach. We recommend to use a long ring forceps, endopath dissector, curved suction, and energy devices to complete the en bloc lymph node dissection (Fig. 9.9).

9.4 Comments

This procedure could be probably performed more successfully in a center in which the double-port technique is already used [1]. It represents the most minimally invasive approach possible. One of the potential advantages of this approach could be less postoperative pain because only one intercostal space is involved instead of three as in the classical 3-port approach [2]. A less immunological response is another potential advantage with possible oncological implications which needs to be studied in the future [3].

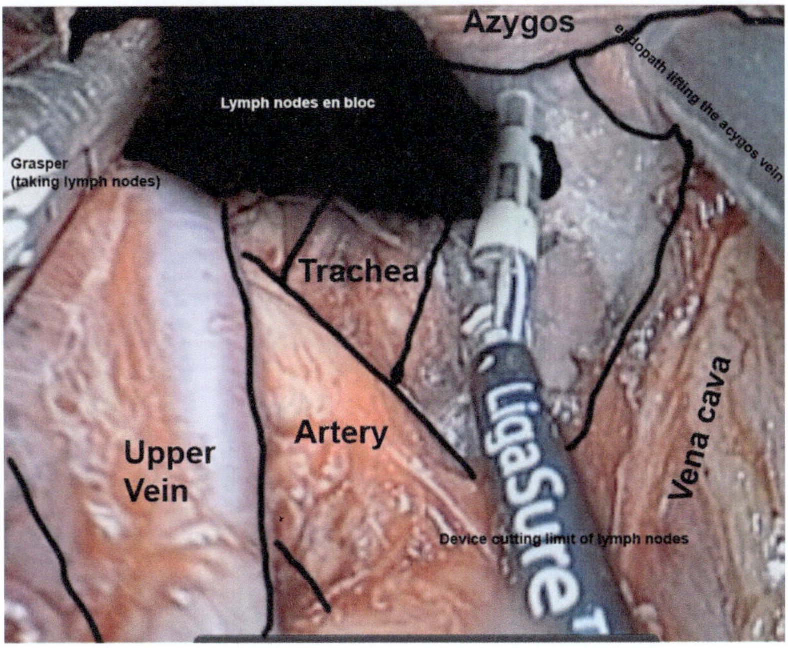

Fig. 9.9 Drawing of paratracheal lymph node dissection

References

1. Burfeind WR, D'Amico TA (2004) Thoracoscopic lobectomy. Oper Tech Thorac Cardiovasc Surg 9:98–114
2. Salati M, Brunelli A, Rocco G (2008) Uniportal video-assisted thoracic surgery for diagnosis and treatment of intrathoracic conditions. Thorac Surg Clin 18:305–310
3. Yim AP, Wan S, Lee TW et al (2000) VATS lobectomy reduces cytokine responses compared with conventional surgery. Ann Thorac Surg 70:243–247

Thoracoscopic Pulmonary Anatomic Segmentectomies

10

Dominique Gossot, Ricard Ramos, and Emmanuel Brian

Contents

D. Gossot, M.D. (✉) • R. Ramos • E. Brian, M.D.
Thoracic Department, Institut Mutualiste Montsouris, 42 Bd Jourdan, Paris F-75014, France
e-mail: dominique.gossot@imm.fr; ricard.ramos@imm.fr; emmanuel.brian@imm.fr

10.1 Introduction

Video-assisted and thoracoscopic major pulmonary resections are gaining popularity, as it becomes more and more evident that minimally invasive surgery is beneficial in terms of reduced postoperative pain, shorter hospital stay, shorter recovery, and better compliance to adjuvant chemotherapy, without compromising oncological principles. The number of publications about video-assisted and thoracoscopic lobectomies is rising [1–5], although these procedures are still considered as technically difficult and their learning curve is steep. This observation is even more valid for anatomic segmentectomies that are complex and encompassing a higher rate of postoperative complications. Very few series of video-assisted pulmonary segmentectomies have been published [6–9] and totally endoscopic – so-called complete VATS – segmentectomies are even more rare [10, 11]. Many different techniques of thoracoscopic major pulmonary resection have been described, depending on the use or nonuse of an accessory mini-thoracotomy and on the use or nonuse of endoscopic instrumentation and video display. One of these techniques is the totally endoscopic approach, in which only endoscopic instruments and monitor control are used. This is the technique that will be described in this chapter. By totally endoscopic, we mean (1) 100% video display, (2) no access incision, and (3) only use of trocars and endoscopic instruments. The aim of this chapter is not to discuss the oncologic validity of segmentectomies for

R.G.C. Inderbitzi et al. (eds.), *Minimally Invasive Thoracic and Cardiac Surgery*, DOI 10.1007/978-3-642-11861-6_10, © Springer-Verlag Berlin Heidelberg 2012

early-stage lung carcinomas – their benefits have been recently underlined [6, 12, 13] – but to describe the technical aspects of totally endoscopic anatomic segmentectomies (TEAS) and their results.

10.2 General Considerations About Endoscopic Segmentectomies

As mentioned by Oizumi et al., thoracoscopic segmentectomy poses some unique challenge to surgeons because – even when done via thoracotomy – the procedure is reputed being complex [10]. Not only the anatomical relationships can be difficult to grasp, especially for the young and less experienced surgeons, but the identification and division of the intersegmental plane is a real concern. Because of the endoscopic vision with its magnification and unusual viewpoints, the anatomical landmarks are changed. In addition, restricted tissue manipulation and use of endoscopic instruments are disturbing.

10.2.1 Ergonomics and Operating Room Setting

It is usually admitted than video-assisted surgery should be done with triangulation of the endoscope and instruments which are positioned opposite one another. This rule is almost impossible to follow during endoscopic major pulmonary resections for the following reasons:

These procedures are lasting 2–4 h. Maintaining an awkward position with both arms spread apart is exhausting and can provoke shoulder pain and stiffness.

In these complex operations, there is not just one but several targets (pulmonary hilum, mediastinum, diaphragm etc.) so that there is not a single ideal position of the scope and instruments. Therefore, whenever possible, we have found it more comfortable manipulating the two working instruments from the back or from the front, depending on the resection to be performed. The opposite side is used for insertion of a lung retractor or a suction device.

The scope is held by a robotic or mechanical scope holder, according to the surgeon preference. Its position should be shrewdly chosen so that it does not conflict with instruments. Endoscopic instruments and trocars are placed on a dedicated rack, and the conventional thoracic instruments are prepared on a separate table.

10.2.2 Trocars

What is the position of trocars is a frequently asked question. Unfortunately, there is no fixed and definite position. It depends not only on the type of resection but also on the patient's morphological type and on the surgeon's habits and preferences. For instance, we prefer performing left resections with the instruments coming from the front, while for right-sided resections, we use a dissection from the back (Figs. 10.1 and 10.2). Other surgeons may feel more comfortable with another approach and different positioning. The only rule we would recommend is inserting the scope in the midaxillary line, in the 6th or 7th intercostal space, depending on the patient's morphological type, because of the need to have an overall view on the whole pleural cavity. Many tasks can be done with micro-instruments. This avoids large ports and, consequently, large scars.

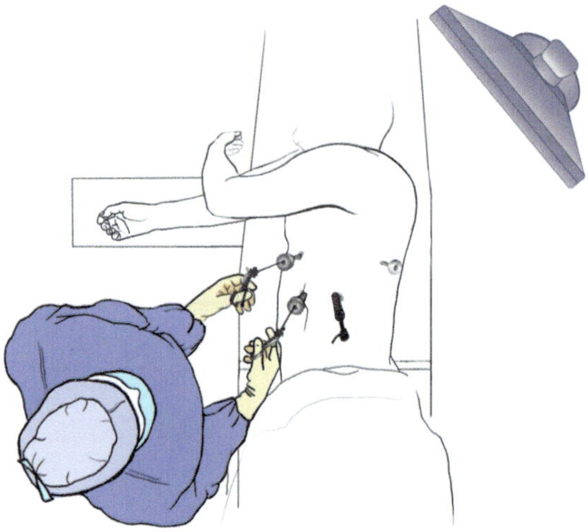

Fig. 10.1 Schematic illustration of port sites during an apical segmentectomy of the left lower lobe

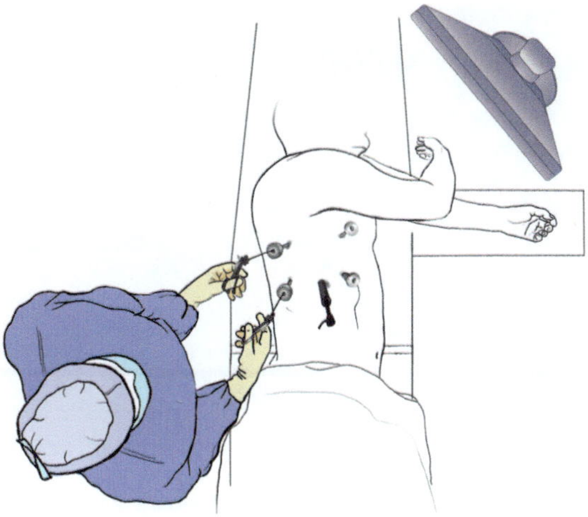

Fig. 10.2 Schematic illustration of port sites during an apicoposterior segmentectomy of the right upper lobe

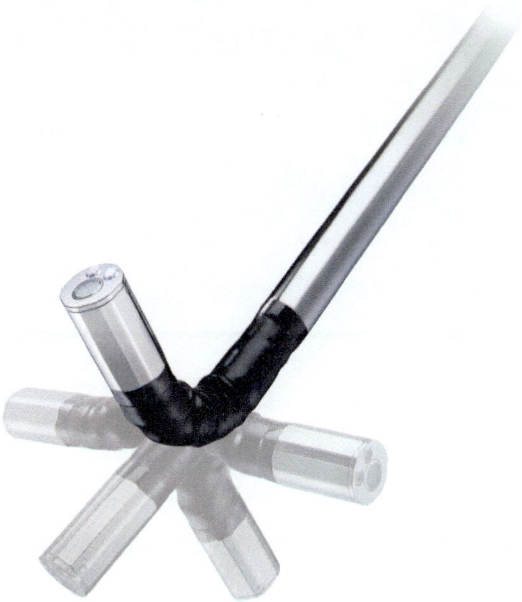

Fig. 10.3 High definition deflectable tip thoracoscope (Olympus LTF™) allows performing the whole procedure with a single endoscope avoids the problems related to tangential vision. Its angle of vision that varies from 0° to 100°

10.2.3 Enhancing Vision and Video Imaging

During open surgery or VATS, the surgeon usually stands at the patient's back because the anatomical landmarks are more familiar to him/her that way. It is sometimes preferable to stand at the patient's front [3], or to switch from behind to the front, according to the operation steps. This means that at least two monitors should be used. The light in the operating room should be reduced as much as possible to enhance the monitors contrast. As working many hours in the dark is tiresome for the staff, the best compromise is to have a blue background lighting which offers a nice contrast and does not oblige working in the dark.

Since the procedure is long lasting, the endoscope tip may be soiled by blood drops sliding down along the trocar sheath [14]. This annoying issue can be partly overcome by using a 12-mm trocar instead of a 10 mm. The port is cleaned with a cotton-tipped applicator. Smoke aspiration can be achieved via a 3-mm suction device that is left in place throughout the procedure.

Maintaining optimal vision of the whole operative field with a single 0° optic is almost impossible. One of the main concerns with a direct viewing scope (0°) is the difficulty in controlling the instrument tip which may be out of the field of vision. Formerly, to overcome this problem, we switched from a direct (0°) to an oblique viewing endoscope (30°) as vision became too tangential. However, these maneuvers were time consuming and tedious. The rigid scope with a deflectable tip (Olympus LTF™, Tokyo, Japan) has an angle of vision that varies from 0° to 100° (Fig. 10.3). The flexibility is controlled by a lever located on the handle. Once chosen, the angulation can be locked. This allows the surgeon to have a bird's-eye view, making dissection more natural and safer. The endoscope tip houses a distal CCD connected to a high definition television standard (HDTV) camera (Exera II™, Olympus) which provides dramatically sharp viewing, thus allowing for close-up vascular dissections [15].

10.2.4 Obtaining a Pathological Diagnosis

Patients who are selected for a totally endoscopic segmentectomy usually present with a clinical stage I tumor. This means the tumor or nodule is

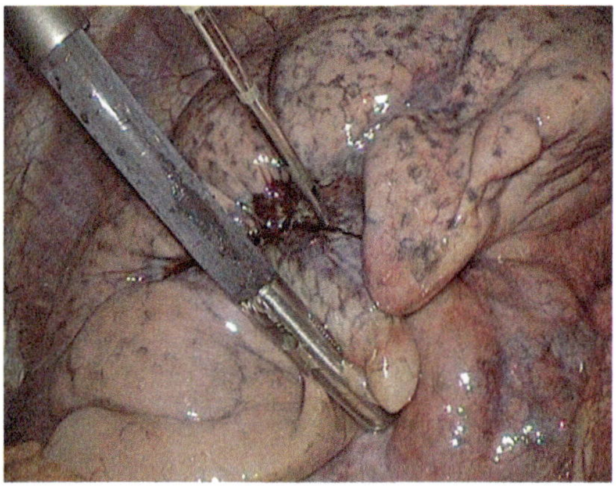

Fig. 10.4 Intraoperative view of a needle biopsy

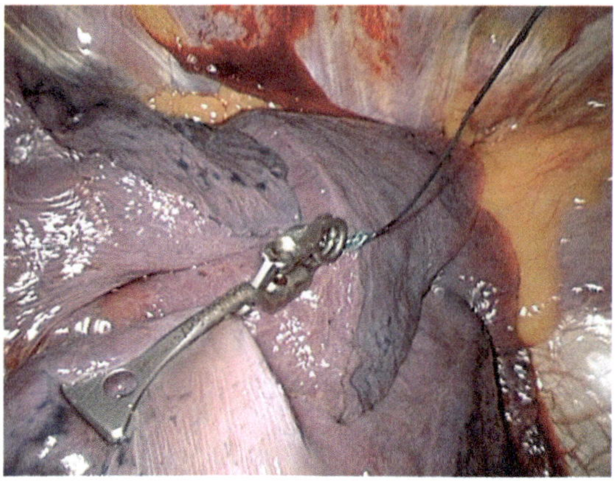

Fig. 10.5 Lung retraction: use of mini-retractors that can be released inside the chest cavity and pulled through the chest wall by a thread

often small and not accessible to a preoperative CT-guided biopsy. Thus, many patients are operated on without confirmed pathological diagnosis. When the nodule is small and subpleural, the easiest way is to perform a wedge resection with frozen section. In other cases, we use a biopsy needle (Bard Monopty®, Covington GA) which provides a pathological diagnosis in most cases (Fig. 10.4).

10.2.5 Exposure and Lung Retraction

The most efficient and most natural way to retract the lung is by mean of a 5- or 10-mm forceps. However, though it is sometimes necessary, the use of a forceps has two drawbacks: (1) it requires an additional port, and (2) it frequently tears the parenchyma, causing oozing or even hemorrhage. Although these minor bleedings are seldom serious, these may be very troublesome. Some have proposed to retract the lung with an endo-loop [16]. When there is no need to retract the lung with force, pushing it back with a simple endoscopic peanut is as effective while being less traumatic.

For long lasting steps where the lung needs to remain retracted, we use either a 3-mm grasping forceps or a miniaturized lung forceps that can be released inside the chest cavity (Aesculap©) [17] (Fig. 10.5). It has a triangular tip, as most lung forceps. A 30-cm-long thread is passed and secured at its ring-shaped basis. Once applied on the portion of the lung to be retracted, the thread is loaded through a 2-mm fascial closure device – whose primary use is port site closure during laparoscopy – and simply passed through the skin. Tension is then adapted by pulling the thread more or less. If needed, two retractors can be used.

10.2.6 Fissures

The access to the branches of the pulmonary artery is easy or difficult depending on whether the fissure is separated or fused. Opening a largely fused fissure may be a tedious step of the procedure. The main concern is that opening and dissecting the fissure can cause some minor oozing that is troublesome during a thoracoscopic operation where the operative field must remain as dry as possible to maintain optimal vision. One of the keys of a bloodless dissection is to progress step by step, from the periphery to the hilum. We have found thin instruments such as ultrasonic (SonoSurg™, Olympus) or electrothermal bipolar shears (LigaSure™, Valleylab) to be less cumbersome and as effective as stapler for the division of the external part of the fissure. For the inner thick part of the fissure, stapling is however required. A guide is usually necessary to drive the stapler jaws without excessive friction and force on the tissue. We use a small diameter silicone suction tube whose base is connected to the stapler tip, or we retract the fissure with a tape.

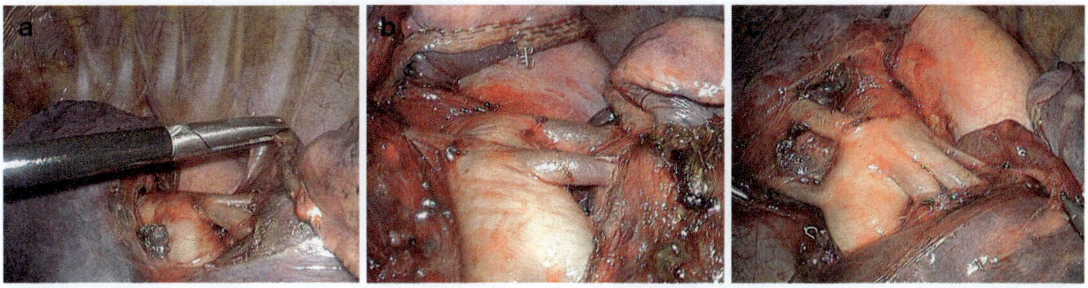

Fig. 10.6 Example of three different arterial supplies to the basilar segment of the left lower lobe, as seen during thoracoscopic left apical segmentectomy. The distribution of the arteries to the apical segment is clear. (**a**) Single apical segmental artery, (**b**) double apical segmental artery, (**c**) triple apical segmental artery. *LUL* left upper lobe, *LLL* left lower lobe

With a direct viewing telescope, the division of the fissure can be difficult because its length may make sharp vision on both of its extremities, almost impossible. A deflectable tip thoracoscope is of great help during this step because it allows a bird's-eye view of the whole fissure throughout the dissection.

In case of fused fissures, identifying some branches of the pulmonary artery (PA) is tedious. This is usually not an issue for lower segmentectomies but can be a real concern for upper segmentectomies since the branching pattern exhibits many variations, especially on the left side. Therefore, preoperative knowledge of vascular anatomy can be helpful. Three-dimensional reconstruction with volume-rendering technique provides an accurate vascular mapping of the lobe or segment to be dissected. This preoperative investigation is time consuming but does not have additional cost or invasiveness since a preoperative CT with injecting contrast medium is needed anyway.

10.2.7 Exposure of Bronchial and Vascular Elements

10.2.7.1 Anatomical Issues

The understanding of anatomy and of the branching pattern of the pulmonary artery can be difficult, since it is highly variable, especially for upper lobes. For lower lobes, anatomical variations do not pose problem and the surgeon can rather easily adjust to an unusual vascular anatomy. For instance, even when there are variations on the vascular pattern of the apical segment of the lower lobe, there is usually no doubt about the distributions of arterial branches (Fig. 10.6). Figure 10.7 shows three different arterial distributions to the left basilar segments, as seen on three-dimensional volume-rendering imaging and on the corresponding thoracoscopic view (Fig. 10.7). These views demonstrate that the anatomy is easily understandable and that the respective branches can be selected according to the segmentectomy performed. Thus, we do not perform anymore a preoperative reconstruction of vessels for lower segmentectomies. However, the issue is more relevant for upper segmentectomies. Not only, the number of arteries arising from the pulmonary artery is variable but their distribution is sometimes difficult to understand because the vessels can usually not been dissected on a sufficient length. This is especially true for the ascending arteries to the right upper lobe. These arteries can supply only the posterior segment of the upper lobe or both the posterior and anterior segments (Fig. 10.8). The study of preoperative computed tomography three-dimensional reconstruction helps asserting the number, size, and direction of these arteries without doubt. For example, knowing preoperatively if the left truncus anterior gives an accessory lingular artery is helpful when embarking in a lingula sparing upper lobectomy (Fig. 10.9). Thus, in our experience, a preoperative assessment of the vessels remains useful for upper segmentectomies. Assessing

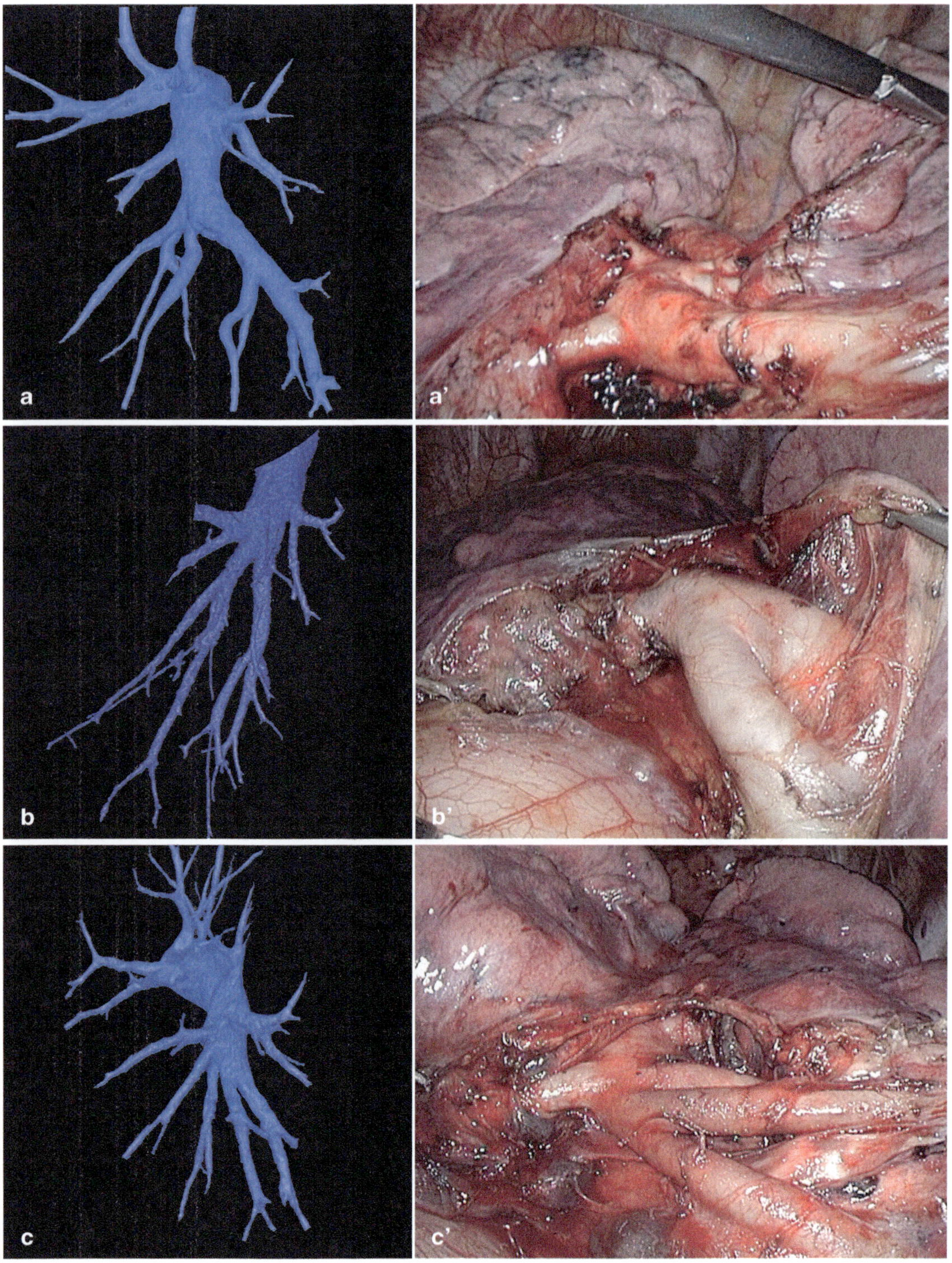

Fig. 10.7 Example of three different arterial supplies to the apical segment of the left lower lobe, as seen during thoracoscopic left basilar segmentectomy. Note the exact correspondence between the computed tomography three-dimensional reconstruction and the thoracoscopic view. (**a**) Single basilar trunk, (**b**) early division of the basilar trunk in two main arterial trunks, (**c**) early division of the basilar trunk in four arteries. *LUL* left upper lobe, *LLL* left lower lobe

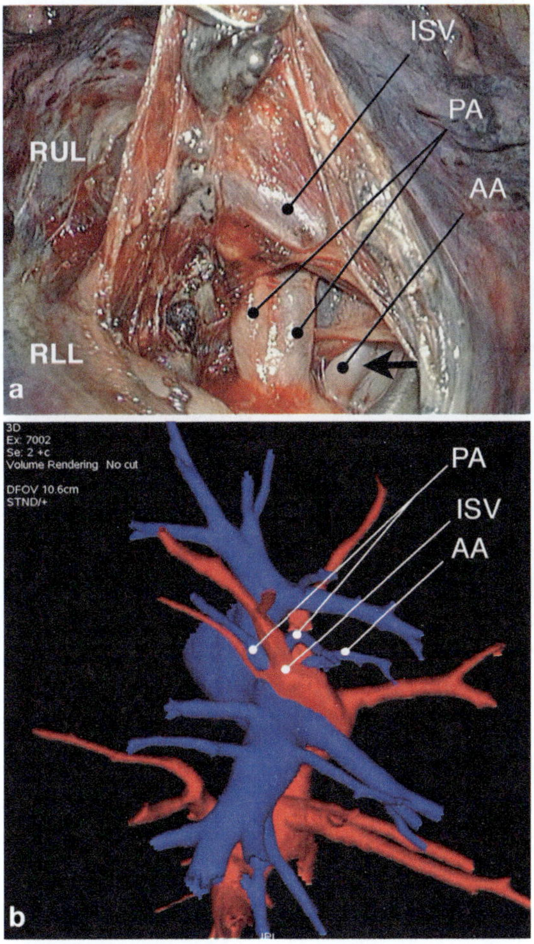

Fig. 10.8 Thoracoscopic view of two ascending arterial branches in the fissure during a right apicoposterior segmentectomy (**a**). Note that the computed tomography three-dimensional reconstruction helps asserting that the smallest artery (*arrow*) supplies the anterior segment (**b**). *RUL* right upper lobe, *RLL* right lower lobe, *PA* posterior artery, *AA* anterior artery, *ISV* intersegmental vein

preoperatively the arterial variations and having the vascular pattern in mind help the surgeon performs a safer dissection of the branches of the pulmonary artery, especially when the fissure is fused and/or when lymph nodes are present. In a series of 49 patients selected for VATS lobectomy, Watanabe et al. found that preoperative three-dimensional computed pulmonary angiography was identifying the PA branches in 95% of the cases [18]. In their series, only some small branches (less than 2 mm in diameter) were missed.

10.2.7.2 Bronchial and Vascular Control

Exposing and retracting a bronchus or a vessel are frequently necessary when it needs to be loaded within the jaws of a clip applier or an endostapler. The latter must be passed as smoothly as possible. One can use some deflectable devices (Endo MiniRetract™, Covidien or Goldfinger™, Ethicon whose tip has the advantage of being atraumatic and has a keyhole for a sling) (Fig. 10.10). These instruments can be used both for retraction and for some blunt dissection to create space around the element to be stapled. If this is not sufficient, a guide can be used. We use a chest tube or a 16 Fr suction tube (Gentle-Flow™, Kendall©). Its base is secured to the anvil by simple pressure. This can be done inside or outside the chest. Its distal end is passed around the structure to be divided and pulled out through the trocar tube. The stapler tip is thus guided around the tissue to be stapled.

Whenever possible, clips should be avoided because they may slip or conflict with staples. However, medium diameter vessels such as some segmental pulmonary branches are too small for an endostapler and too large to be coagulated with electrocautery or ultrasounds. When clips are used, they are doubled or even tripled. Another solution is to apply a clip at the origin of the vessel and complete division with bipolar sealing, so that only one clip is present in the operative field. For all other minor vessels, we use ultrasonic shears (US) (EndoSurg™, Olympus) or a bipolar vessel sealing device (VSD) (Ligasure™, Covidien). Large vessels are stapled. Complications related to stapling of bronchus or parenchyma are rare but have been reported while accidents with vascular stapling are extremely rare [19]. However, the stapler must load the vessel without any force or friction, which implies a perfect vascular dissection. Lymphadenectomy is done only with VSD, and clips are almost never used. A suction device can be activated all over the dissection time for immediate evacuation of smoke and mist.

10.2.7.3 Vascular Injuries

Avoiding bleeding and massive vascular injury is a constant concern throughout the procedure.

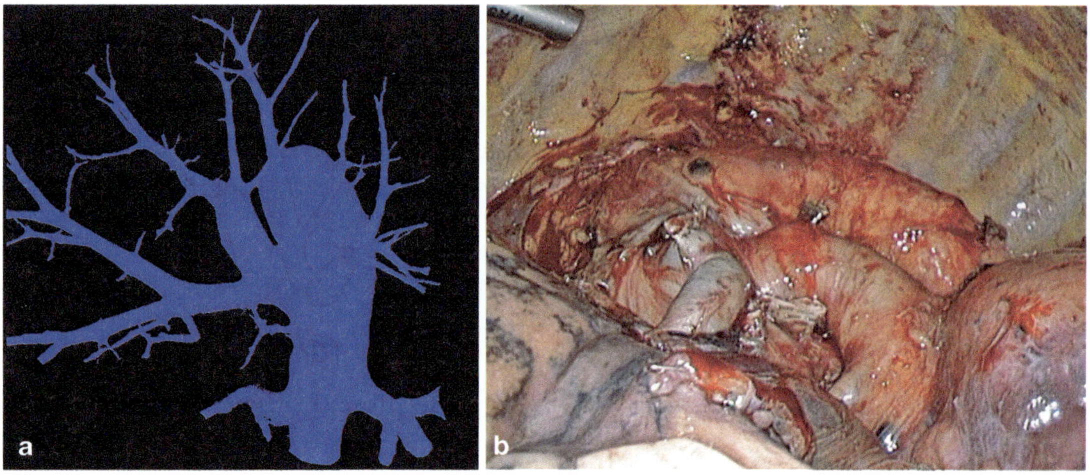

Fig. 10.9 (**a**) Computed tomography three-dimensional reconstruction of the left pulmonary artery demonstrating an independent apicoposterior and accessory lingular artery, (**b**) corresponding thoracoscopic view after completion of a lingula sparing upper lobectomy

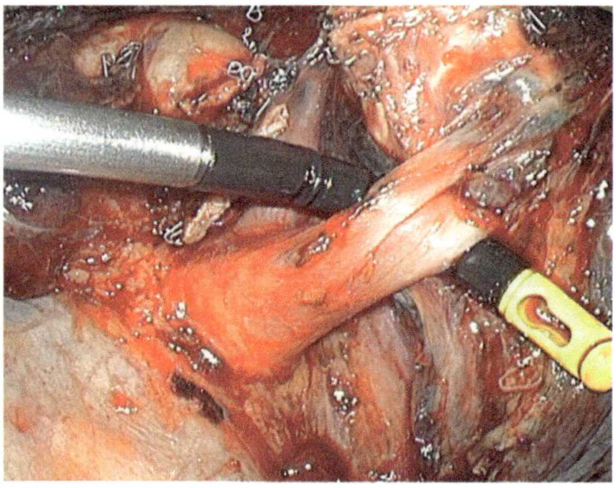

Fig. 10.10 Example of dissection and retraction of the basilar segmental vein using a deflectable retractor during a left basal segmentectomy

Some authors have advocated clamping the main pulmonary artery using a silk suture in order to control any bleeding [20]. This maneuver can be easily achieved during conventional open procedure or even during some VATS procedures through a utility mini-thoracotomy. But it seems at risk to be done via a totally endoscopic approach, because a tear of the main pulmonary artery could not be controlled. This is one of the limitations of the endoscopic approach. However, in patients presenting with a regular anatomy, the risk of major vascular injury is minimal due to the close-up dissection and the camera magnification. Dissection becomes more risky when neoplastic or inflammatory lymph nodes are present and prevent opening the vascular sheath which is adherent to the underlying vessel. These situations should lead to abandon and convert to an open procedure.

Massive Hemorrhage: Although it never occurred in our experience, a massive bleeding that is not controllable by thoracoscopy should lead to introduce gauzes through the larger port and temporary control bleeding by pressure, while the surgeon convert to thoracotomy. This outlines the importance of having the conventional thoracic instruments ready on a separate operative table.

Minor Hemorrhage: A 5-mm clamp must be available. An alternate solution is the use of throw-off vascular bulldog clips (Aesculap©). They are used for controlling a hemorrhage or during the temporary occlusion of a vessel. They are inserted through a 12-mm trocar using a dedicated applier that is withdrawn after the device has been applied. The same instrument is used for retrieving the device.

10.2.8 Intersegmental Plane and Division of the Parenchyma

Another difficulty faced during thoracoscopic segmentectomy is the identification and division of the intersegmental plane. When performed through a thoracotomy, this step is facilitated by the use of manual inspection and palpation which are not possible via thoracoscopy. Several methods have been described. The most common is the creation of a ventilated-deflated line by reventilating the operated lung once the segmental bronchus has been stapled. This technique has two drawbacks: (1) reventilation obscures the vision, a much more troublesome problem than during thoracotomy; (2) the segments to be resected can be partly reventilated through the collateral canals, leading to an unclear demarcation line. Therefore, some authors have suggested acting reverse, i.e., reventilating the whole lung once the segmental bronchus has been divided and then collapsing it, so that only the diseased segments remain inflated [18]. Others have suggested using selected jet ventilation in the segmental bronchi to be divided [8]. We have used a similar method by injecting air through the channel of a bronchofiberscope, after selective endoscopy of the segmental bronchus. In our experience, the technique resulted in some inflation of adjacent segments and was eventually disappointing.

Once the intersegmental plane has been determined, the last issue is the choice of the division method. Some authors use a combination of blunt dissection, electrocautery, and application of fibrin sealant [8] (Table 10.1). When air leaks are observed, some surgeons applied mattress suture with pledgets [18]. These methods have the advantage of sparing parenchyma but comprise a risk of postoperative air leak. Actually, most authors use staplers [6, 9, 21, 22] (Table 10.1). Stapling is however not that easy. First, it may require using many cartridges, up to five in the series of Watanabe [18]. Second, the limited opening of the endostaplers and the thickness of the parenchyma expose to disruption of the staples line [23], an adverse event that occurred twice in our series. The consequences are not serious but lead to troublesome blood loss and require suturing.

10.2.9 Specimen Retrieval

It would not be recommended to morcellate the specimen as done in other fields of surgery, since it is of utmost importance to analyze the bronchus, the peribronchial lymph nodes, and to check that all margins are free. The segment must be retrieved en bloc. For a segmentectomy, enlarging a port on a 2–3 cm length is sufficient. The use of a retractor is never necessary. A solid and large specimen bag must be used. The incision should be done at a site where the intercostal space is soft, preferably in the lower part of the chest on the anterior axillary line or in the axilla.

10.3 Technique

Only the right apicoposterior segmentectomy will be described in details and illustrated as many technical principles can be applied to other resections. A detailed description of all types of anatomic segmentectomy has been given in another work [24].

10.3.1 Right Upper Lobe: Apicoposterior Segments

The right upper lobe comprises three segments: apical (S1), posterior (S2), and anterior (S3). The three segmentectomies of the right upper lobe are feasible. With respect to the anterior segment, dissection is considered as one of the most challenging for the following reasons: the segmental bronchus is not easily accessible, the anterior segmental artery is covered by the apical vein, and the preservation of the anterior segmental vein is tedious. For these reasons, only the apicoposterior segmentectomy will be described thereafter. As mentioned above, this is one of the procedures where the surgeon takes profit of a preoperative three-dimensional reconstruction of the vascular anatomy (Fig. 10.11).

Table 10.1 Technical data available for published series of VATS or totally endoscopic segmentectomies

First author (year)	N	VATS/TT	Number of trocars	Utility incision (cm)	Optics	Op. time[a] (min)	Op. blood loss[a] (ml)	Division of intersegmental plane
Shiraishi (2004) [27]	34	TT	6	None	Rigid 30°	240 ± 72	169 ± 68	Ultrasonic shears
Okada (2007) [8]	52	VATS	1	6.5 (4–12)	NS	155 (85–225)	60 (10–210)	Electrocautery + fibrin sealant
Atkins (2007) [6]	48	VATS	1	4	NS	136 ± 45	250 ± 200	Stapling
Oizumi (2009) [10]	29	TT	4	None	Rigid 30°	216 (146–425)	100 (3–305)	Stapling
Yamada (2009) [11]	9	TT	3–4	None	Rigid 30°	NS	NS	Stapling
Schuchert (2009) [9]	104	VATS	3	4	Rigid 0°	136 (120–152)	171 (133–209)	Stapling
Watanabe (2009) [18]	41	VATS	2	4 (3.5–6)	NS	220 (100–306)	183 (30–770)	Electrocautery + stapling + fibrin sealant
Shapiro (2009) [22]	31	VATS	2	NS	NS	NS	NS	Stapling
Leshnower (2010) [28]	15	VATS	3	NS	Rigid 30°	145 ± 55	NS	Stapling
This series	71	TT	4–5	None	Deflectable	181 ± 52	77 ± 69	Stapling

N number, *VATS* video-assisted, *TE* totally endoscopic, *cm* centimeter, *min* minutes, *ml* milliliter, *NS* not stated
[a]Expressed as mean and range or mean ± standard deviation

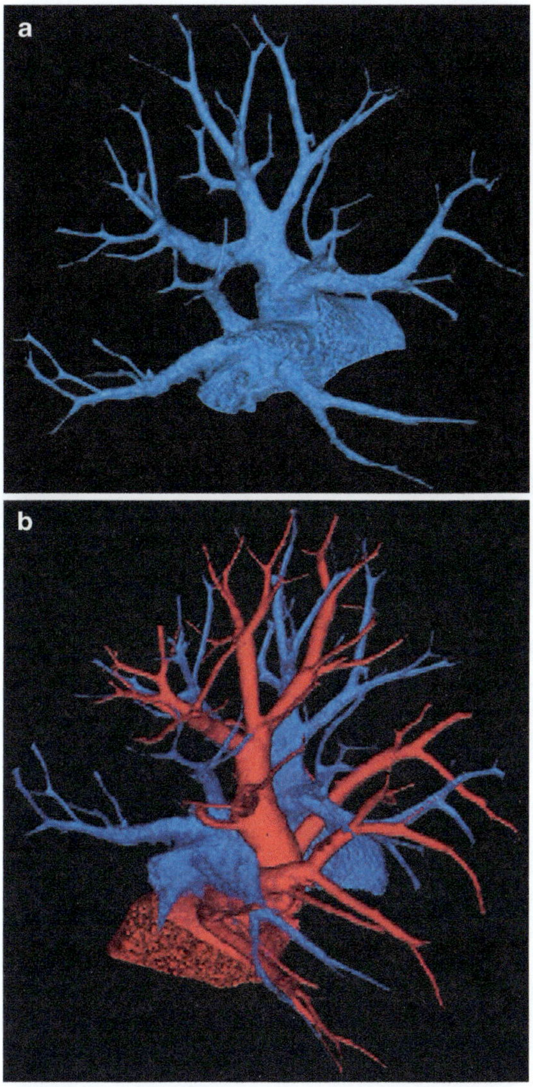

Fig. 10.11 Vascular landmarks as demonstrated by three-dimensional reconstruction: (**a**) arterial supply to the apicoposterior segments (anterior view), (**b**) relationships between veins and arteries of the apicoposterior segments (anterior view) (*dotted lines* level of division, *a* artery, *v* vein)

10.3.1.1 Fissure and Ascending Posterior Artery

As for some right upper lobectomies, it is more convenient to start the resection by controlling and dividing the bronchi. However, this can be done only if the ascending posterior artery, which hides the upper lobe bronchus, is severed. The posterior aspect of the oblique fissure is opened. This is achieved by stretching the upper lobe or lower lobe anteriorly, until the posterior mediastinum is fully exposed. The pleura facing the inferior aspect of the upper bronchus is opened using either cautery or blunt dissection or both. A dissecting forceps is then passed from the hilum – at the level of the posterior aspect of the pulmonary artery – to the periphery under vision control, thanks to the deflectable scope. A 60-mm endostapler can then be applied. This helps expose the posterior artery (Fig. 10.12a) which is then dissected and clipped or severed after bipolar sealing. Dissection of this artery can be tedious if multiple venous branches run within the fissure (Fig. 10.12b).

10.3.1.2 Segmental Bronchi

Once the ascending posterior arterial branch has been divided, the anterior surface of the right upper bronchus is fully exposed. The tissues overlying its superior aspect are freed using a cautery hook. Clearing of the upper lobe bronchus must be pursued forward until the apical segmental bronchus becomes apparent.

Dissection of the segmental bronchi is continued by a combination of gentle traction of the upper lobe and blunt dissection. This is best achieved by an Endo Peanut while any oozing or minor bleeding from small peribronchial arteries is immediately controlled. Finally, the trifurcation is exposed: the anterior segmental bronchus which is the lowest branch and the posterior and apical bronchi which can take off independently or as a common stem (Fig. 10.13).

At this stage, two different situations can be faced: (1) dissection is easy because tissues are soft and anatomy is clear, and (2) dissection is uneasy. In the later situation, getting around the bronchi is at risk of tearing the arteries which run anterior to the bronchi. One should prefer controlling the truncus anterior and the apical artery from the mediastinal side. But if the dissection is smooth, turning around the apical and posterior bronchi from the back is possible, always keeping in mind that the arteries run anteriorly to the bronchi. A blunt tip retractor is used to retract the bronchi backward and move them away from the arteries (Fig. 10.14). The bronchi can then be stapled one by one or as a stem.

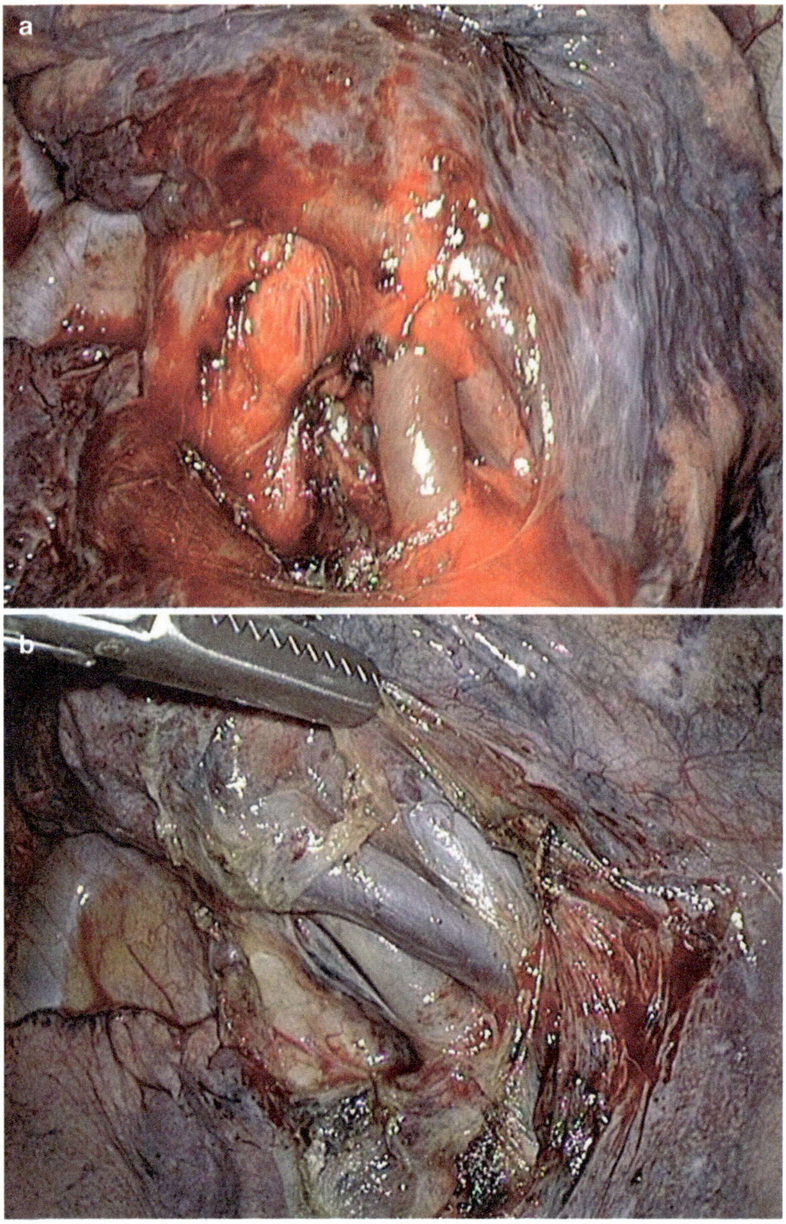

Fig. 10.12 Exposure of the ascending artery to the posterior segment after division of the posterior part of the oblique fissure. (**a**) On a patient without venous branches in the fissure, (**b**) on a patient with venous branches crossing the posterior ascending artery. *RUL* right upper lobe, *RLL* right lower lobe

10.3.1.3 Apical Artery

This maneuver liberates the apicoposterior segments which unfold forward, thus exposing the apical artery, which is the uppermost tributary of the truncus anterior. Dissection of its posterior and lateral aspects can be done from behind. If necessary, its anterior aspect can be freed from the front after exposure of the truncus anterior by retracting the upper lobe backward (Fig. 10.15). The apical artery is stapled.

10.3.1.4 Apical Vein

The superior pulmonary vein is exposed by retracting the upper lobe backward and incising the

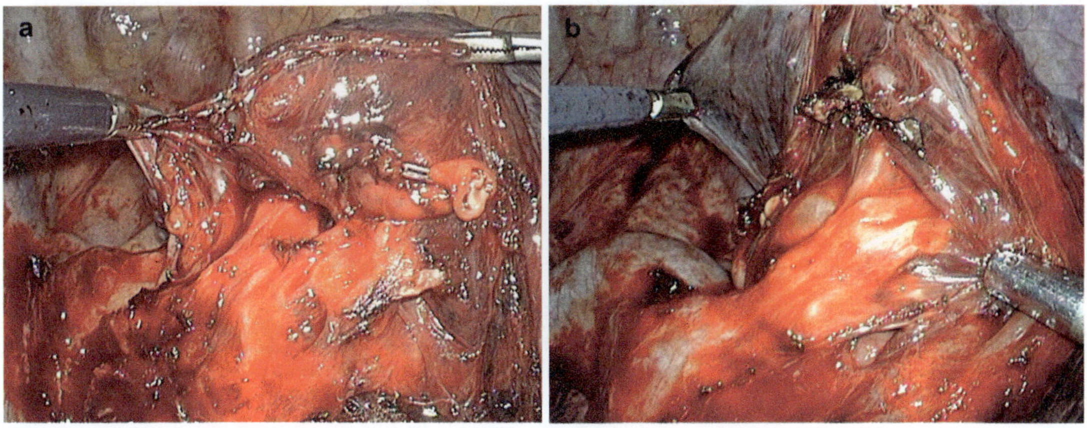

Fig. 10.13 Exposure of the segmental bronchi of the right upper lobe. (**a**) Independent bronchi, (**b**) common apicoposterior stem

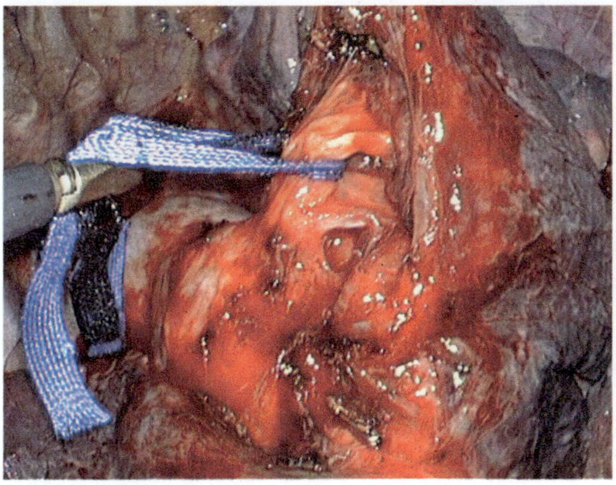

Fig. 10.14 Retraction of the apicoposterior bronchus

mediastinal pleura posterior to the phrenic nerve (Fig. 10.16a). Its dissection is achieved by a combination of bipolar cautery and gentle sweeping motion with an Endo Peanut. The three segmental branches of the upper root of the superior pulmonary vein are exposed as well as the origin of the middle lobe vein. Theoretically, both the apical and posterior venous branches should be divided. However, even if the segmental pattern of the vein is clear, it seems advisable to divide only its uppermost tributary (Fig. 10.16b), since one cannot be certain that the branch in the middle of the trifurcation does only drain the posterior segment.

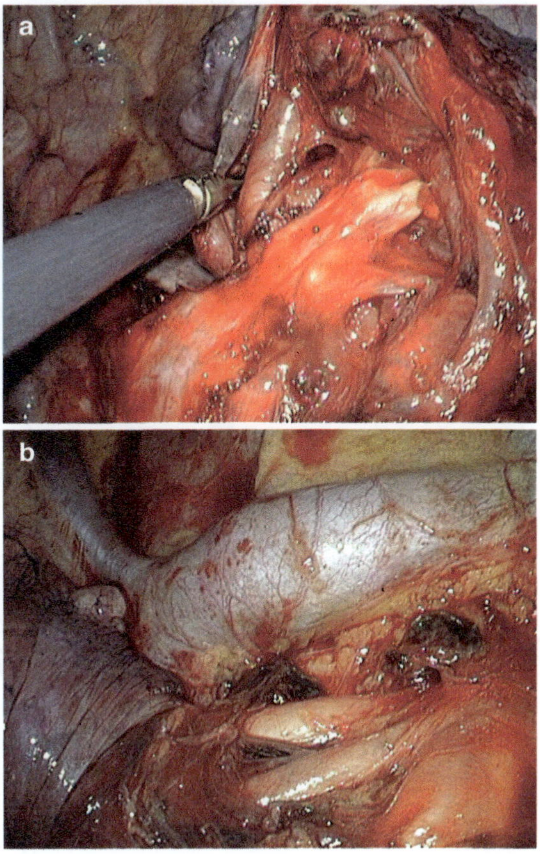

Fig. 10.15 Exposure of the apical artery. (**a**) From the back by retracting the upper lobe forward, (**b**) from the front by retracting the upper lobe backward

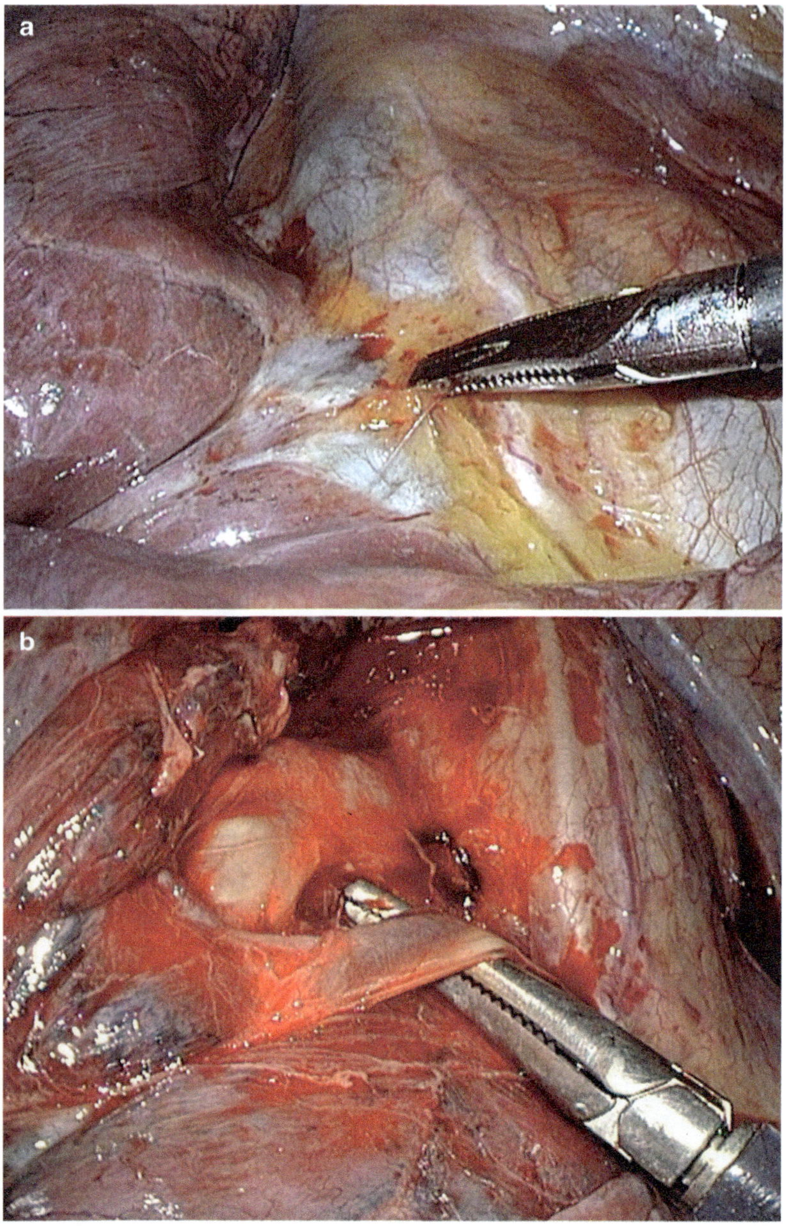

Fig. 10.16 Dissection of the superior branch of the superior pulmonary vein. (**a**) Approach to the superior pulmonary vein using bipolar diathermy, (**b**) dissection of the superior branch

10.3.1.5 Division of the Parenchyma

Once all segmental vascular and bronchial elements have been divided, the lobe can be lifted up and a clamp is applied on the parenchyma (Fig. 10.17a). Low volume and low pressure reventilation help determine the intersegmental plane while the clamp is repositioned on the demarcation line between ventilated and non-ventilated zones. Some force is applied on the clamp to crush and flatten the parenchyma. The 60-mm endostapler with 4.8-mm cartridge can then be applied (Fig. 10.17b). The specimen is placed into an endobag and retrieved after minor enlargement of a port. The pulmonary ligament is freed to facilitate reexpansion, a chest tube is placed, and the lung is reventilated (Fig. 10.18).

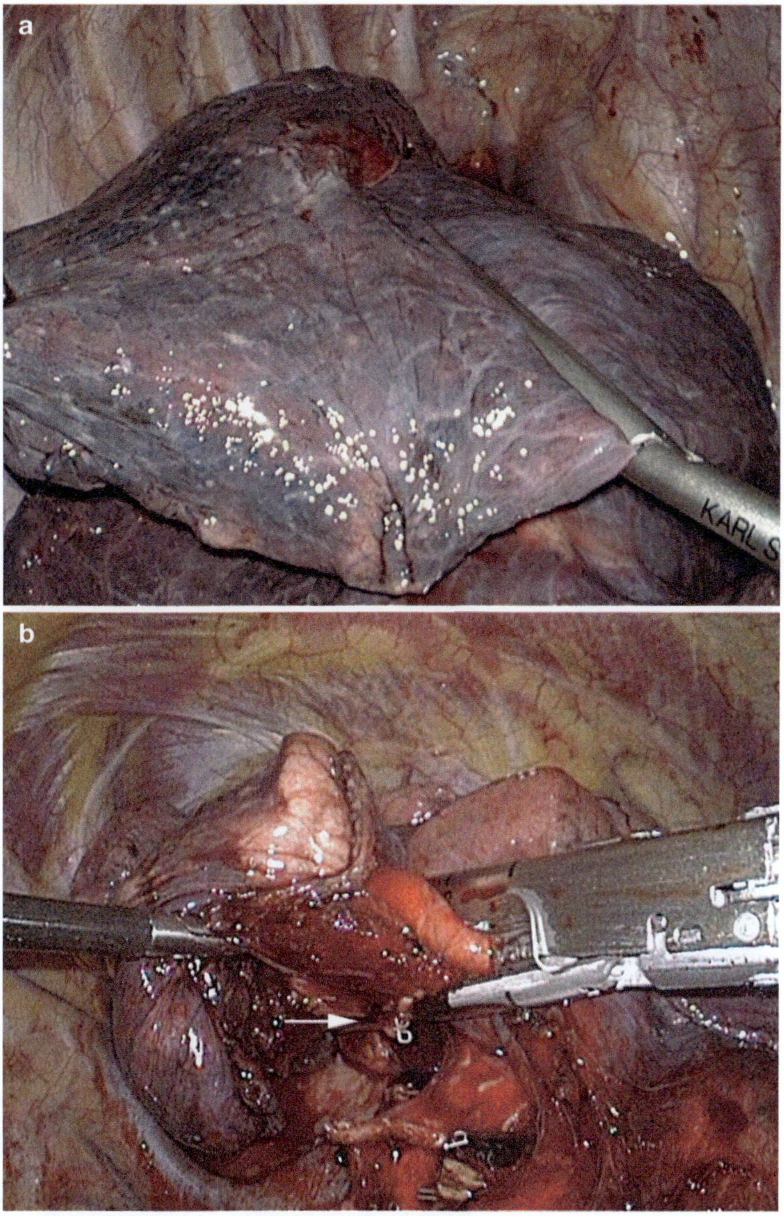

Fig. 10.17 Division of the parenchyma. (**a**) Delineation of the intersegmental plane by clamping, (**b**) stapling. The bronchial stump (*white arrow*) must be kept remote of the stapler jaws

10.3.2 Right Lower Lobe: Superior Segment

Resection of the superior segment (S6) of the right lower lobe is reasonably easy, thanks to the constant anatomical landmarks. However, as for a right lower lobectomy, the exposure of the pulmonary artery and its segmental branch can be tedious in case of fused fissure.

10.3.2.1 Fissure and Artery

This step is similar to the dissection of the fissure during a right lower lobectomy. The pulmonary artery may be visible or hidden if the fissure is fused. Depending on the difficulty in identifying the arterial pattern, it can be advisable to first open the posterior part of the fissure or, on the contrary, to first dissect the pulmonary artery.

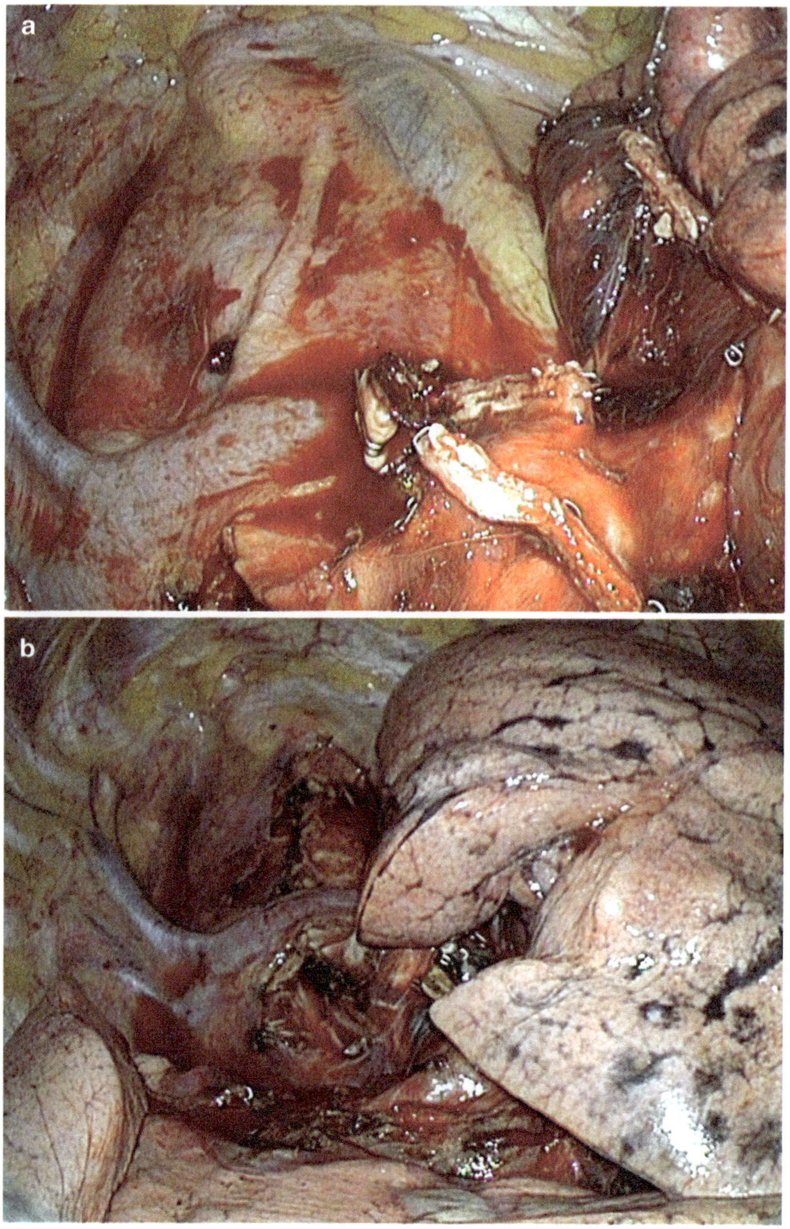

Fig. 10.18 Final view before reventilation. (**a**) Close-up view of the bronchial trifurcation, (**b**) final aspect after specimen retrieval and reventilation

The posterior fissure is opened, as for a right lower lobectomy. Once the pulmonary artery has been identified, a dissecting forceps is introduced from the posterior surface of the artery toward the posterior mediastinum. This may require retracting the lobes forward in order to expose the posterior mediastinal pleura. The pleura is incised at the level of the intermediate bronchus. An oblique viewing endoscope or a deflectable scope is helpful to control this maneuver. The posterior fissure is then stapled.

The pulmonary artery is dissected in the fissure. It is not necessary to expose the whole arterial crossroad, but the origin of the posterior ascending branch to the upper lobe and the origin of the basal trunk should at least been made out, making sure that no accessory branch originates from the superior artery. The superior segmental artery, which runs anteriorly to the segmental bronchus, is usually single. It is dissected, clipped, or stapled, depending on its size.

10.3.2.2 Bronchus

The division of the segmental artery gives access to the segmental bronchus which is cleared of peribronchial tissues and stapled.

10.3.2.3 Vein

The pulmonary ligament is incised up to the lower vein using both diathermy and gentle traction on the lower lobe. The inferior vein is cleared from the surrounding tissues, until its uppermost tributary is identified. It lies usually inferior to the bronchus. It can be clipped or divided after application of bipolar sealing.

10.3.3 Right Lower Lobe: Basal Segments

In addition to the superior segment (S6), the lower lobe comprises four basal segments: medial (S7), anterior (S8), lateral (S9), and posterior (S10). These segments are usually removed together since they depend from a single bronchial trunk. The main steps of the procedure are similar to those of a right lower lobectomy. The main concern is the preservation of the elements of the superior segment, especially the superior segmental vein.

10.3.3.1 Fissure and Artery

The dissection starts as for a lower lobectomy. The pulmonary artery is identified at the junction of the oblique and transverse fissure. When the fissure is incomplete or inflammatory, this step can be tedious. Opening the fissure can lead to pulmonary tears and troublesome oozing. Thorough progression using a combination of bipolar diathermy and blunt dissection is required until the artery is discovered. There is no need to divide the posterior portion of the oblique fissure. Access to the basal trunk is facilitated by the division of the anterior portion of the oblique fissure between the middle lobe and lower lobe. This part of the fissure is usually thin and can be split by bipolar or ultrasonic dissection. If its central portion is too thick, stapling can be necessary.

The sheath of the artery is entered. The artery to the middle lobe and the posterior segmental artery to the upper lobe must be clearly visible before any division. The basal trunk can then be stapled.

10.3.3.2 Bronchus

Division of the basilar trunk gives access to the basal bronchus which is cleared and divided, with avoidance of impingement on the segmental superior bronchus. If any doubt, a reventilation test can be helpful.

10.3.3.3 Vein

The pulmonary ligament is incised up to the lower vein using both diathermy and gentle traction on the lower lobe. The inferior pulmonary vein is cleared from the surrounding tissues, and its basal branches are dissected. They can join the inferior pulmonary vein, either via multiple segmental branches or via two trunks. Demonstration of the segmental veins is achieved by using a combination of gentle traction of the lobe and blunt dissection with an Endo Peanut. All branches are isolated and clipped, taking care to preserve the superior segmental vein.

10.3.3.4 Division of the Parenchyma

A long clamp is applied on the parenchyma. A reventilation test allows delineating the intersegmental plane. The parenchyma is compressed by the clamp to ease stapler application.

During stapling, the bronchial and arterial stumps should be pushed away so that they stay on the specimen side and remote from the stapler jaws. A constant watch should be kept on the superior segmental vein.

10.3.4 Left Upper Lobe: Superior Segments

Segmental resections involving the left upper lobe are the following: upper division (S1 + 2 and S3) (lingular sparing lobectomy), apicoposterior segmentectomy (S1 + 2), and lingulectomy (S4 and S5).

10.3.4.1 Upper Division

The procedure is similar to a left upper lobectomy apart from the lingular vessels which are preserved and the anterior portion of the fissure which does not require splitting. As for an upper lobectomy, part of the dissection can be carried out from behind.

Veins

The superior branches of the superior pulmonary vein partly hide the truncus anterior and should be divided first. The upper lobe is pulled backward. The mediastinal pleura is incised posterior to the phrenic nerve. Dissection of the vein is achieved by a combination of bipolar diathermy and gentle sweeping motion with an Endo Peanut. The lowermost tributary which drains the lingula is preserved. Only the two superior branches are divided using either a stapler or clips or a vessel sealing device, depending on their diameter.

Truncus Anterior

Division of the veins gives access to the anterior surface of apicoposterior and anterior branches of the truncus anterior. Clearing of their posterior and superior surfaces require a posterior dissection which is achieved by retracting the upper lobe downward and forward. The apicoposterior and anterior branches are stapled.

Fissure and Posterior Arteries

Both lobes are spread apart to expose the middle portion of the fissure. The upper lobe is gently pulled forward, avoiding any undue traction which could lead to injury to the vessels. Dissection is conducted cephalad, and all encountered posterior arteries are divided by turn. Traction helps expose the first segmental artery whose dissection is usually easy. It is controlled by clipping or with a vessel sealing device or with a combination of both.

As the posterior segmental arteries are gradually divided, the upper lobe unfolds and uncovers the posterior aspect of the truncus anterior which can be approached posteriorly. It is then also dissected from above and from the front, using various visions, thanks to the deflectable scope. Gentle blunt dissection is used to clear the origin of the trunk. If the trunk bifurcates into two large branches, these are dissected with caution and stapled independently.

Bronchi

Once the arteries and veins have been divided, traction on the parenchyma helps expose the segmental bronchi. The origin of the lingular bronchus is visualized, and the upper trunk – which separates into an anterior bronchus and an apicoposterior bronchus – is exposed, cleared using a blunt tip dissector, and stapled as a stem.

10.3.4.2 Apicoposterior Segmentectomy

From the vascular aspect, the procedure is simpler since only the apical and posterior arteries are divided, and this can be done from behind by stretching the upper lobe anteriorly. But, from the bronchial aspect, the dissection of the segmental bifurcation can be difficult, especially in case of peribronchial nodes, because of the shortness of the segmental bronchi.

Fissure and Arteries

This step is similar to the posterior control of arteries during a lingular sparing upper lobectomy. The only difference is that only the uppermost branch of the truncus anterior requires division. This can be achieved through a total posterior approach or partially through an anterior dissection of the hilum for the control of the apical artery.

Vein

When the superior pulmonary vein receives multiples radiating branches, making the venous pattern difficult to grasp, only the uppermost vein should be divided, thus making sure to preserve the middle branch which drains the anterior segment.

Bronchi

As above mentioned, the segmental bronchi are concealed by arteries which should always be divided before dissection of the segmental bronchi. Once the posterior segmental arteries have been divided, the posterior surface of the bronchi appears. Gentle retraction of the upper lobe and blunt dissection with an Endo Peanut progressively expose the segmental trifurcation: the anterior segmental bronchus (the lowermost and the most anterior one) which will be preserved and the apicoposterior trunk. Although the arteries have already been divided, it is advisable to keep flush with the bronchi as the dissection of their anterior surface is pursued. Since these bronchi are short, a guide for the stapler can be helpful.

10.3.5 Left Upper Lobe: Lingula

Although a lingulectomy (S4 and S5) is equivalent to a middle lobectomy with respect to pulmonary function and anatomy, it is actually technically more difficult because of the variable anatomical relationships.

10.3.5.1 Fissure and Artery

The anterior portion of the oblique fissure is open from the periphery to the hilum. The peripheral portion is usually thin so that the division can be initiated with either ultrasonic shears or a bipolar sealing device. When the fissure is thick and large, it is preferable to first staple its peripheral portion, always keeping an eye on the pulmonary artery.

The anterior aspect of the pulmonary artery is approached, and its sheath is opened. The lingular artery – its trunk or the two segmental branches – is divided after clipping or stapling, depending on its diameter.

10.3.5.2 Bronchus

The division of the lingular artery allows identification of the upper lobe bronchus and the lingular bronchus which is its lowest and most anterior branch. It is dissected, taking care to the artery of the anterior segment which runs behind the bronchus. The lingular bronchus has a short course and the peribronchial space is very narrow so that a guide can be helpful for passing the stapler anvil smoothly.

10.3.5.3 Vein

The lowest tributary of the superior pulmonary vein is transected. It can be difficult asserting that the adjacent venous branch drains the lingula. When in doubt, this branch must not be divided until the lingula has been fully mobilized, and the intersegmental plane has been initiated.

10.3.6 Left Lower Lobe: Superior Segment

Resection of the superior segment (S6) of the left lower lobe is more or less similar to the resection of the superior segment of the right lower lobe but even simpler because the segmental artery is usually readily identified in the fissure.

10.3.6.1 Fissure and Artery

This step is similar to the dissection of the fissure during a left lower lobectomy. The posterior fissure is opened by inserting the tip of a dissecting forceps from the posterior aspect of the pulmonary artery to the posterior mediastinum. This may require retracting the lobes forward in order to expose the posterior mediastinal pleura. An oblique viewing endoscope or a deflectable scope is helpful to control this maneuver. The posterior fissure is then stapled. The superior segmental artery, which runs anteriorly to the segmental bronchus, is usually single, sometimes double. It is dissected and clipped.

10.3.6.2 Bronchus

Division of the segmental artery gives access to the segmental bronchus which is cleared and divided, with avoidance of impingement on the basilar bronchus. If any doubt, a reventilation test can be helpful.

10.3.6.3 Vein

The pulmonary ligament is incised up to the lower vein using both diathermy and gentle traction on the lower lobe. The inferior vein is cleared from the surrounding tissues, until its uppermost tributary is identified. It lies usually inferior to the bronchus. It can be clipped or divided with a vessel sealing device.

10.3.7 Left Lower Lobe: Basilar Segments

In addition to the superior segment (S6), the lower lobe comprises four basal segments: anterior (S7), medial (S8), lateral (S9), and posterior (S10). Although the medial and anterior (S7+8) and the posterior and lateral (S9+10) segments can sometimes be individualized, it is usual to remove all basal segments together. The procedure is similar to a left lower lobectomy. Only the demonstration of the basilar vein and the recognition of the intersegmental plane may be difficult.

10.3.7.1 Fissure and Artery

The dissection starts as for a lower lobectomy. Once the peripheral portion of the fissure has been divided, it becomes easier to display the reflection of the mediastinal pleura, between the two pulmonary veins. The pleura is opened with electrocautery, and a right angle dissector can then be passed toward the pulmonary artery. This allows completing the division of the anterior fissure.

Completion of the anterior fissure division helps expose the pulmonary artery whose sheath is opened. The basilar trunk is dissected. There is no need to isolate the superior segmental artery, but the latter must be identified before stapling the basilar artery which can present as a common trunk or with multiple branches. The posterior part of the fissure does not need to be stapled.

10.3.7.2 Bronchus

Division of the basilar trunk gives access to the basal bronchus which is cleared and divided, with avoidance of impingement on the segmental superior bronchus. If any doubt, a reventilation test can be helpful.

10.3.7.3 Vein

The pulmonary ligament is incised up to the lower vein using both diathermy and gentle traction on the lower lobe. Demonstration of the segmental vein is achieved by using a combination of gentle traction of the lobe and blunt dissection with an Endo Peanut. The vein is cleared from the surrounding tissues, and its inferior root is dissected, isolated, and clipped, with care taken to preserve the superior segmental vein.

10.4 Experience (Table 10.2)

From January 2008 to June 2011, TEAS was attempted in 71 patients (34 males and 37 females) ranging in age from 25 to 81 years (mean, 56). The indication was either a benign lesion (18 patients), a solitary metastasis (12 patients), or a suspicion of clinical stage I non-small-cell lung carcinoma (NSCLC) (41 patients). For the patients operated on for a suspicion of primary lung carcinoma, the reason for performing a segmentectomy was an impaired lung function and/or a previous history of pulmonary resection (segmentectomy in 1 patient and lobectomy in 2 patients).

Intraoperative and postoperative data were recorded in a prospective manner. The data were the following: need for conversion to open thoracotomy, duration of the surgical procedure as noted on the operating room records, operative blood loss, intraoperative complications, number

Table 10.2 Resected segments

Right	*N*	Left	*N*
Apicoposterior (S1+S2)	16	Upper division (S1–3)	11
Superior (S6)	6	Apicoposterior (S1+S2)	4
Basilar segments (S7–10)	11	Lingula (S4–5)	4
		Superior (S6)	11
		Basilar segments (S7–10)	8

of collected lymph nodes and of dissected lymph node stations for patients operated on for NSCLC, duration of chest drainage, postoperative stay, and postoperative complications. We did not include in the series the 31 thoracoscopic right middle lobectomies (segments S4 and S5) which were performed in the same period of time, as other authors did [12] basing on the anatomic and functional similarity between the middle lobe and the lingula.

10.4.1 Technical Aspects

All patients candidate to an upper segmentectomy had a multidetector row preoperative computed tomography (CT) angiography with three-dimensional volume-rendering reconstruction of arterial and venous anatomy [11, 25, 26]. CT reconstruction was not done for the lower segments since anatomical variations of the vascular supply to the lower lobes have less impact on the surgical technique and can be easily managed. A radical lymphadenectomy was performed for all patients operated on for a suspicion of lung carcinoma. No utility incision was used. On completion of the pulmonary resection, the specimen was wrapped into an endobag and retrieved through one of the port sites that was enlarged to a length of 2–4 cm (Fig. 10.1b), depending on the specimen size [11]. The use of a rib spreader was never required for this task. Depending of the type of resection, one or two chest tubes were placed through the port sites. Their removal was decided according to usual rules, i.e., no air leakage and output inferior to 150 cc/day.

10.4.2 Results

There were three conversions to thoracotomy (4.2%) for a noncontrollable hemorrhage from the apical artery during a right apicoposterior segmentectomy. All three patients had a simple postoperative course and were discharged before the eighth postoperative day. In the 68 other patients who had a totally endoscopic procedure, there were two intraoperative complications, i.e., a partial disruption of the staple line during division of the intersegmental plane. It required endoscopic suturing. The postoperative course of these two patients was simple, and they were discharged at days 4 and 5. The operation time ranged from 92 to 315 min (mean, 181 ± 52 min). The estimated blood loss ranged from 0 (nonmeasurable) to 450 ml (mean, 77 ± 69 ml). No patient needed blood transfusion. All but six patients had an uneventful postoperative course (12%). The complications were minor and were the following: prolonged air leak (>6 days) (2), pneumothorax requiring chest drainage (2), sputum retention requiring bronchoscopy (2), and neurologic disorder (1). The drainage duration ranged from 1 to 7 days (mean: 3.1 ± 1.8 days) and the hospital stay from 2 to 14 days (mean: 5.6 ± 2.4 days). For the 41 patients who were operated on for a suspicion of primary lung carcinoma and who had an additional lymphadenectomy, the mean number of collected lymph nodes from station 10 ranged from 0 to 6 (mean: 3 ± 2) and from station 11 ranged from 1 to 9 (mean: 3 ± 2). The mean number of collected mediastinal lymph nodes was 18 ± 8, and the mean number of dissected lymph node stations was 3.5 ± 1. In lung cancer cases, the tumors were staged pathological N0 in all but two cases which were upstaged N2.

Conclusion

Although a totally endoscopic approach to anatomic segmentectomies can seem challenging and difficult, the operation time was reasonable in our series and the morbidity rate was low, as in other recent series (Table 10.3). Experience and improvements of some instruments such as endostaplers will facilitate the procedure. Combining the advantages of an endoscopic approach and an anatomic limited resection could be highly beneficial for those of the patients who fulfill the criteria of a sublobar resection [22].

Table 10.3 Results for published series of VATS or totally endoscopic segmentectomies

First author (year)	N	VATS/TT	Conversion rate (%)	Morbidity (%)	Chest tube duration[a] (days)	Postoperative stay[a] (days)
Shiraishi (2004) [27]	34	TT	0	11.7	4.5 ± 3.2	12.7 ± 3.6
Okada (2007) [8]	52	VATS	NS	13.5	3 (2–13)	NS
Atkins (2007) [6]	48	VATS	0	31.3	3.5 ± 4	4.3 ± 3
Oizumi (2009) [10]	29	TT	0	10	1 (1–7)	NS
Yamada (2009) [11]	9	TT	0	11	1.6	7.6 (5–11)
Schuchert (2009) [9]	104	VATS	NS	26	NS	5
Watanabe (2009) [18]	41	VATS	0	10	3 (1–9)	NS
Shapiro (2009) [22]	31	VATS	13	26	2 (1–33)	4 (1–98)
Leshnower (2010) [28]	15	VATS	0	0	2.8 ± 1.3	3.5 ± 1.4
This series	71	TT	4.2	11.3	3.1 ± 1.8	5.6 ± 2.4

N number, *VATS* video-assisted, *TE* totally endoscopic, *NS* not stated
[a]Expressed as mean and range or mean ± standard deviation

References

1. McKenna R, Houck W, Fuller C (2006) Video-assisted thoracic surgery lobectomy: experience with 1100 cases. Ann Thorac Surg 81:421–426
2. Yamamoto K, Ohsumi A, Kojima F, Imanishi N, Matsuoka K, Ueda M, Miyamoto Y (2010) Long-term survival after video-assisted thoracic surgery lobectomy for primary lung cancer. Ann Thorac Surg 89:353–359
3. Seder C, Hanna K, Lucia V, Boura J, Kim S, Welsh R, Chmielewski G (2009) The safe transition from open to thoracoscopic lobectomy: a 5-year experience. Ann Thorac Surg 88:216–226
4. Yan T, Black D, Bannon P, McCaughan B (2009) Systematic review and meta-analysis of randomized and nonrandomized trials on safety and efficacy of video-assisted thoracic surgery lobectomy for early-stage non-small-cell lung cancer. J Clin Oncol 27:2553–2562
5. Paul S, Altorki N, Sheng S, Lee P, Harpole D, Onaitis M, Stiles B, Port J, D'Amico T (2010) Thoracoscopic lobectomy is associated with lower morbidity than open lobectomy: a propensity-matched analysis from the STS database. J Thorac Cardiovasc Surg 139:366–378
6. Atkins B, Harpole D, Mangum J, Toloza E, D'Amico T, Burfeind W (2007) Pulmonary segmentectomy by thoracotomy or thoracoscopy: reduced hospital length of stay with a minimally-invasive approach. Ann Thorac Surg 84:1107–1113
7. Yamashita S, Chujo M, Kawano Y, Miyawaki M, Tokuishi K, Anami K, Yamamoto S, Kawahara K (2011) clinical impact of segmentectomy compared with Lobectomy Under Complete Video-Assisted thoracic surgery in the treatment of stage I non-small cell lung cancer. J Surg Res 166:46–51
8. Okada M, Mimura T, Ikegaki J, Katoh H, Itoh H, Tsubota N (2007) A novel video-assisted anatomic segmentectomy technique: selective segmental inflation via bronchofiberoptic jet followed by cautery cutting. J Thorac Cardiovasc Surg 133:753–758
9. Schuchert M, Pettiford B, Pennathur A, Abbas G, Awais O, Close J, Kilic A, Jack R, Landreneau J, Landreneau J, Wilson D, Luketich J, Landreneau R (2009) Anatomic segmentectomy for stage I non-small-cell lung cancer: comparison of video-assisted thoracic surgery versus open approach. J Thorac Cardiovasc Surg 138:1318–1325
10. Oizumi H, Kanauchi N, Kato H, Endoh M, Takeda S, Suzuki J, Fukaya K, Sadahiro M (2009) Total thoracoscopic pulmonary segmentectomy. Eur J Cardiothorac Surg 36:374–377
11. Yamada S, Suga A, Inoue Y, Inoue H (2009) Use of multi-detector rox angiography for the arrangement of video-assisted modified segmental resection. Eur J Cardiothorac Surg 36:727–730
12. Schuchert MJ, Pettiford BL, Keeley S, D'Amato TA, Kilic A, Close J, Pennathur A, Santos R, Fernando HC, Landreneau JR, Luketich JD, Landreneau RJ (2007) Anatomic segmentectomy in the treatment of stage I non-small cell lung cancer. Ann Thorac Surg 84:926–933
13. Wisnivesky J, Henschke C, Swanson S, Yankelevit D, Zulueta J, Marcus S, Halm E (2010) Limited resection for the treatment of patients with stage IA lung cancer. Ann Surg 251:550–554
14. Schoofs J, Gossot D (2004) A neglected but frustrating ergonomic issue: the thoracoscopic trocar. Minim Invasive Ther Allied Technol 13:133–137
15. Gossot D (2008) Technical tricks to facilitate totally endoscopic major pulmonary resections. Ann Thorac Surg 86:323–326
16. Ikeda Y, Tamura M, Umezu H, Karube Y, Seki N, Kobayashi S, Nagai S, Miyoshi S (2003) Usefulness of mini loop retractor in video-assisted thoracic surgery. Kyobu Geka 56:199–202
17. Gossot D, Pryschepau M, Martinez Berenys C, Magdeleinat P (2009) Throw-off instruments for advanced thoracoscopic procedures. Interact Cardiovasc Thorac Surg 10:159–160

18. Watanabe A, Ohori S, Nakashima S, Mawatari T, Inoue N, Kurimoto Y, Higami T (2009) Feasibility of video-assisted thoracoscopic surgery segmentectomy for selected peripheral lung carcinomas. Eur J Cardiothorac Surg 35:775–780
19. Gossot D, Girard P, Stern J, Raynaud C, Caliandro R, Debrosse D, Magdeleinat P (2009) Totally endoscopic major pulmonary resections for stage I bronchial carcinoma: initial results. Rev Mal Respir 26:961–970
20. Watanabe A, Koyanagi T, Nakashima S, Higami T (2007) How to clamp the main pulmonary artery during video-assisted thoracoscopic surgery lobectomy. Eur J Cardiothorac Surg 31:129–131
21. D'Amico TA (2008) Thoracoscopic segmentectomy: technical considerations and outcomes. Ann Thorac Surg 85:S716–S718
22. Shapiro M, Weiser T, Wisnivesky J, Chin C, Arustamyan M, Swanson S (2009) Thoracoscopic segmentectomy compares favorably with thoracoscopic lobectomy for patients with small stage I lung cancer. J Thorac Cardiovasc Surg 137:1388–1393
23. Gossot D, Merlusca G, Tudor A, Boudaya M, Radu C, Magdeleinat P (2009) Pitfalls related to the use of endostaplers during video-assisted thoracic surgery. Surg Endosc 23:189–192
24. Gossot D (2010) Atlas of endoscopic major pulmonary resections. Springer, Paris
25. Fukuhara K, Akashi A, Nakane S, Tomita E (2008) Preoperative assessment of the pulmonary artery by three-dimensional computed tomography before video-assisted thoracic surgery lobectomy. Eur J Cardiothorac Surg 34:875–877
26. Nakamoto K, Omori K, Nezu K (2010) Superselective segmentectomy for deep and small pulmonary nodule under the guidance of three-dimensional reconstructed computed tomographic angiography. Ann Thorac Surg 89:877–884
27. Shiraishi T, Shirakusa T, Miyoshi T, Hiratsuka M, Yamamoto S, Iwasaki A (2006) A completely thoracoscopic lobectomy/segmentectomy for primary lung cancer: technique, feasibility and advantages. Thorac Cardiovasc Surg 54:202–207
28. Leshnower B, Miller D, Fernandez F, Pickens A, Force S (2010) Video-assisted thoracoscopic surgery segmentectomy: a safe and effective procedure. Ann Thorac Surg 89:1571–1576

Non-anatomical Resections of the Lung

11

Rolf G.C. Inderbitzi

Contents

R.G.C. Inderbitzi, M.D.
Thoraxzentrum Zurich, Witellikerstrasse 40,
CH-8008, Zurich, Switzerland
e-mail: r.inderbitzi@thoraxzentrum.ch

11.1 Indications

The so-called non-anatomical lung resection, which essentially describes a simple wedge resection of the peripheral lung parenchyma using a stapler (Fig. 11.1), is one of the most common thoracoscopic procedures in the everyday life of the surgeon. Its introduction into clinical practice meant a fundamental extension of the feasibilities of diagnosis for thoracic surgery and pneumology. Besides ensuring a generously measured tissue sample – the findings can usually be resected in toto, with sufficient clear zone to the surrounding tissue, i.e. a local radical resection – the direct exploration of the thoracic space and its structures

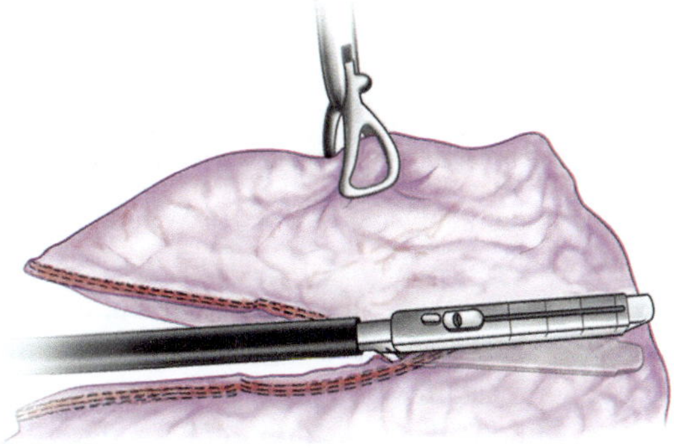

Fig. 11.1 Lung wedge resection using a stapling device

R.G.C. Inderbitzi et al. (eds.), *Minimally Invasive Thoracic and Cardiac Surgery*,
DOI 10.1007/978-3-642-11861-6_11, © Springer-Verlag Berlin Heidelberg 2012

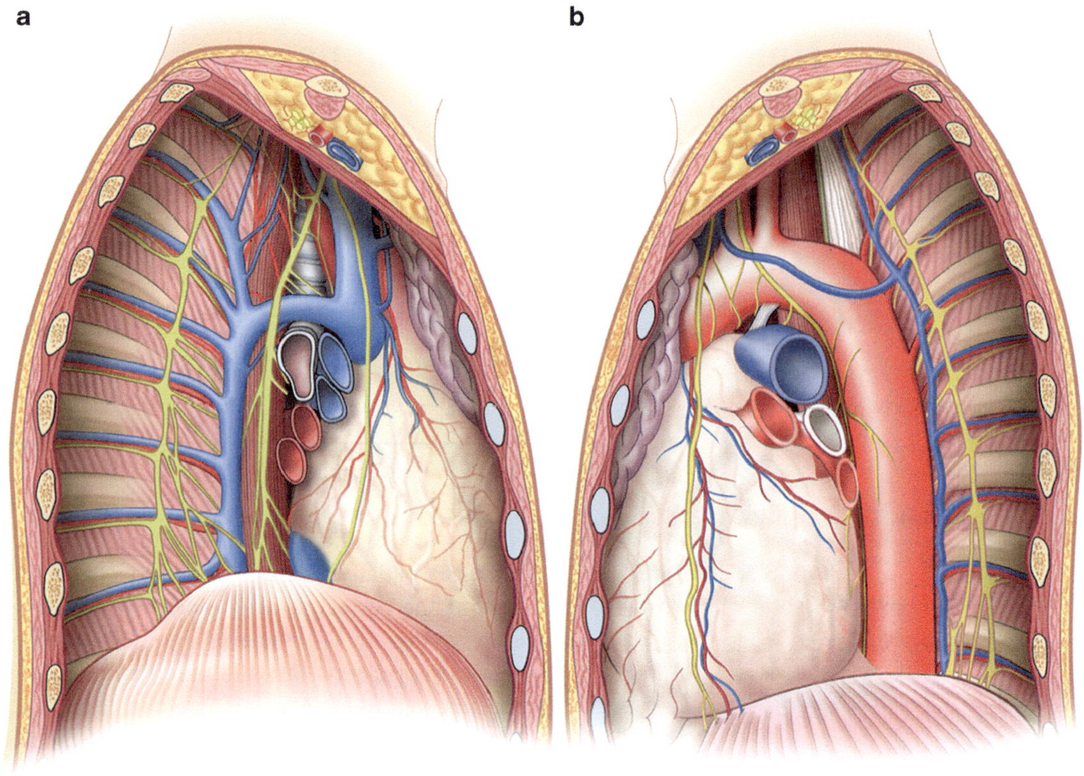

Fig. 11.2 (**a–b**) Endoscopic overview of the right (**a**) and left (**b**) thoracic cavity with their relevant anatomical structures

(Fig. 11.2a, b) allows a comprehensive anatomical pathological assessment. Even an extensive thoracotomy cannot achieve a comparably complete overview of the thoracic space. As a result of thoracoscopic access, a wedge resection of the lung represents a valuable diagnostic context: Specific biopsy, swab and sampling of effusion throughout the thoracic space allow comprehensive cytological, histological, microbiological, immunological and chemical analysis [2, 6, 8, 9]. When carrying out a diagnostic wedge resection in a context where bronchial carcinoma is suspected, a thoracoscopy also becomes a significant part of the "staging procedure" (see following section).

An additional application of here described techniques is commonly used in the treatment of spontaneous primary and secondary pneumothorax (Fig. 11.3a–d) as well as for lung volume reduction surgery (q.v. Chap. 15).

11.2 Surgical Procedure

The patient undergoes the operation under general anaesthetic with pulmonary ventilation in the lateral decubitus (Fig. 11.4). The approaches are established beforehand by means of the target findings in the preoperative computer tomography; three mini-incisions usually suffice (Fig. 11.5). The pulmonary ligament can be released thoracoscopically without problem for better mobilisation of the lower lung sections. The lung resection is performed with a stapling device; the choice of these has become large meanwhile and depends on the location of the target finding (bendable stapler device) and the tissue composition of the lung. If the lung tissue is friable, crumbly or of varying consistency, it is sensible to strengthen it with the use of a biocompatible material for reinforced suture lines

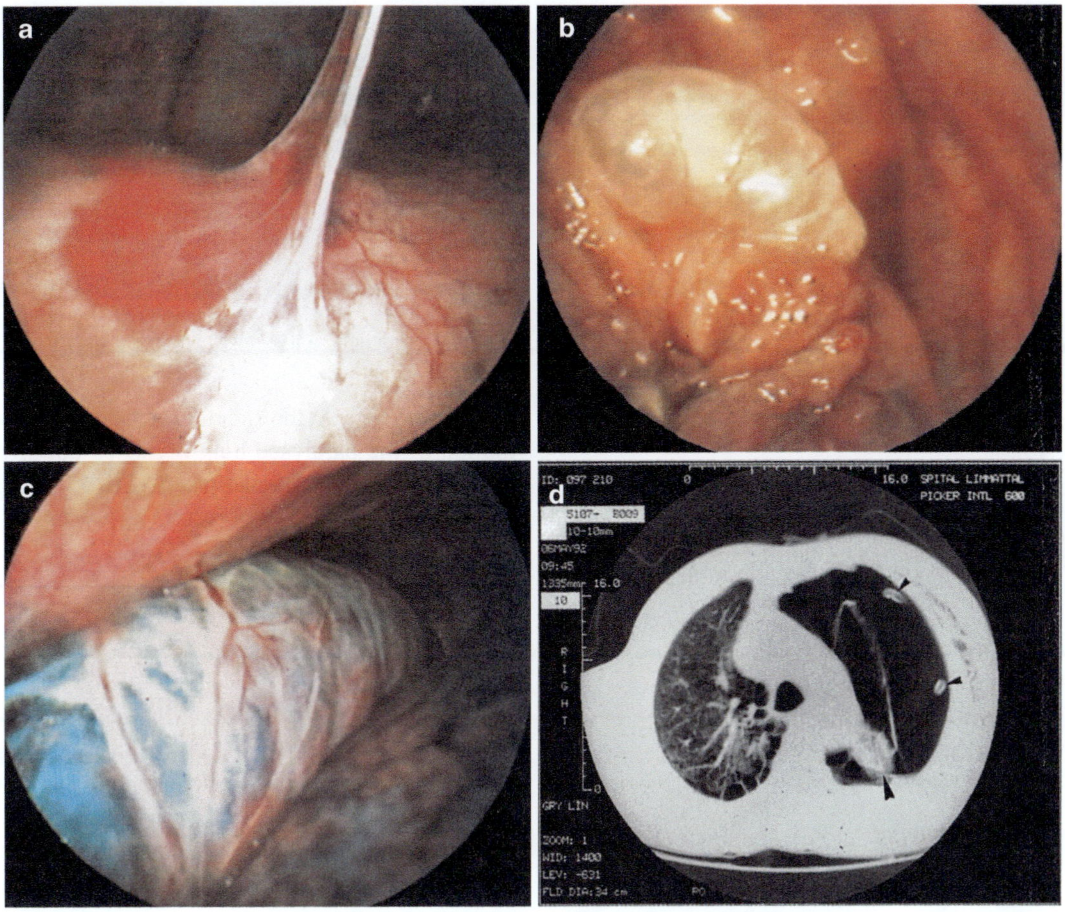

Fig. 11.3 (**a–d**) All pictured examples have to be removed by a wedge resection altogether with healthy underlying lung tissue: (**a**) (Abb. 26.21 S 352 Nakhosteen/Inderbitzi) The sanguineous inhibition of the adhesion points a recent event. The adhesion is formed from a burst bulla responsible for pneumothorax. (**b**) (Abb. 26.22 S 352 Nakhosteen/Inderbitzi) Bulla (2.5 cm in diameter) with underlying collapsed lung tissue in a young healthy patient according to a primary spontaneous pneumothorax. (**c**) (Abb. 26.23 S 352 Nakhosteen/Inderbitzi) Huge bulla alteration of a patient with secondary spontaneous pneumothorax. Alteration is positioned between lung parenchyma and parasternal thoracic wall. (**d**) (Abb. 26.24 S 352 Nakhosteen/Inderbitzi) Thoracic CT scan of aforementioned patient

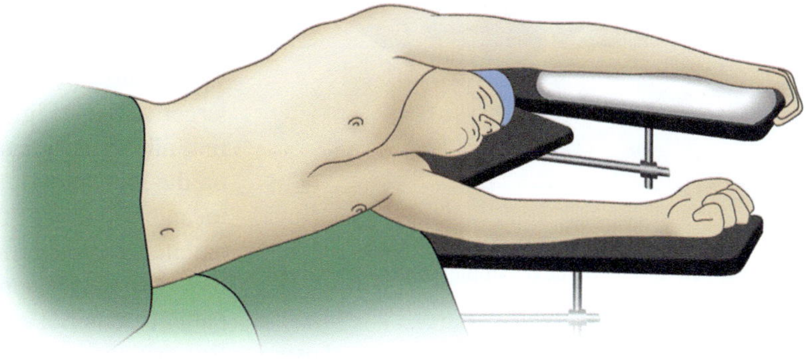

Fig. 11.4 Lateral position of the patient for non-anatomical thoracoscopic resection

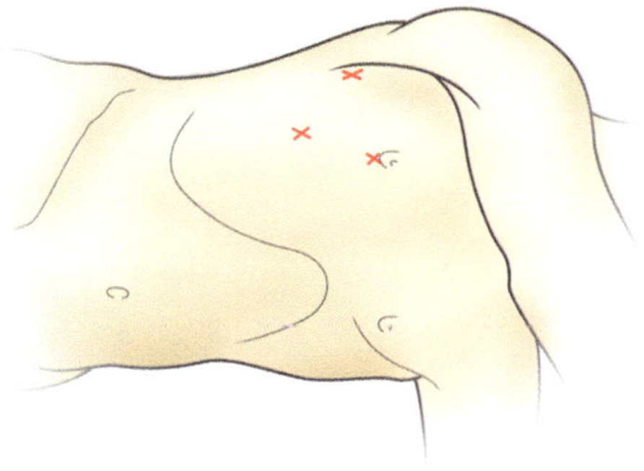

Fig. 11.5 The three mini-incisions are made in a low-muscle triangle when possible

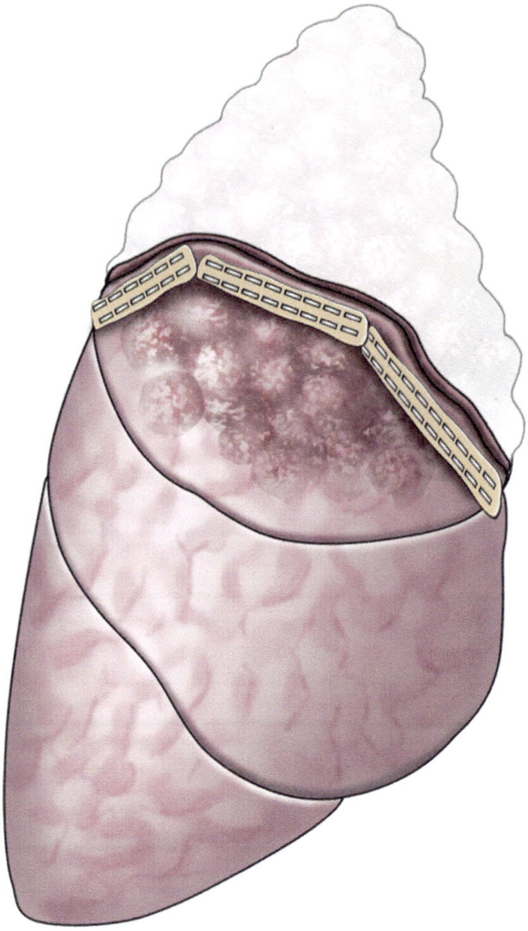

Fig. 11.6 Reinforcement material of suture lines in emphysematous lung tissue (example: Seamguard Gore)

(Fig. 11.6). The resected tissue is evacuated using a specimen pouch to prevent implantation metastasis (Fig. 11.7). At the end of the procedure, ventilation of the paralysed lung is carried out after prior insertion of drainage (see Chap. 15) using endoscopic guidance.

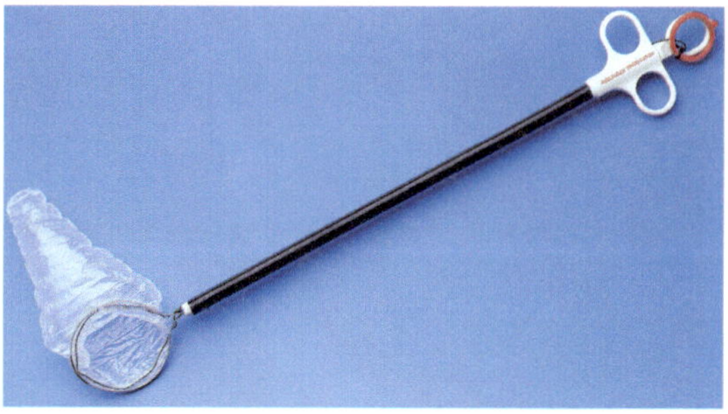

Fig. 11.7 Example of a one-way specimen pouch

11.3 Diffuse, Interstitial Pneumopathies

The majority of *diffuse, interstitial pneumopathies* (Fig. 11.8) can only be diagnosed using bioptic procedures. It is true that sputum analysis and bronchoalveolar lavage often produce positive cytological and microbiological evidence, but these findings do not allow a conclusive diagnosis in more than 50% of cases [3, 4]. The standard procedure for ensuring a diagnosis is a sufficiently large lung biopsy. The open lung biopsy via a thoracotomy has been replaced by a minimally invasive procedure in the last few years. The meaningfulness of the thoracoscopic lung wedge resection is crucially dependent on the removal technique. With a diffuse interstitial pneumopathy, the pathologist is directed to a representative tissue sample. For this, the excised wedge must contain central parts of lung tissue with assessable bronchial structures and parts of larger vessels (Fig. 11.9). A wedge resection like this allows a precise diagnosis. When deciding on the indication, therefore, it is not the brilliant meaningfulness of the test compared to a differentiated consideration which is compelling but the definitely increased co-morbidity in the patient material with diffuse pneumopathies. Besides the changed lung tissue, which often leads to technical malfunction of the stapler with

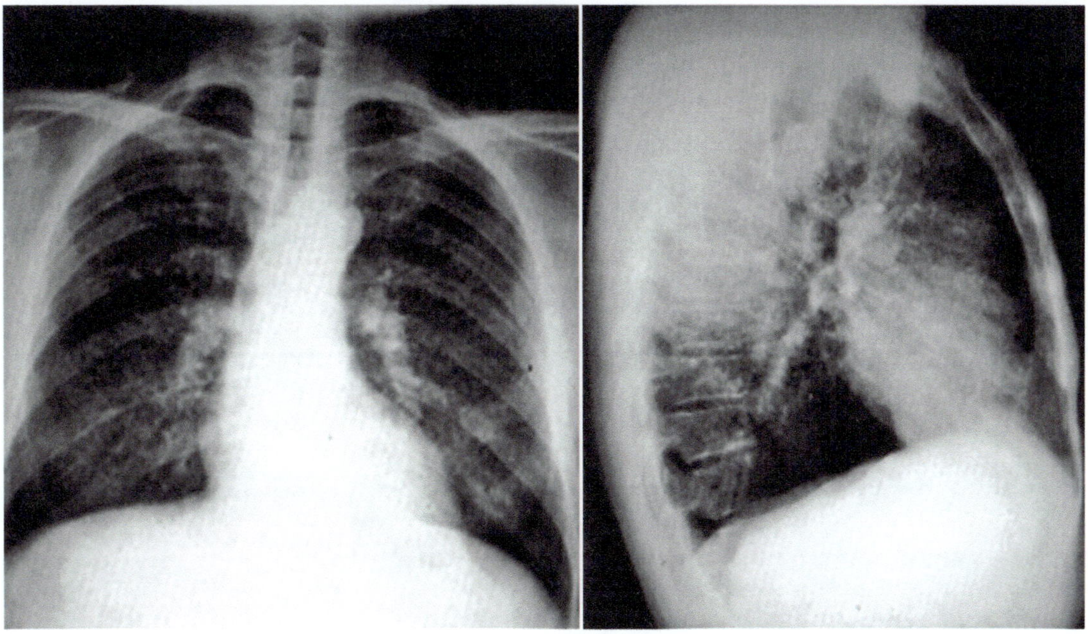

Fig. 11.8 (Abb. 26.1, S 342 Nakhosteen/Inderbitzi): Diffuse, interstitial pneumopathy. The X-ray image does not allow closer aetiological differentiation; *left* p.a., *right* lateral position

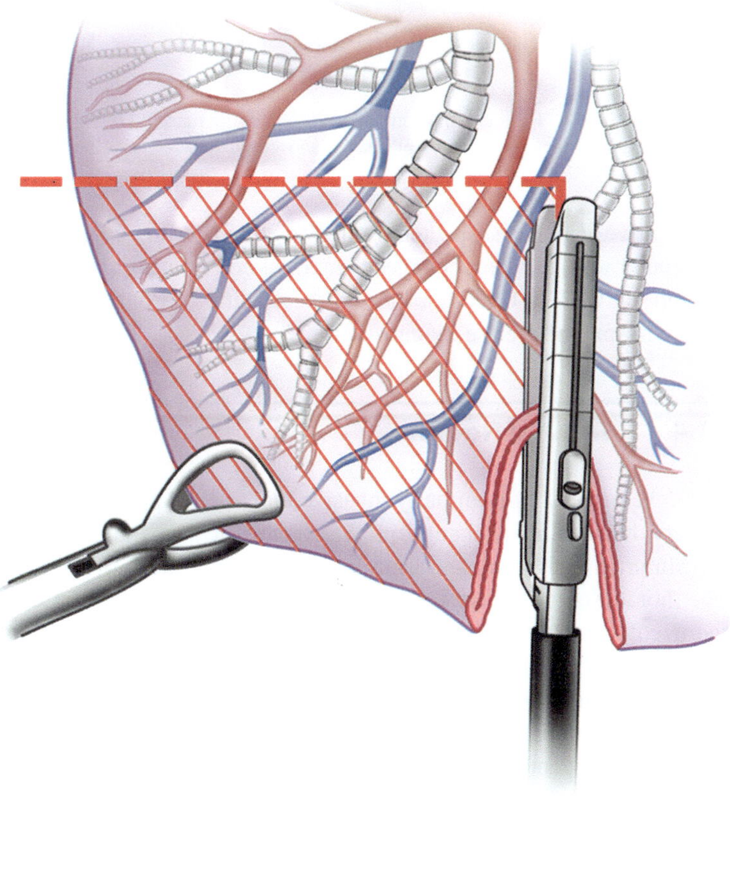

Fig. 11.9 Wedge excision for diagnosis of diffuse pneumopathies. The excised wedge must contain central parts of lung tissue, bronchial structures and vessel parts

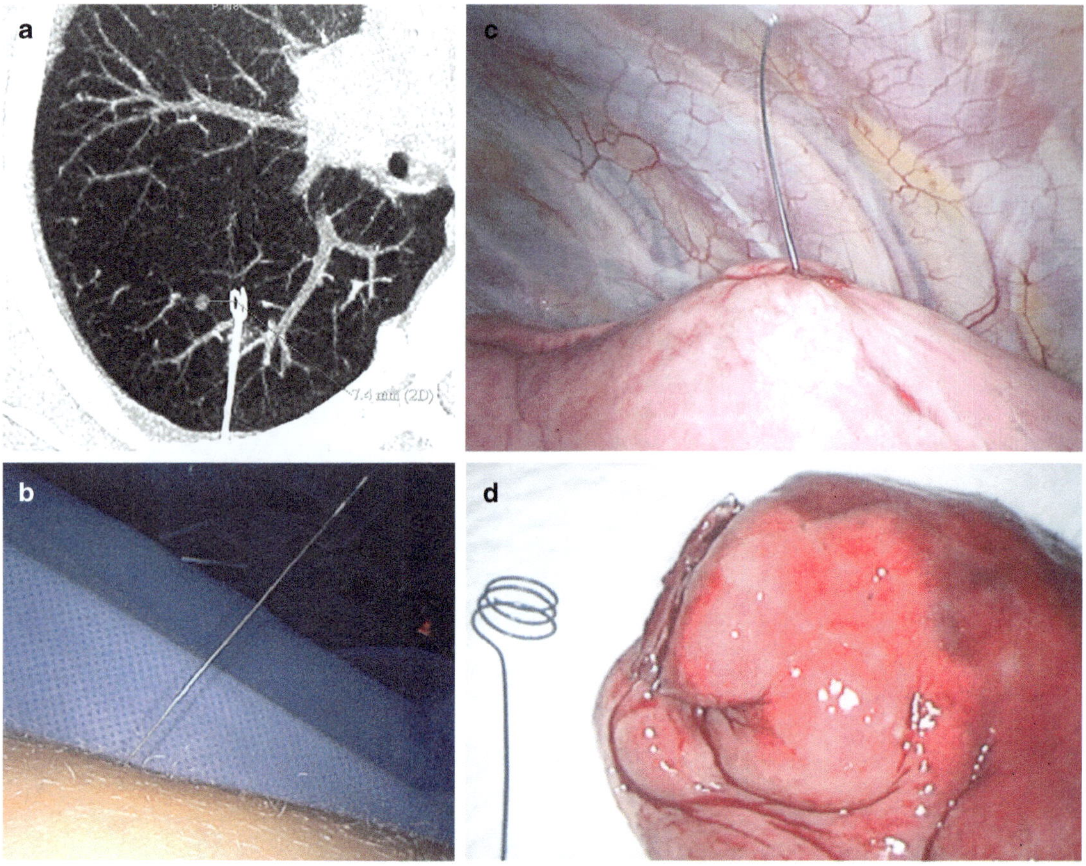

Fig. 11.10 (**a–d**) CT-guided, transcutaneous lung nodule marking using marker wire. (**a**) Marked CT findings. (**b**) Wire in place, external view. (**c**) Wire in place, thoracoscopic view. (**d**) Excised lung wedge with removed marker wire

consecutive airholes, suspected limited treatment associated with the lung changes should be considered, as well as the often limited therapeutic results in spite of precise diagnosis [5].

11.4 The Lung Nodule

The development of minimally invasive thoracic surgery has led to a change in the diagnostic algorithm in lung nodules requiring diagnosis. The thoracoscopic wedge resection has replaced the needle and punch biopsy as the method of choice. Lung parenchyma tumours where cytological and histological assessment is inclusive or still outstanding can be removed in toto for further assessment. The low mortality and morbidity, the simple process of the thoracoscopic procedure, the excellent diagnostic meaningfulness and bearable costs have led to its triumphant progress [13].

The intraoperative location must be given for resection of the target findings. If nodules are sufficiently large and in a subpleural location, thoracoscopic positioning is easy after study of the preoperative computer tomography; an unventilated collapsed lung allows systematic palpation of the tissue between two instruments in the outer third of the parenchyma. If the findings are small or deeply situated (<1 cm diameter) and cannot be palpated with thoracoscopic instruments, preoperative CT marking is required [7, 11]. The series of images Fig. 11.10a–d explains this technique. This preoperative nodule marking is of increasing importance within the framework of CT screening for early recognition of lung cancer [1].

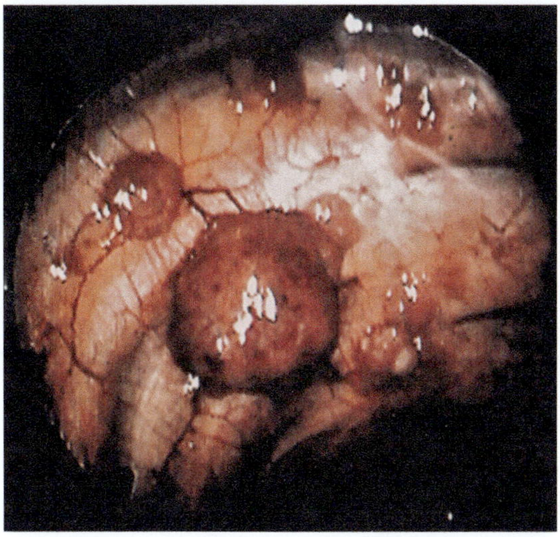

Fig. 11.11 Pleural metastases which could not be visualised using imaging techniques. The thoracoscopy carried out because of persistent myasthenia symptoms in spite of radical thymectomy showed not only the larger nodule visible in the CT but also several more tiny offspring on the thoracic wall and the diaphragm

If a bronchial carcinoma is the cause of a lung nodule, the thoracoscopic diagnosis via tissue sampling is often of crucial significance. Even when the histological diagnosis is certain, the resectability cannot in the end be established until a thoracotomy has been carried out: A small-nodule pleural tumour metastasis, tumour infiltration in the surrounding structures such as the vena cava, oesophagus, vertebral column, etc., cannot always be proven with imaging techniques in every case (Fig. 11.11 = Abb 26.54, S 377, Nakhosteen, Inderbitzi). Of the metastases of a malignant thymoma shown here, only the nodes in the middle of the picture were demonstrated in the CT. The small nodal changes around it and on the diaphragm remained invisible. With about 5% of all patients for whom an anatomical resection is planned, this is unnecessary and can be avoided by means of a prior thoracoscopic evaluation [10].

References

1. Dijkman JH, van der Meer JW, Bakker W, Wever AM, van der Broek PJ. et al (2011) The national lung screening trial: overview and study design. Radiology 258(1):243–253, Epub 2010 Nov 2
2. Dijkman JH, van der Meer JWM, Bakker W, Wever AMJ, van der Broek PJ (1982) Transpleural lung biopsy by the thoracoscopic route in patients with diffuse interstitial pulmonary disease. Chest 82:76–83
3. Gaensler EA, Carrington CB (1980) Open biopsy for chronic diffuse infiltrative lung disease. Ann Thorac Surg 30:411–426
4. Gaensler EA, Moister MVB, Hamm J (1964) Open lung biopsy in diffuse pulmonary disease. N Engl J Med 270:1319–1331
5. Lachappelle KJ, Morin JE (1995) Benefit of open lung biopsy in patients with respiratory failure. Can J Surg 38:316–321
6. Light RE (1990) Pleural diseases, 2nd edn. Lea & Febiger, Philadelphia
7. Mack MJ, Gordon MJ, Postma TW, Berger MS, Aronoff RJ, Acuff TE, Ryan WH (1992) Percutaneous localization of pulmonary nodules for thoracoscopic lung resection. Ann Thorac Surg 53:1123–1124
8. Menzies R, Charbonneau M (1991) Thoracoscopy for the diagnosis of pleural disease. Ann Intern Med 114:271–276
9. Miller JI, Hatcher CR (1978) Thoracoscopy: a useful tool in the diagnosis of thoracic disease. Ann Thorac Surg 26:68–72
10. Roviaro G, Varoli F, Rebuffat C, Vergani C, Maciocco M, Scalambra SM, Sonnino D, Gozi G (1995) Videothoracoscopic staging and treatment of lung cancer. Ann Thorac Surg 59:971–974
11. Templeton PA, Krasna M (1993) Localization of pulmonary nodules for thoracoscopic resection: use of needle/wire breast biopsy system. AJR Am J Roentgenol 160:761–762
12. Voellmy W (1981) Résultats diagnostiques de la thoracoscopie dans les affections du poumon et de la plèvre. Poumon Coeur 37:67–73
13. Walker WS, Leaver HA (2007) Immunologic and stress responses following video-assisted thoracic surgery and open pulmonary lobectomy in early stage lung cancer. Thorac Surg Clin 17:241–249

Robotic Lobectomy

12

Franca M.A. Melfi, Federico Davini, Olivia Fanucchi,
Ralph Alexander Schmid, and Alfredo Mussi

Contents

F.M.A. Melfi, M.D.
Department of Cardio-Thoracic Surgery,
University of Pisa, Via Paradisa 2, Pisa 56100, Italy
e-mail: f.melfi@med.unipi.it

F. Davini, M.D. • O. Fanucchi, M.D. • A. Mussi, M.D.
Department of Cardio-Thoracic and Vascular Surgery,
University of Pisa, Via Paradisa 2, Pisa 56124, Italy
e-mail: davinifederico@gmail.com;
o.fanucchi@med.unipi.it; a.mussi@dc.med.unipi.it

R.A. Schmid, M.D. (✉)
Division of General Thoracic Surgery,
University Hospital Berne, Freiburgstrasse, Berne
CH-3010, Switzerland
e-mail: ralph.schmid@insel.ch

12.1 Introduction

The rapid development of minimally invasive surgery (MIS) in the last decades has allowed surgeons to perform an increasing number of operations with minimal tissue trauma and a progressive broadening of the indications. In thoracic surgery, several studies have suggested improvements in postoperative pain control, earlier discharge, lower levels of perioperative inflammatory cytokine levels, lower complication rates and earlier return to normal activities compared with open thoracotomy procedures [1–4].

However, for lung cancer treatment, unanswered questions still remain among surgeons who have not accepted this technique as appropriate oncologic procedure. Concerns include: safety of anatomical hilum's dissection, adequacy of clearance (oncological resection with a curative intent) unclear long-term benefits over open surgery [5–8].

In addition, technical-mechanical limitations of equipment, such as to two-dimensional image (2D), limited instrument's manoeuvrability (due to poor dexterity for long instruments and the fulcrum effect) unstable camera platform and poor ergonomics for surgeon, still exist. Advanced engineering technology makes it possible to overcome several of these difficulties.

Robotic surgery is the most recent and advanced stage of this process, thanks to "micromecratronic" instruments introduced through traditional trocars. It is the resulting transformation of the minimally invasive surgical evolution.

R.G.C. Inderbitzi et al. (eds.), *Minimally Invasive Thoracic and Cardiac Surgery*,
DOI 10.1007/978-3-642-11861-6_12, © Springer-Verlag Berlin Heidelberg 2012

Currently different types of robotic devices are used in clinical practice [8–11].

However, the da Vinci™ Robotic System (*Intuitive Surgical, Inc., CA, US*) represents the only complete surgical system currently applied in a wide range of surgical procedures. Although there is a real difference between thoracic surgery and other surgical disciplines, an application in this field seemed realistic. In the last years, an increasing number of thoracic surgeons have been used the robot to perform a wide range of thoracic procedures ranging from simplest operations to complex ones such as lobectomies for treatment of non-small cell lung cancer (NSCLC) [12–20].

This chapter describes technical aspects, indications and surgical sequences of this new technique to perform robotic major lung resections for treatment of NSCLC patients.

12.1.1 Historical Notes

The early robot systems employed in surgery were relatively simple – programmed to handle the scope only or to maintain an endoscopic instrument in a fixed position during surgery.

In 1994, the US Food and Drug Administration (FDA) approved the first Automated Endoscopic System for Optimal Positioning (AESOP) arm to be used in laparoscopic surgery [21]. The device is controlled through voice activation to provide a flexible view of the surgical field. Around the same time, the TISKA Endoarm became available, and it could act as a camera guided by electromagnetic friction and could work as a tissue retractor [22]. While foot pedals were being replaced by voice-activated systems, other manufacturers were designing cameras that moved in synchrony with the movements of the surgeon's head. To combat dexterity problems, the master–slave telemanipulator concept was developed for medical use in the early 1990s. The first master–slave manipulator for medical use was developed at Stanford Research Institute by SRI International, a research and defence contractor in Palo Alto, California. The da Vinci Robotic Surgical System has been cleared by the FDA for laparoscopy, thoracoscopy and intracardiac mitral valve repair surgery. In parallel, the ZEUS Surgical System was developed and cleared for sale by the FDA for general and laparoscopic surgery. The two systems were similar, with some minor differences. However, after few years, Zeus was completed replaced by da Vinci System.

In 1995, Intuitive Surgical licensed the rights to patents from SRI, International Business Machines and the Massachusetts Institute of Technology and commenced work on a telerobotic system [23].

The da Vinci™ System creates an immersive operating environment for the surgeon by providing both high-quality stereo visualization and a man–machine interface that directly connects the surgeon's hands to the motion of the surgical tool tips inside the patient's body. The surgeon visualizes the stereoscopic images by a 3D display located above the hands, restoring hand-eye coordination and providing an intuitive correspondence with manipulations. Furthermore, the controller transforms the spatial motion of the instruments into the camera frame of reference, so that the surgeon feels as if his hands are inside the patient's body. The da Vinci system restores the degrees of freedom lost in conventional laparoscopy by placing a three DOF wrist inside the patient, enabling natural wrist pronation/supination and providing a total of seven DOF for control of the instrument tip (three orientation, three translation and grip). The system also uses its control system to filter out surgeon tremor, making the instrument tips steadier compared to the unassisted hand. Also, the system allows for variable motion scaling from each master (moved by surgeon's hands) to each slave. Since the first version (robot received FDA approval in 2000) the system has been modified, however, the master console and the slave robot mechanisms have remained essentially the same (the changes made relate only to their mechanical design).

Human robotic surgery was introduced by Cadiere's team in March 1997 [24]. A thoracic procedure was performed using a voice-controlled robot (ZeusTM, Computer Motion Inc.,

Goleta, CA, USA) [25, 26], and in the same period, a different robotic device was used by other surgical teams [27, 28].

Robotic pulmonary lobectomy was first performed in 2002 [13]. Subsequently, other centres confirmed that this technique is feasible and safe, although technical differences from various centres are reported [13–28].

12.2 Technique

12.2.1 Robot System in the Operating Room

The system employed to perform robot lobectomy (VRL) is the da Vinci™ Robotic System (*da Vinci, Intuitive Surgical, Sunnyvale, California*). This is a complete surgical robot which comprehends a master remote console, a computer controller and a four-arm surgical manipulator with fixed remote centre kinematics connected via electrical cables and optic fibres.

The master console (Fig. 12.1) is connected to a surgical manipulator with three instrument arms and a central arm to guide the endoscope. Two master handles at the surgeon's console are manipulated by the user. The position and the orientation of the surgeon's hands on the handles trigger highly sensitive motion sensors which transfer the surgeon's movements to the tip of the instrument at a remote location.

The surgical arm cart provides three degrees of freedom (pitch, yaw, insertion). Attached to the robot arm is the surgical instrument, the tip of which is provided by a mechanical cable-driven wrist (EndoWrist TM). This adds four more degrees of freedom (internal pitch, internal yaw, rotation and grip). To increase precision, the system uses downscaling from the motion of the handles to that of the surgical arms. In addition, unintended movements caused by human tremor are filtered by a 6-Hz motion filter.

This robotic device requires meticulous preparation in terms of set-up of the system and its placement at the operating table. The main body of the system (surgical cart) and the robotic arms are placed, in relation to the side of the lesion. Only when the surgical cart has been positioned appropriately and the patient placed in the chosen position can the robotic arms be brought into the operative field (Fig. 12.2).

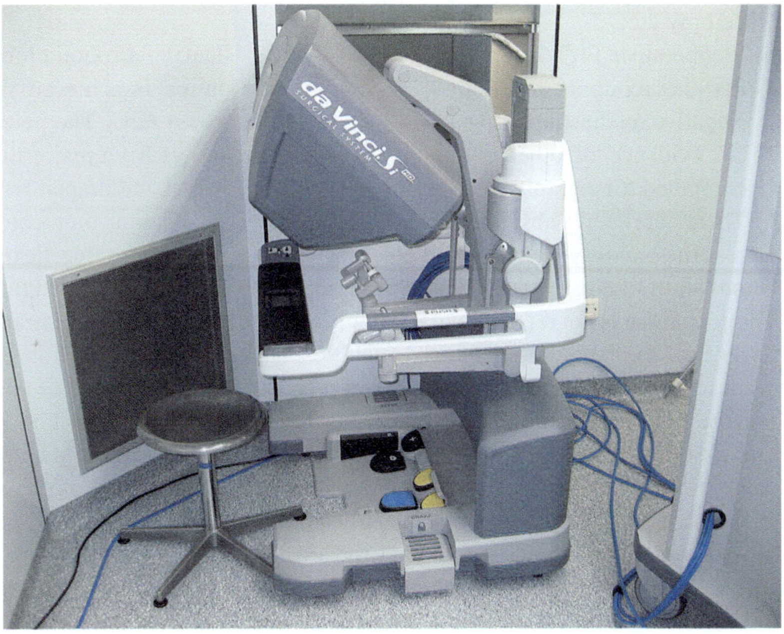

Fig. 12.1 Master console

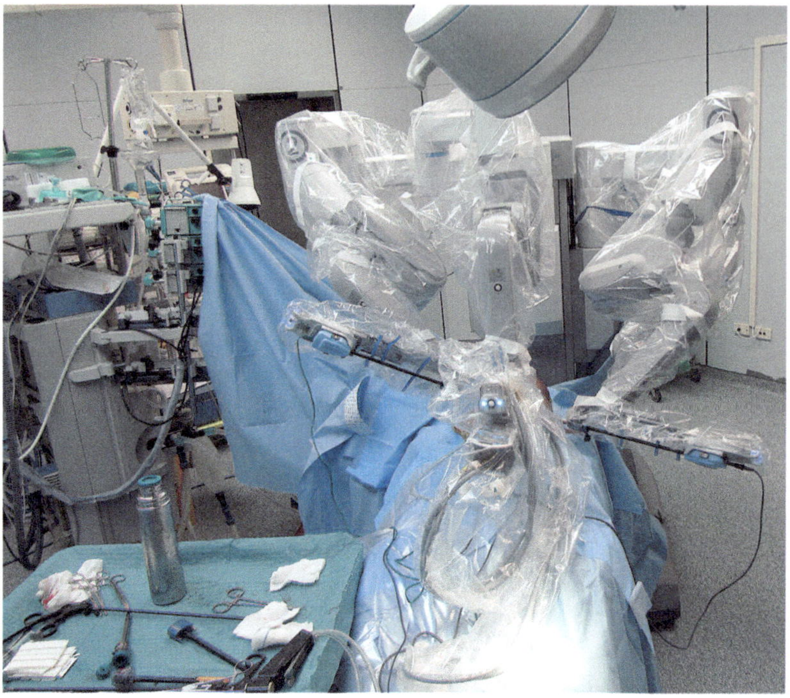

Fig. 12.2 Surgical cart

12.3 Robotic Lobectomy (RL)

12.3.1 Indications

Currently, the indications to perform a robotic lobectomy are:

- Preoperative T1/T 2, N0/N 1
- Peripheral pulmonary lesion
- Negative mediastinoscopy
- No evidence of other pulmonary lesions on computed tomography (CT) scan

There are few absolute contraindications. Except the inability to tolerate single-lung ventilation, all of them are anatomical considerations. This technique is not recommendable for tumours larger than 4 cm, not for technical difficulties, but because ribs have to be excessively spread to retrieve the specimen. Thick adhesion is not a real absolute contraindication. Once a space is created when the correct plane in the pleural space is entered, endoscopic adhesiolysis can proceed quickly and safely. Robot has the advantage over conventional thoracotomy in visualizing details the apex and base of the hemithorax with high resolution. Fused fissure is a technical challenge to robot surgery. However, with increased experience, successful lobectomy can be accomplished.

12.3.2 Anaesthesia and Positioning

During a robotic lobectomy, a single-lung ventilation is achieved via a double lumen endotracheal tube. The general standards of monitoring are as for a major thoracotomy. Patients are prepared and draped for a formal thoracotomy (posterolateral thoracotomy) (Fig. 12.3) with the operating table flexed at 30° at the level of the scapula tip so that the procedure can be converted in the event of intraoperative complications such as bleeding, or for technical reasons.

Insufflation of low pressure of carbon dioxide (CO_2 = 5–8 mmHg) into the pleural cavity can be useful to facilitate lung collapse and wash out intrapleural smoke.

12.3.3 Port Mapping

The location of the incisions is critical for the successful of the procedure. The best positioning

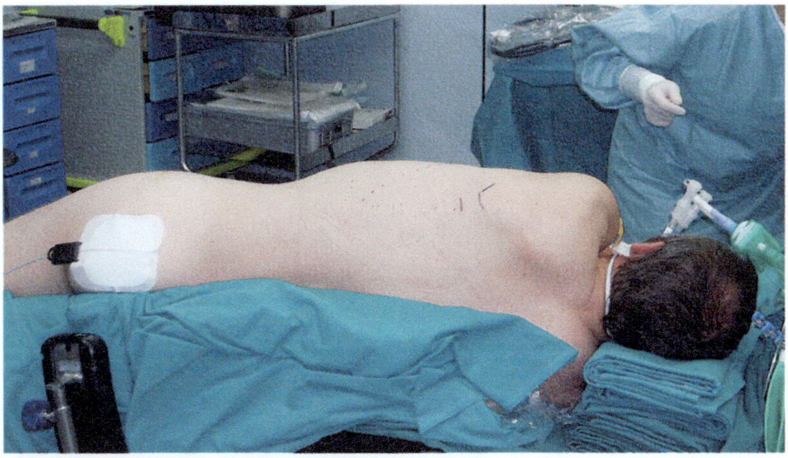

Fig. 12.3 Patient's position

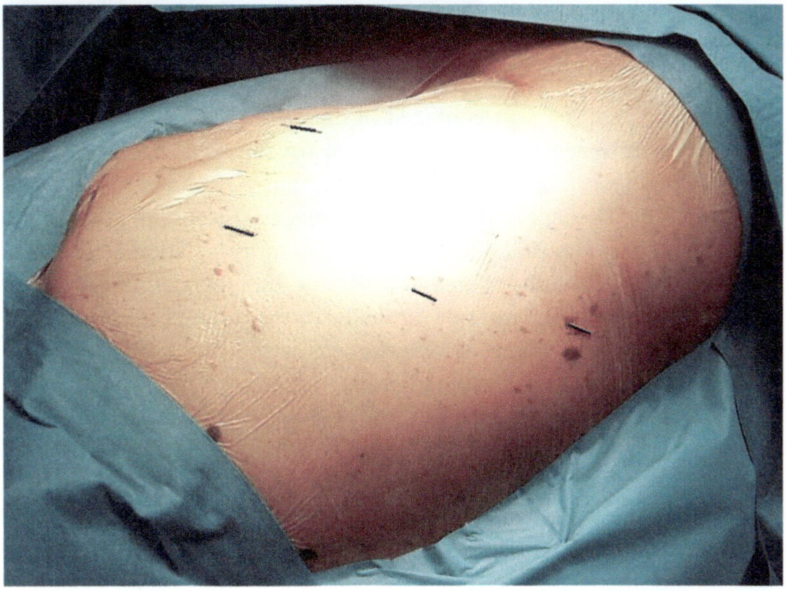

Fig. 12.4 Incision

of the main body (*surgical cart*) and arms is well established in relation to the site of the lesion in order to have an excellent, unobstructed view of the chest cavity without arm impingement and interference (Figs. 12.4 and 12.5). However, the exact position of the operating ports is best assessed during the operation when suitable points of entry in relation to the shape of each patient's chest cavity are made.

A video exploration prior to the operation could yield important information that would markedly alter the treatment strategy. If there is no contraindication to proceed, the da Vinci (surgical cart) is positioned at posterior, and the patient's head is brought into position from the posterior aspect of the patient, with the centre column at an approximately 45° angle with respect to the longitudinal axis of the patient. This is mandatory in order to avoid arm impingement.

A 30° scope angled down (generally preferred) is introduced through a 12-mm trocar and secured to the camera arm. The positioning of the instrument arms and the remaining access incisions are accomplished under direct vision.

Only when the robotic cart has been positioned appropriately and the patient placed in the chosen position, the robotic arms can be brought into the operative field. The standard layout is the same for right and left side.

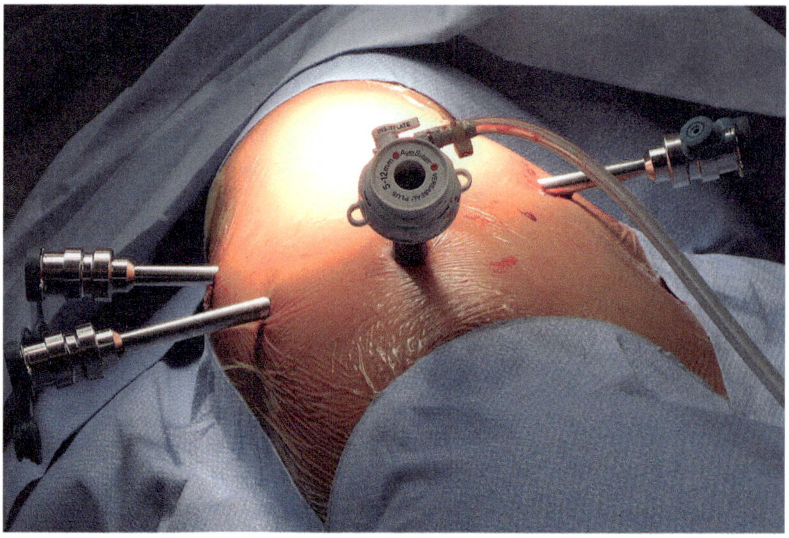

Fig. 12.5 Port mapping

Currently, the first port is placed in the 7th–8th intercostal space at mid-axillary line (over the mid to posterior axillary line), for the camera port (30° 3D scope). The others are placed in the 6th–7th intercostal space at post-axillary line and in the *auscultatory area* (usually for the 4th arm). The anterior incision is made in the 4th–5th intercostal space at anterior axillary line. However, this port mapping varies. Instead of the small anterior incision, a 'service entrance' can be made (16, 18, 20). This or an additional small incision can be a useful access for the assistant surgeon. Accessory conventional endoscopic instruments can be inserted and, in addition, facilitate later retrieval of the specimen.

12.3.4 Instruments

Currently, few robotic instruments are used:

- *Cadiere Forceps (Intuitive R, EndoWrist TM)*
- *Fenestrated Bipolar Forceps (Intuitive R, EndoWrist TM)*
- *Permanent Cautery Hook (Intuitive R, EndoWrist TM)*
- *Curved Scissors (Intuitive R, EndoWrist TM)*
- *Large Clip Applier (Intuitive R, EndoWrist TM)*
- *Endovascular Staplers*

12.3.5 Surgical Steps

Robotic lobectomy follows the standard surgical steps of open thoracic surgery and implies the isolation and resection of the vascular and bronchial hilar elements. This approach implies to dissect the hilar structures and control each in turn in an entirely analogous technique to an open procedure.

12.3.5.1 Hilum Dissection

The dissection is performed by using 1 or 2 Cadiere forceps and the permanent spatula or hook (preferably) attached to the electrocautery. Individual isolation of the hilar structures proceeds with dissection around the hilar vessels and bronchi performed through a combination of cautery and sharp and blunt dissection.

12.3.5.2 Arterial Phase

Dissecting around the pulmonary vessels is basically the same as in conventional open surgery.

When the fourth arm is available, a Cadiere forceps (EndoWrist) for lung retraction (through port 2), a Bipolar fenestrated forceps (EndoWrist) (through port 3) and a monopolar hook or Spatula-Endowers (through the utility incision) are used for the artery dissection. If the interlobar fissure is complete or nearly complete, the incision of the visceral pleura with electrocautery or blunt dissection with a pledget mounted on the Cadiere forceps allows the pulmonary artery to be easily identified. When the vessels are sufficiently dissected, two blunt-tipped Cadiere forceps are used to isolate the pulmonary artery. Then, a sling is passed. The dissection begins after vein isolation for upper and middle lobectomies; the arteries are isolated and often taken separately, for lower lobectomies. Thanks to the wrist instruments, the suture may be performed by using double-tie linen 2.5 or by vascular stapler introduced through the posterior access incision, when an upper or middle lobectomy is performed or through the anterior utility incision for the lower lobectomy. Innovative robotic clips are now available for pulmonary vessels (Hem-o-lok, WECK, TFX Medical, High Wycombe, UK). These clips may be delicately applied by the surgeon who can position the vascular clip with a safe and precise manoeuvre.

Currently all elements are isolated and surrounded with a sling. Usually all vessels are taken separately and resected by stapling or when particularly thin, managed by ligation (with linen 2.5 or silk) and secured with clips. In this case, the large clip applier (*Intuitive R*, *EndoWrist TM*) is particularly useful.

12.3.5.3 Vein Phase

Usually the surgical time sequence implies treating the vein as a second step. Vein isolation is generally performed with Cadiere forceps on the left arm and hook or spatula on the right arm. For lower lobectomies, the vein identification begins from the pulmonary ligament that is incised. For upper and middle lobectomies, a good exposure of the mediastinum is required to clear the vein from the surrounding tissues. Again, a sling is passed and a double tie (with linen 2.5 or silk) is placed to close the vessel; when necessary, an additional transfected suture can be added. When the vein wall is particularly thick, it is advisable to use a mechanical stapler. Another way of handling the vein is to place a vascular curved clamp through the utility incision and stitch it by using the robot Debakey forceps and a large needle holder (polypropylene monofilament 4/0). This is more difficult and not safe, considering that both the stapler and the clamp have to be placed by the assistant surgeon whose hand-eye orientation (bidimensional vision) is less precise compared with the surgeon who, at the console, has a different depth perception and optical resolution. Consequently, poor coordination between the surgeon and the assistant can jeopardize the success of the operation.

12.3.5.4 Bronchus Phase

The last step consists of dissecting the lobar bronchus so that lobar bronchial nodes can be completely removed with the specimen. A sling is used to encircle bronchus, which is subsequently stapled (Endopath ATB45 *Ethicon Endo-Surgery, INC*). This manoeuvre is necessarily performed by the assistant surgeon. This is the only possible way to resect and suture the bronchus. Although the robot wrists are able to simulate even fine physiologic movements, the surgeon cannot make a running stitch when dealing with the bronchus, because the robotic instruments in current use are too small to handle such a thick structure.

When feasible, the completion of the fissure is performed last, just before removing the specimen. Ultimately, the specimen is placed in a sterile plastic bag and removed through the utility incision without rib spearing. The bronchial stump is then tested under water for air leaks with 20 cm of positive airway pressure.

The bronchial stump is then tested under water for air leaks with 20 cm of positive airway pressure. Ultimately, the specimen is placed in a sterile plastic bag and removed through the anterior incision enlarged no more than 3 cm without rib spearing.

12.3.5.5 Lymph Node Sampling

At the end of the operation, all the accessible nodal stations are systematically sampled to ensure proper staging of the lung cancer. Currently, the lymph node samplings are made at stations that are more likely involved for tumour originating from a particular lobe (Naruke 1999) [29]. Right upper lobe (prevascular and tracheal N3 and lower paratracheal N4R), middle lobe (N3 and subcarinal N7), right lower lobe (N7), left upper lobe (sub aortic N5 and para-aortic N6), left lower lobe (N7). If a complete lymph node dissection is considered necessary, it should be done through a thoracotomy. Unlike VATS approach, there are no limitations regarding accurate lymph node sampling, given this is carried out at the end of the operation when a part of the lung has been removed. One chest drain, through the previous camera port, completes the operation.

12.4 Left Side Lobectomies

12.4.1 Technique

Usually the artery is dealt with before the vein and eventually the bronchus is resected. However, priorities are not strictly set. Frequently, as is the case of open thoracic surgery, due to surgical strategies, the ligature of the vein precedes that of the artery. In some cases, it is preferable to resect the bronchus before resecting the artery branch.

12.4.1.1 Left Upper Lobectomy

The lingular branches are first divided. The dissection continues up to the pulmonary artery so that the posterior, apical and anterior branches can be divided separately. In this phase the 4th arm which allows to obtain the right tension of the upper lobe is particularly helpful. The dissection proceeds on the anterior mediastinum in order to expose the superior vein which is divided. The bronchus can be cleared and resected easily.

Suggestions: When possible, it is recommendable to firstly manage the artery's branches in the fissure, then the vein, the bronchus and the apical artery.

12.4.1.2 Left Lower Lobectomy

The pulmonary ligament is incised and the pulmonary vein cleared and encircled by sling. The appropriate traction of the lung helps the surgeon to position the lobes so that the hilum and the vessels can be easily accessed. Currently, the apical and main-stem lower vessels are taken separately, surrounded with a sling. Usually they are tied with linen 2.5 or silk and secured by Ha-e-mo clips or divided by stapling through the anterior port. The vein is divided by stapling through the anterior incision.

The bronchus is the last element cleaned of surrounding tissue and divided by the mechanical stapler used by the assistant surgeon through the anterior port.

Suggestions: we recommend to decrease the CO_2 pressure during the vein phase to obtain the right plane of dissection.

12.5 Right Side Lobectomies

12.5.1 Technique

12.5.1.1 Right Upper Lobectomy

The upper lobe vein is cleaned and encircled with a sling which is ensured with a clip. The posterior segmental artery is divided and the upper lobe bronchus cleared and surrounded with a sling. The lobe is retracted forward and pulmonary artery cleaned to expose the apical and anterior segmental vessels, which can be dealt separately by legation or by stapling.

When all is ready, the vein is divided by stapling inserted through the posterior port (6th–7th at posterior axillary line), following the artery and finally the bronchus.

12.5.1.2 Right Lower Lobectomy

The pulmonary ligament is incised and the pulmonary vein cleared and encircled by sling.

The apical lower segmental artery and the main trunk are divided (by ligation or stapling trough the posterior incision). The lower lobe is retracted inferiorly, and the anterior portion of the oblique fissure between the middle and lower lobes is divided by stapler or by hook when the fissure is near complete. Finally, the lower bronchus is divided with care taken to preserve the middle lobe origin.

12.5.1.3 Middle Lobectomy

The oblique fissure between the middle and lower lobes is divided by stapler or by hook when it is near complete. The vein is exposed and cleared so that can be divided by ligation. The second step is to deal the bronchus that is resected by stapler. This allows the exposure of the artery that can be easily divided by ligation or stapling inserted through the posterior incision.

12.6 Personal Experience

Since February 2001, *372* patients (median age 56 years, range 19–81) were selected for various surgical robotic procedures ranging from the simplest operations, such as benign tumour enucleations and excisions, to very complex procedures, such as major lung resections. Robot lobectomy was performed in 181 (*87 M, 67 F; range 40–85*) (*mean age 63.5*) good-risk patients with cardiopulmonary function demonstrating an adequate pulmonary reserve (forced expiratory volume in 1 s O1.5 L) and arterial blood gases within normal limits. In accordance with protocols at that time, mediastinoscopy was not performed for small lesions without mediastinal lymphadenopathy identified on CT or PET scan. The patients were judged to have clinical stage I NSCLC (non-small cell lung cancer). In all patients, an anatomic major lung resection with lymphadenectomy was performed. Specific consent was obtained to attempt a robotic resection.

12.7 Results

In this highly selected group of patients, no technical operative mishaps related to manoeuvres of the instrument arms occurred. None of the patients had problems related to operative bleeding. Summarizing the results, a median of 22 lymph nodes were removed. Most of the series had adenocarcinoma (103 pts), and the most representative postoperative stage was stage I (147 pts: 103 IA and 39 IB) in a higher number of the cases. The other postoperative stages were stage II in 24 patients (15 IIA and 9IIB), stage III in 8 (4 stage IIIA and 4 stage IIIB) and IV in 2 pts.

In ten cases (9.4%), the procedure was converted to thoracotomy because of pleural adhesions in two patients and because of fused fissure in six. In two cases, the lobectomies were begun by isolating and stitching the transected lower vein with the robot. The operations had to be completed using the service entrance (enlarged by about 2 cm) because of hilar calcified lymph nodes, however, because these rendered the dissecting of the pulmonary artery unsafe. Ten patients had air leaks greater than seven postoperative days. In all patients, mechanical staplers were used to complete the fissure. There was one death on the twelfth postoperative day (not related to the surgical technique) because of pulmonary embolus. After an initial excellent postoperative recovery, the patient had acute kidney failure on the fourth postoperative day, which led to a worsening of the clinical condition.

Operative time (median operative time) was 215 min (range, between 130 and 250 min), of which 60 min was used to do the self-test of the machine and instrument set-up. Chest tubes were removed in mean 2.1 postoperative days (range, 2–28), and the patients were discharged in mean three postoperative days.

All patients were discharged in good condition and returned to preoperative levels of physical activity within 10 days of the operation.

12.8 Comments and Technical Considerations

As far as is known, few robotic lobectomies are performed; consequently, few surgeons have experience in this field (16–20). Currently, many of the limitations of robotics surgery are related to the imperfections of the system. At present, the greatest difficulties are associated with the available arm instruments, which are still not adequate for thoracic surgery. Consequently, some procedures become more complicated especially for the major lung resection. It is desirable that more devices, like the robotic stapler, be developed to permit the surgeon at the console to perform various phases of the procedure, increasing the safety and reducing the operative time.

Other limitations are system related. The surgeon does not receive information on the amount of force applied to tissue or sutures and therefore is dependent on visual feedback. This is sufficient in the majority of manoeuvres, but not when the surgeon wants to distinguish tissue characteristics. This poor tactility impairs surgeon's ability to judge the amount of tension applied during the manoeuvres of suture/legation tensioning [12].

Considering all these aspects, robotic procedures may be technically feasible but only in highly selected cases and in the hands of an experienced thoracic surgeon. Beside, adequate training is required for surgeons to acquire and master the new skills to improve surgical performance. Like the VATS, this new surgical technique should only be undertaken by surgeons trained in thoracic surgery. Moreover, a perfect knowledge of topographical anatomy and broad experience in conventional surgery and training in specific thoracoscopic skills, are required.

Nonetheless, we believe that many of the current limitations can be overcome in the near future and that, as the da Vinci System is improved and its instruments better adapted to thoracic surgery, their application will be extended to a wider range of operations.

References

1. Yim APC, Wan S, Lee TW, Arifi AA (2000) VATS lobectomy reduces cytokine responses compared with conventional surgery. Ann Thorac Surg 70:243–247
2. Walker WS, Leaver HA, Craig SR, Yap PL (2000) The immune response to surgery: conventional and VATS lobectomy. In: Yim APC, Hazelrigg SR, Izzat MB et al (eds) Minimal access cardiothoracic surgery. WB Saunders, Philadelphia, pp 152–167
3. Yamashita JI, Kurusu Y, Fujino N (2000) Detection of circulating tumor cells in patients with non-small cell lung cancer undergoing lobectomy by video-assisted thoracic surgery: a potential hazard for intraoperative hematogenous tumor cell dissemination. J Thorac Cardiovasc Surg 119:899–905
4. Nakajima J, Takamoto S, Kohno T, Ohtsuka T (2000) Costs of video thoracoscopic surgery versus open resection for patients with lung carcinoma. Cancer 89:2497–2501
5. Roberts JR, DeCamp MM, Mentzer MD, Sugarbaker DJ (1996) Prospective comparison of open and video assisted lobectomy. Chest 110:45S
6. Kirby TJ, Mack MJ, Landraneau RJ, Rice TW (1995) Lobectomy – video-assisted thoracic surgery versus muscle-sparing thoracotomy:a randomized trial. J Thorac Cardiovasc Surg 109:997–1002
7. Nomori H, Horio H, Naruke T, Suemasu K (2001) What is the advantage of a thoracoscopic lobectomy over a limited thoracotomy procedure for lung cancer surgery? Ann Thorac Surg 72:879–884
8. Hazelrigg SR, Mulder DS, Naunheim KS, Sugarbaker DJ (1993) Session IX: panel discussion on thoracoscopic lobectomy. Ann Thorac Surg 56:787–791
9. LaPietra A, Grossi EA, Derivaux CC, Applebaum RM, Hanjis CD, Ribakove GH, Galloway AC, Buttenheim PM, Steinberg BM, Culliford AT, Colvin SB (2000) Robotic-assisted instruments enhance minimally invasive mitral valve. Ann Thorac Surg 70:835–838
10. Rininsland HH (1993) Basics of robotics and manipulators in endoscopic surgery. Endosc Surg Allied Technol 1:154–159
11. Reichenspurner H, Damiano RJ, Mack M, Boehm DH, Gulbins H, Detter C, Meiser B, Ellgass R, Reichart B (1999) Use of the voice-controlled and computer-assisted surgical system ZEUS for endoscopic coronary artery bypass grafting. J Thorac Cardiovasc Surg 118:11–16
12. Okada S, Tanaba Y, Yamauchi H, Sato S (1998) Single-surgeon thoracoscopic surgery with a voice-controlled robot. Lancet 351:1249
13. Melfi FM, Menconi GF, Mariani AM, Angeletti CA (2002) Early experience with robotic technology for thoracoscopic surgery. Eur J Cardiothorac Surg 21:864–868
14. Okada S, Tanaba Y, Sugawara H, Yamauchi H, Ishimori S, Satoh S (2000) Thoracoscopic major lung resection for primary lung cancer by a single surgeon with a voice-controlled robot and an instrument retraction system. J Thorac Cardiovasc Surg 120:414–415
15. Morgan JA, Ginsburg ME, Sonett JR, Morales DLS, Kohmoto T, Gorenstein LA, Smith CR, Argenziano M (2003) Advanced thoracoscopic procedures are facilitated by computer-aided robotic technology. Eur J Cardiothorac Surg 23:883–887
16. Bodner J, Wykypiel H, Wetscher G, Schmid T (2004) First experiences with the da VinciTM operating robot in thoracic surgery. Eur J Cardiothorac Surg 25:844–851
17. Melfi FMA, Ambrogi MC, Lucchi M, Mussi A (2011) Video robotic lobectomy. MMCTS. doi:10.1510/mmcts.2004.000448. Available at: http://mmcts.ctsnetjounals.org/cgi/content/full/2005/0628/mmcts.2004.000448. Accessed 1 May 2011
18. Veronesi G, Galetta D, Maisonneuve P, Melfi F, Schmid RA, Born A et al (2010) Fourarm robotic lobectomy for the treatment of early-stage lung cancer. J Thorac Cardiovasc Surg 140:19–25
19. Park BJ, Melfi F, Mussi A, Maisonneuve P, Spaggiari L, Caetano Da Silva RK, Veronesi G (2012) Robotic lobectomy for non–small cell lung cancer (NSCLC): long-term oncologic results. J Thorac Cardiovasc Surg 143(2):383–389
20. Cerfolio RJ, Bryant AS, Skylizard L, Minnich DJ (2011) Initial consecutive experience of completely portal robotic pulmonary resection with 4 arms. J Thorac Cardiovasc Surg 142:740–746
21. Osmote K, Feussner H, Ungeheurer A, Arbter K, Wey GQ, Siewert JR (1999) Self-guided robotic camera control. Am J Surg 177:321–324

22. Schurr MO, Arezzo A, Neisius B et al (1999) Trocar and instrument positioning system TISKA: an assist device for endoscopic solo surgery. Surg Endosc 13: 528–531
23. Ballantyne GH, Moll F (2003) The da Vinci telerobotic surgical system: the virtual operative field and telepresence surgery. Surg Clin North Am 83:1293–1304, vii
24. Cadiere GB, Himpens J, Vertruyen M, Favretti F (1999) The world's first obesity surgery performed by a surgeon at a distance. Obes Surg 9:206–209
25. Vassiliades TA Jr, Nielsen JL (2000) Alternative approaches in off-pump redo coronary artery bypass grafting. Heart Surg Forum 3:203–206
26. Stephenson ER, Sankholkar S, Ducko CT, Damiano RJ (1998) Robotically assisted microsurgery for endoscopic coronary artery bypass grafting. Ann Thorac Surg 66:1064–1067
27. Loulmet D, Carpantier A, D'attelis N, Berrebi A, Cardon C, Ponzio O (1999) Endoscopic coronary artery bypass grafting with the aid of robotic assisted instruments. J Thor Cardiovasc Surg 118: 4–10
28. Falk V, Diegeler A, Walther T, Bannusch J, Autschbach R, Mohr FW (2000) Total endoscopic coronary artery bypass grafting. Eur J Cardiothorac Surg 17:38–45
29. Naruke T, Tsuchiya R, Kondo H, Nakayama H, Asamura H (1999) Lymph node sampling in lung cancer: how should it be done? Eur J Cardiothorac Surg 16:S17–S24

Minimally Invasive Robotic Assisted Sleeve Lobectomy

13

Thomas Schmid, Johannes Bodner
and Florian Augustin

Contents

T. Schmid, M.D. (✉) • J. Bodner, M.D.
F. Augustin, M.D.
Department of Visceral, Transplant and Thoracic Surgery, Innsbruck Medical University, Anichstrasse 35, A-6020 Innsbruck, Austria
e-mail: thomas.schmid@i-med.ac.at; johannes.bodner@i-med.ac.at; florian.augustin@i-med.ac.at

13.1 Introduction

Bronchoplastic procedures involve resections of the airway distal to the tracheal carina. Sleeve resections are the most common bronchoplastic procedures; it is a circumferential airway resection with end-to-end anastomosis of the remaining airways. The first successful bronchoplastic procedure was completed in 1947 [1]. It was introduced as alternative to pneumonectomy for patients with disease involving proximal bronchi and a decreased pulmonary reserve. Although initial indications for sleeve resections were for lung parenchyma-sparing purposes, sleeve lobectomy has become accepted for anatomically suitable tumors, regardless of pulmonary function [2].

As indications for thoracoscopic procedures are expanding to more complex operations, the first minimally invasive bronchoplastic operation was reported in 2002 [3, 4]. Even though benefits of a minimally invasive approach like shorter hospital stay, faster rehabilitation, less pain, etc., apply to a minimally invasive sleeve lobectomy, too, its application has been limited due to concerns about safety, technical feasibility, and oncologic equivalence to conventional open resections.

13.2 Indications

Sleeve lobectomy is most commonly indicated for benign or low-grade malignant neoplasms involving the main or lobar bronchi [2]. Low-

R.G.C. Inderbitzi et al. (eds.), *Minimally Invasive Thoracic and Cardiac Surgery*,
DOI 10.1007/978-3-642-11861-6_13, © Springer-Verlag Berlin Heidelberg 2012

grade neuroendocrine carcinomas of the lung, also called carcinoid tumors, account for more than 80% of these low-grade neoplasms.

13.3 Contraindications

Absolute contraindications include inability to tolerative single lung ventilation and patients with advanced lung cancer, specifically invasion to surrounding structures like the pericardium, superior vena cava, aortic arch, thoracic wall, etc. Even though nodal involvement (N1, N2) does not contraindicate a sleeve lobectomy, it may be difficult in a minimally invasive setting, and long-term outcome is impaired by systemic recurrences [2]. For minimally invasive sleeve lobectomies, all relative contraindications for a VATS lobectomy apply, too: previous surgery (VATS or thoracotomy), pleural adhesions, fused intralobar fissures and large tumors (diameter > 4 cm) [5].

13.4 VATS Versus Robotic Approach

Theoretically, the da Vinci Surgical System should be very helpful in performing a bronchial anastomosis. Its EndoWrist® instruments allow for 7° of freedom and human wrist-like movements; this is clearly its greatest potential improvement over straight instruments employed in conventional VATS procedures. Waseda et al. performed a controlled trial of airway reconstruction in rabbits in 2007 [6]. Bronchoplasty was performed by means of conventional VATS, robotically assisted or through an open approach. Regarding the time to perform an anastomosis, the robotic approach was significantly faster than the VATS approach. Anastomosis time did not differ between the robotic and open approaches.

13.5 Operative Technique

We performed a robotic assisted bronchoplastic procedure in a 30-year-old woman. A low-grade neuroendocrine carcinoma was diagnosed, occluding the orifice of her right upper lobe bronchus. We started off with a conventional VATS approach for hilar dissection, since operative time for a robotic lobectomy was longer than for a VATS approach in our own experience. Three incisions were created as for a regular VATS lobectomy: The first incision was created in the eighth intercostal space at the site of the posterior axillary line and is the site of the camera insertion. Under direct vision, the second incision (1.5 cm) was created below the inferior angle of the scapula, usually in the seventh intercostal space. For the anterior access incision (4.5 cm), the upper lobe vein was used as landmark; the incision was made exactly above the vein. The upper lobe vein, the arterial branches, and the fissure were divided using staplers. The upper lobe bronchus was then stapled distally to the tumor to gain more space for determining the borders of the bronchial sleeve resection. The lobe was removed through the anterior incision using an endobag. The bronchial sleeve containing the tumor was resected in the next step. The bronchus was cut distally with conventional scissors, introduced through the anterior access incision. This allowed for direct view on the tumor and facilitated the meticulous dissection of the subcarinal lymph nodes. Then the right main bronchus was transected completing the sleeve resection. Again, the specimen was removed in an endobag and sent for frozen section to confirm tumor-free margins. Subcarinal and mediastinal lymph node dissection was performed. For bronchial reanastomosis, the da Vinci robotic cart was approached to the patient from cephalad using the preexisting incisions to introduce the robotic instruments. An additional thoracocentesis was created at this point to introduce a suction device or clamps to retract stay sutures (Fig. 13.1).

The main bronchus was shaped with the robotic scissors (Figs. 13.2 and 13.3). The anastomosis was performed in a three-step fashion. As a first step, three interrupted stay sutures (Biosyn 3.0, Ethicon) were placed, one in the middle of the pars cartilaginea and the others at the two corners of the pars cartilaginea to the pars

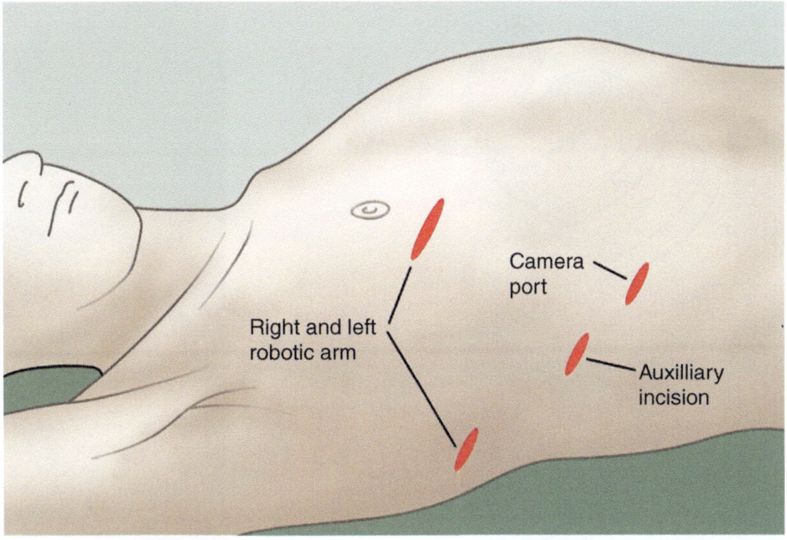

Fig. 13.1 Patient positioning and port placement

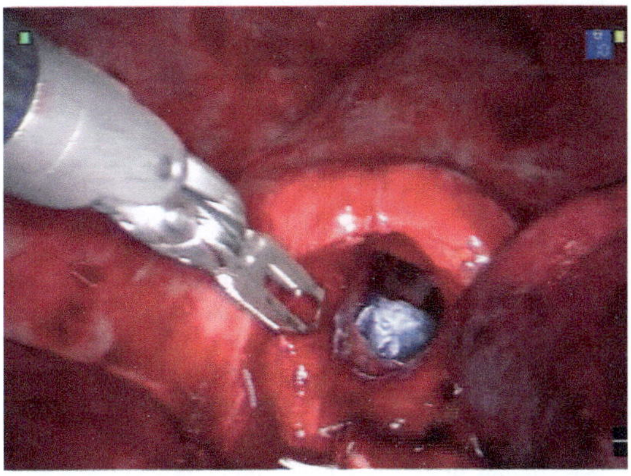

Fig. 13.2 Transected right main bronchus

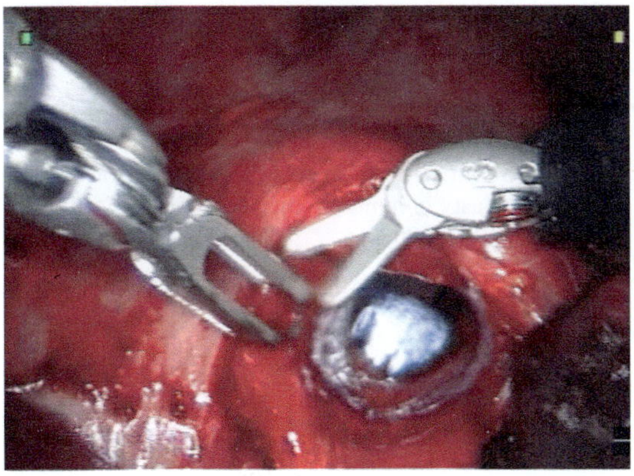

Fig. 13.3 Modelling of the right main bronchus

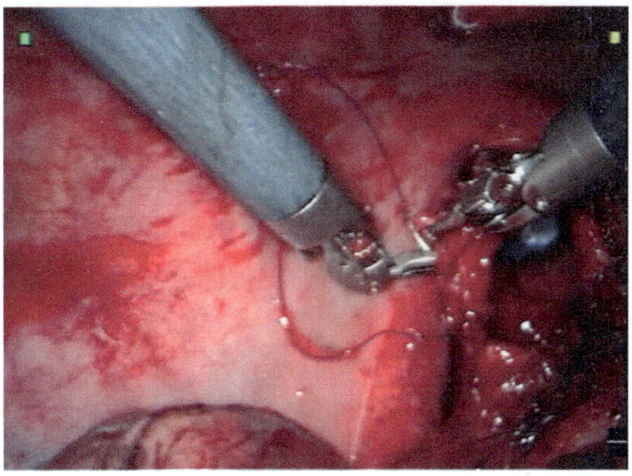

Fig. 13.4 Running suture for bronchial anastomosis

membranacea. Next, the anastomosis of the pars cartilaginea was completed with two running sutures (Fig. 13.4). These running sutures were kept loose until the stay sutures were tightened and fixed with clamps introduced through the anterior incision. The running suture for the pars membranacea was performed as a final step (Fig. 13.5).

The patient was extubated at the end of the procedure (Fig. 13.6). Postoperative course was without any major complication, and bronchoscopy 4 weeks after the procedure showed a patent anastomosis (Fig. 13.7).

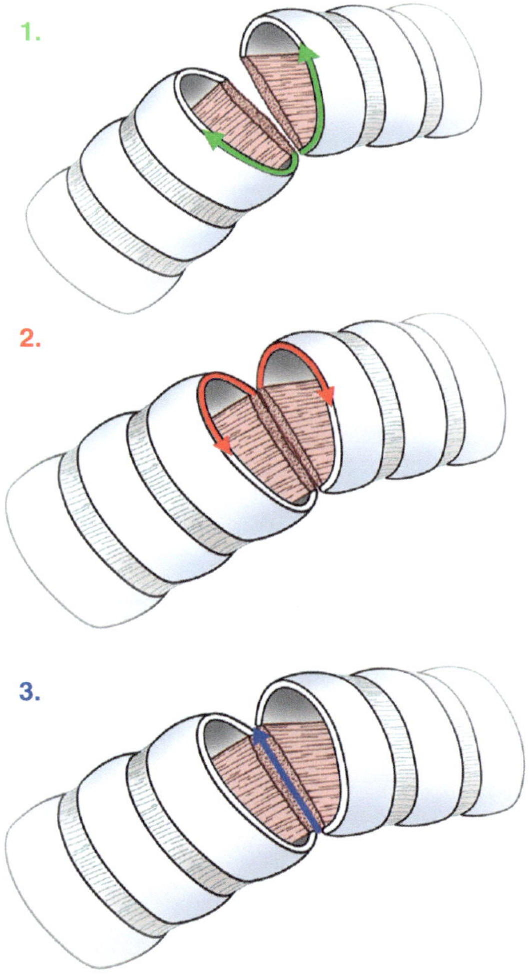

Fig. 13.5 Sequence of sutures to complete the anastomosis

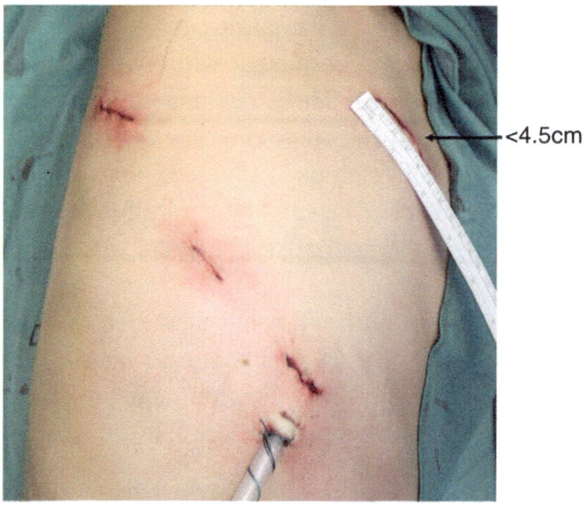

Fig. 13.6 Postoperative view of incisions

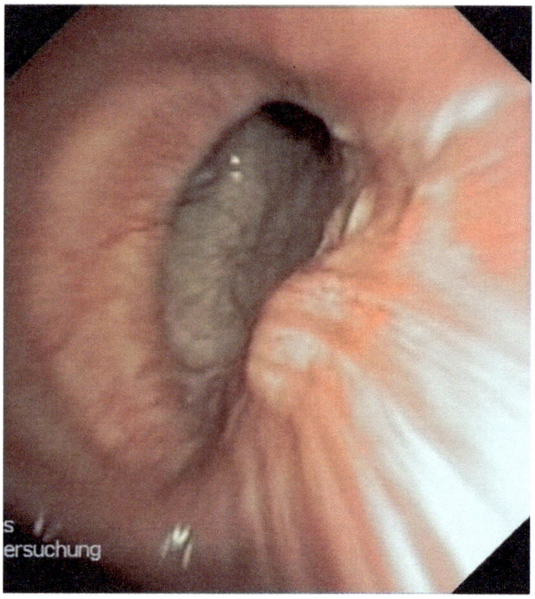

Fig. 13.7 Bronchoscopic view of the anastomosis 4 weeks after the procedure

References

1. Thomas CP (1956) Conservative resection of the bronchial tree. J R Coll Surg Edinb 1:169–186
2. Predina JD, Kunkala M, Aliperti LA et al (2010) Sleeve lobectomy: current indications and future directions. Ann Thorac Cardiovasc Surg 16:310–318
3. Santambrogio L, Cioffi U, De Simone M et al (2002) Video-assisted sleeve lobectomy for mucoepidermoid carcinoma of the left lower lobar bronchus: a case report. Chest 121:635–636
4. Nwogu CE, Yendamuri S, Demmy TL (2010) Does thoracoscopic pneumonectomy for lung cancer affect survival? Ann Thorac Surg 89:2102–2106
5. Yim AP (2002) VATS major pulmonary resection revisited – controversies, techniques, and results. Ann Thorac Surg 74:615–623
6. Waseda R, Ishikawa N, Oda M et al (2007) Robot-assisted endoscopic airway reconstruction in rabbits, with the aim to perform robot-assisted thoracoscopic bronchoplasty in human subjects. J Thorac Cardiovasc Surg 134:989–995

Robotically Assisted Pneumonectomy for Lung Cancer

14

Lorenzo Spaggiari, Giulia Veronesi,
and Ruy Fernando Kuenzer Caetano da Silva

Contents

L. Spaggiari, M.D. • G. Veronesi, M.D. (✉)
R.F.K.C. da Silva
Division of Thoracic Surgery, European Institute of Oncology, Via Ripamonti 435, 20141 Milan, Italy

Division of Thoracic Surgery, European Institute of Oncology, Via Ripamonti 435, 20100 Milan, Italy

Division of Thoracic Surgery, University of Milan School of Medicine, Milan, Italy
e-mail: lorenzo.spaggiari@ieo.it; giulia.veronesi@ieo.it; rfkcs@bol.com.br

14.1 Introduction

Minimally invasive surgery is becoming more popular. In the field of general thoracic surgery, muscle-sparing thoracotomy [1], VATS surgery [2, 3], and active limited resections [4, 5] have been introduced. A video-assisted thoracoscopic (VATS) lobectomy with mediastinal node dissection for primary lung cancer was first reported in 1995 by McKenna and associates [6]. Benefits in terms of analgesic requirements, chest pain, and reduced postoperative release of proinflammatory and anti-inflammatory cytokines compared with the open approach have been reported by different authors [7–9]. Although minimally invasive surgery certainly sounds good and its role in treating thoracic disease has grown, due to concerns of complete oncologic resection, technical difficulties, and safety, its use for treatment of lung cancer has proceeded cautiously.

In addition, the application of these techniques to larger resections such as pneumonectomy and chest wall or sleeve resections has been limited, owing to concerns about safety, technical feasibility, and oncologic equivalence to conventional, open resections. But there is a growing body of literature that suggests that more radical pulmonary resections can be safely accomplished by use of minimally invasive incisions [11–17].

However, thoracic surgeons seem reluctant to embrace video-assisted thoracic surgery (VATS) owing to the limited maneuverability and unsatisfactory ergonomic characteristic of the

R.G.C. Inderbitzi et al. (eds.), *Minimally Invasive Thoracic and Cardiac Surgery*,
DOI 10.1007/978-3-642-11861-6_14, © Springer-Verlag Berlin Heidelberg 2012

instruments, the limitations of the two-dimensional view of the operating field, and persisting controversy regarding oncologic efficacy [18, 19].

The da Vinci Robotic System (Intuitive Surgical, Inc, Mountain View, Calif) for thoracoscopic surgery overcomes many of the disadvantages of traditional VATS in that it has a superior range of motion and improved ergonomic characteristics, as well as offering three-dimensional visibility. In addition, surgeons appear to adapt quicker to the surgical robot, and the technology may provide a greater probability of oncologic radicality. This system includes a master remote console, a computer controller, and a three- to four-arm surgical manipulator with fixed remote center kinematics connected by electrical cables and optic fibers. At present, very few centers use the da Vinci System to treat lung cancer. Nevertheless, published early experience is encouraging, although the series were small and not compared with open procedures [20–23].

Robotic surgery in humans was first described by Cadiere and associates [24] in 1997. Today, the commonest indication for robotic thoracic oncology is resection of mediastinal masses [25], with relatively few publications on robotic lobectomy for lung cancer [19–25]. In this chapter, we describe the technique or robotic assisted pneumonectomy and discuss indications and results.

14.2 Indications

The indications for this procedure are quite narrow. Primary lesions or associated lymphadenopathy abutting a significant length of the main pulmonary artery necessitate a pneumonectomy for complete oncologic resection, when vascular reconstructions are not feasible. Selected patients with synchronous ipsilateral upper and lower lobe malignancies or isolated tumors extending into multiple lobes are also appropriate candidates when diameter is less than 5–6 cm.

Lesions with extensive chest wall or mediastinal invasion are probably unsuitable for minimally invasive pneumonectomy; however, endoscopic rib cutters (Sofamor Danek, Medtronic Corp, Minneapolis, MN) allow limited en bloc resections.

A safe resection mandates full visualization and control of the proximal hilar vessels. Lesions larger than 5 cm may be difficult to extract through a small incision without significant rib spreading, although tumors have a wide range of compressibility. Thus, the value of minimally invasive pneumonectomy in such cases is unclear and requires careful judgment before undertaking.

14.3 Surgical Technique

14.3.1 Anesthesia, Patient Positioning, and Port Placement

The single-lung anesthesia is achieved via a double lumen endotracheal tube. Operative setup is comparable to management of robotic lobectomy; a central venous access and invasive blood pressure control are installed. The patient is positioned in a lateral decubitus with the arms in front of the patient and flexion of the thoracic part of spine in order to stretch the thoracic cage of the upper side (Fig. 14.1). Patient is draped in a standard way. If conversion to open surgery is required without urgency, the arm is moved up and lateral muscle-sparing thoracotomy is performed. The robot cart is positioned at the head of the patient, slightly posteriorly, with the console in the same or separate operating room (Fig. 14.2).

The camera port is introduced in the seventh intercostal space at the midaxillary line after exclusion of the lung by the anesthetist. Exploration of the pleural cavity is performed to evaluate adhesions, pleural or parenchyma nodules, degree of lung exclusion, and any other possible contraindication to surgical resection. Under vision, a 4-cm utility incision is performed at the level of the superior vein, usually in the fourth intercostal space anteriorly (Fig. 14.3) trying to follow the mammary sulcus. No rib spreading is performed. A skin retractor (Weitlaner – 16.5 cm) allows to separate soft tissue (anterior serratus muscle and subcutaneous tissue) and favor

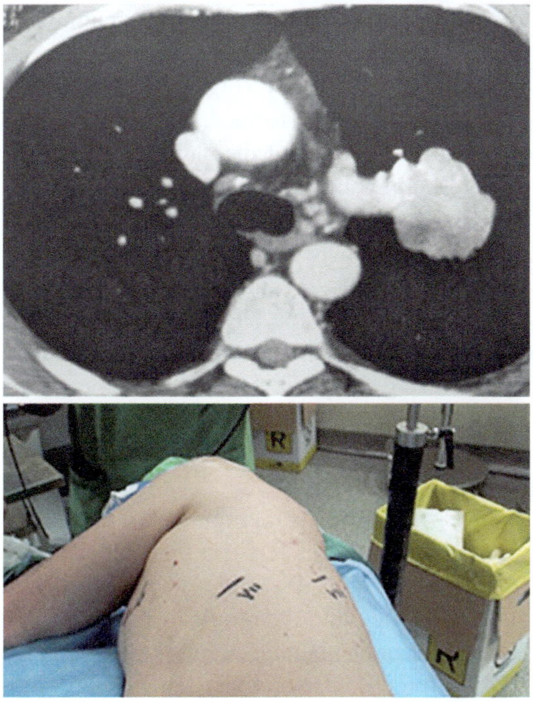

Fig. 14.1 Patient position in a lateral decubitus. CT scan with lesion involving left pulmonary artery

instrument insertion in the utility incision. Two other 7-mm ports are placed in the 8th–9th intercostal space 1–3 cm anteriorly the tip of the scapula and in the seventh intercostal space 3 cm posteriorly the tip of the scapula.

The robot is docked. The port for the anterior robotic arm is usually inserted under vision at one edge of the utility incision after docking the robotic arm with the port. The camera is introduced, and the robotic instruments are inserted under vision.

The hook cautery is manipulated by the right arm of the robot introduced through the utility thoracotomy for right side dissections or through the posterior trocar in the eighth intercostal space for left side procedures. One Cadiere forceps is manipulated by the fourth robotic arm to retract the lung and expose structures. The other Cadiere is manipulated by the left arm of the robot and used to grip structures during dissection: it is introduced through the utility incision for left side procedures or through the posterior trocar in the eighth intercostal space for right side cases.

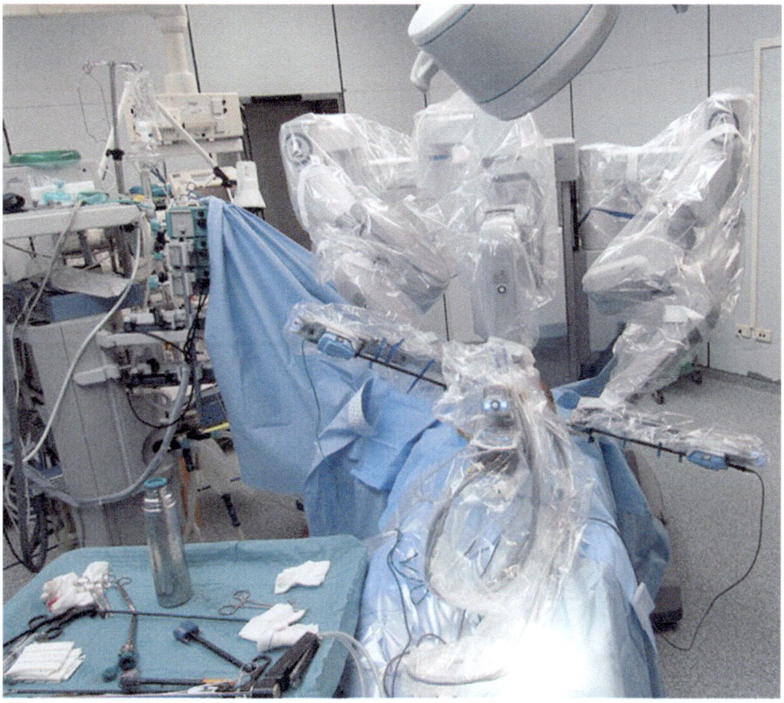

Fig. 14.2 Positioned patient together with robotic equipment in the operating room disposed for robotic anatomic resection

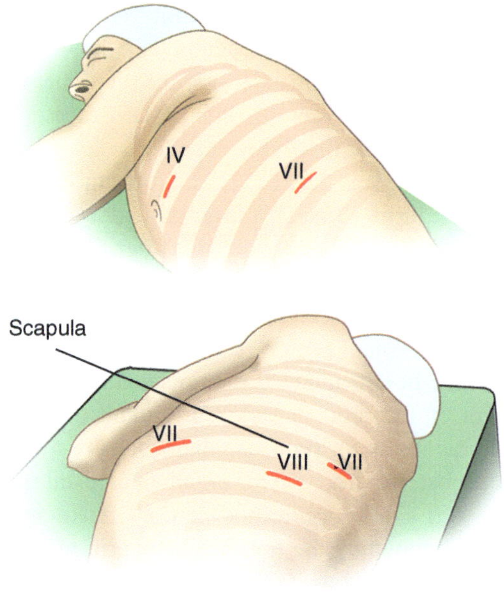

Fig. 14.3 Incisions for left robotic pneumonectomy

14.3.2 Left Pneumonectomy

14.3.2.1 The Veins

At the left side, the camera port is positioned 2 cm posteriorly compared with right side to avoid the heart obscure the vision of hilar structures. The dissection starts with vein isolation. The lung is retracted upward, and the ligament is put in tension (Fig. 14.4). The lower ligament is resected with the hook cautery. The inferior vein is surrounded with a vessel loop for stapler introduction. To better complete this maneuver, a third Cadiere forceps is usually inserted instead of the hook trough the utility incision. The vein is sectioned with Endogia vascular cartridge inserted through the utility incision, after removal of the robotic arm (Fig. 14.5). The upper vein is prepared with the hook cautery and the Cadiere forceps with the lung retracted posteriorly to expose the hilar structure (Fig. 14.6). The vessel is encircled and transacted with the endostapler introduced trough the posterior trocar incision after removal of the robotic arm.

14.3.2.2 The Artery

Once the pulmonary veins have been divided, the main artery is easily visualized (Fig. 14.6b). Lymph node dissection of the aortopulmonary window station is performed to complete liberation of the main artery (Fig. 14.7). Dissection of the artery is performed, incising the tissue with the hook until the entire artery can be seen. Manipulation of the 30° scope allows visualization of the superior aspect of the hilum and the junction between artery and bronchus (Fig. 14.8).

The isolation of the left pulmonary artery is performed with the hook cautery and the Cadiere by dissecting the plane with the main bronchus. The artery can be encircled using the monofilament suture as a guide and a third Cadiere forceps to pass the suture. The stapling device is introduced by the posterior trocar after removal of the robotic arm, and it is passed between the artery and the bronchus and fired. We prefer to use articulated staplers as they allow more flexibility. The lung retraction can be maintained by a grasper and the Cadiere forceps introduced trough the fourth posterior robotic arm.

14.3.2.3 The Bronchus

The bronchus is isolated last. Lymph nodes are removed from subcarinal station retracting the lung anteriorly and exposing the posterior mediastinum. Mediastinal pleura is incised, and the posterior aspect of the main bronchus is dissected and isolated, paying attention to avoid devascularization. Lymph nodes of the tracheobronchial angle are removed following the same steps of open surgery.

The nodes of the subcarinal station are removed after resection of the pulmonary ligament and retraction of the lung toward the anterior mediastinum to expose the posterior mediastinum. Bronchial arteries could usually be avoided, thanks to the good visibility, otherwise they are simply coagulated or clipped.

When the bronchus is ready to be surrounded, the hook is substituted with a Cadiere (Fig. 14.9). The stapler is introduced through the posterior thoracoscopic port by the assistant surgeon after removal of a robotic arm. The green cartridge of 45 mm should be an adequate length.

The lung is extracted through the anterior utility incision of 4–5 cm with no rib spreading using an

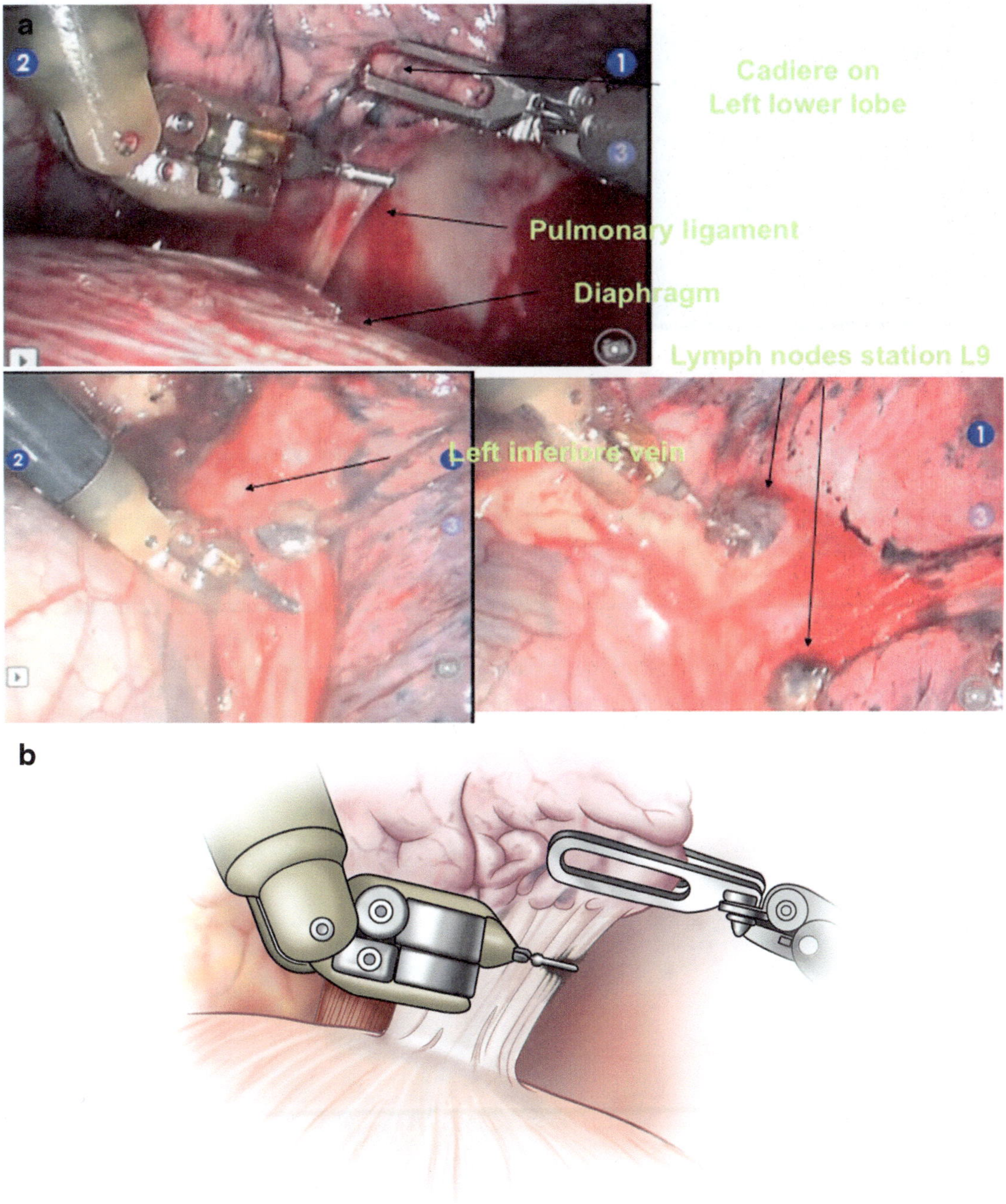

Fig. 14.4 (**a**) Operation field: section of pulmonary ligament, extirpation of lymph node ATS 8. (**b**) Transection of pulmonary ligament

EndoCatch (Autosuture, Covidien) (Fig. 14.10). One 28F (Tyco Healthcare, Switzerland) pleural drain is positioned at the end of the operation in the port of the camera.

14.3.3 Right Pneumonectomy

The steps of the right pneumonectomy do not differ from the contralateral procedure.

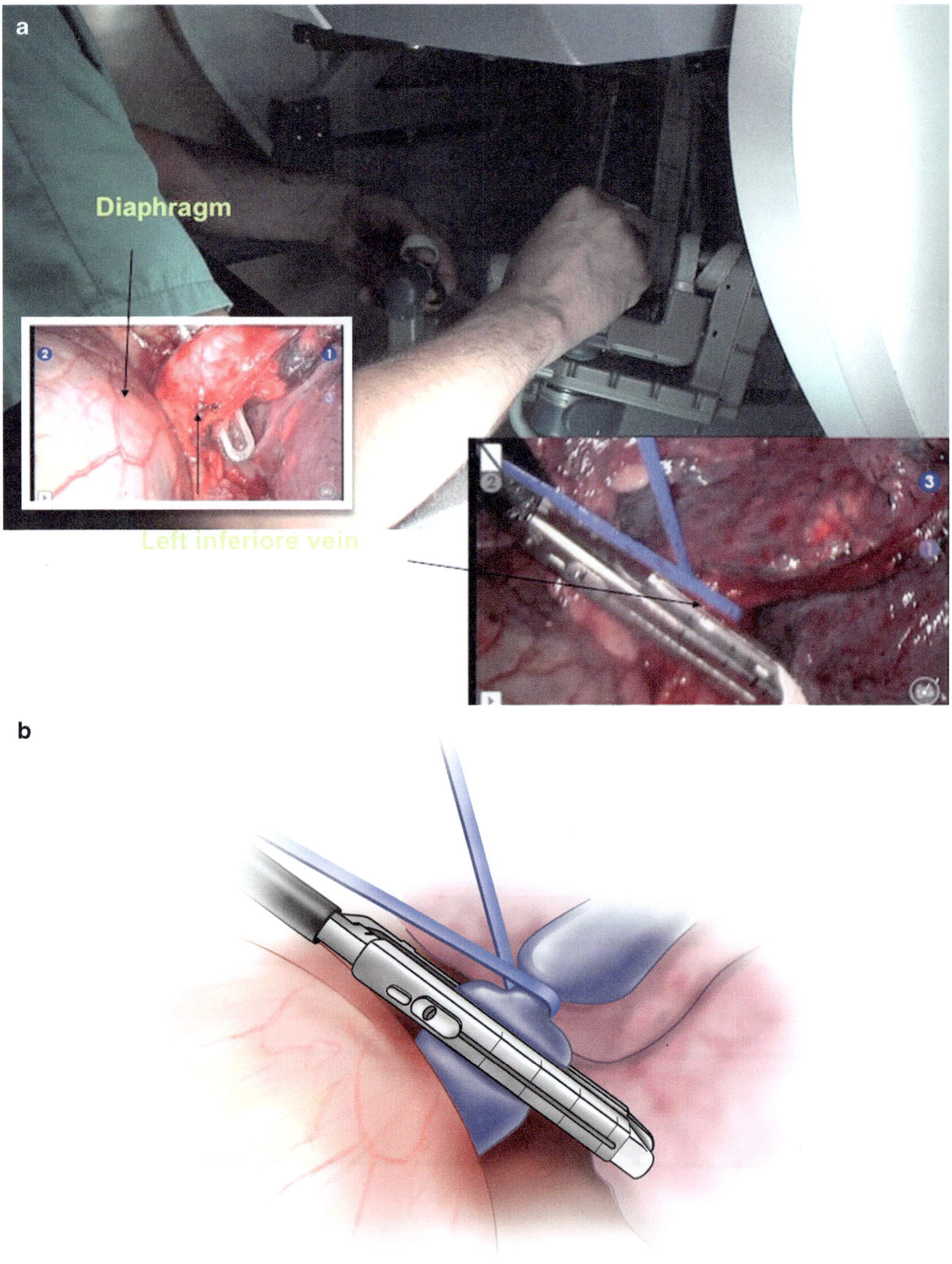

Fig. 14.5 (**a**) Operative field: preparation and cutting of inferior pulmonary vein. (**b**) Schematic: cutting of inferior pulmonary vein by stapler.

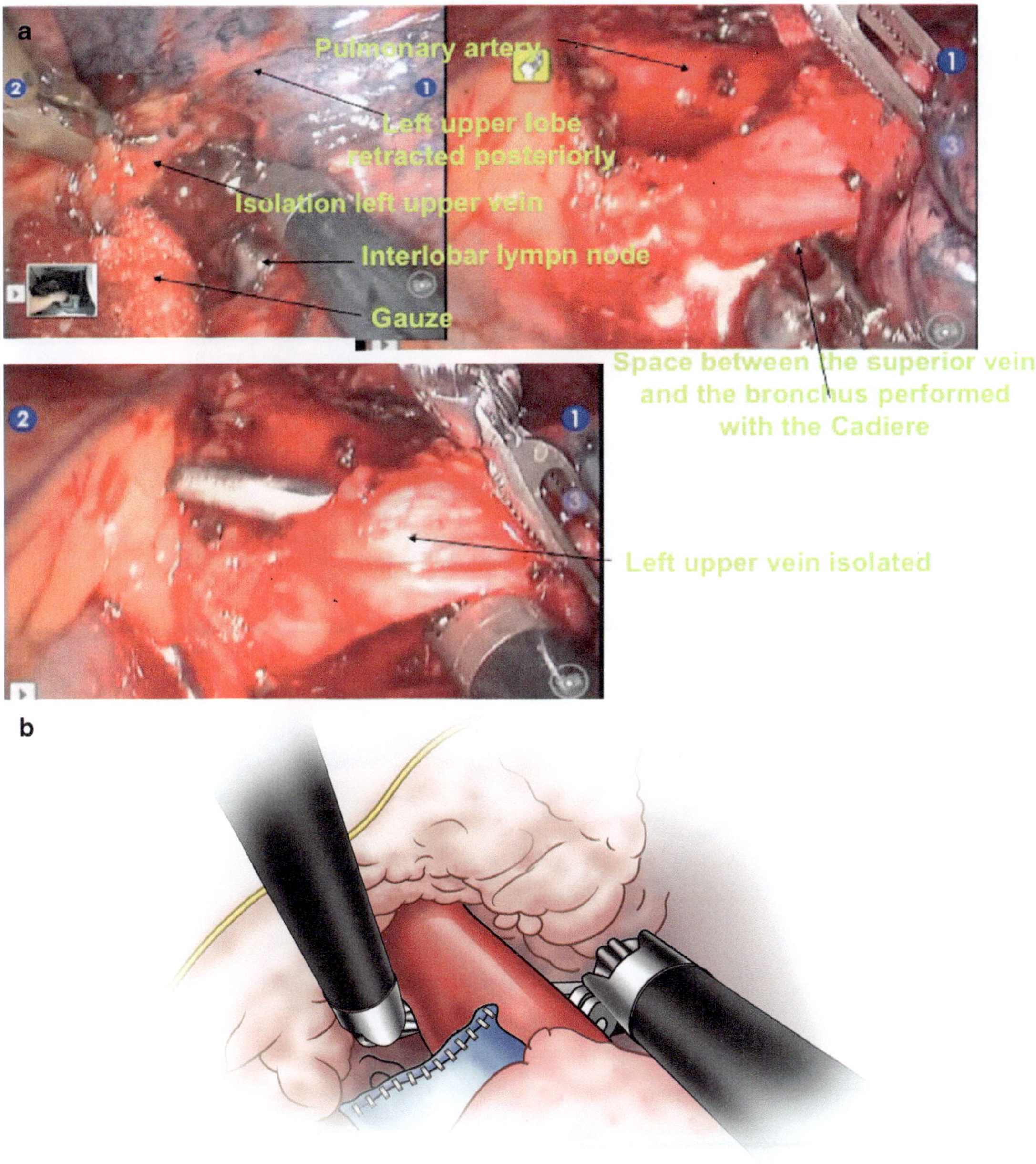

Fig. 14.6 (**a**) Isolation and section of the left upper vein during a robotic pneumonectomy. (**b**) Schematic: robotic aspect of left main artery after transecting of upper pulmonary vein

The dissection starts with the vein isolation using the Cautery hook introduced through the utility incision for the right hand, two Cadiere forceps through 8th intercostal space and through the 7th intercostal space by the fourth arm to retract the lung for better exposure. If phrenic nerve is attached to hilar structures, we use Maryland bipolar forceps instead the Cautery hook to dissect the tissue around the superior vein. After the pulmonary ligament is dissected, the inferior vein is isolated and sectioned with endostapler introduced through the utility incision. The superior

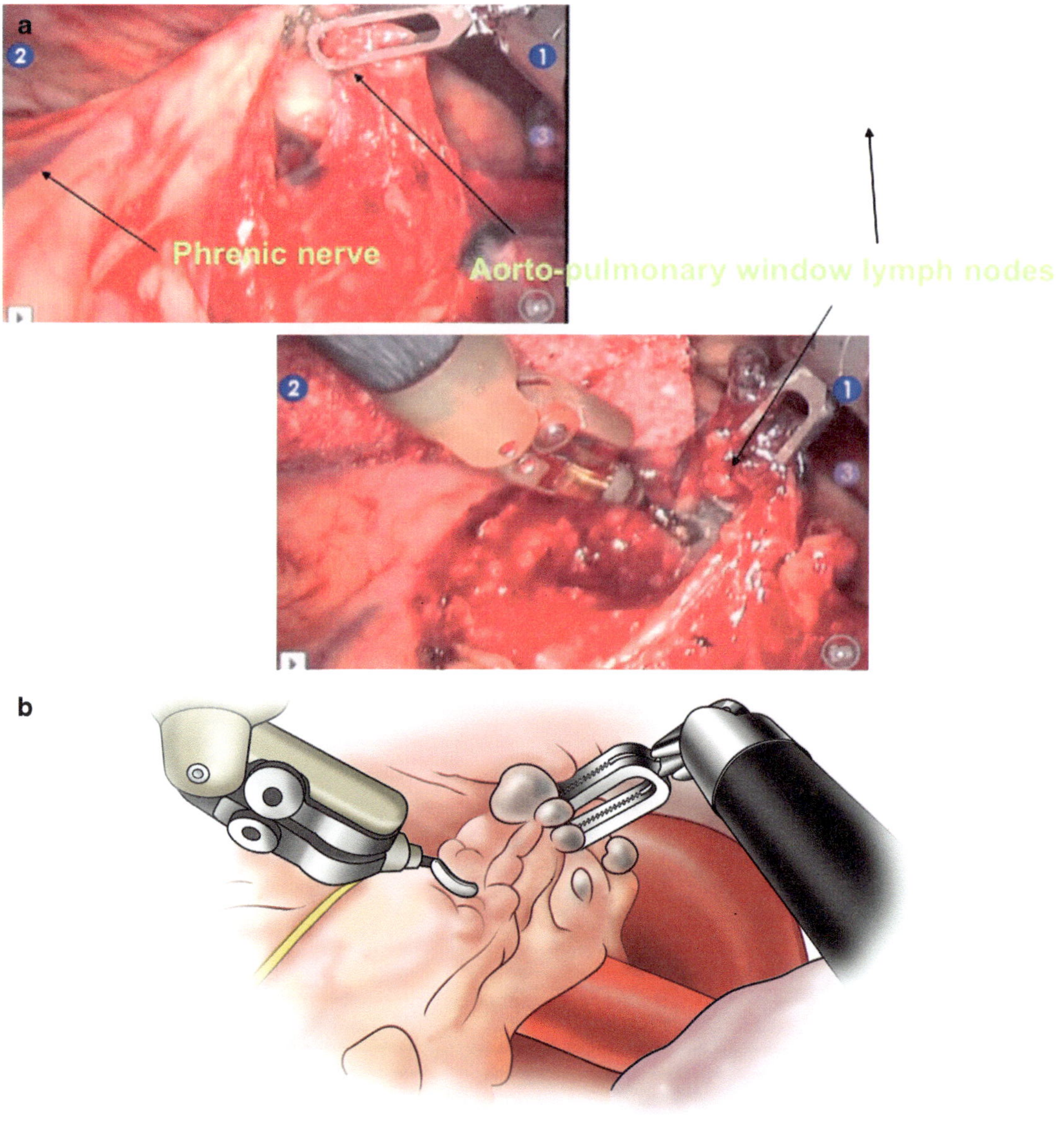

Fig. 14.7 (**a**) Operative field: dissection of aortopulmonary lymph node (ATS 5). (**b**) Schematic: dissection of aortopulmonary lymph node (ATS 5)

vein is then isolated and resected with the same technique with the stapler introduced through the posterior port in the 8th intercostal space. The conjunction of the truncus arteriosus and the main artery is isolated, and hilar lymph station 10 removed if present. Once the artery is freed by sharp and blunt dissection, it is encircled and resected with endostapler introduced through the 8th intercostal space posterior port.

The right main bronchus is prepared and the lung retracted with the Cadiere to introduce and fire the endostapler in the proximal part of the bronchus next to the carina.

The operation is completed with the dissection of paratracheal lymph node stations R2 and R4. The mediastinal pleura between the superior vena cava and the azygos vein is incised. The lymph nodes, together with the fatty soft tissue of

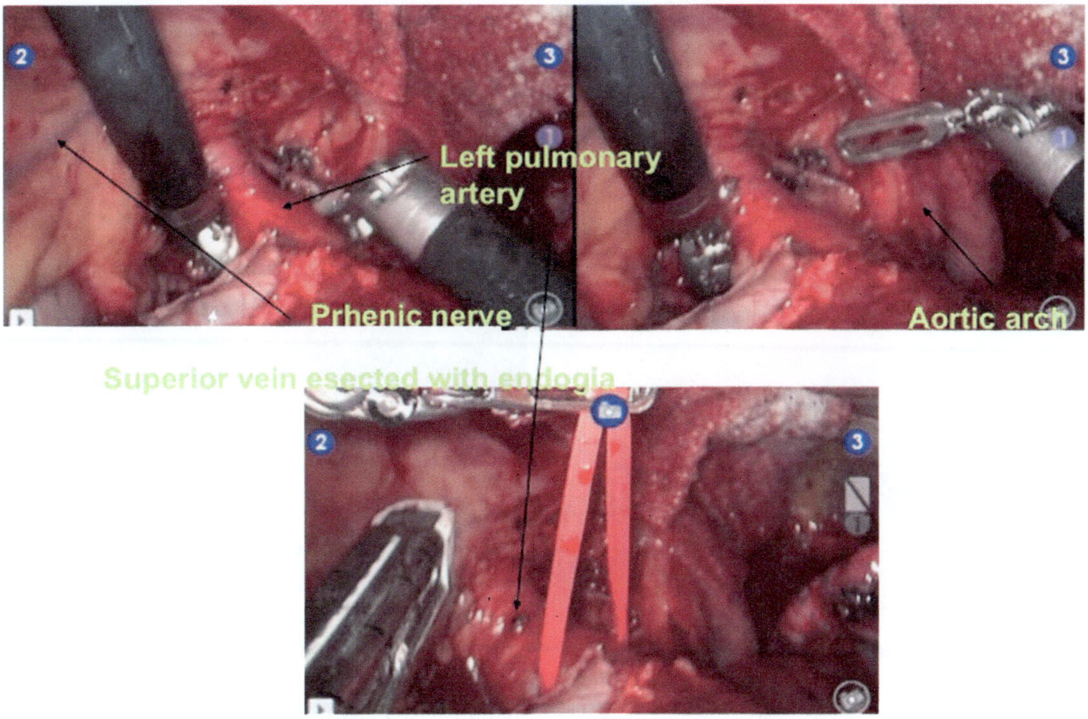

Fig. 14.8 Operative field: robotic preparation of left main pulmonary artery

the region of Barety, are removed en bloc using the hook and a Cadiere. Sometimes a PK system or ultracision is used in patients with large quantities of mediastinal fat to reduce bleeding and lymphatic leakage. Fibrin sealant (Tissucol, Baxter, Italy) is applied to lymphadenectomy sites to reduce lymphorrhea, to the bronchial stump, and lymph node station after dissection.

14.4 Results and Discussion

Numerous advances in surgical techniques and video instrumentation have enabled minimally invasive pneumonectomy. Recent studies have reported on the feasibility and safety of minimally invasive oncologic operations compared with conventional thoracotomy for early-stage lung cancer [26]. Benefits have included shorter hospital stay [27], decreased pain [8, 9, 28, 29], decreased blood loss [30], earlier return to normal activities, tolerance of adjuvant chemotherapy [31, 32], and improved quality of life [33, 34].

Some authors have reported improved patient survival after thoracoscopic lobectomies compared with similar procedures through thoracotomy [7, 35–39]. Immunologic mechanisms may account for this putative improved survival [10, 27, 36], and this has been explained by the reduced immunosuppression from the minimally invasive approach. It could improve a patient's ability to scavenge residual tumor cells or cells shed at the time of resection from tumor manipulation [35]. It has also been reported that numbers of circulating natural killer and T cells, T-cell oxidative activity, and levels of immunochemokines such as insulin-like growth factor-binding protein-3 are higher after VATS than after thoracotomy [36]. Furthermore, by postoperative day 7, NK cell numbers were found to be significantly higher following VATS lobectomy compared to the open approach, suggesting that minimally invasive surgery is associated with a quicker NK cell recovery than conventional thoracotomy [40, 41]. In the context of lung tumor surgery, less suppressed cellular immunity during the early

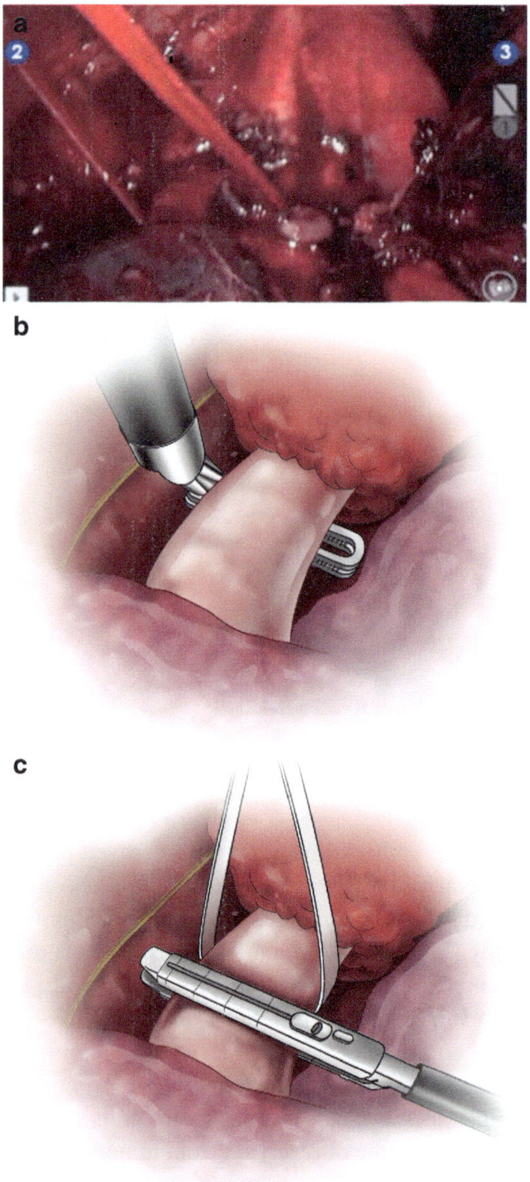

Fig. 14.9 (**a**) Intraoperative view on left main bronchus neighbored to aortic arch. (**b**, **c**) Schematic: preparing, looping, and transecting of left main bronchus

postoperative period may confer a lower predisposition to tumor growth and recurrence.

However, it should be noted that this apparent survival advantage has not been consistently demonstrated [30, 42].

There are still questions about whether the use of thoracoscopic surgery can be expanded to the

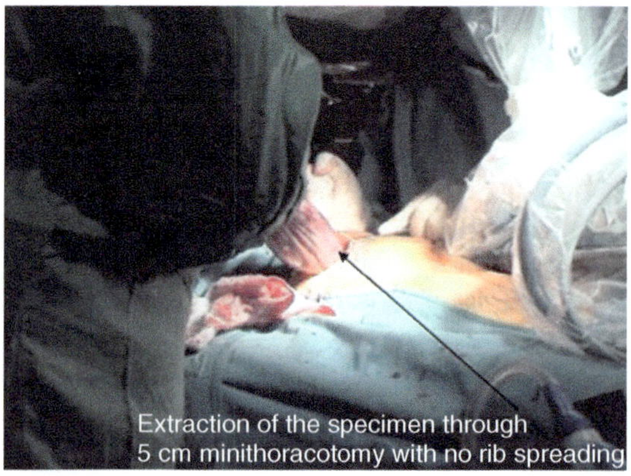

Fig. 14.10 Extraction of the lung through the anterior utility incision of 5 cm with no rib spreading

treatment of more advanced disease, such as lung cancer requiring a pneumonectomy. Minimally invasive pneumonectomy is performed rarely and only in very selected centers, some case reports of thoracoscopic pneumonectomies for malignant disease exist in the literature [16, 43–45], or small series for a single surgeon are often included with lobectomy results [46] or less frequently in a separate setting [11–13].

There are no reports of intraoperative complications of VATS pneumonectomy, and only one case of conversion to open surgery to facilitate a bronchoplastic procedure is described [16]. It is unknown whether intraoperative conversion leads to an adverse short-term or long-term disadvantage compared with patients whose initial planned operation was through an open thoracotomy.

Lesions with extensive chest wall or mediastinal invasion are probably unsuitable for minimally invasive pneumonectomy; however, endoscopic rib cutters (Sofamor Danek, Medtronic Corp, Minneapolis, MN) allow limited en bloc resections. A safe resection mandates full visualization and control of the proximal hilar vessels. Lesions larger than 5 cm may be difficult to extract through a small incision without significant rib spreading, although tumors have a wide range of compressibility. Thus, the value of VATS pneumonectomy in such cases is unclear and requires careful judgment before undertaking.

Thoracoscopic procedures can attain benefit in selected patients with lung cancer, but they are uncomfortable and difficult (long learning curves) for the surgeon, with visual information limited to two dimensions, and instruments having restricted maneuverability mainly because of the rigid axes that are fixed to the thoracic wall by the entry trocar [22, 47]. The advanced engineering embodied in the da Vinci System has now made it possible to overcome many of these disadvantages, without compromising oncologic radicality or patient safety. Robotic surgery for thoracic disease is therefore likely to become widespread, provided that the high costs of the early robotic systems can be significantly reduced.

The system is designed so that the surgeon's tremor can be compensated on the end-effector motion through appropriate hardware and software filters. Moreover, this robotic system eliminates the fulcrum effect, making instrument manipulation more intuitive. These technology proponents underscore greater technical ease owing to the advantages of a stable camera platform, the elimination of tremor, and instrumentation that provides motion with seven degrees of freedom.

A further advantage is the surgeon's ability directly to control a stable visual field with increased magnification and maneuverability. All of this creates images with increased resolution that, combined with the increased degrees of freedom and enhanced dexterity, greatly enhances the surgeon's ability to identify and dissect anatomic structures [21].

The disadvantages include the lack of tactile feedback, the requirement of another surgeon experienced in VATS, because the assistant has to place the endoscopic staplers under bidimensional vision and the operating surgeon is seated at the console, away from the patient, and increased nursing support. In addition, the robotic arms must be continuously removed to allow stapling of structures during the venous, arterial, bronchial, and fissural phases of the procedure. Another disadvantage is the size of this system. This is an important disadvantage in today's already crowded operating rooms [21]. Moreover, one of the potential disadvantages identified is a lack of compatible instruments and equipment. Lack of certain instruments increases reliance on tableside assistants to perform part of the surgical operation [21].

One of the most important differences in the robotic technique compared with VATS is that it requires the surgeon to abandon the operating table and sit at a control console, so that all tactile feedback is lost, and a new set of manual and eye-hand coordination skills must be acquired [22].

According to Park et al., the current data suggest that robotic-assisted VATS resection is feasible but unlikely to be universally adopted unless significant technologic advancements are made that make it more suitable [20]. During these last few years, new robotic clips for vessels (Hem-o-lok) were developed making some procedures safer and more straightforward, above all pulmonary resections. It is desirable that more robotic devices, like the robotic stapler, were already developed to permit the surgeon at the console to perform every phase of the procedure, increasing the safety of the procedure and reducing the operative time.

We believe indications to lung cancer surgery may expand in the near future to patients with cardiologic comorbidities and those who have been pretreated. However, patients with functional impairment seem at increased risk of postoperative acute respiratory distress syndrome [48], probably in relation to the long duration of the operation during which operated lung is excluded from ventilation.

As it has been shown in many minimally invasive procedures, there is definitely a learning curve with thoracoscopic lobectomy and pneumonectomy [49, 50]. We believe the progression to robotic pneumonectomy is a natural next step once the thoracic surgeon reaches the point on the learning curve where the majority of patients requiring lobectomy can expect a robotic approach without conversion. At this point, the same skills developed for difficult dissections and management of modest bleeding without conversion can be used for tumors that require pneumonectomy.

Robotic major lung resection surgery required about an hour more to complete than open surgery, even at the end of the learning curve. Median duration of robotic surgery is 218–221 min as reported by Park et al. [20] and Veronesi et al. [23].

Regarding oncologic radicality, complete mediastinal lymphadenectomy can be accomplished in a minimally invasive fashion, although this remains controversial [51]. Many general thoracic surgeons have thought that nodal dissection (ND) for primary lung cancer by VATS or robot is inferior to that through open thoracotomy. It is difficult to perform standard ND by VATS for primary lung cancer without any devices or instruments. The use of robot is related to an easier and more radical lymph node dissection due to improved quality of vision and instrument maneuverability. According to a recent paper, an equal number of lymph nodes was removed during robotic and open lobectomies providing some indication of the likely oncologic radicality [23].

Intraoperative conversion rates to open thoracotomy range up to 13% in reports of thoracoscopic lobectomy for treatment of early-stage lung cancer [9, 22, 28, 46]. Although, previous published series have commented that converted patients have no increase in perioperative morbidity and mortality compared with patients who had a successful VATS procedure [28, 46].

Conclusions

As long as oncologic principles are maintained, minimally invasive pneumonectomy represents an advancement that surgeons have a responsibility to explore if it offers to frail patients the opportunity for surgical cure. In addition, the faster recovery may allow more patients to start adjuvant chemotherapy in a more timely fashion. However, the expected decrease in morbidity is worthwhile only if there is no compromise to the curative potential in patients who can tolerate thoracotomy. The robotic technique is still evolving, and more studies on a large population are necessary. The current literature and our experience showed, however, that this procedure is feasible and safe. Although these studies suffer from the limitations of being nonrandomized analysis, they revealed several key technical points that are essential for a successful procedure. First, the patient's position and the site of arm incisions are critical and have to be chosen to avoid arm impingement and interference. For this reason, a minimum distance of 8–10 cm is advisable.

Patients with anatomic characteristics that would allow minimally invasive pneumonectomies are uncommon. There is definitely a learning curve for these procedures. However, it is feasible to perform such resections using current robotic technique. Short-term results are encouraging, but prospective long-term outcome data are required to properly assess the role of minimally invasive pneumonectomy in the contemporary care of lung cancer patients.

References

1. Bettencourt DM, Holmes EC (1988) Muscle-sparing posterolateral thoracotomy. Ann Thorac Surg 45: 337–339
2. Daniel TM, Kern JA, Tribble CG, Kron IL, Spotnitz WB, Rodgers BM (1993) Thoracoscopic surgery for diseases of the lung and pleura. Effectiveness, changing indications, and limitations. Ann Surg 217:566–575
3. Kirby TJ, Mack MJ, Landreneau RJ, Rice TW (1993) Initial experience with video-assisted thoracoscopic lobectomy. Ann Thorac Surg 56:1248–1253
4. Yoshikawa K, Tsubota N, Kodama K, Ayabe H, Taki T, Mori T (2002) Prospective study of extended segmentectomy for small lung tumors: the final report. Ann Thorac Surg 73:1055–1059
5. Koike T, Yamato Y, Yoshiya K, Shimoyama T, Suzuki R (2003) Intentional limited pulmonary resection for peripheral T1 N0 M0 small-sized lung cancer. J Thorac Cardiovasc Surg 125:924–928
6. McKenna R Jr (1995) Vats lobectomy with mediastinal lymph node sampling or dissection. Chest Surg Clin N Am 5:223–232
7. Yim AP (2002) VATS major pulmonary resection revisited – controversies, techniques, and results. Ann Thorac Surg 74:615–623
8. Giudicelli R, Thomas P, Lonjon T, Ragni J, Morati N, Ottomani R, Fuentes PA, Shennib H, Noirclerc M (1994) Video-assisted minithoracotomy versus muscle-sparing thoracotomy for performing lobectomy. Ann Thorac Surg 58:712–718
9. Nomori H, Horio H, Naruke T, Suemasu K (2001) What is the advantage of a thoracoscopic lobectomy

over a limited thoracotomy procedure for lung cancer surgery? Ann Thorac Surg 72:879–884
10. Yim AP, Wan S, Lee TW, Arifi AA (2000) VATS lobectomy reduces cytokine responses compared with conventional surgery. Ann Thorac Surg 70:243–247
11. Conlan AA, Sandor A (2003) Total thoracoscopic pneumonectomy: indications and technical considerations. J Thorac Cardiovasc Surg 126:2083
12. Craig SR, Walker WS (1995) Initial experience of video assisted thoracoscopic pneumonectomy. Thorax 50:392
13. Roviaro G, Varoli F, Vergani C et al (1999) Techniques of pneumonectomy: video-assisted thoracic surgery pneumonectomy. Chest Surg Clin N Am 9:419
14. Roviaro G, Varoli F, Rebuffat C et al (1993) Major pulmonary resections: pneumonectomies and lobectomies. Ann Thorac Surg 56:779–783
15. Walker WS, Carnochan FM, Mattar S (1994) Video-assisted thoracoscopic pneumonectomy. Br J Surg 81:81–82
16. Nwogu CE, Glinianski M, Demmy TL (2006) Minimally invasive pneumonectomy. Ann Thorac Surg 82:e3–e4
17. Sahai RK, Nwogu CE, Yendamuri S, Tan W, Wilding GE, Demmy TL (2009) Is thoracoscopic pneumonectomy safe? Ann Thorac Surg 88:1086–1092
18. Cerfolio RJ, Bryant AS (2008) Is palpation of the nonresected pulmonary lobe(s) required for patients with non–small cell lung cancer? A prospective study. J Thorac Cardiovasc Surg 135:261–268
19. Flores RM, Alam N (2008) Video-assisted thoracic surgery lobectomy (VATS), open thoracotomy, and the robot for lung cancer. Ann Thorac Surg 85: S710–S715
20. Park BJ, Flores RM, Rusch VW (2006) Robotic assistance for video-assisted thoracic surgical lobectomy: technique and initial results. J Thorac Cardiovasc Surg 131:54–59
21. Melfi FMA, Mussi A (2008) Robotically assisted lobectomy: learning curve and complications. Thorac Surg Clin 18:289–295
22. Gharagozloo F, Margolis M, Tempesta B (2008) Robot-assisted thoracoscopic lobectomy for early-stage lung cancer. Ann Thorac Surg 85:1880–1886
23. Veronesi G, Galetta D, Maisonneuve P, Melfi F, Schmid RA, Borri A, Vannucci F, Spaggiari L (2010) Four-arm robotic lobectomy for the treatment of early-stage lung cancer. J Thorac Cardiovasc Surg 140(1):19–25
24. Cadiere GB, Himpens J, Vertruyen M, Favretti F (1999) The world's first obesity surgery performed by a surgeon at a distance. Obes Surg 9:206–209
25. Rea F, Marulli G, Bortolotti L, Feltracco P, Zuin A, Sartori F (2006) Experience with the "da Vinci" robotic system for thymectomy in patients with myasthenia gravis: report of 33 cases. Ann Thorac Surg 81: 455–459
26. Swanson SJ, Herndon JE 2nd, D'Amico TA et al (2007) Video-assisted thoracic surgery lobectomy: report of CALGB 39802 – a prospective, multi-institution feasibility study. J Clin Oncol 25:4993–4997
27. Whitson BA, Andrade RS, Boettcher A et al (2007) Video-assisted thoracoscopic surgery is more favorable than thoracotomy for resection of clinical stage I non-small cell lung cancer. Ann Thorac Surg 83: 1965–1970
28. Walker WS, Codispoti M, Soon SY et al (2003) Long-term outcomes following VATS lobectomy for non-small cell bronchogenic carcinoma. Eur J Cardiothorac Surg 23:397
29. Sugiura H, Morikawa T, Kaji M, Sasamura Y, Kondo S, Katoh H (1999) Long-term benefits for the quality of life after video-assisted thoracoscopic lobectomy in patients with lung cancer. Surg Laparosc Endosc Percutan Tech 9:403–408
30. Shigemura N, Akashi A, Funaki S et al (2006) Long-term outcomes after a variety of video-assisted thoracoscopic lobectomy approaches for clinical stage IA lung cancer: a multi-institutional study. J Thorac Cardiovasc Surg 132:507–512
31. Petersen RP, Pham D, Burfeind WR et al (2007) Thoracoscopic lobectomy facilitates the delivery of chemotherapy after resection for lung cancer. Ann Thorac Surg 83:1245–1250
32. Nicastri DG, Wisnivesky JP, Litle VR et al (2008) Thoracoscopic lobectomy: report on safety, discharge independence, pain, and chemotherapy tolerance. J Thorac Cardiovasc Surg 135:642–647
33. Aoki T, Tsuchida M, Hashimoto T, Saito M, Koike T, Hayashi J (2007) Quality of life after lung cancer surgery: video-assisted thoracic surgery versus thoracotomy. Heart Lung Circ 16:285–289
34. Balduyck B, Hendriks J, Lauwers P, Van Schil P (2007) Quality of life evolution after lung cancer surgery: a prospective study in 100 patients. Lung Cancer 56:423–431
35. Whitson BA, Groth SS, Duval SJ, Swanson SJ, Maddaus MA (2008) Surgery for early-stage non-small cell lung cancer: a systematic review of the video-assisted thoracoscopic surgery versus thoracotomy approaches to lobectomy. Ann Thorac Surg 86: 2008–2018
36. Ng CS, Wan IY, Yim AP (2009) Impact of video-assisted thoracoscopic major lung resection on immune function. Asian Cardiovasc Thorac Ann 17: 426–432
37. Shiraishi T, Shirakusa T, Hiratsuka M, Yamamoto S, Iwasaki A (2006) Video-assisted thoracoscopic surgery lobectomy for c-T1N0M0 primary lung cancer: its impact on locoregional control. Ann Thorac Surg 82:1021–1026
38. Kaseda S, Aoki T, Hangai N, Shimizu K (2000) Better pulmonary function and prognosis with video-assisted thoracic surgery than with thoracotomy. Ann Thorac Surg 70:1644–1646
39. Sawada S, Komori E, Yamashita M, Nakata M, Nishimura R, Teramoto N et al (2007) Comparison in prognosis after VATS lobectomy and open lobectomy

for stage I lung cancer. Retrospective analysis focused on a histological subgroup. Surg Endosc 21:1607–1611
40. Ng CS, Whelan RL, Lacy AM, Yim AP (2005) Is minimal access surgery for cancer associated with immunologic benefits? World J Surg 29:975–981
41. Leaver HA, Craig SR, Yap PL, Walker WS (2000) Lymphocyte responses following open and minimally invasive thoracic surgery. Eur J Clin Invest 30:230–238
42. Yamashita JI, Kurusu Y, Fujino N, Saisyoji T, Ogawa M (2000) Detection of circulating tumor cells in patients with non-small cell lung cancer undergoing lobectomy by video-assisted thoracic surgery: a potential hazard for intraoperative hematogenous tumor cell dissemination. J Thorac Cardiovasc Surg 119:899–905
43. Nakanishi R, Hirai A, Yamashita T, Oka S (2008) Video-assisted thoracoscopic completion pneumonectomy for a second primary cancer: a case report. J Thorac Cardiovasc Surg 135:945–946
44. Suda T, Kitamura Y, Hasegawa S, Negi K, Hattori Y (2007) Video-assisted thoracoscopic extrapleural pneumonectomy for malignant pleural mesothelioma. J Thorac Cardiovasc Surg 134:1088–1089
45. Anselmo DM, Perez IA, Shaul DB (2008) Thoracoscopic pneumonectomy for severe bronchiectasis in a 9-year-old female. J Laparoendosc Adv Surg Tech A 18:775–777
46. McKenna RJ Jr, Houck W, Beeman Fuller C (2006) Videoassisted thoracic lobectomy: experience with 1100 cases. Ann Thorac Surg 81:421–426
47. Kernstine KH (2008) Computer-assisted surgical systems in cardiothoracic surgery: why are we reluctant to accept the future? Ann Thorac Cardiovasc Surg 14:203–204
48. Bernard GR, Artigas A, Brigham KL, Carlet J, Falke K, Hudson L et al (1994) The American European Consensus Conference on ARDS. Definition, mechanisms, relevant outcomes, and clinical trial coordination. Am J Respir Crit Care Med 149:818–824
49. Ng T, Ryder BA (2006) Evolution to video-assisted thoracic surgery lobectomy after training: initial results of the first 30 patients. J Am Coll Surg 203:551–557
50. Ferguson J, Walker W (2006) Developing a VATS lobectomy programme can VATS lobectomy be taught? Eur J Cardiothorac Surg 29:806–809
51. Sagawa M, Sato M, Sakurada A, Matsumura Y, Endo C, Handa M, Kondo T (2002) A prospective trial of systematic nodal dissection for lung cancer by video-assisted thoracic surgery: can it be perfect? Ann Thorac Surg 73:900–904

Video-Assisted Thoracic Surgery for Emphysema: Lung Volume Reduction Surgery, Concomitant Cancer Resection, and Volume Reduction Surgery and Bullectomy

15

Cliff K.C. Choong, Julian A. Smith,
Joel David Copper, and Rolf G.C. Inderbitzi

Contents

C.K.C. Choong, MBBS, FRACS, FRCS (✉)
Department of Surgery (MMC), Monash University, Level 5, Block E, Monash Medical Centre, 246 Clayton Road, Clayton, Melbourne, VIC 3168, Australia
e-mail: cliffchoong@hotmail.com

J.A. Smith, MB, MS, FRACS, FACS, FCSANZ
Department of Surgery (MMC), Monash Medical Centre, Monash University, Level 5, Block E, 246 Clayton Road, Clayton, Melbourne, VIC 3168, Australia

Department of Cardiothoracic Surgery, Southern Health, Monash Medical Centre, Clayton, Melbourne, VIC, Australia

Specialty Program, Southern Health, Monash Medical Centre, Clayton, Melbourne, VIC, Australia

J.D. Copper, M.D., FACS
Division of Thoracic Surgery, University of Pennsylvania Health System, 3400 Spruce Street 6 Silverstein, Philadelphia, PA 19104, USA

R.G.C. Inderbitzi, M.D.
Thoraxzentrum Zurich, Hirslanden Clinic, Witellikerstrasse 40, CH-8008 Zurich, Switzerland
e-mail: r.inderbitzi@thoraxzentrum.ch

15.1 Bilateral Lung Volume Reduction Surgery

15.1.1 Introduction

Surgery for emphysema was first introduced by Brantigan and colleagues in 1957. It however did not gain acceptance due to high morbidity, mortality and a lack of objective results [1]. Cooper and colleagues at Washington University in St. Louis revived surgery for emphysema by reporting on their initial experience in 20 patients in 1995, and subsequently on the early outcomes (up to 2 years) in 150 patients in 1996, and the long-term outcomes (up to 5 years) in 250 patients in 2003 [2–4]. The surgery was termed as lung volume reduction surgery (LVRS). Cooper and colleagues showed that in appropriately selected patients, bilateral LVRS can produce significant functional improvement lasting at least 5 years

R.G.C. Inderbitzi et al. (eds.), *Minimally Invasive Thoracic and Cardiac Surgery*,
DOI 10.1007/978-3-642-11861-6_15, © Springer-Verlag Berlin Heidelberg 2012

Table 15.1 Preoperative evaluation for LVRS

History taking with emphasis on symptoms from emphysema and effects on quality of life, cessation of smoking, careful evaluation of patient comorbidity, realistic goals regarding medical and surgical treatment for emphysema, and social support
Physical examination with emphasis on respiratory and cardiovascular examinations
Radiology: Chest X-ray, CT chest, ventilation-perfusion (VQ) radionuclide scan
Lung function tests including pre- and post-bronchodilator spirometry assessments, diffusion capacity, 6-min walk test, and arterial blood gas
Cardiac assessment: ECG and transthoracic echocardiography
Questionnaires assessing quality of life and dyspnea

for most of these patients and a low inhospital mortality rate of 4.8% [4]. The National Emphysema Treatment Trial (NETT) investigators confirmed the efficacy of bilateral LVRS over medical therapy in a prospective randomized multicentre study [5–7]. Lung volume reduction surgery for emphysema is now a proven therapy despite earlier concerns and controversies regarding the efficacy.

15.1.2 Selection of Patients for LVRS

Patients for LVRS are highly selected [3, 4, 6, 7]. Patients for consideration of LVRS are carefully investigated (Table 15.1) and assessed in a multidisciplinary team setting consisting of a respiratory physician, surgeon, radiologist and other team members with interests and experience in the treatment of emphysema. The strict patient selection criteria are outlined in Table 15.2. A lack of suitable target areas for surgical resection is the most common reason for exclusion [4]. Preoperative pulmonary rehabilitation program, usually for 3 months, and optimization of medical therapy are important preoperative preparations before surgery.

15.1.3 Operative Considerations

Lung volume reduction surgery (LVRS) requires an experienced thoracic anaesthetist to place a double lumen endotracheal tube, manage single lung ventilation and provide anaesthetic and monitoring of the patient during surgery. Bilateral LVRS is performed either through bilateral video-assisted thoracic surgery (VATS) (Fig. 15.1) or alternatively via a median sternotomy. Rarely, it is performed via bilateral thoracotomy. Twenty percent to thirty-five percent of each lung is removed using lung stapler reinforcement with buttressing material [4, 6, 7] (Fig. 15.2a). This usually involves removing 75% or more of the right upper lobe, and about half of the left upper lobe. The technique performed involves successive applications of the stapler removing almost most of the upper lobe (Fig. 15.2b). In patients with lobar destruction and complete fissures, an anatomic lobectomy can be considered rather than wedge resections [4]. Lobectomy in emphysema patient is an outstanding indication for thoracoscopic approach. In the VATS approach, LVRS can generally be performed via mini-incisions without the use of rib spreaders.

15.1.4 Post-operative Management

Patients are generally extubated in the operating room or shortly thereafter in the recovery room. During the early post-operative period, the patients are monitored and managed in a high dependency unit. Review by the hospital pain service team on a regular basis is essential to provide optimal post-operative pain management with minimal respiratory depressants, thereby allowing the patient to satisfactorily perform breathing exercises and undergo physiotherapy. In some centres, adequate post-operative pain relief is facilitated by the use of continuous analgesia through a thoracic epidural catheter positioned with its tip at the T4 level [4]. It is important that the patients are cared for by experienced thoracic surgical nurses and physiotherapists to provide vigorous chest physiotherapy and ambulation. Post-operative bedside bronchoscopy and mini-tracheostomy placement to clear secretions are rarely required. They should however be considered in patients who are unable to clear their secretions, particularly in the presence of thick secretions, mucus plugging and complications such as lobar collapse [4].

Table 15.2 Guidelines on selection criteria for LVRS

	Inclusion criteria	Exclusion criteria
General	Symptomatic with adverse quality of life despite maximal medical therapy and pulmonary rehabilitation Cessation of smoking for 6 months Reasonable expectations regarding treatment Motivated with good social support	Asymptomatic or minimal symptoms Recurrent chest infections Significant sputum production Continued smoking Inability to complete pulmonary rehabilitation program Pleural or interstitial disease that precludes surgery, significant bronchiectasis Significant comorbidity Previous pleurodesis or thoracotomy Markedly underweight or overweight Poorly motivated or inadequate social support
Radiographic/ anatomic	Marked thoracic hyperinflation CT scan showing marked emphysema, with suitable target areas of upper zone severe emphysema (heterogenous emphysema) and better preserved lower zone lungs Poorly perfused upper zone lungs on VQ scan	Minimal radiographic evidence of severe emphysema Homogenous emphysema with no suitable target zone and no preserved lung tissue Bronchiectasis Thoracic cage or chest wall abnormalities
Physiological evaluation	Marked airflow obstruction FEV1 > 20% predicted Marked hyperinflation (TLC ≥ 100% predicted & RV ≥ 150% predicted) $PaO_2 \geq 45$ mmHg and $PaCO_2 \leq 60$ mmHg DLCO > 20% predicted 6 MWD > 140 m with oxygen requirement ≤6 L to maintain $SaO_2 \geq 90\%$ Good cardiovascular function with normal cardiac ejection fraction	FEV1 ≤ 20% predicted Alveolar gas exchange DLCO ≤ 20% predicted Significant comorbidity Cardiac dysfunction with left ventricular ejection fraction <45% Significant coronary artery disease Pulmonary hypertension with mean pulmonary arterial pressure ≥35 mmHg

Post-operative optimal medical management of emphysema is provided within a multidisciplinary team setting by the respiratory physician, the surgeon and other team members. The important points in the post-operative management of LVRS are outlined in Table 15.3.

15.1.5 Outcomes of Bilateral LVRS

The important findings of the National Emphysema Treatment Trial (NETT) and other LVRS publications are summarized below [4, 6–12].

(A) Cooper and colleagues from Washington University in St. Louis reported on 250 consecutive patients (mean age 62 ± 8 years) who underwent bilateral LVRS between January 1993 and June 2000 through median sternotomy (except one) with a follow-up ranged 1.8–9.1 years (median 4.4 years). The study found that there were significant improvements of FEV1 and RV between preoperative values and each follow-up time point. There was also significant post-operative improvement in health-related quality of life and with time correlated well with the improvement in FEV1. The most common complication following surgery was prolonged air leaks (>7 days) 45.2% and other complications were re-exploration for air leak 3.2%, bleeding 1.2%, re-intubation and mechanical ventilation 7.2%, pneumonia 9.6% and tracheostomy 4%. The inhospital mortality was 4.8% (post-operative deaths due to respiratory failure except 1 due to pulmonary embolism), and there was no intra-operative death. The median length of hospitalization was 9 days (range 4–168 days). At follow-up (median 4.4 years), 38.4% of 250 patients have died and mostly (65%) due to respiratory failure. The Kaplan-Meier survival after LVRS at 1, 3 and 5 years were 93.6%, 84.4% and 67.7%, respectively. 7.2% of patients subsequently underwent lung transplantation (median interval 4.3 years) [4].

(B) The National Emphysema Treatment Trial (NETT) evaluated 3,777 patients between January 1998 and July 2007. One thousand two hundred and eighteen patients underwent randomization (608 to LVRS and 610 to medical therapy). Eventually, only 580 underwent LVRS as 21 declined surgery and 7 were deemed unsuitable. The important findings from the NETT study included:

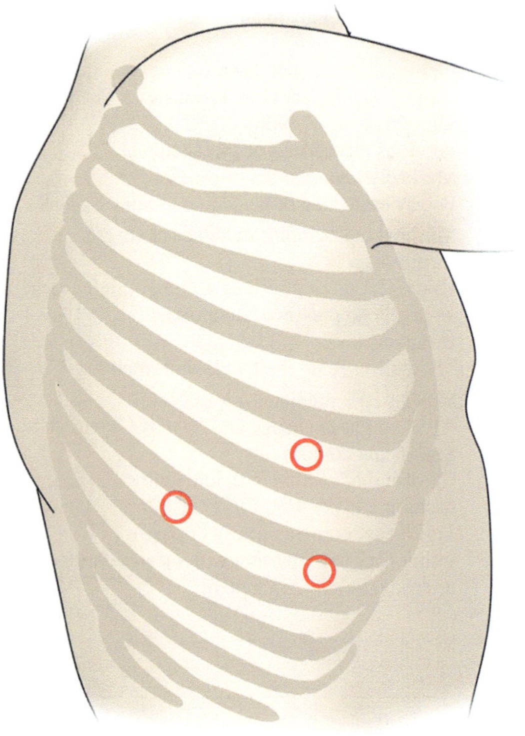

Fig. 15.1 Placement of mini-incisions for thoracoscopic LVRS

1. The findings of patients at high risks of death after LVRS. By June 2001, 1,033 patients were randomized. The 30-day mortality rate after surgery was 16% for 69 patients with FEV1 ≤ 20% and either a homogeneous distribution of emphysema on CT or a DLCO ≤ 20% as compared with a rate of 0% among 70 medically treated patients. Following these findings, these patients were considered high risk for death after LVRS, with little chance of functional benefit and were no longer eligible for randomization [8].
2. Following the exclusion of the high-risk subgroup in 2001, 1,078 patients without high risk were analyzed and reported in 2003. These patients were divided into four subgroups on the basis of combinations of upper lobe or non-upper lobe emphysema and low or high exercise capacity at base line [6].
   - *Subgroup 1* consisted of 290 patients with upper lobe disease and low exercise capacity. The LVRS patients had a lower risk of death than patients in the

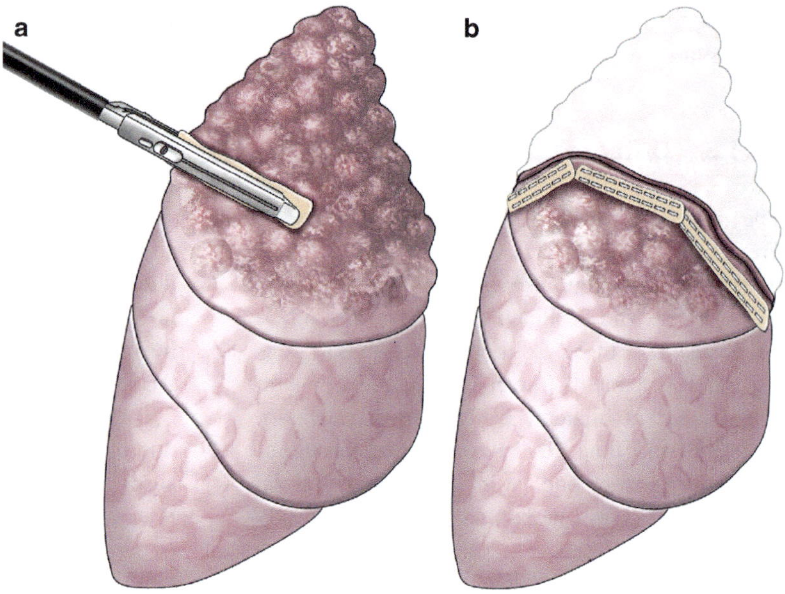

Fig. 15.2 (**a**) Stapling technique: the lung stapler is reinforced with buttressing material and sequentially stapling across the target area. (**b**) Careful sequential applications of stapler under direct vision and strict thoracoscopic control to avoid lung damage or tension which may lead to air leakage at the suture lines

Table 15.3 Summary of post-operative management for LVRS

Early extubation in the operating room or recovery area to avoid prolonged intubation and mechanical ventilation
Multidisciplinary team management by high dependency unit physicians, pain service team, respiratory physicians, experienced physiotherapists, and thoracic surgical nurses
Optimal pain relief
Ability to satisfactorily perform breathing exercises, cough, and early ambulation
Vigorous physiotherapy
Optimal medical management of emphysema in a multidisciplinary setting

medical-therapy group and were more likely to have an improvement of more than 10 W in the maximal workload at 24 months (30% vs. 0%, $P<0.001$). The LVRS patients were also more likely to have an eight-point improvement in the St. George's Respiratory Questionnaire score at 24 months (48% vs. 10%, $P<0.001$).

- *Subgroup 2* consisted of 419 patients with upper lobe disease and high exercise capacity. The LVRS patients were however more likely than those in the medical-therapy group to have improvement of more than 10 W in the maximal workload at 24 months (15% vs. 3%, $P=0.001$). The LVRS patients also had an eight-point improvement in the health-related quality-of-life score at 24 months (41% vs. 11%, $P<0.001$). The mortality between LVRS and the medical group was similar in the two groups. However, it should be noted that the mortality for the LVRS group in the high exercise capacity group was identical to that in the low exercise capacity group and the difference was the fact that mortality in the high exercise medical group was, as would be expected, considerably less in the first few years, then it was for the medical group in the low-exercise group. Since mortality, and not quality of life, exercise tolerance or measured pulmonary function was the primary endpoint, the NETT concluded that only patients with low exercise capacity and upper lobe disease were proven to derive benefit from bilateral LVRS.
- *Subgroup 3* consisted of 149 patients with non-upper lobe disease and low exercise capacity. The mortality between LVRS and medical group was similar, and both groups had similar chances of improvement of more than 10 W in the maximal workload at 24 months. The LVRS patients had a greater chance than patients in the medical-therapy group of an eight-point improvement in health-related quality of life at 24 months (37% vs. 7%, $P=0.001$).
- *Subgroup 4* consisted of 220 patients with non-upper lobe disease and high exercise capacity. The LVRS patients had a higher risk of death than those in the medical-therapy group (risk ratio, 2.06; $P=0.02$). Both groups had a similarly low chance of improvement of more than 10 W in the maximal workload at 24 months (3% in both groups, $P=1.00$) and a similar chance of an eight-point improvement in health-related quality of life (15% vs. 12%, $P=0.61$).

3. In 2006, the NETT Research Group reported an updated analysis with median of 4.3 years follow-up in comparison to 2.4 years median follow-up published in 2003, including 40% more patients with functional measures 2 years after randomization [7]. The intention-to-treat analysis of 1,218 randomized patients demonstrates an overall survival advantage for LVRS, with a 5-year risk ratio (RR) for death of 0.86. The improvement was more likely in the LVRS than in the medical group for maximal exercise through 3 years and for health-related quality of life (St. George's Respiratory Questionnaire [SGRQ]) through 4 years. The updated comparisons of survival and functional improvement were consistent with the initial results for

the four clinical subgroups of non-high-risk patients defined by upper lobe predominance and exercise capacity. After LVRS, the upper lobe patients with low exercise capacity (subgroup 1) demonstrated improved survival (5-year RR, 0.67), exercise throughout 3 years, and symptoms (SGRQ) through 5 years. The upper lobe-predominant and high exercise capacity LVRS patients (subgroup 2) obtained no survival advantage but were likely to improve exercise capacity (years 1–3) and SGRQ (years 1–4). The effects of LVRS were found to be durable and could be recommended for upper lobe-predominant emphysema patients with low exercise capacity (subgroup 1) and should be considered for palliation in patients with upper lobe emphysema and high exercise capacity (subgroup 2).

4. The NETT Research Group also evaluated the predictors of operative mortality and cardiopulmonary morbidity in 511 LVRS patients in the non-high-risk group [9]. The incidence of operative mortality (death within 90 days of the operation) was 5.5% and major pulmonary morbidity (tracheostomy, failure to wean, re-intubation, pneumonia and ventilator for ^{3}3 days) occurred in 29.8% of patients. The cardiovascular morbidity (infarction, pulmonary embolus or arrhythmia requiring treatment) occurred in 20.0% of patients. The predictor for operative mortality was non-upper lobe predominance assessed by radiologist (RR 2.99), and the predictors for pulmonary morbidity were age in years (RR 1.05), FEV1 predicted (RR 0.97), and DLCO% predicted (0.97). Pulmonary morbidity can be expected in elderly patients who have a low diffusing capacity for carbon monoxide and low forced expiratory volume in 1 s. The predictors for cardiovascular morbidity were age in years (RR 1.07), oral steroid use (RR 1.72) and non-upper lobe predominance (RR 2.67). The authors concluded that LVRS can be performed in selected patients with acceptable mortality; the incidence of major cardiopulmonary morbidity however remains high.
5. The NETT Research Group also evaluated the safety and efficacy of median sternotomy versus video-assisted thoracic surgery (VATS) [10]. LVRS was performed by median sternotomy only at eight centres and video-assisted thoracoscopy only at three centres. There were six centres which randomized the approach to LVRS. In the nonrandomized comparison, 359 patients received LVRS by median sternotomy, and 152 patients received LVRS by VATS. No significant difference in the 90-day mortality (5.9% for median sternotomy and 4.6% for VATS) was found. The overall mortality was 0.08 deaths per person-year for median sternotomy and 0.10 deaths per person-year for VATS. The complication rates were low and not statistically different for the two approaches. The median hospital length of stay was longer for median sternotomy than for VATS (10 vs. 9 days). By 30 days after surgery, 70.5% of median sternotomy patients and 80.9% of VATS patients were living independently. Functional outcomes were similar for both groups at 12 and 24 months. Costs for the operation and the associated hospital stay and costs in the 6 months after surgery were both less for the VATS patients than for median sternotomy. Similar results were noted for the randomized comparison. The authors concluded that morbidity and mortality were comparable after LVRS by VATS or median sternotomy, as were functional results. The VATS approach to LVRS allowed earlier recovery at a lower cost than median sternotomy.
6. Detailed air leak data were available and analyzed for 552 of 580 patients receiving bilateral stapled LVRS in the NETT [11]. Within 30 days of LVRS, 90% of patients developed air leak (median duration 7 days). The occurrence was more common and duration prolonged in patients with lower diffusing capacity, upper lobe disease, and important pleural adhesions. Duration was

also protracted in Caucasians, patients using inhaled steroids, and those with lower FEV1. Surgical approach, buttressing, stapler brand, and intra-operative adjunctive procedures were not associated with fewer or less prolonged air leaks. Post-operative complications occurred more often in matched patients experiencing air leak (57% vs. 30%), and post-operative stay was longer (11.8+6.5 vs. 7.6+4.4 days). The analysis found that air leak accompanied LVRS in 90% of patients, is often prolonged, and is associated with a more complicated and protracted hospital course. Its occurrence and duration are associated with characteristics of patients and their disease, and not with a specific surgical technique.

7. In 2010, Sanchez and co-authors under the Freedom of Information Act obtained the follow-up data of the NETT to determine the long-term outcome for "a heterogeneous distribution of emphysema with upper lobe predominance", postulated by the NETT hypothesis to be optimal candidates for LVRS [12]. The results of LVRS were compared with those of patients receiving medical management. The authors also compared the results of the NETT LVRS group with a previously reported consecutive case series of 250 patients reported by the St. Louis Group undergoing bilateral LVRS using similar selection criteria [4]. Of the 1,218 patients enrolled into NETT, 511 (42%) conformed to the NETT hypothesis selection criteria and received the randomly assigned surgical or medical treatment (surgical=261; medical=250). LVRS resulted in a 5-year survival benefit (70% vs. 60%; P=0.02). Results at 3 years compared with baseline data favoured surgical reduction in terms of residual volume reduction (25% vs. 2%; P<0.001), University of California San Diego dyspnea score (16 vs. 0 points; P<0.001), and improved St. George Respiratory Questionnaire quality-of-life score (12 vs. 0 points; P<0.001). For the 513 patients with a homogeneous pattern of emphysema randomized to surgical or medical treatment, LVRS produced no survival advantage and very limited functional benefit. The authors concluded that patients most likely to benefit from LVRS have heterogeneously distributed emphysema involving the upper lung zones predominantly. Such patients in the NETT Trial had results nearly identical to those previously reported in a nonrandomized series of similar patients undergoing LVRS. The analysis of data obtained from the NETT improves the ability to understand and clarify the current role of LVRS. The analysis confirms that the NETT hypothesis was indeed correct and that patients with heterogeneously distributed upper lobe predominant emphysema achieved significant benefit in terms of survival and functional improvement. It is also concluded that for patients with a homogeneous pattern of emphysematous destruction, bilateral LVRS offers no survival advantage and produces much less functional improvement than in the heterogeneous upper lobe predominant group. This analysis of the NETT results confirms, with remarkable concordance, the previous report by Ciccone and associates of the St. Louis Group on a 250 consecutive case series of bilateral LVRS [4]. The similarity of results will contribute to the ongoing debate as to the relative merits of case-controlled series versus randomized clinical trials for surgical procedures.

15.1.6 Conclusions on Bilateral LVRS

Successful LVRS requires a multidisciplinary team approach and involves careful patient selection, rigorous preoperative preparation, and detailed operative and perioperative care. LVRS can provide a significant improvement in pulmonary function and quality of life, increased exercise tolerance, and decreased requirement for supplemental oxygen. Persistent objective benefits appear to last at least 5 years for most patients [4]. In patients with upper lobe emphysema and low exercise capacity at baseline, LVRS also provides a survival benefit over medical therapy alone [6, 7].

15.2 Unilateral LVRS

Unilateral LVRS is utilized in two different clinical settings. The first setting is in patients whom bilateral LVRS is contraindicated [13]. The relative contraindications to bilateral LVRS include marked asymmetrical unilateral distribution of emphysema, previous unilateral thoracotomy or pleurodesis, or both, previous unilateral thoracic radiotherapy, intra-operative findings of dense pleural adhesions in one side and a decision to avoid LVRS on that side, or findings of bilateral dense pleural adhesions and a decision to perform LVRS on just one side, as attempting to divide dense adhesions can lead to substantial air leaks. The intra-operative strategies utilized for unilateral LVRS is generally wedge resections of approximately 80% of the upper lobe for procedures on the right and approximately 60% of the upper lobe on the left [13]. The lingula is spared as it is usually better preserved than the superior subdivisions of the left upper lobe. In patients with severe lobar parenchymal destruction and complete fissures, an anatomic lobectomy can be performed rather than wedge resections. Meyers et al. from Washington University in St. Louis reported on 43 such patients and found that unilateral LVRS produces improvements in pulmonary function, exercise capacity, and quality of life with an acceptable morbidity and mortality [13]. The study found that after unilateral LVRS, the mean increase in FEV1 was 32% at 6 months and 28% at 3 years. The FEV1 was not significantly improved at 5 years. The 90-day mortality was 0%, and Kaplan-Meier survival was 97.7%, 80.9%, and 45.5% at 1, 3, and 5 years. The benefits of unilateral LVRS are however of lower magnitude than those achieved with bilateral LVRS [13].

The second clinical setting of performing unilateral LVRS is surgeon preference. The rationale include: (1) unilateral LVRS may have a reduced incidence of post-operative morbidity and mortality in comparison to bilateral LVRS, and (2) although bilateral LVRS results in greater physiological improvements than unilateral surgery, it may be associated with a more rapid decline in its physiological benefits in comparison to a staged unilateral approach [14]. The staged unilateral approach involves initially performing unilateral LVRS and at a later time, usually several years later, performing unilateral LVRS on the other side [14]. Some surgeons advocate unilateral staged approach as it may not only reduce the operative risk but also prolong the benefits of LVRS [14]. The first lung to be reduced will usually be the one with worse emphysematous disease and the timing of the second side operation being dependent on a combination of surgeon and patient decisions, as well as the duration of initial unilateral LVRS benefits and rate of physiological decline back to baseline [14].

15.3 Concomitant LVRS and Cancer Resection

Cigarette smoking is an important cause of both lung cancer and emphysema. Early-stage non-small cell lung cancer is best treated by complete anatomic resection. Patients with resectable lung cancer but with associated advanced emphysema are often precluded from surgery due to severe respiratory limitation. Certain highly selected patients with clinically resectable lung cancer and severe respiratory limitation due to emphysema may have an acceptable operative risk and functional improvements by combining a suitable lung cancer resection with LVRS [15, 16]. This combination would provide the best treatment for early-stage lung cancer while at the same time be a palliative treatment for the symptoms of emphysema. Several groups have evaluated their experience of combined lung cancer resection and LVRS and have reported beneficial early and long-term results [15, 16]. Several evaluative processes have been reported for the selection of suitable patients for combined surgery [15, 16]. Despite these various methods, no single test has been found to best define the patients who will and who will not tolerate resection. Instead, these investigations, together with the performance status of the patient and the surgeon's experience, help to select patients suitable for combined surgical resection. Patients who are offered concomitant surgery are very highly selected and must satisfy the strict criteria set out for both LVRS and cancer surgery.

Various intra-operative strategies have been employed in performing the combined surgery. The decision to perform either a wedge resection or a lobectomy depends upon the size and location of the tumour and the distribution and severity of the emphysema [15, 16].

The intra-operative strategies for a concomitant cancer resection and lung volume reduction surgery include (Fig. 15.3a–g):

1. Lobectomy only. This is usually performed in the setting of an upper lobe lung cancer in a patient with upper lobe predominant severe emphysema where the lobe has been severely destroyed by the emphysematous process and is virtually functionless. A lobectomy in such instance serves to treat both diseases well. Rarely, a lower lobectomy is performed in a patient with a lower lobe lung cancer who also has lower lobe predominant emphysema. It is however rare to have lower lobe predominant severe emphysema as the smoking-related emphysematous process usually, predominantly affects both the upper lobes.
2. Lobectomy and contralateral LVRS (Fig. 15.3a). This is performed in the setting of an upper lobe lung cancer in patients with bilateral upper lobe predominant severe emphysema. In the VATS approach, thoracoscopic lobectomy should be performed followed by minimally invasive contralateral LVRS in the same surgical setting. Alternatively, a median sternotomy can be utilized as this surgical approach provides access to both lungs through a single incision. Apart from upper lobectomy, middle or lower lobectomy in combination with contralateral LVRS can also be undertaken and has been reported previously. The decision to perform either an upper lobectomy alone or lobectomy in combination with contralateral LVRS depends on the distribution and severity of the emphysematous disease and the surgeon's personal preference and experience.
3. Ipsilateral middle lobectomy and LVRS (Fig. 15.3b). This is utilized in patients with a right middle lobe lung cancer with upper lobe predominant emphysema. The middle lobectomy in combination with ipsilateral upper lobe LVRS in such patients allows for treatment of both diseases through a right-sided surgical approach.
4. Unilateral LVRS (Fig. 15.3c). This is a useful and simple strategy in the treatment of an upper lobe lung cancer that is situated within the resection target area of an upper lobe LVRS. A large wedge resection of the upper lobe serves to remove both the lung cancer and a significant part of the upper lobe emphysematous disease. This is a simple and relatively quick operation to perform. It however has the disadvantage that only a wedge resection is performed for the lung cancer whereas lobectomy is considered a better oncological operation and is currently the gold standard in the treatment of lung cancer. The decision to perform either an upper lobectomy or just a large upper lobe wedge resection would depend on the size of the tumour, the location of the tumour, and the distribution of the upper lobe emphysematous disease. A large tumour or a tumour situated outside the usual resection area of an upper lobe LVRS may not be amendable to a large wedge resection and would be better treated by a lobectomy. An upper lobe which is virtually destroyed and functionless would also be served by a lobectomy rather than a large wedge resection.
5. Ipsilateral lower lobe wedge resection and upper lobe LVRS (Fig. 15.3d). When the cancer is located in a well-preserved lower lobe in a patient with an upper lobe predominant emphysema, a wedge resection of the lower lobe lung cancer in combination with an ipsilateral upper lobe LVRS can be performed.
6. Bilateral LVRS (Fig. 15.3e). This is particularly suitable in patients with a small upper lobe lung cancer that is situated within the target resection area for LVRS. A bilateral LVRS

in such instance would remove the upper lobe lung cancer and also palliate the emphysematous diseases on both lungs. A less aggressive approach in the management of the emphysema can be considered and adopted by performing a unilateral LVRS.

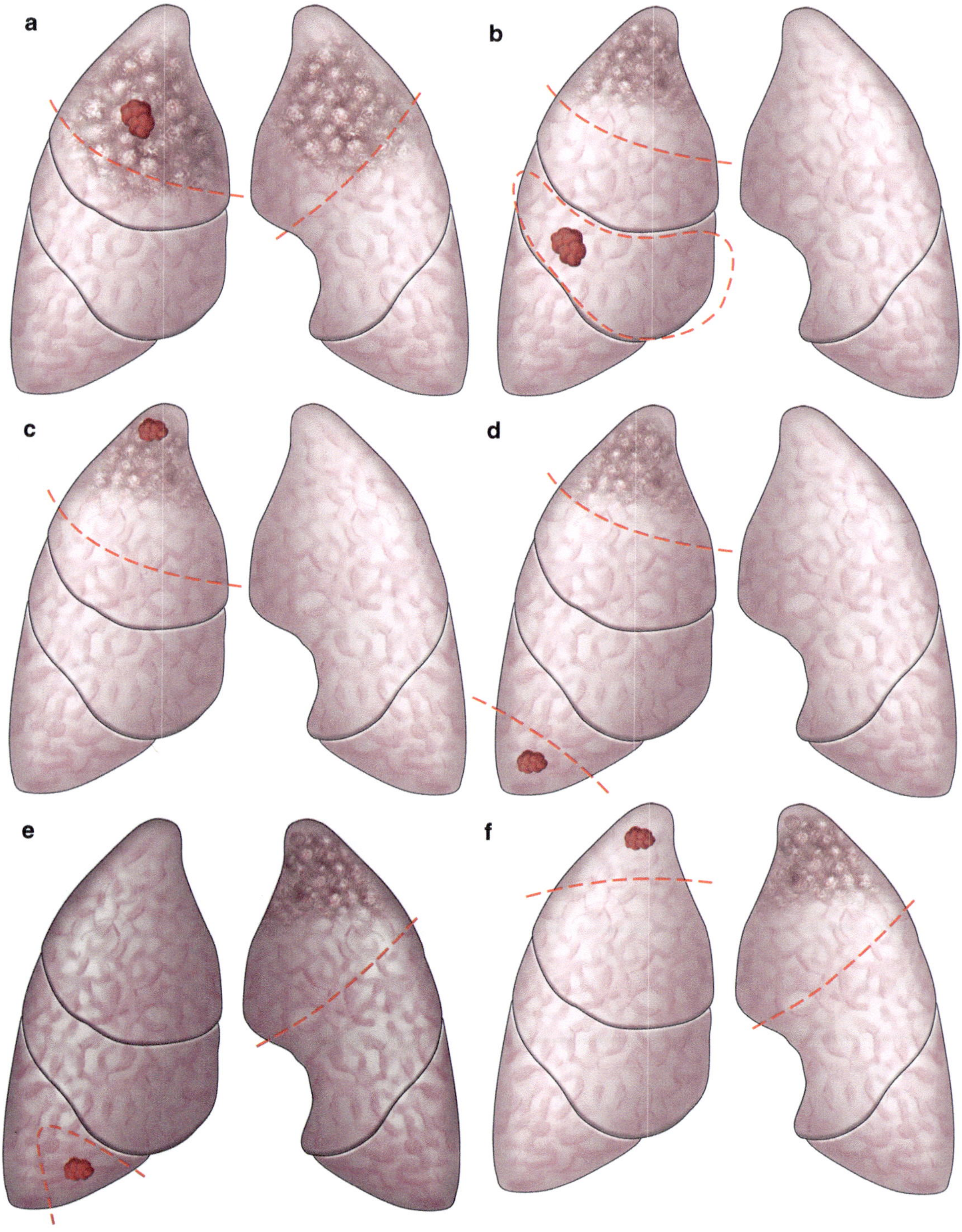

Fig. 15.3 (**a**) Lobectomy and contralateral LVRS. (**b**) Ipsilateral middle lobectomy and LVRS. (**c**) Unilateral LVRS. (**d**) Ipsilateral lower lobe wedge resection and upper lobe LVRS. (**e**) Bilateral LVRS. (**f, g**) Wedge resection and contralateral LVRS

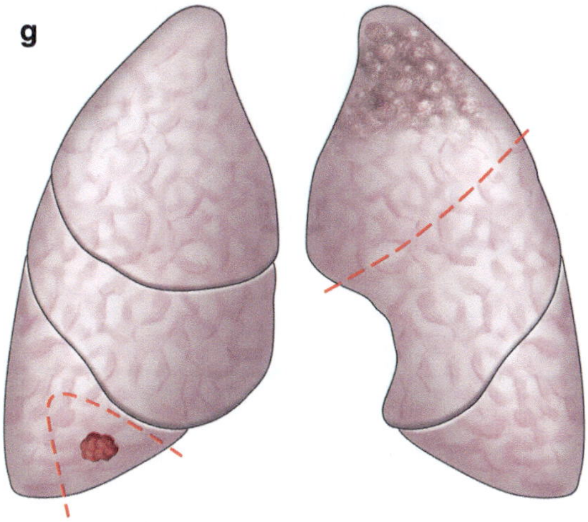

Fig. 15.3 (continued)

7. Wedge resection and contralateral LVRS (Fig. 15.3f, g). This is rarely performed and is in the setting of an apical lower lobe lung cancer in patients with predominant contralateral upper lobe severe emphysema. Alternative to bilateral thoracoscopic procedures, a median sternotomy may provide adequate access to both lungs and allows for wedge resection of a peripheral lower lobe lung cancer and contralateral LVRS. The scenario of predominant contralateral upper lobe emphysema is generally quite rare as the emphysematous disease from smoking-related aetiology is generally a bilateral process.

Thus, it can be seen that they are several potential options in dealing with a patient who has a concomitant lung cancer and severe emphysema. The choice of technique applied depends on the location and size of the tumour, the severity and distribution of the emphysema and the surgeon's preference and experience. The combination of lung cancer resection with LVRS offers selected patients, who have concomitant early lung cancer and severe emphysema, the opportunity to undergo resection of their cancer with improvement rather than further reduction in their pulmonary function [15, 16]. By traditional criteria, these patients would otherwise be considered unsuitable surgical candidates because of the limited pulmonary function.

15.4 Combined LVRS and Cardiac Surgery

Most patients with end-stage emphysema have a history of smoking and are therefore at increased risk for coronary artery disease (CAD). CAD is prevalent in patients with severe emphysema who are being considered for LVRS. Significant cardiac comorbidity is generally considered a contraindication to LVRS. Successful combined bilateral LVRS and cardiac surgery in the form of coronary bypass surgery or aortic valve replacement however have been achieved through multidisciplinary strategies [17–19]. These patients are highly selected fulfilling the strict criteria for LVRS apart from cardiac comorbidity. The perioperative approach has involved the usage of a thoracic epidural catheter placed 4 h before the scheduled surgery to minimize the risk of epidural hematoma related to the impending systemic anticoagulation required for cardiopulmonary bypass (CPB) [17–19]. A satisfactory thoracic epidural analgesia is considered important in the patient's good compliance with post-operative physiotherapy and breathing exercises, thereby reducing the risks of post-operative sputum retention and chest infection. A double-lumen endotracheal tube is placed, and a median sternotomy is utilized for both cardiac and LVRS. The cardiac surgery is performed first. At the completion of cardiac surgery, while still on CPB, pleural adhesions on the deflated lungs are divided using electrocautery. The patient is then weaned off CPB, and the anticoagulation is fully reversed. Following satisfactory cardiorespiratory stability and hemostasis, bilateral LVRS is then performed utilizing single-lung ventilation. The rationale to perform the cardiac surgery first followed by reversal of anticoagulation prior to LVRS is to ensure there was normal hemostasis during LVRS to minimize the risk of pulmonary haemorrhage. It is also useful to divide the pleural adhesions while both lungs were deflated during CPB. It is important that satisfactory cardiorespiratory stability and hemostasis are achieved before proceeding with the LVRS. Following surgery, the patient undergoes a planned early extubation. Careful anaesthetic and intensive care

Table 15.4 Symptoms and pulmonary function measurements before and after combined bilateral LVRS and aortic valve replacement surgery

	Preoperative baseline	Four-month post-operative	Percentage improvement
NYHA symptoms	Class III	Class I	
Modified Medical Research Council Dyspnea Scale (degree of dyspnea)	Category 4 (Severe)	Category 1 (Slight)	
SF-36 Physical Function Score	20	70	
Supplemental oxygen therapy	15 h a day	None	
FEV_1 (% predicted)	0.44 L (20)	0.85 L (38)	93
FVC (% predicted)	1.42 L (54)	2.35 L (89)	65
TLCO mmolCO/kPa/min (% predicted)	2.09 (28)	3.39 (46)	62
FRC (% predicted)	5.19 L (204)	2.90 L (114)	44
RV (% predicted)	4.47 L (267)	1.81 L (108)	60
TLC (% predicted)	6.27 L (139)	4.16 L (92)	34
RV/TLC (%)	71	44	38
6-min walk	190 m	432 m	127
Oxygen saturation on room air (%)	89	97	9

Reprinted from Choong et al. [18]

NYHA New York Heart Association, *SF-36* Short-Form 36, *FEV1* forced expiratory volume in 1 s, *FVC* forced vital capacity, *TLCO* transfer factor for carbon monoxide, *FRC* functional residual capacity, *RV* residual volume, *TLC* total lung capacity

management is important for executing a planned early extubation, thereby minimizing the risks associated with mechanical ventilation and maintenance of perioperative cardiorespiratory stability. The post-operative management of these patients is otherwise similar to the post-operative care specific for LVRS and cardiac surgical patients. A multidisciplinary team approach together with careful perioperative planning, highly selected patients can undergo successful combined LVRS and cardiac surgery resulting in quality of life, functional, cardiopulmonary, and prognostic benefits (Tables 15.4 and 15.5) [17–19].

15.5 Endoscopic Treatment of Emphysema

Novel bronchoscopic treatment of severe emphysema has emerged over the past few years. The aims of these minimally invasive approaches are to provide a lung volume reduction effect without the morbidity, mortality, and costs of LVRS. There are two concepts.

The first concept is the usage of one way valves which are placed within the lumen of airways allowing air to flow only unidirectionally out of the airways (i.e. air flow in the direction of expiration) but does not allow air to be inspired through the valves. The endobronchial valves are of variable sizes to allow placement within different bronchial lumen sizes [20, 21]. The aim is to completely collapse a hyperinflated segment or lobe of the lung by placing several endobronchial valves to occlude all the segmental or subsegmental airways supplying the specific segment or lobe of the lung. The valves are placed through the working channel of a flexible bronchoscope and are removable if necessary. This treatment is targeted at patients with heterogeneous emphysema, a similar population as those for consideration of LVRS. There are two different companies which produce these one way endobronchial valves. The valve designs are different; however, they both share the above common features. The first company is Pulmonx producing the Zephyr Endobronchial Valve (EBV) [22]. The second company is Spiration Inc., producing the IBV® Valve [23]. The second concept is the usage of airway bypass stents [24–27]. The ability of gas to move from one part of the lung to another part (within the lung) through non-anatomic pathways is termed "collateral ventilation" and was first observed by Van Allen and colleagues in 1930 [28]. The importance of collateral

Table 15.5 Symptoms and pulmonary function measurements before and after combined bilateral LVRS and coronary artery bypass grafting surgery

	Preoperative baseline	Six-month post-operative	Percentage improvement (%)
Modified Medical Research Council Dyspnea Scale (degree of dyspnea)	Category 4 (Severe)	Category 1 (Slight)	
SF-36 Physical Function Score	30	70	
Normal full-time work (office-based with intermittent travelling)	Unable	Back to normal full-time work	
FEV_1 (% predicted)	1.40 L (45)	2.60 L (84)	85
FER (% predicted)	42 (52)	73 (90)	72
TLCO mmolCO/kPa/min (% predicted)	3.26 (36)	3.68 (41)	4
KCO (% predicted)	0.71 (49)	0.85 (59)	14
FRC (% predicted)	4.81 L (147)	4.13 L (126)	16
RV (% predicted)	4.43 L (212)	3.22 L (153)	38
RV/TLC (%)	65	47	27
6-min walk	195 m	360 m	84
Oxygen saturation on room air (%)	90	98	9

Reprinted from Choong et al. [17]

SF-36 Short-Form 36, *FEV1* forced expiratory volume in 1 s, *FER* forced expiratory ratio, *TLCO* transfer factor of carbon monoxide, *KCO* carbon monoxide transfer coefficient, *FRC* functional residual capacity, *RV* residual volume, *TLC* total lung capacity

ventilation is minimal in normal lungs because the resistance to air flow is higher in collateral channels than in the airway. The resistance of air flow in collateral channels is however low in patients with emphysema in comparison to that of normal lungs. In emphysematous lungs, collateral ventilation provides important channels for gas distribution and may be therapeutically useful. Experimental and clinical work has demonstrated that creation of direct passages between emphysematous pulmonary parenchyma and bronchial airways (airway bypass) could take advantage of the extensive collateral ventilation present in emphysema to provide improvement in expiratory flow and volume which is otherwise limited by the collapse of the small, peripheral airways during expiration [27]. A hole is made through the bronchial wall (transbronchial fenestration or airway bypass) followed by placement of an airway bypass stent [24–27]. Airway bypass stent is made of stainless steel embedded within silicone rubber impregnated with paclitaxel (paclitaxel-eluting airway bypass stent). The stent is mounted on a delivery device and is delivered bronchoscopically through a 2-mm working channel of a flexible bronchoscope. The expanded stent is 3 mm long × 3 mm wide in the mid-portion but expands out to a 5.5-mm flange on either side that helps to secure the stent on the bronchial wall [25–27]. The stent is placed through segmental or subsegmental airway to provide an extra-anatomic airway to allow for trapped gas to escape and thereby reduce hyperinflation [27]. The airway bypass treatment is targeted at patients with severe homogenous emphysema. The airway bypass stent is manufactured by Broncus Technologies Inc., Mountain View, California, USA, producing the "Exhale® Emphysema Treatment System" (http://www.broncus.com/default.asp) [29]. The company funded the EASE (exhale airway stents for emphysema) trial which was a randomized, double-blind, sham-controlled study which recruited 315 patients in 38 specialist respiratory centres worldwide. The results were published in the Lancet in 2011 [27]. The study found that at 6 months, there was no difference between treatment arms with respect to co-primary efficacy endpoint. The 6-month composite primary safety endpoint was 14.4% for airway bypass versus 11.2% for sham control. The EASE trial study group concluded that the findings showed safety and transient improvements; however, no sustainable benefit was recorded with airway bypass in patients with severe homogenous emphysema [27].

The United States Food and Drug Administration (FDA) has presently not approved the use of the above endoscopic treatments for emphysema as the benefits have not been found to be sufficiently durable. It is therefore unlikely that they will become a significant therapeutic option for the management of emphysema.

15.6 Bullae

Bullous disease is often found with relatively normal underlying tissue and characterized either by bleb or bulla formation. A bleb is a subpleural collection of air within the layers of the visceral pleura caused by ruptured alveolus. The air dissects through the interstitial tissue into the thin fibrous layer of the visceral pleura, where it enlarges to form a bleb. Blebs characteristically occur at the lung apices and may produce a pneumothorax when it ruptures. Small blebs may coalesce to form larger ones, or they may appear as multiple and discrete blebs scattered over the upper surface of the lungs. The management of blebs should be as those for the management of spontaneous pneumothoraces.

A bulla is an air-filled space within the lung parenchyma, usually more than 2.5 cm in size, resulting from a deterioration of alveolar tissue. Bullae have fibrous walls and are trabeculated by the remnants of alveolar septa. Majority of patients are generally asymptomatic and do not require surgical intervention. The patients who benefit from surgical excision of bullae have large space-occupying non-functioning air spaces encroaching on normal or near normal adjacent lung. Excision removes the space-occupying bulla, allows the compressed lung to expand, permits better ventilation and perfusion, and decreases both dead space and residual volume. The general indications for surgical intervention on bullae include: (1) very large bullae occupying more than one-third of the lung field, (2) symptoms of dyspnea attributed to the bullae while other causes have been carefully excluded, (3) complications of bullous disease such as pneumothorax, persistent infection in a bulla despite maximal medical therapy or hemoptysis (recurrent or significant first episode), and suspicion of carcinoma in a bulla. The most common operation performed is bullectomy either via a VATS approach or a thoracotomy approach depending on the size, location and number of bullae, patient factors, and surgeon preference. Bullectomy is performed by initially opening the bulla by an incision into it to deflate and decompress the bulla. The wall of the bulla, made up of visceral pleura, can then either be excised or folded onto the base of the bulla to be incorporated by the stapler. Lung staplers reinforced with buttressing material are generally utilized, and the stapler is carefully placed to incorporate an adjacent area of normal lung tissue so as to optimize pneumostasis. It is however important to preserve as much of the adjacent compressed normal lung tissue by avoiding unnecessary excessive removal. Following bullectomy, pleurodesis is generally advocated. Bullectomy is the most common operation performed for bulla. Other less common procedures have been described and performed in poor-risk patients who are considered unsuitable to bullectomy surgery. These procedures have included the Monaldi procedure (intra-cavity suction and drainage), Brompton technique, and laser therapy [30–33]. Lobectomy is generally not recommended in the management of bulla so as to avoid excessive removal of normal compressed lung tissue. Patients who have undergone successful bullectomy experience functional and quality-of-life benefits.

References

1. Brantigan OC, Mueller E (1957) Surgical treatment of pulmonary emphysema. Am Surg 23:789–804
2. Cooper JD, Trulock EP, Triantafillou AN et al (1995) Bilateral pneumonectomy (volume reduction) for chronic obstructive pulmonary disease. J Thorac Cardiovasc Surg 109:106–119
3. Cooper JD, Patterson GA, Sundaresan RS, Trulock EP, Yusen RD, Pohl MS, Lefrak SS (1996) Results of 150 consecutive bilateral lung volume reduction

procedures in patients with severe emphysema. J Thorac Cardiovasc Surg 112:1319–1329
4. Ciccone AM, Meyers BF, Guthrie TJ, Davis GE, Yusen RD, Lefrak SS, Patterson GA, Cooper JD (2003) Long-term outcome of bilateral lung volume reduction in 250 consecutive patients with emphysema. J Thorac Cardiovasc Surg 125:513–525
5. The National Emphysema Treatment Trial Research Group (1999) Rationale and design of the National Emphysema Treatment Trial (NETT): a prospective randomized trial of lung volume reduction surgery. J Thorac Cardiovasc Surg 118:518–528
6. Fishman A, Martinez F, Naunheim K, National Emphysema Treatment Trial Research Group (2003) A randomized trial comparing LVRS with medical therapy for severe emphysema. N Engl J Med 348:2059–2073
7. Naunheim KS, Wood DE, Mohsenifar Z, Sternberg AL, Criner GJ, DeCamp MM, Deschamps CC, Martinez FJ, Sciurba FC, Tonascia J, National Emphysema Treatment Trial Research Group (2006) Long-term follow-up of patients receiving lung-volume-reduction surgery versus medical therapy for severe emphysema by the national emphysema treatment trial research group. Ann Thorac Surg 82:431–443
8. National Emphysema Treatment Trial Research Group (2001) Patients at high risk of death after LVRS. N Engl J Med 345:1075–1083
9. Naunheim KS, Wood DE, Krasna MJ, DeCamp MM, Ginsburg ME, McKenna RJ, Criner GJ, Hoffman EA, Sternberg AL, Deschamps C, National Emphysema Treatment Trial Research Group (2006) Predictors of operative mortality and cardiopulmonary morbidity in the National Emphysema Treatment Trial. J Thorac Cardiovasc Surg 131:43–53
10. National Emphysema Treatment Trial Research Group (2004) Safety and efficacy of median sternotomy versus video-assisted thoracic surgery for lung volume reduction surgery. J Thorac Cardiovasc Surg 127:1350–1360
11. DeCamp MM, Blackstone EH, Naunheim KS, Krasna MJ, Wood DE, Meli YM, McKenna RJ, NETT Research Group (2006) Patient and surgical factors influencing air leak after lung volume reduction surgery: lessons learned from the national emphysema treatment trial. Ann Thorac Surg 82:197–207
12. Sanchez PG, Kucharczuk JC, Su S, Kaiser LR, Cooper JD (2010) National Emphysema Treatment Trial redux: accentuating the positive. J Thorac Cardiovasc Surg 140:564–572
13. Meyers BF, Sultan PK, Guthrie TJ, Lefrak SS, Davis GE, Patterson GA, Cooper JD, Yusen RD (2008) Outcomes after unilateral lung volume reduction. Ann Thorac Surg 86:204–211
14. Waller D, Oey I (2009) Staged lung volume reduction surgery. Rationale and experience. Thorac Surg Clin 19:187–192
15. Choong CK, Meyers BF, Battafarano RJ, Guthrie TJ, Davis GE, Patterson GA, Cooper JD (2004) Lung cancer resection combined with lung volume reduction in patients with severe emphysema. J Thorac Cardiovasc Surg 127:1323–1331
16. Choong CK, Mahesh B, Patterson GA, Cooper JD (2009) Concomitant lung cancer resection and lung volume reduction surgery. Thorac Surg Clin 19:209–216
17. Choong CK, Naylor J, Vuylsteke A, Hardy I, Screaton N, Porter JN, Davies M (2009) Successful combined bilateral lung volume reduction and coronary artery bypass grafting surgery: implications and advantages. J Thorac Cardiovasc Surg 137:1552–1554
18. Choong CK, Agarwal A, Pulimood T, Screaton N, Hardy I, Vuylsteke A, Davies M (2009) Concomitant bilateral lung volume reduction surgery and aortic valve replacement: multidisciplinary strategies in achieving a successful outcome. J Thorac Cardiovasc Surg 137:1551–1552
19. Choong CK, Schmid RA, Miller DL, Smith JA (2009) Combined cardiac and lung volume reduction surgery. Thorac Surg Clin 19:217–221
20. Venuta F, Rendina EA, Coloni GF (2009) Endobronchial treatment of emphysema with one-way valves. Thorac Surg Clin 19:255–260
21. Springmeyer SC, Bollinger CT, Waddell TK, Gonzalez X, Wood DE (2009) Treatment of heterogeneous emphysema using the Spiration IBV valves. Thorac Surg Clin 19:247–253
22. Pulmonx website: http://www.pulmonx.com/index.php
23. Spiration website: http://www.spiration.com/index.asp
24. Choong CK, Haddad FJ, Gee EY, Cooper JD (2005) Feasibility and safety of airway bypass stent placement and influence of topical mitomycin C on stent patency. J Thorac Cardiovasc Surg 129:632–638
25. Choong CK, Phan L, Massetti P, Haddad FJ, Martinez C, Roschak E et al (2006) Prolongation of patency of airway bypass stents with use of drug-eluting stents. J Thorac Cardiovasc Surg 131:60–64
26. Choong CK, Cardoso PFG, Sybrecht GW, Cooper JD (2009) Airway bypass treatment of severe homogenous emphysema: taking advantage of collateral ventilation. Thorac Surg Clin 19:239–245
27. Shah PL, Slebos DJ, Cardoso PFG, on behalf of the Ease trial study group et al (2011) Bronchoscopic lung-volume reduction with Exhale airway stents for emphysema (EASE trial): randomised, sham-controlled, multicentre trial. Lancet 378:997–1005
28. Van Allen C, Lindskog G, Richter H (1930) Gaseous interchange between adjacent lung lobules. Yale J Biol Med 2:297–300
29. Website airway bypass: http://www.broncus.com/index.asp
30. Monaldi V (1947) Endocavitary aspiration: its practical applications. Tubercle 28:223
31. MacArthur AM, Fountain SW (1977) Intracavity suction and drainage in the treatment of emphysematous bullae. Thorax 32:668
32. Goldstraw P, Petrou M (1995) The surgical treatment of emphysema: the Brompton approach. Chest Surg Clin North Am 5:777
33. Wakabayashi A (1993) Thoracoscopic technique for management of giant bullous lung disease. Ann Thorac Surg 56:708

Part III

Minimally Invasive Thoracic Surgery: The Pleura

The Pleura: General Aspects

16

Rolf G.C. Inderbitzi

Contents

R.G.C. Inderbitzi, M.D.
Thoraxzentrum Zurich, Hirslanden Clinic,
Witellikerstrasse 40,
CH-8008 Zurich, Switzerland
e-mail: r.inderbitzi@thoraxzentrum.ch

16.1 Topography and Anatomy

The pleura comprises the visceral and the parietal pleura, and this forms two layers which merge into each other in the hilum of the lung. The reflective surfaces of the healthy pleura (Fig. 16.1) are separated from each other by the capillary

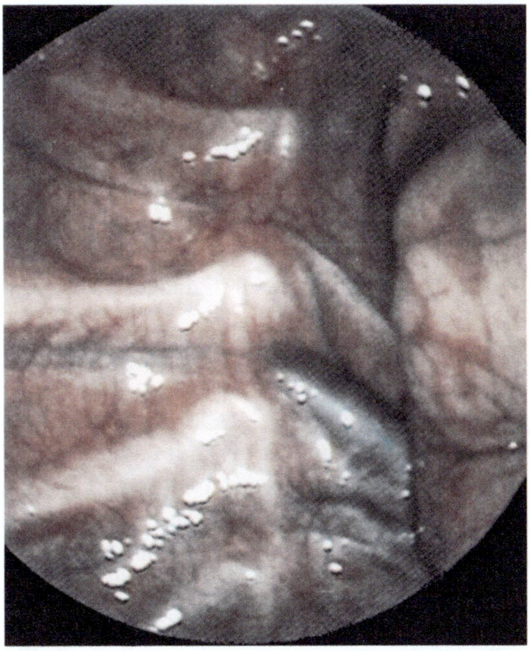

Fig. 16.1 Thoracoscopic view of a healthy, right-sided parietal pleura from a young 20-year-old male patient with spontaneous pneumothorax. The ribs are visible in *white* covered with sympathic striations and the venous confluence which forms the start of the azygos vein (Nakhosteen and Inderbitzi 1994)

R.G.C. Inderbitzi et al. (eds.), *Minimally Invasive Thoracic and Cardiac Surgery*,
DOI 10.1007/978-3-642-11861-6_16, © Springer-Verlag Berlin Heidelberg 2012

space filled with approximately 3 ml of pleural fluid. The visceral pleura is attached directly to the lung and is about 100–200 μm thick. The superficial mesothelium (covering cell layer) is formed by the mesothelial cells which are joined with desmosomes and demonstrate microvilli on their surface. On the inside are three layers of connective tissue delineated by a basal membrane. The main connective tissue layer of the pleura is formed by an external and internal border lamina with a fibrous layer in between, which controls the blood vessels. The internal lamina borders on the alveolar wall and is connected to the interstitial connective tissue of the lung in the area of the lobular septum. The parietal pleura borders on the intercostal muscles and ribs over the endothoracic fascia.

The vessels run through the pleura's main connective tissue layer. The visceral pleura is supplied in the costal and diaphragm area by the pulmonary arteries and in the other sections by branches of the bronchial arteries with anastomoses to the pulmonary arteries. The parietal pleura is supplied in the costal area by branches of the intercostal arteries and the intercostal branches of the internal thoracic artery.

The lymph vessels of the pulmonary pleura run close to the lungs in the main connective tissue layer. In the parietal pleura, lymphatic stomata of 2–8-μm diameter are of particular significance. In these zones, the pleural space is connected directly to the lymph vessel drainage system [6].

16.2 Pleural Diagnostics

In 80% of post-mortems of adult cases, there is evidence of residues from previous predominantly inflammatory pleural processes. These changes are most likely the results of disease processes of the neighbouring organs, although it is not uncommon for systemic diseases to lead to non-specific concomitant inflammation of the pleura. The acute, non-specific pleurisy usually occurs as a reaction to lung disease (pneumonia, infarction, tumours). If disease persists, the formation of an effusion follows the initial oedema of the main connective tissue layer, with intrapleural vascular dilation (Fig. 16.2), as the balance between the physiological circulation of exudation and absorption is disturbed due to lung processes.

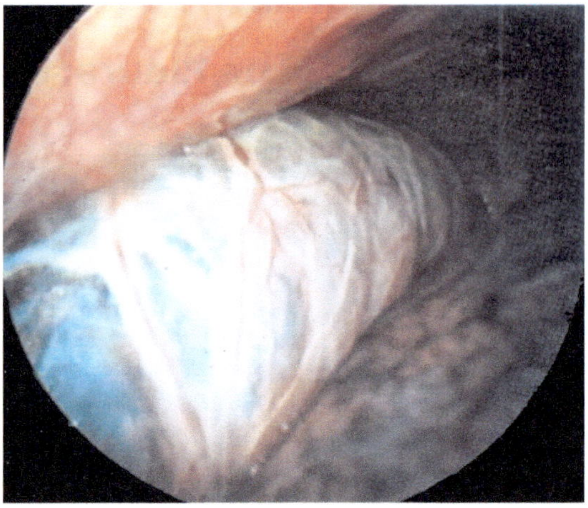

Fig. 16.2 Both the extended capillaries of the parietal pleura and the visceral pleural (here bullous) form a typical checkerboard pattern (Nakhosteen and Inderbitzi 1994)

Transudates are usually the consequence of increased hydrostatic pressure, which may be caused by a cardiac problem, or a reduction in colloid osmotic pressure such as protein deficiency.

Exudates predominantly develop due to underlying inflammatory or neoplastic diseases as a result of increased capillary permeability. If fibrin deposits occur, these lead primarily to a netlike pattern of the pleura and later to microscopic and macroscopic netlike adhesions (Fig. 16.3). Fibrin exudate causes pain. If there is only a small amount of effusion, this leads to a picture of painful pleuritis sicca [dry pleurisy] with audible pleural rub on auscultation. With exudative pleurisy, protective hypoventilation quickly supports the rapid organisation of a fibrinopurulent empyema (Fig. 16.4) which later becomes fibrosing empyema (Fig. 16.5). Forty-seven percent of cases of pleural empyema occur as a result of a respiratory tract infection, 33% are caused by a prior operation, 10% by an intra-abdominal source of infection and another 10% by non-surgical, iatrogenic measures [8]. At its most impressive, this event drains away if caused by a bacterial infection.

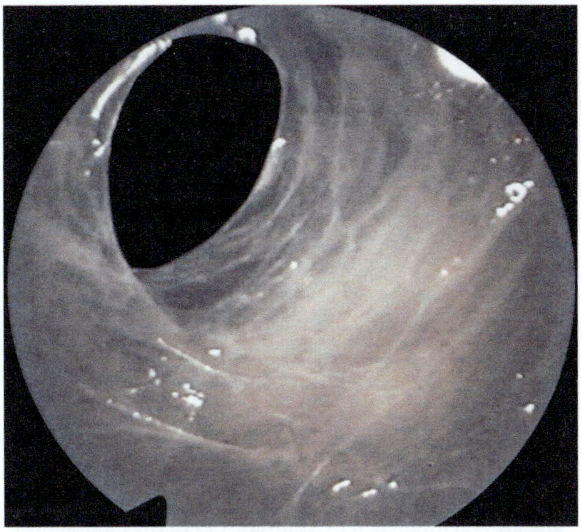

Fig. 16.3 Delicate, easily separable, fibrinous adhesions in a patient with incipient empyema formation (Nakhosteen and Inderbitzi 1994)

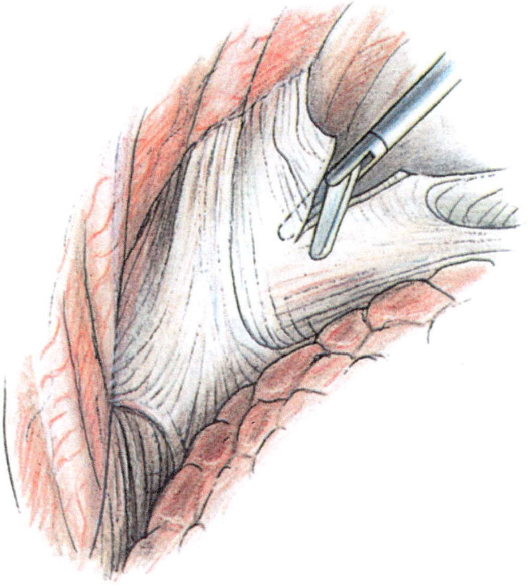

Fig. 16.4 Fibrinopurulent phase of an empyema with incipient granulation (Nakhosteen and Inderbitzi 1994)

Almost any form of pleurisy leads to significant reactions in the acute or subacute stage, involving mesothelial cells, cell enlargement and the formation of polynuclear giant cells, and then in the chronification phase to development of vessel-rich granulation tissue. The main diseases which form granulomatous pleurisy are tuberculosis,

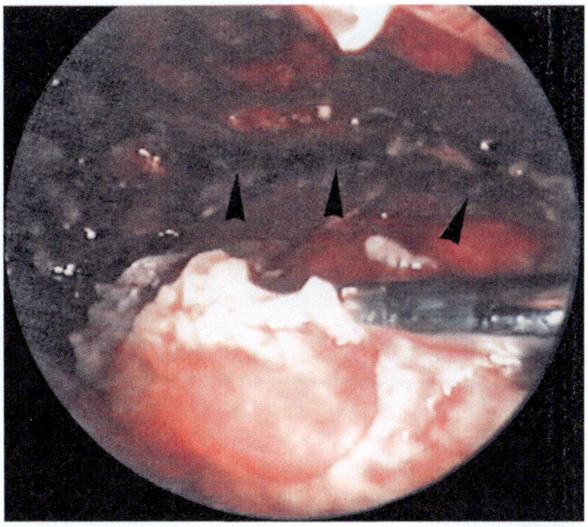

Fig. 16.5 Organised fibrin coating on the diaphragm after opening of the costodiaphragmatic recess (*arrow*) (Nakhosteen and Inderbitzi 1994)

sarcoidosis, a picture of rheumatic disease and foreign body reactions after iatrogenic measures.

If there is a transudative, ipsilateral formation of effusion, a differential diagnosis of a malignant event must always be considered; this is usually of a secondary origin and rarely of a primary origin, such as in malignant mesothelioma of the pleura. This is the case in over 50% of cases among those over 60 years of age [5]: with breast carcinoma, it occurs in 26–49%, bronchial carcinoma in 10–24%, ovarian carcinoma in 16–17% and malignant lymphomas in 7–15% [2, 3]. In over 80%, both pleural layers are involved when an effusion occurs, though parietal tumour manifestations are more commonly visible macroscopically (Fig. 16.6) [3, 4, 10, 11]. The colonisation of the pleural space by malignant cells is substantiated in half of the cases by cytological evidence of malignant cells in the aspirate from the needle biopsy. In the chest X-ray, there is evidence of fluid from an effusion in the postero-anterior view from 175 cm^3 and in the lateral view from 100 cm^3 [1, 3, 9, 12]. Often, the symptoms of breathlessness, cough and chest pain caused by effusion are the first evidence of disease, and yet they are always late signs of it as well. After a diagnosis has been made, the survival time for a malignant effusion is usually less than 1 year [2, 11].

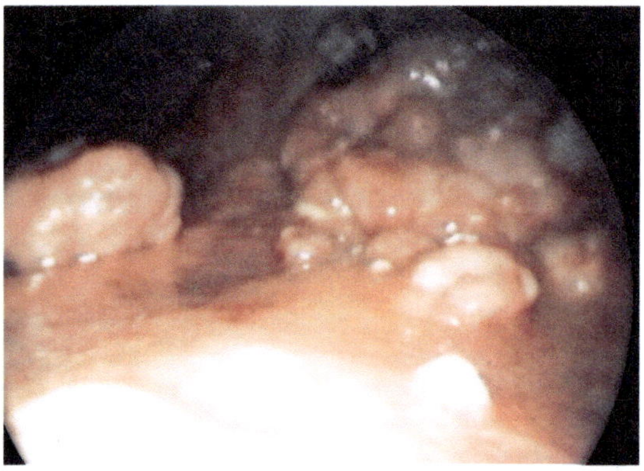

Fig. 16.6 Pleural dissemination of a breast carcinoma on the thoracic wall, cytologically negative (Nakhosteen and Inderbitzi 1994)

16.3 Surgery of the Pleural Space

Videothoracoscopy of the pleural space allows precise assessment and diagnosis of both pleural layers and the associated anatomical structures. Overview, search for a focus and sufficient targeted tissue samples for molecular biological, microbiological and histological examination are possible. The procedure is frequently carried out as combined diagnosis and therapy. The Chap. 2 gives more detailed information on the technical procedure. The imaging documentation of the findings is also significant. Besides the lung biopsy – for more detail, see in chapter "10. "Non-anatomical Resections" – the treatment of the chronic pleural effusion, whether transudate or exudate, has priority (especially malignant effusion and pleural empyema): The different techniques used for this are described later.

References

1. Austin EH, Flye MW (1979) The treatment of recurrent malignant pleural effusion. Ann Thorac Surg 28:190–203
2. Chernow B, Sahn SA (1977) Carcinomatous involvement of the pleura. Am J Med 63:695–702
3. Hausheer FH, Yabro JW (1985) Diagnosis and treatment of malignant pleural effusion. Semin Oncol 12:54–75
4. Leff A, Hopeweöö PC, Costello J (1978) Pleural effusion from malignancy. Ann Intern Med 88:532–537
5. Moore DWO (1991) Malignant pleural effusion. Semin Oncol 18:59–61
6. Müller KM (1994) Erkrankungen der Pleura – pathologische Anatomie. In: Nakhosteen JA, Inderbitzi R (eds) Atlas und Lehrbuch der thorakalen Endoskopie: Bronchoskopie, Thorakoskopie. Springer Verlag, Berlin/Heidelberg, p S 325
7. J. Nakhosteen, R. Inderbitzi: Atlas und Lehrbuch der thorakalen Endoskopie 3. Auflage, Springer-Verlag 1994
8. Orringer MB (1988) Thoracic empyema – back to basics. Chest 93:901–902
9. Peterson JA (1984) Recognition of infrapulmonary pleural effusion. Radiology 74:34
10. Rosato FE, Wallach MW, Rosato GF (1974) The management of malignant effusions from the breast cancer. J Surg Oncol 6:441–449
11. Sahn SA (1981) Pleural manifestations of pulmonary disease. Hosp Pract 16:73–79, 83–85, 89
12. Woodring JH (1984) Recognition of pleural effusion on supine radiographs: how much fluid is required? Am J Roentgenol 142:59–64

Talc Poudrage

17

Giuseppe Cardillo, Luigi Carbone,
Francesco Carleo, Anna Rita Forcione,
and Massimo Martelli

Contents

G. Cardillo, M.D., FRCS, FETCS (✉)
L. Carbone, M.D. • F. Carleo, M.D.
A.R. Forcione, M.D. • M. Martelli, M.D.
Department of Thoracic Surgery, Azienda Ospedaliera S. Camillo-Forlanini, Carlo Forlanini Hospital,
Via Portuense 332, Rome 00149, Italy
e-mail: gcardillo@scamilloforlanini.rm.it;
lcarbone@scamilloforlanini.rm.it;
fcarleo@scamilloforlanini.rm.it;
aforcione@scamilloforlanini.rm.it;
mmartelli@scamilloforlanini.rm.it

17.1 Indications

17.1.1 Primary and Secondary Spontaneous Pneumothorax (Fig. 17.1a)

Amending the focussed treatments (ablation of blebs and bullae), pleurodesis represents a cornerstone of the treatment of spontaneous pneumothorax. Thus, in thoracoscopic literature, various techniques for such treating spontaneous pneumothorax have been reported. In addition to more circumscribed procedures like pleural abrasion (Chap. 19) or parietal pleurectomy (Chap. 20), chemical pleurodesis effects a secure obliteration of pleural space and therefore prophylaxis of relapse of pneumothorax. First and foremost, used techniques of chemical pleurodeses is talc poudrage [5, 13, 22], achieving impressive results with a recurrence rate below 8%. However, in adolescents and young adults with primary spontaneous pneumothorax talc, pleurodesis remains a standby procedure contrary to patients with secondary spontaneous pneumothorax and extended pulmonary tissue lesions without generalized emphysema treatable by lung volume reduction surgery (Chap. 15).

17.1.2 Malignant and Benign Pleural Effusion (Fig. 17.1b)

In patients aged over 60 years, malignant disease is the cause of exudative pleural effusions in more

R.G.C. Inderbitzi et al. (eds.), *Minimally Invasive Thoracic and Cardiac Surgery*,
DOI 10.1007/978-3-642-11861-6_17, © Springer-Verlag Berlin Heidelberg 2012

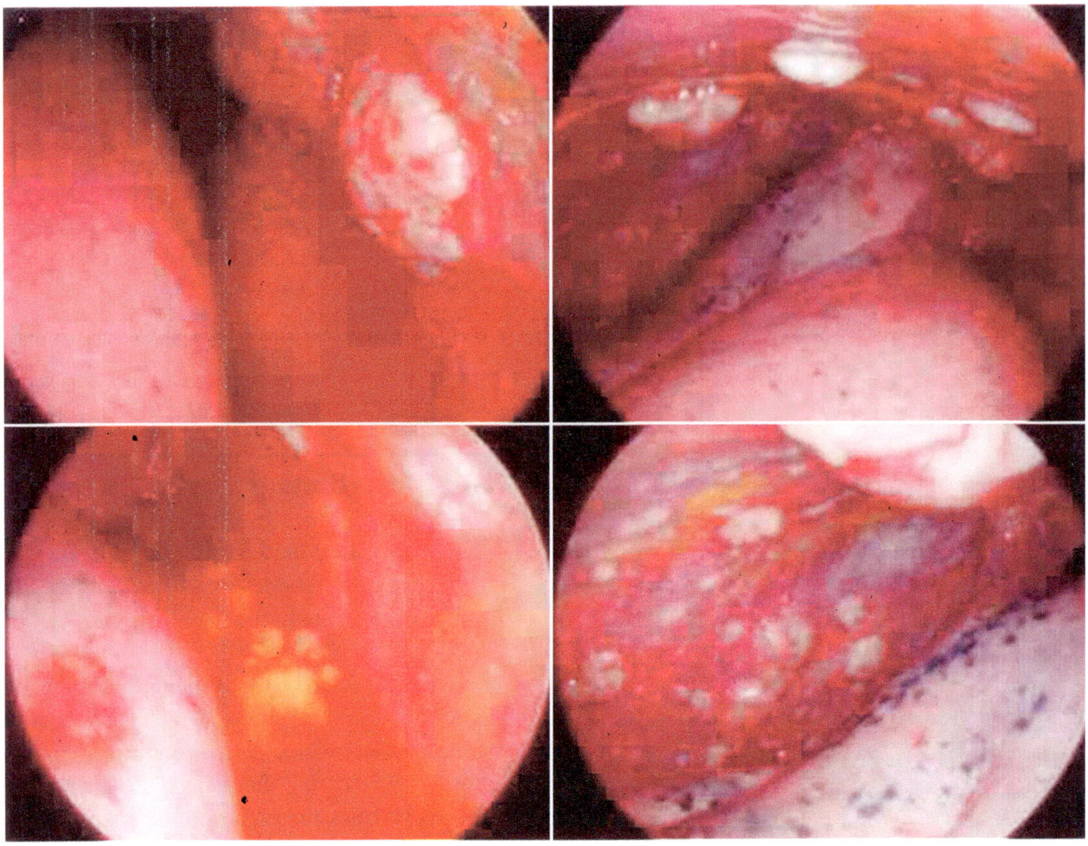

Fig. 17.1 Metastasis of pleural pleura of a patient with breast cancer

than 50% of cases [18]. The formation of malignant pleural effusions can be expected during the course of the disease in 26–49% of patients with carcinoma of the breast, 10–24% with bronchial carcinoma, 16–17% with ovarian carcinoma and 7–15% with malignant lymphomas [9, 15]. The pleural cavity is almost always infiltrated by tumour cells, which in turn can be confirmed diagnostically in more than half the cases by the cytological examination of aspirated fluid (Fig. 17.2). The effusion results either from increased capillary permeability owing to distended or destroyed capillary endothelium or is caused by tumorous lymph drainage [15]. It is also not uncommon for a hypoalbuminaemia in cachectic patients to be the sole or contributive cause of pleural effusions. In over 80% of cases, both pleural membranes are involved in the exudation [15, 17].

Malignant pleural effusions often cause shortness of breath, coughing and thoracic pain. The clinical examination leads to a suspected diagnosis based on weakened breathing sounds, a dull percussion note and reduced respiratory mobility of the diaphragm. Fluid can be detected on X-rays in the posteroanterior (PA) view when there is more than 175 cm^3, or in the lateral view with as little as 100 cm^3 [1, 19, 25]. The symptoms arising from the effusion are often the first indications of disease. They are the dominant cause of the patient feeling ill and further restrict the quality of life of this group of tumour patients whose prognosis is already extremely poor. The survival time after diagnosis of malignant effusion is usually less than 1 year [9, 20].

After excluding the possibility of successful systemic oncological therapy, the aim of any

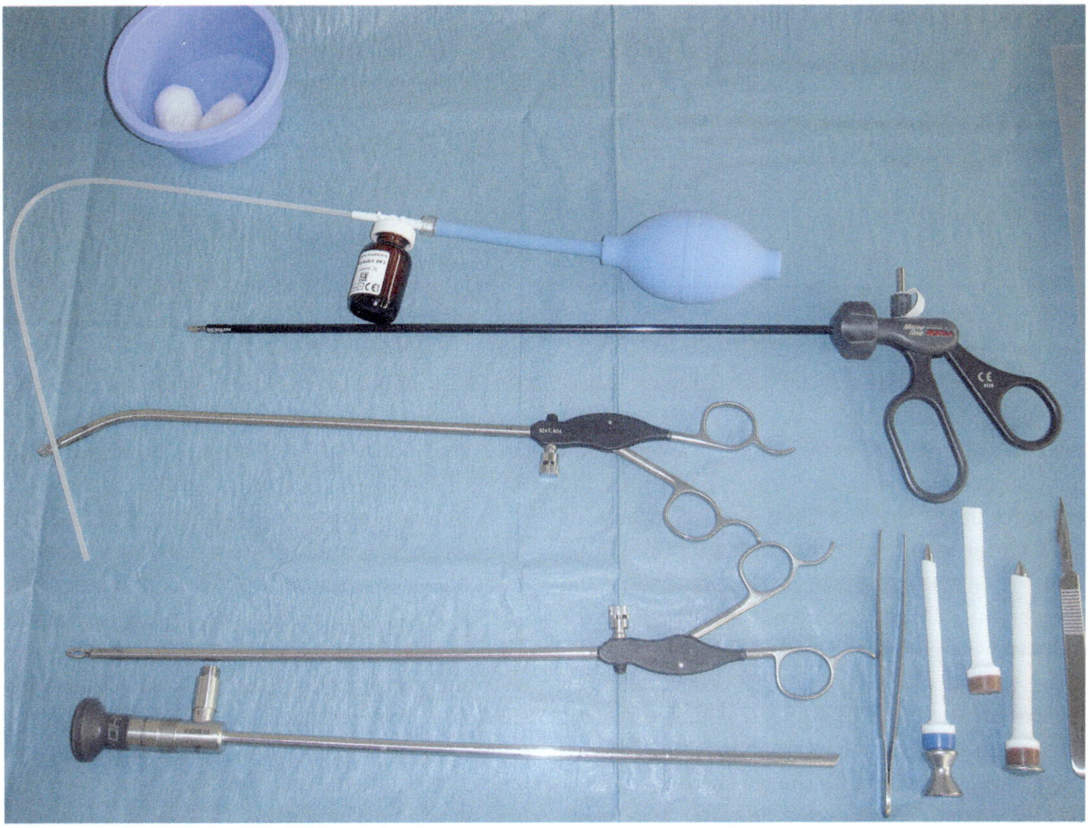

Fig. 17.2 Basic instrument set for thoracoscopic talc peurodeseis. Disposable powder atomizer (Steritalc PF3; Novatech SA, France), forceps, cautery forceps, thoracoscope (0–30°), trocar sleeves (5, 7 mm diameter)

treatment must be fast, effective and lasting alleviation of the respiratory symptoms. The therapeutic strategies must be orientated towards the pathophysiological features of the disease. The obliteration of the pleural cavity with chemical pleurodesis by local instillation of sclerosing substances is the most common method but has recurrence rates of up to 30% [5, 12]. Thoracoscopic pleurodesis was first proposed by Béthune in France in 1935 and is still mainly propagated today in French-speaking countries. Guérin and Boniface have a series of 792 cases, 630 malignant and 162 non-neoplastic effusions. They report no recurrences in 90% of cases [3, 14]. The results of Boutin in Marseilles are equally impressive, with personal experience of 300 cases of malignant effusion and a success rate of over 90% after talc pleurodesis [5]. Boutin also reviews the literature covering a total of 1,244 patients treated with talc pleurodesis with an average success rate of 87%.

The success of pleurodesis depends primarily on the careful evaluation of the patient [4, 12]. Not all patients with malignant effusions can be treated by thoracoscopic pleurodesis. The following conditions must be met when the therapy is commenced:

1. The compressed lung must be shown clinically and radiologically to be fully expanded following drainage of the effusion
2. The evacuation of the pleural cavity and the decompression of the lung must lead to a significant alleviation of the respiratory symptoms

The possible *surgery-related complications* of thoracoscopic talc pleurodesis are those inherent in thoracoscopy. They include surface lung injuries when inducing the pneumothorax, slight bleeding of the thoracic wall and local infection. The possibility of local tumour propagation in the area of the thoracoscopic entry site is known and occurs primarily with pleural mesothelioma [5, 20].

17.2 Talc

Talc is a mineral defined as hydrated magnesium silicate in its pure form. Talc was used for pleurodesis for the first time in 1935 by the Canadian lung surgeon Norman Bethune who helped the sufferers in the Spanish Civil War regardless of their uniform and first organized a mobile blood transfusion service [2]. In the second half of the last century, talc became increasingly popular for induction of pleurodesis in various pleural diseases, such as spontaneous pneumothorax, benign pleural effusion and malignant pleural effusion. Compared to other agents for chemical pleurodesis, talc appeared to give the best results in terms of efficacy and recurrence, both after talc poudrage, and after instillation of talc slurry through a chest tube. The superior effectiveness of talc pleurodesis compared to other forms of pleurodesis has also been confirmed in different studies. In addition, talc is inexpensive and widely available [16, 21, 22].

The mechanism of action of talc in pleurodesis has not been fully elucidated, although it is thought to stimulate a typical local inflammatory response, with reduced fibrinolytic activity, mesothelial cell injury and fibroblast proliferation. This acute-phase inflammatory response is dose related and is inhibited by glucocorticoids. Talc may also have an adhesion-stimulating quality.

Some authors have claimed concern regarding the use of talc in young patients. As regards as oncological risk, it can be ruled out in the light of a survey of Chappel and co-authors which showed the safety of asbestos-free talc [8]. As regards as the possibility of empyema, with the use of sterile talc, the risk should approach zero as long as aseptic technique is employed. As regards as the risk of ARDS, very few cases have been reported in the world literature [7]. The evaluation of such reported cases of ARDS shows that all of these cases are reported from studies performed in the USA and Brazil and not in Europe or Israel. Ferrer in 2001 showed that talc preparations varied markedly from one preparation to others and from country to country [10].

The median particle size of the talc preparation used in our study is 25.6 μ: the distribution curve of talc particles shows that the concentration of small particles (<5 μ) in this talc is 11%, compared to up to 82% in some of the Brazilian talcs analysed, and 54% in one sample of USA talc [10, 24].

In order to assess the distribution of talc deposition in the lung parenchyma and other organs as a possible explanation for ARDS and other complications, various animal studies have been performed. Deposition of talc in the lung parenchyma and other organs was found in studies from the USA and Brazil, whereas talc deposition in other organs was absent in a study from Europe. In animal studies in the same species of rats, distribution of talc was found in 100% of animals in a study from Brazil versus 2% in a European study. In the European study, the authors proposed that the occurrence of talc in 4/198 organs was most probably caused by contamination during storage of the organs [10, 11, 16].

Only in recent years, attention has been drawn to the possible role of talc particle size as a major contributing factor of the side effects, as well as an explanation for the fact that talc deposition in other organs occurred in some studies, while it was absent in others [6, 7].

The use of large size talc particles seems to be a protective factor. As a matter of fact, no case of ARDS has been reported in the largest published experience (861 cases treated by videothoracoscopic talc poudrage for primary spontaneous pneumothorax) [6].

Chest pain and fever are the most common *adverse effects of talc pleurodesis*. The intensity of chest pain ranged from non-existent to severe but, generally, has been minimal with an incidence of 7%. Fever (usually <38°C) occurred in 16–69% of cases characteristically 4–12 h after talc instillation and no longer than 72 h [16, 23].

There are no data to assess the optimal dosage schedule of talc. The reported dosage ranges from 2 to 10 g. There are no controlled trials to state that higher dosages of talc are more effective in inducing pleurodesis. In our experience, we nebulized in the pleural cavity 2–4 g of talc, and we believe there is no reason to use a higher dosage of talc with such technique [6, 7].

Most of concerns regarding the use of talc are related to a misunderstanding of the chemical properties of talc: most of the thoracic surgeons believe that talc is always the same. But it is not true [7].

17.3 Surgical Techniques

Talc can be insufflated into pleural space in a powder form (talc poudrage) (Fig. 17.2) or can be mixed with normal saline and instilled through a standard chest tube (talc slurry). More often, talc poudrage is performed with the patient under general anaesthesia and one lung ventilation; nevertheless, it can be used with the patient under local anaesthesia. Talc pleurodesis needs a basic instrument set only (Fig. 17.2). The patient is placed in the lateral position with the arm held abducted to allow maximum superior displacement of the scapula. The first incision is always placed in the fifth or sixth intercostal space in the midaxillary line, and a 0° thoracoscope connected to a video camera is introduced through a 10.5/5.5-mm trocar sleeve (Fig. 17.3a, b). Any adhesions are completely lysed for complete thoracoscopic overview. Entire visceral pleural surface is coated with the talc. Dry asbestos-free talc is then insufflated into the pleural cavity, and the camera is used to ensure uniform, complete coverage of both visceral and parietal pleural surfaces with a thin coating of talc (Figs. 17.4 and 17.5). At the completion of the procedure, one or two chest tubes are positioned through the trocar sites under thoracoscopic guidance (Fig. 17.6). The pleural drain is left in situ for around 4 days. Steroid and nonsteroid drugs after the intrapleural administration of talc markedly lower the initial inflammatory response and the effectiveness of pleurodesis [26].

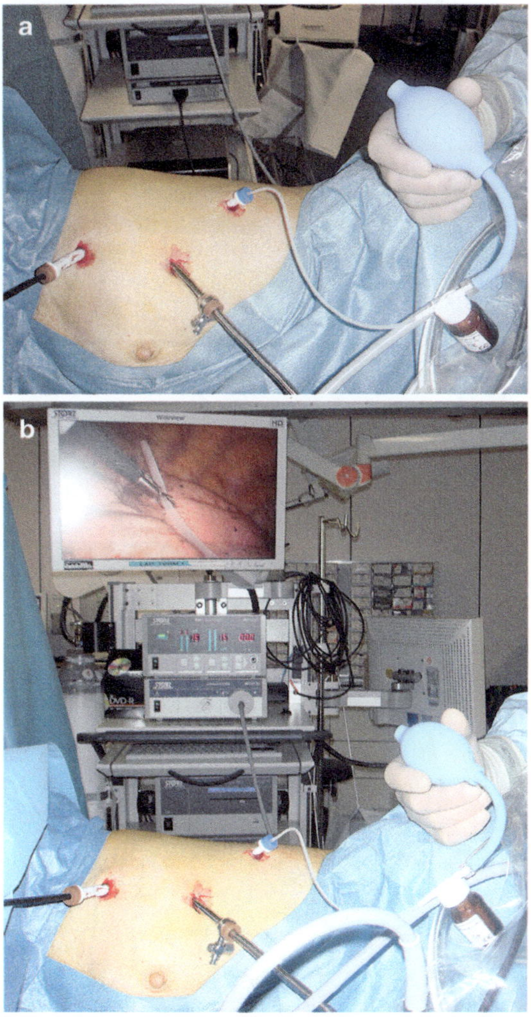

Fig. 17.3 (**a**) Incisions for surgical videothoracoscopic talc poudrage. Thoracoscope is positioned in the central trocar sleeve. Through left port, a forceps directs the tip of powder atomizer (Fig. 17.4). (**b**) Standard arrangement in the operation theatre with patient in lateral position. Surgical team stand ventral to the patient, TV screen is positioned on the opposite

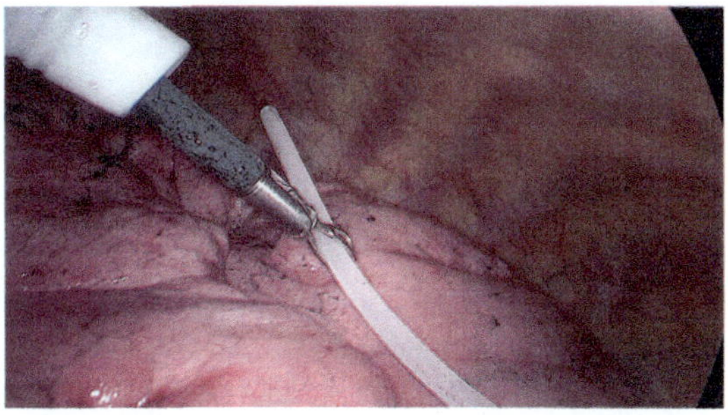

Fig. 17.4 Endoscopic view. Forceps directs the tip of powder atomizer

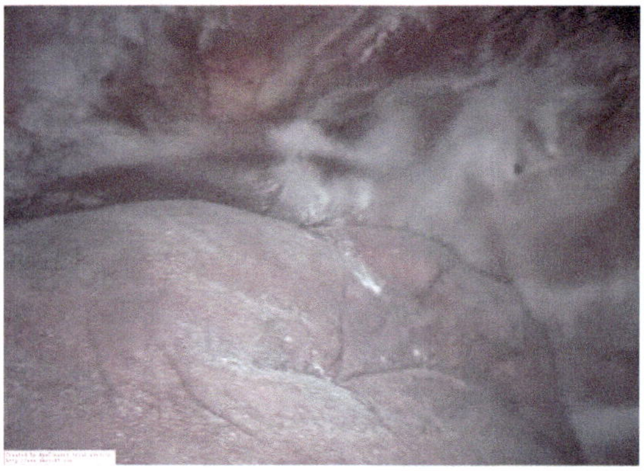

Fig. 17.5 Entire surface of visceral and parietal pleura is covered with talc

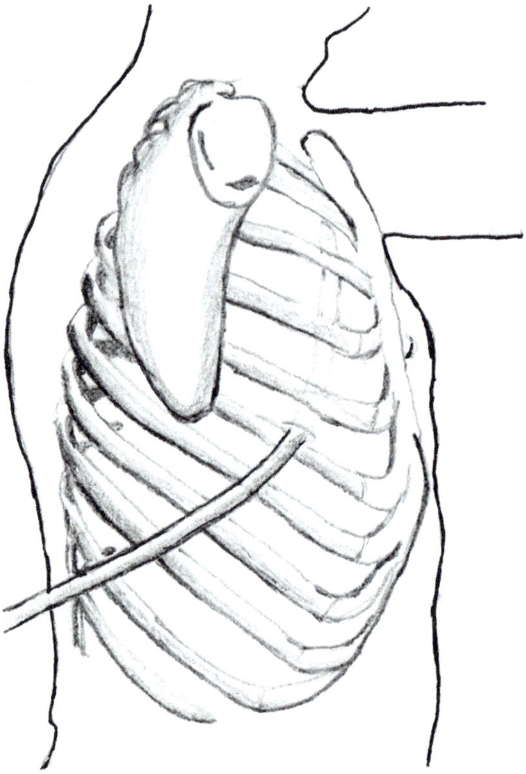

Fig. 17.6 Common position of drainages

References

1. Austin EH, Flye MW (1979) The treatment of recurrent malignant pleural effusion. Ann Thorac Surg 28:190–203
2. Bethune N (1935) Pleural drainage. A new technique for the deliberate production of pleural adhesions as a preliminary to lobectomy. J Thorac Surg 4:251–261
3. Boniface E, Guerin JC (1989) Intérêt du talcage par thoracoscopie dans les traitement symptomatique des pleurésies récidivantes. A propos de 302 cas. Rev Mal Respir 6:133–139
4. Boutin C, Astoul P, Seitz B (1990) The role of thoracoscopy in the evaluation and management of pleural effusions. Lung 168(Suppl):1113–1121
5. Boutin C, Viallat JR, Aclony Y (1991) Practical thoracoscopy. Springer, Berlin/ Heidelberg/ New York/ Tokyo
6. Cardillo G, Carleo F, Giunti R, Carbone L, Mariotta S, Salvadori L, Petrella L, Martelli M (2006) Videothoracoscopic talc poudrage in primary spontaneous pneumothorax: a single-institution experience in 861 cases. J Thorac Cardiovasc Surg 131(2):322–328, Epub 2006 Jan 18
7. Cardillo G et al (2007) Long-term function following videothoracoscopic talc poudrage for primary spontaneous pneumothorax. Eur J Cardiothorac Surg 31: 803–806
8. Chappel AG et al (1979) A survey of the long-term effects of talc and kaolin pleurodesis. Br J Dis Chest 73:285–288
9. Chernow B, Sahn SA (1977) Carcinomatous involvement of the pleura. Am J Med 63:695–702
10. Ferrer J, Villarino MA, Tura JM, Traveria A, Light RW (2001) Talc preparations used for pleurodesis vary markedly from one preparation to another. Chest 119:1901–1905
11. Fraticelli A, Robaglia-Schlupp A, Riera H et al (2002) Distribution of calibrated talc after intrapleural administration: an experimental study in rats. Chest 122: 1737–1741
12. Furrer M, Inderbitzi R (1992) Pleurodeseverfahren beim malignen Pleuraerguss. Schweiz Med Wochenschr 122:181–188
13. Guerin JC, Champel F, Biron E, Kalb IC (1985) Talcage pleural par thoracoscopie dans le traitement du pneumothorax. Etude d'une série de 109 cas traités en 3 ans. Rev Mal Respir 2:25–29
14. Guerin JC, Boniface E (1990) Les méthodes de pleurodèse. Rev Prat 40:1854–1856
15. Hausheer FH, Yabro JW (1985) Diagnosis and treatment of malignant pleural effusion. Semin Oncol 12: 54–75
16. Kennedy L, Sahn SA (1994) Talc pleurodesis for the treatment of pneumothorax and pleural effusion. Chest 106:1215–1222
17. Leff A, Hopeweöö PC, Costello J (1978) Pleural effusion from malignancy. Ann Intern Med 88:532–537
18. Moore DWO (1991) Malignant pleural effusion. Semin Oncol 18:59–61
19. Peterson JA (1984) Recognition of infrapulmonary pleural effusion. Radiology 74:34
20. Rosato FE, Wallach MW, Rosato GF (1974) The management of malignant effusions from the breast cancer. J Surg Oncol 6:441–449
21. Sahn SA, Light RW (2000) Pro/con editorial: talc should/should not be used for pleurodesis. Am J Respir Crit Care Med 162:2023–2026

22. Vanderschueren RG (1981) Le talcage pleural dans le pneumothrax spontané. Poumon Coeur 37:273–276
23. Walker-Renard PB, Vaughan LM, Sahn SA (1994) Chemical pleurodesis for malignant pleural effusions. Ann Intern Med 120:56–64
24. Werebe EC, Pazetti R, Milanez de Campos JR et al (1999) Systemic distribution of talc after intrapleural administration in rats. Chest 115:190–193
25. Woodring JH (1984) Recognition of pleural effusion on supine radiographs: how much fluid is required? Am J Roentgenol 142:59–64
26. Xie C, Teixeira LR, Mc Govern JP, Light RW (1998) Systemic corticosteroid decrease the effectiveness of talc pleurodesis. Am J Respir Crit Care Med 157: 1441–1444

18 Pleural Abrasion

Uliano Morandi, Alessandro Stefani,
and Christian Casali

Contents

18.1 Introduction

Pleural abrasion represents a surgical technique employed to obtain pleural symphysis in spontaneous pneumothorax. In 1941, Tyson described excision of blebs and gauze abrasion of the pleura as a procedure to prevent recurrence in spontaneous pneumothorax [42]. Gaensler, in 1956, reported the first series of patients with recurrent spontaneous pneumothorax treated with pleurectomy [17]. In 1968, Clagett proposed the use of abrasion instead of pleurectomy, considered a too-radical method [12]. Nowadays, though it can be used also for secondary spontaneous pneumothorax (SSP), pleural abrasion is largely applied in the treatment of primary spontaneous pneumothorax (PSP).

The peculiar feature of spontaneous pneumothorax is the possibility to present recurrences. The recurrence rate after nonsurgical treatment of PSP (conservative treatment so-called bed rest, thoracentesis, chest drain insertion) is considerably high: 30% after the first episode and more than 60% after the first recurrence [14]. The aim of the definitive treatment of spontaneous pneumothorax is the prevention of recurrences. The discussion of indications to surgical treatment of spontaneous pneumothorax is beyond the purposes of this chapter.

Prevention of recurrences is achieved by a surgical operation that permits to excise the offending blebs or bullae and to promote adhesion formation. Pleural symphysis can be accomplished by various methods, such as pleural

U. Morandi, M.D. (✉) • A. Stefani, M.D.
C. Casali, M.D.
Division of Thoracic Surgery, Department of General Surgery and Surgical Specialties, University of Modena and Reggio Emilia, Policlinico of Modena,
Largo del Pozzo 71, Modena 41100, Italy
e-mail: morandi.uliano@unimore.it;
stefani.alessandro@unimore.it;
casali.christian@unimore.it

R.G.C. Inderbitzi et al. (eds.), *Minimally Invasive Thoracic and Cardiac Surgery*,
DOI 10.1007/978-3-642-11861-6_18,

abrasion, pleurectomy or chemical irritation by talc or tetracycline. All these procedures can be performed through an open procedure (thoracotomy) or video-assisted thoracic surgery (VATS).

18.2 Technique

Pleural abrasion represents a step in the surgical operation for the treatment of spontaneous pneumothorax, and it is usually performed after the excision of blebs/bullae. This operation is undertaken under general anaesthesia and single-lung ventilation, and the patient is placed in the lateral decubitus position. The surgical approach can be either by thoracotomy or by VATS.

Pleural abrasion is obtained by scrubbing the parietal pleura until a uniform aspect of bloody pleura is achieved (Fig. 18.1). Lacerations of the mesothelial layer lead to the formation of adhesions and subsequent pleurodesis. The exact mechanism responsible for the formation of adhesions remains unclear. The development of an early inflammatory process has been demonstrated, with ingrowth of capillaries, influx of inflammatory cells and activation of fibroblasts [20, 27, 36]. In animal models, some authors found that fibrosis with scar tissue between visceral and parietal pleura is present 3–4 weeks after pleurodesis, without a significant inflammatory reaction [13, 26]. These findings supports the hypothesis that formation of adhesions is dependent on an initial and transient inflammatory reaction but not on a persistent chronic inflammation.

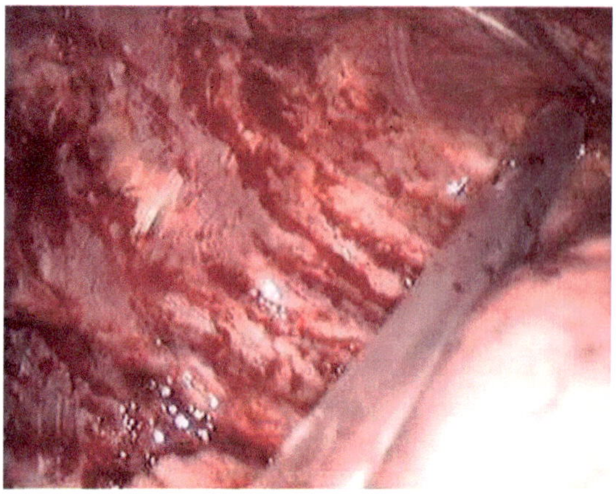

Fig. 18.1 The intraoperative picture shows the bloody aspect of the parietal pleura after videothoracoscopic pleural abrasion. The abrasion was accomplished from the apex to the sixth rib

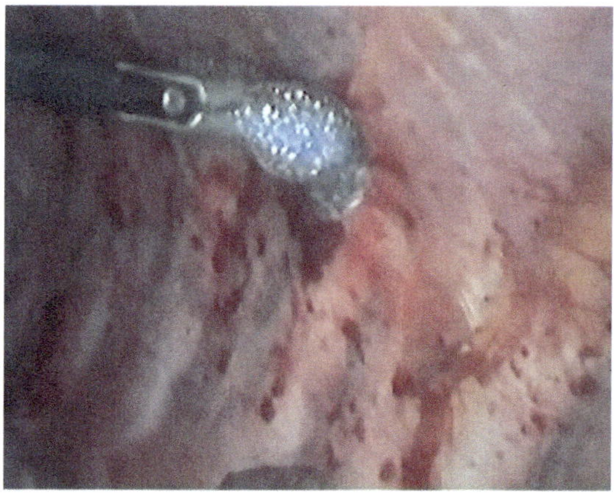

Fig. 18.2 Intraoperative picture showing the procedure of pleural abrasion performed with an electrosurgical tip cleaner attached to the tip of an endoscopic grasper

Various tools can be used for mechanical pleural abrasion: polyglactin [19], polypropylene [8, 22, 37] or nylon [15] meshes, polyglycolic acid gauze [25], plastic sponge [23] or the electrosurgical tip cleaner [26, 41]. Meshes or gauzes should be dry, to warrant a more effective abrasion. When abrasion is performed through thoracotomy, the mesh is put on the hand and abrasion is directly accomplished by the surgeon's hand. For abrasion by VATS, a swab or a pladget of mesh or gauze is attached to the tip of an endoscopic grasper or long vascular clamp and introduced into the pleural cavity through a thoracoport (Fig. 18.2). The support for the pad should be curved, in order to reach the whole pleural circumference. Pleural abraders especially fit for VATS have been developed, such as the one reported in Figs. 18.3 and 18.4. Some authors argued that the limit of endoscopic pleural abrasion, with respect to abrasion performed by thoracotomy, is the limited surface of the small abrading swab [19, 30]. This may make the manoeuvre tiresome and lengthy, and it may be difficult to create a homogeneous pleural irritation, since pressure is exerted on small areas; moreover, pads get soaked with blood quickly and have to be changed. Thereafter, alternative

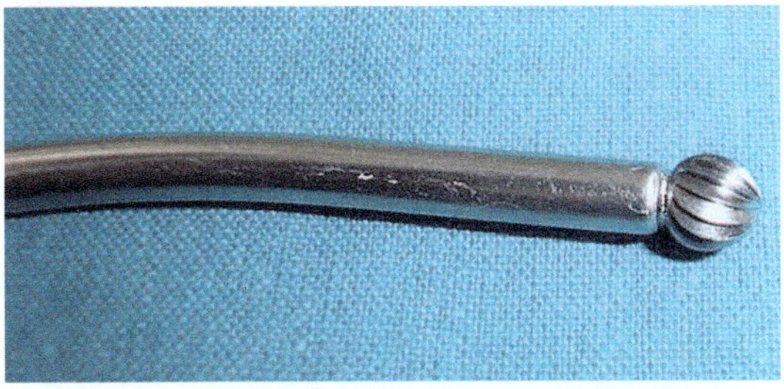

Fig. 18.3 The picture shows the abrader used at our institute (Richard Wolf GmbH, Knittlingen, Germany). It is a metal tool with a 50-cm-long stick, having a diameter of 4.5 mm. The tip is curved and endowed with a milled sphere of the same diameter than the stick

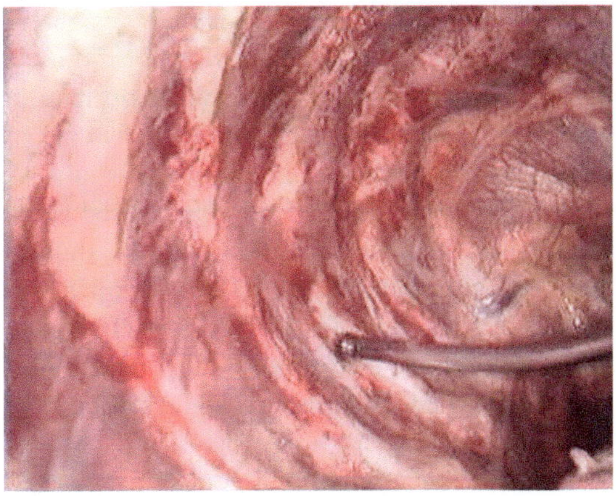

Fig. 18.4 Intraoperative picture showing pleural abrasion performed with the endoscopic abrader described in Fig. 18.3

solutions have been proposed, such as disposable curved plastic brushes or an electrical rotating brush [30]. In effect, when performing pleural abrasion through thoracoscopic approach, the appreciation of the proper level of pressure to exert on the instrument for achieving an appropriate abrasion requires some experience. Furthermore, the ability to distinguish between bloody pleura and mere diffusion of oozing along the pleural surface requires experience too, as well as optimal video equipment. As reported by some authors, the diffuse oozing observed after videothoracoscopic abrasion can be deceptive at the beginning of the surgeon's experience (19). Waller found a significant decrease in recurrence rate with increasing experience, thus suggesting the existence of a learning curve for thoracoscopic pleural abrasion [45].

Regarding the pleural surface to be abraded, the apex is the most important area to treat. Most surgeons recommend to carry out the abrasion from the apex downward to the fifth-sixth rib, as also stated by the American College of Chest Physicians consensus conference on management of spontaneous pneumothorax [5]. In this document, a good consensus for a pleurodesis limited to the upper half of the haemithorax is reported. However, some surgeons prefer to extend the abrasion to the entire parietal pleura [8, 19] or, further, to the diaphragmatic pleura [25], with the aim to prevent partial recurrence in the lower part of the pleural cavity. The abrasion should be extended along the whole pleural circumference, from the internal mammary artery anteriorly to the sympathetic nerve chain posteriorly. Caution must be paid to avoid abrading on the first sympathetic ganglion and on the vascular structures of the apex. Pleural abrasion does not be performed on visceral and mediastinal pleura and pericardium.

18.3 Results

Table 18.1 shows the results of pleural abrasion in the treatment of spontaneous pneumothorax. Results of pleural abrasion must be evaluated both in terms of effectiveness in achieving pleural symphysis and in terms of complications, in comparison with other techniques of pleurodesis, such as chemical pleurodesis, pleural coagulation or pleurectomy.

There are no controlled trials comparing talc and tetracycline instilled through the chest tube, but recurrence rates seem to be unacceptably high, at 10–20% [1, 4, 31]. Thus, this approach can be proposed only for patients who present increased surgical risk or who refuse surgery, as suggested in the ACCP consensus conference [5].

Talc poudrage is the most effective technique of chemical pleurodesis, yielding recurrence rates of about 2% in spontaneous pneumothorax. In two experimental studies, talc poudrage showed results comparable to mechanical abrasion [9, 13]. However, some concerns limited the use of

Table 18.1 Recurrence rates after pleural abrasion for spontaneous pneumothorax

Author	Year	Pts (*n*)	Surgical access	Recurrence (%)
Thomas et al. [40]	1993	107	Open	0
Bertrand et al. [7]	1996	87	Open	1.3
Kim et al. [24]	1996	66	VATS	11.1
Jimenez-Merchal et al. [23]	1997	627	Open	0
Dumont et al. [15]	1997	237	Open	0.4
Lang-Ladzunski et al. [25]	2003	182	VATS	3
Gossot et al. [19]	2004	185	VATS	3.6
Sawada et al. [38]	2005	154	VATS	11.7
Bobbio et al. [8]	2006	60	VATS	3.4
Rena et al. [37]	2008	112	VATS	6.2

talc in PSP: the creation of tight adhesions, difficult to free if thoracotomy become necessary in the future, the risk of pleural infection, the possibility that mesothelioma may develop as a late effect (which has been suggested but never demonstrated) and a mild to moderate restrictive impairment of pulmonary function [18, 43]. British Thoracic Society guidelines for the management of spontaneous pneumothorax recommend that talc pleurodesis should not be considered as initial treatment for PSP [21].

Parietal pleura diathermy or laser coagulation has been also proposed as methods of pleurodesis in spontaneous pneumothorax. The presumed benefit of these procedures is to obtain an inflammatory response on the pleural surface without pleural bleeding. Argon beam coagulation has been used in PSP, but it was found less effective than mechanical abrasion [8, 9].

Partial excision of the apical portion of the parietal pleura (partial pleurectomy) has been performed for a long time to achieve pleurodesis in spontaneous pneumothorax. Its use as an alternative to pleural abrasion is still debated. Experimental studies have demonstrated that pleurectomy obtains a more intense pleurodesis than pleural abrasion [13]. In fact, results of pleurectomy are excellent, with recurrence rates <2%, so there seems to be an advantage to pleurectomy over pleural abrasion in terms of effectiveness. Unfortunately, most comparative clinical studies on the treatment of spontaneous pneumothorax compared the surgical approaches (VATS versus thoracotomy) and not the techniques of pleurodesis. Moreover, many studies had few patients; in some studies, patients with PSP and SSP were mixed or different techniques of pleurodesis were employed, and blebs excision was not routinely performed in all studies. This makes difficult to evaluate the role of the employed technique of pleurodesis in the achievement of the results. A recent meta-analysis of 25 nonrandomised and 4 randomised studies, from 1993 to 2006, showed an overall recurrence rate of 1.1% for open surgery (0–6.8%) and 5.4% for VATS (0–16%) [3]. Table 18.2 reports the results of the 4 randomised studies and the 8 uncontrolled studies with more than 100 patients.

The only randomised trial comparing pleurectomy and pleural abrasion was published by Rena and colleagues in 2008 [37]: in a series of 208 patients with PSP operated by VATS, a nonsignificant difference was found in recurrence rates between pleural abrasion (6.2%) and pleurectomy (4.6%). Conversely, in a nonrandomised study on 65 patients with PSP operated by VATS, Chang and colleagues reported that pleurectomy was significantly more effective than pleural abrasion (recurrence rates of 0% vs. 8.6% respectively) [10].

Of course, recurrence rate alone is not the sole determinant that can affect the choice of form of access and pleurodesis: early and late morbidity, length of hospital stay and recovery and costs must be also taken into account. In the study of Rena [37], postoperative morbidity and haemothorax rates were significantly higher in the pleurectomy group; these patients complained greater chest pain and discomfort at long-term follow-up, whereas no difference was found with respect to early postoperative pain, chest drain

Table 18.2 Comparative results of VATS and open surgery in the prevention of recurrent pneumothorax

			Surgical access		Recurrence (%)	
Author	Year	Pts (*n*)	VATS	Open	VATS	Open
Waller et al. [44]	1994	60	Pleurectomy	Pleurectomy	6.7	3.3
Ayed and Al-Din [2]	2000	60	Pleurectomy	Pleurectomy	10	0
Freixenet et al. [16]	2004	90	Pleural abrasion	Pleural abrasion	4.3	0
Li et al. [29]	2006	143	Pleural abrasion	Pleurectomy Pleural abrasion	0	0
Cheynel et al. [11]	1994	111	Pleurectomy Pleural abrasion	Pleurectomy Pleural abrasion	2.1	0
Dumont et al. [15]	1996	338	Pleural abrasion	Pleural abrasion	3	0.4
Jimenez-Merchan et al. [23]	1997	737	Pleural abrasion	Pleural abrasion	1.8	0
Passlick et al. [35]	1997	122	Pleurectomy Pleural abrasion	Pleurectomy Pleural abrasion	6.9	0
Matzusoe et al. [32]	1999	336	NR	NR	11.5	2.9
Sawada et al. [38]	2005	187	Pleural abrasion	NR	11.7	3
Ben-Nun et al. [6]	2006	121	Pleural abrasion	Pleural abrasion	3.4	0
Ingolfsson et al. [22]	2006	240	Pleurectomy Pleural abrasion Talc	Pleurectomy Pleural abrasion Talc	6.3	0

NR not reported

and hospital stay duration. In the work of Chang [10], no difference was observed with respect to postoperative pain, complication rate, chest tube duration, hospital stay and postoperative pulmonary function, while a significantly longer operative time was required for pleurectomy (103 min vs. 78 min, respectively). Although the morbidity of pleurectomy remains acceptably low, this procedure seems to carry a risk of bleeding and late fibrothorax higher than pleural abrasion [28, 33, 37, 39]. Another drawback of pleurectomy is that tight adhesions created by this procedure may make reintervention extremely difficult, due to the lack of a dissection plane. On the contrary, mechanical abrasion is less aggressive and allows to preserve an extrapleural plane for dissection, in case thoracotomy needs to be done later on for other reasons.

The differences observed for other variables, such as postoperative pain, complications other than bleeding, length of hospital stay, postoperative recovery and costs, seem to be related to the surgical access rather than to the technique of pleurodesis. In fact, several authors have suggested that VATS offers significant advantages over open procedures, including less postoperative pain, shorter hospital stay, faster recovery, better pulmonary function in the postoperative period and better cosmetic results [3, 21]. However, these benefits are not unequivocally established [24].

At the Division of Thoracic Surgery of the University of Modena and Reggio Emilia, VATS with blebs excision and mechanical pleurodesis was performed on 272 patients affected by PSP, starting from 1994. One-hundred and ninety-eight patients (73%) were operated for a recurrent pneumothorax; the remaining 74 were treated, at the first episode, for a persistent pneumothorax after chest drainage. The surgical technique of pleurodesis has changed over the years: in our early experience with the first 21 patients, we employed conventional monopolar diathermy, but the high rate of early recurrences in this group of patients (3 patients, 21%) induced us to abandon its use. In the remaining 251 patients, a mechanical pleural abrasion was performed using an electrosurgical tip cleaner attached to the tip of a long vascular clamp or, alternatively, the abrader described in Fig. 18.3. We usually extend pleural abrasion from the apex to the fifth or sixth rib. In our experience, pleural abrasion takes about 10 min to be appropriately performed. Perioperative mortality was absent and postoperative complications were recorded in 32 patients (12%): 18 prolonged air leaks, 13 haemothoraces and 1 pleural empyema. One patient was reoperated for a prolonged air leak whereas no patients required reintervention for major postoperative bleeding. Fifteen of the 251 patients treated with pleural abrasion developed recurrence (recurrence rate of 5.9%). Of note, recurrence rate has significantly reduced throughout the investigated period: 7% (9/128 patients) and 4.8% (6/123 patients) in the years 1995–2002 and 2003–2010, respectively. Such improvement in effectiveness was likely due to the learning curve.

Conclusions

Nowadays, pleural abrasion performed by videothoracoscopic approach is considered by most surgeons as the procedure of choice for the treatment of spontaneous pneumothorax.

The ACCP consensus conference [5] stated that thoracoscopy represents the preferred approach for preventing PSP recurrence (very good consensus) and pleurodesis should be performed in most patients with pleural abrasion (good consensus). For SSP, thoracoscopy is the preferred management (very good consensus), although an axillary thoracotomy represents an acceptable alternative (good consensus); pleural abrasion or pleurectomy are both satisfying methods for producing pleural symphysis in these patients (good consensus).

The BTS guidelines [21] stated that, in the absence of clear evidence of superiority of VATS over thoracotomy, thoracotomy associated with pleurectomy remains the procedure with the highest efficacy. It represents the method of choice in patients with SSP, who may have extensive parenchymal disease, requiring more extensive bullectomy and strong pleurodesis. Nevertheless, a survey conducted in 2006 by the Royal Society of Medicine showed that, in Great Britain, the VATS approach with pleural abrasion is three times more common than an open approach [34].

All in all, advantages and drawbacks of the two different surgical approaches and methods of pleurodesis have to be balanced for each individual patient, to reach the best compromise between the lowest risk of recurrence but highest morbidity of thoracotomy + pleurectomy and the highest risk of recurrence but lowest morbidity of VATS + pleural abrasion. For young fit people with PSP, we think that pleural abrasion through VATS is appropriate. For patients with a targeted 0% recurrence rate, such as aviators, scuba divers or other military or civilian personnel with special professional requirements, pleurectomy through VATS should be preferred. For patients with SSP, an open approach is often necessary to accomplish the required extensive bullectomy; in these cases, pleural abrasion or pleurectomy may be both acceptable methods of pleurodesis.

Finally, it would be pertinent to emphasise to patients, especially those with PSP, the various possibilities, with the risks and potential advantages, so that the final decision will be based not only on the surgeon's preference but also on the choice of an informed patient.

References

1. Almind M, Lange P, Viskum K (1989) Spontaneous pneumothorax: comparison of simple drainage, talc pleurodesis and tetracycline pleurodesis. Thorax 44:627–630
2. Ayed AK, Al-Din HJ (2000) Video-assisted thoracoscopy versus thoracotomy for primary spontaneous pneumothorax: a randomized controlled trial. Med Princ Pract 9:113–118
3. Barker A, Maratos EC, Edmonds L et al (2007) Recurrence rates of video-assisted thoracoscopic versus open surgery in the prevention of recurrent pneumothoraces: a systematic review of randomised and non-randomised trials. Lancet 370:329–335
4. Baumann MH, Strange C (1997) Treatment of spontaneous pneumothorax: a more aggressive approach? Chest 112:789–804
5. Baumann MH, Strange C, Heffner JE et al (2001) Management of spontaneous pneumothorax. An American College of Chest Physicians Delphi Consensus Statement. Chest 119:590–602
6. Ben Nun A, Soudack M, Best LA (2006) Video-assisted thoracoscopic surgery for recurrent spontaneous pneumothorax: the long-term benefit. World J Surg 30:285–290
7. Bertrand PC, Regnard JF, Spaggiari L et al (1996) Immediate and long-term results after surgical treatment of primary spontaneous pneumothorax. Ann Thorac Surg 61:1641–1645

8. Bobbio A, Ampollini L, Internullo E et al (2006) Thoracoscopic parietal pleural argon beam coagulation versus pleural abrasion in the treatment of primary spontaneous pneumothorax. Eur J Cardiothorac Surg 29:6–8
9. Bresticker MA, Oba J, LoCicero J et al (1993) Optimal pleurodesis: a comparison study. Ann Thorac Surg 55:364–367
10. Chang YC, Chen CW, Huang SH et al (2006) Modified needlescopic video-assisted thoracic surgery for primary spontaneous pneumothorax: the long-term effects of apical pleurectomy versus pleural abrasion. Surg Endosc 20:757–762
11. Cheynel N, Bernard A, Belichard C et al (1994) Comparative study of thoracoscopy and thoracotomy in spontaneous pneumothorax. Lyon Chir 90:193–196
12. Clagett OT (1968) The management of spontaneous pneumothorax. J Thorac Cardiovasc Surg 55:761–762
13. Colt HG, Russack V, Chiu Y et al (1997) A comparison of thoracoscopic talc insufflation, slurry and mechanical abrasion pleurodesis. Chest 111:442–448
14. DeHoyos A, Fry WH (2009) Pneumothorax. In: Shields TW, Locicero J III, Reed CE, Feins RH (eds) General thoracic surgery. Lippincott Williams and Wilkins, Philadelphia
15. Dumont P, Diemont F, Massard G et al (1997) Does a thoracoscopic approach for surgical treatment of spontaneous pneumothorax represent progress? Eur J Cardiothorac Surg 11:27–31
16. Freixenet JJG, Rodriguez P, Santana N (2001) Axillary thoracotomy versus video-assisted thoracoscopy in the surgical treatment of primary spontaneous pneumothorax. Eur Respir J 18:524
17. Gaensler EA (1956) Parietal pleurectomy for recurrent spontaneous pneumothorax. Surg Gynecol Obstet 102:293–308
18. Globbel WG, Rhea WG, Nelson IA (1963) Spontaneous pneumothorax. J Thorac Cardiovasc Surg 46:331–334
19. Gossot D, Galetta D, Stern JB et al (2004) Results of thoracoscopic pleural abrasion for primary spontaneous pneumothorax. Surg Endosc 18:466–471
20. Haws MJ, Kucan JO, Roth AC et al (1996) The effects of chronic ketorolac tromethamine (toradol) on wound healing. Ann Plast Surg 37:147–151
21. Henry M, Arnold T, Harvey J (2003) BTS guidelines for the management of spontaneous pneumothorax. Thorax 58(suppl II):ii39–ii52
22. Ingolfsson I, Gyllstedt E, Lillo-Gil R et al (2006) Reoperations are common following VATS for spontaneous pneumothorax: study of risk factors. Interact Cardiovasc Thorac Surg 5:602–607
23. Jimenez-Merchan R, Garcia-Diaz F, Arenas Linares C et al (1997) Comparative retrospective study of surgical treatment of spontaneous pneumothorax. Thoracotomy vs thoracoscopy. Surg Endosc 11:919–922
24. Kim KH, Kim HK, Han JY et al (1996) Transaxillary minithoracotomy versus video-assisted thoracic surgery for spontaneous pneumothorax. Ann Thorac Surg 61:1510–1512
25. Lang-Lazdunski L, Chapuis O, Bonnet PM et al (2003) Videothoracoscopic bleb excision and pleural abrasion for the treatment of primary spontaneous pneumothorax: long-term results. Ann Thorac Surg 75:960–965
26. Lardinois D, Vogt P, Yang L et al (2004) Non-steroidal anti-inflammatory drugs decrease the quality of pleurodesis after mechanical pleural abrasion. Eur J Cardiothorac Surg 25:865–871
27. Lee YC, Malkerneker D, Devin CJ et al (2001) Comparing transforming growth factor beta2 and fibronectin as pleurodesing agents. Respirology 6:281–286
28. Leo F, Pastorino U, Goldstraw P (2000) Pleurectomy in primary pneumothorax: is extensive pleurectomy necessary? J Cardiovasc Surg (Torino) 41:633–636
29. Li ZJ, Zhang Y, Fu T et al (2006) Evaluation of curative effects of axillary thoracotomy and videothoracoscopy in treatment for primary spontaneous pneumothorax. J Jilin Univ Med Ed 32:711–713
30. Maier A, Anegg U, Renner H et al (2000) Four-year experience with pleural abrasion using a rotating brush during video-assisted thoracoscopy. Surg Endosc 14:75–78
31. Massard G, Thomas P, Wihlm JM (1998) Minimally invasive management for first and recurrent pneumothorax. Ann Thorac Surg 66:592–599
32. Matsuzoe D, Iwasaki A, Okabayashi K et al (1999) Recurrence after thoracoscopic surgery for spontaneous pneumothorax. Int Surg 84:111–114
33. Nkere UU, Griffin SC, Fountain SW (1991) Pleural abrasion. A new method for pleurodesis. Thorax 46:596–598
34. Treasure T (2007) Minimally invasive surgery for pneumothorax: the evidence, changing practice and current opinion. J R Soc Med 100:419–422
35. Passlick B, Born C, Thetter O (1997) Results of video-assisted thoracic surgery (VATS) in patients with recurrent or persisting primary spontaneous pneumothorax. Pneumologie 51:1135–1139
36. Perez RL, Roman J (1995) Fibrin enhances the expression of IL-1 beta by human peripheral blood mononuclear cells. Implications in pulmonary inflammation. J Immunol 154:1879–1887
37. Rena O, Massera F, Papalia E et al (2008) Surgical pleurodesis for Vanderschueren's stage III primary spontaneous pneumothorax. Eur Respir J 31:837–841
38. Sawada S, Watanabe Y, Moriyama S (2005) Video-assisted thoracoscopic surgery for spontaneous pneumothorax: evaluation of indications and long-term outcome compared with conservative treatment and open thoracotomy. Chest 127:2226–2230
39. Sing SV (1982) The surgical treatment of spontaneous pneumothorax by partial pleurectomy. Scand J Thorac Cardiovasc Surg 16:75
40. Thomas P, Le Mee F, Le Hors H et al (1993) Results of surgical treatment of recurrent pneumothorax. Ann Chir 47:136–140
41. Tschopp JM, Rami-Porta R, Noppen M et al (2006) Management of spontaneous pneumothorax: state of the art. Eur Respir J 28:637–650

42. Tyson MD, Crandall WB (1941) The surgical treatment of recurrent idiopathic spontaneous pneumothorax. J Thorac Surg 10:566
43. Viskum K, Lange P, Mortenson J (1989) Long-term sequelae after talc pleurodesis for spontaneous pneumothorax. Pneumologie 43:105–106
44. Waller DA, Forty J, Morritt GN (1994) Video-assisted thoracoscopic surgery versus thoracotomy for spontaneous pneumothorax. Ann Thorac Surg 58:372–376
45. Waller D (1999) Video-assisted thoracoscopic surgery for spontaneous pneumothorax: a 7-year learning experience. Ann R Coll Surg Engl 81:1387–1392

19 Video-Thoracoscopic Parietal Pleurectomy

Paul E.Van Schil, Jeroen M. Hendriks,
Chantal Vandenbroeck, and Patrick R. Lauwers

Contents

P.E. Van Schil, M.D., Ph.D. (✉) • J.M. Hendriks, M.D., Ph.D.
C. Vandenbroeck, M.D. • P.R. Lauwers, M.D.
Department of Thoracic and Vascular Surgery,
Antwerp University Hospital, Wilrijkstraat 10,
Edegem (Antwerp), B-2650, Belgium
e-mail: paul.van.schil@uza.be; jeroen.hendriks@uza.be;
chantal.vandenbroeck@uza.be; patrick.lauwers@uza.be

19.1 Introduction

Pleurectomy implies removal of the parietal and/or visceral pleura in order to obtain tight adherence of the lung to the chest wall or better expansion of a trapped lung which is not able to expand due to an inflamed, thickened visceral pleura. In the latter case, the procedure is called decortication as the lung is covered by a tough fibrous pleural peel.

Due to further refinements in minimally invasive techniques, pleurectomy can be performed by video-assisted thoracic surgery (VATS) in many cases providing a superb view of the entire pleural cavity from the apex to the diaphragm.

Indications for pleurectomy are listed in Table 19.1. The extent of pleurectomy is variable and depends on the specific indication: it can be performed in the apical part only, as, e.g. in primary spontaneous pneumothorax; partially over a variable degree of the chest cavity, as, e.g. in secondary spontaneous pneumothorax; or fully over the entire rib cage as in malignant disorders.

Table 19.1 Indications for pleurectomy

Pneumothorax
Primary spontaneous
Secondary spontaneous
Empyema, trapped lung
Recurrent pleural effusion (inflammatory disorders)
Metastatic pleuritis
Malignant pleural mesothelioma

R.G.C. Inderbitzi et al. (eds.), *Minimally Invasive Thoracic and Cardiac Surgery*,
DOI 10.1007/978-3-642-11861-6_19, © Springer-Verlag Berlin Heidelberg 2012

Table 19.2 Levels of evidence

Level	Description
A	Randomised controlled trials with a consisted pattern and rich body of data
B	Randomised controlled trials with a limited number of patients or inconsistent results
C	Nonrandomised trials, observational studies
D	Panel consensus judgement

Table 19.3 Indications for invasive treatment (level C evidence)

Recurrent or persisting pneumothorax
Bronchopleural fistula with air leak 5–7 days
Haemopneumothorax
Bilateral pneumothorax
First contralateral pneumothorax
Professions at risk (aircraft personnel, divers)

Regarding the specific technique of pleurectomy in our centre, we first delineate with cautery the borders of the planned parietal pleurectomy. Subsequently, with an endodissector, we strip off the parietal pleura twisting and rotating it on the instrument. This makes it fairly easy to remove the parietal pleura. Specifically designed pleural strippers, sponge sticks or peanut dissectors may also be helpful and facilitate the procedure.

When dealing with thickened parietal pleura, it is sometimes easier to start an extrapleural dissection with the index finger through a thoracoport incision at some distance from the camera, especially when additional biopsies have to be taken. With a grasper and cautery, the pleurectomy can then be continued at the inside of the chest.

For pleural abrasion, a piece of mesh can be mounted on a forceps to scarify the parietal pleura and obtain a slightly haemorrhagic surface. More extensive bleeding can usually be controlled thoracoscopically by careful cauterization or by putting haemostatic clips on bleeding vessels as the intercostal or internal mammary arteries.

In cases of chronic empyema and malignant pleural mesothelioma, usually a formal decortication is necessary. As this is discussed in another chapter, we will focus in this chapter on pneumothorax, recurrent pleural effusion and metastatic pleuritis with main emphasis on pneumothorax. As much as possible, levels of evidence are indicated (Table 19.2).

19.2 Spontaneous Pneumothorax

19.2.1 Treatment of Pneumothorax by VATS

Indications for invasive treatment of pneumothorax are summarised in Table 19.3. With the introduction of VATS in the early 1990s, the interest in early definitive treatment of spontaneous pneumothorax has rekindled to avoid a large lateral thoracotomy incision and to obtain a minimally invasive treatment for pneumothorax. There is a difference between a so-called medical pleuroscopy performed by pulmonary physicians and a VATS procedure. Medical pleuroscopy is often done under local anaesthesia and is limited to an intervention on the pleural space. A chemical pleurodesis is easy to perform under direct vision. In contrast, a VATS procedure requires general anaesthesia with double lumen intubation and single lung ventilation [30]. In this way, also, an intervention on the lung itself is possible as, e.g. a bullectomy with the aid of endostaplers (Fig. 19.1a-b). Many series have been published on VATS treatment for pneumothorax, and specific ones are summarised in Table 19.4 [4–8, 10–12, 17, 18, 21, 22, 25, 27, 28, 32]. However, level A evidence is lacking, so the results of these studies should be interpreted with caution.

19.2.1.1 Treatment of Lung

Although the exact cause of a pneumothorax remains unknown, most authors advocate to resect any blebs or bullae that are visible during

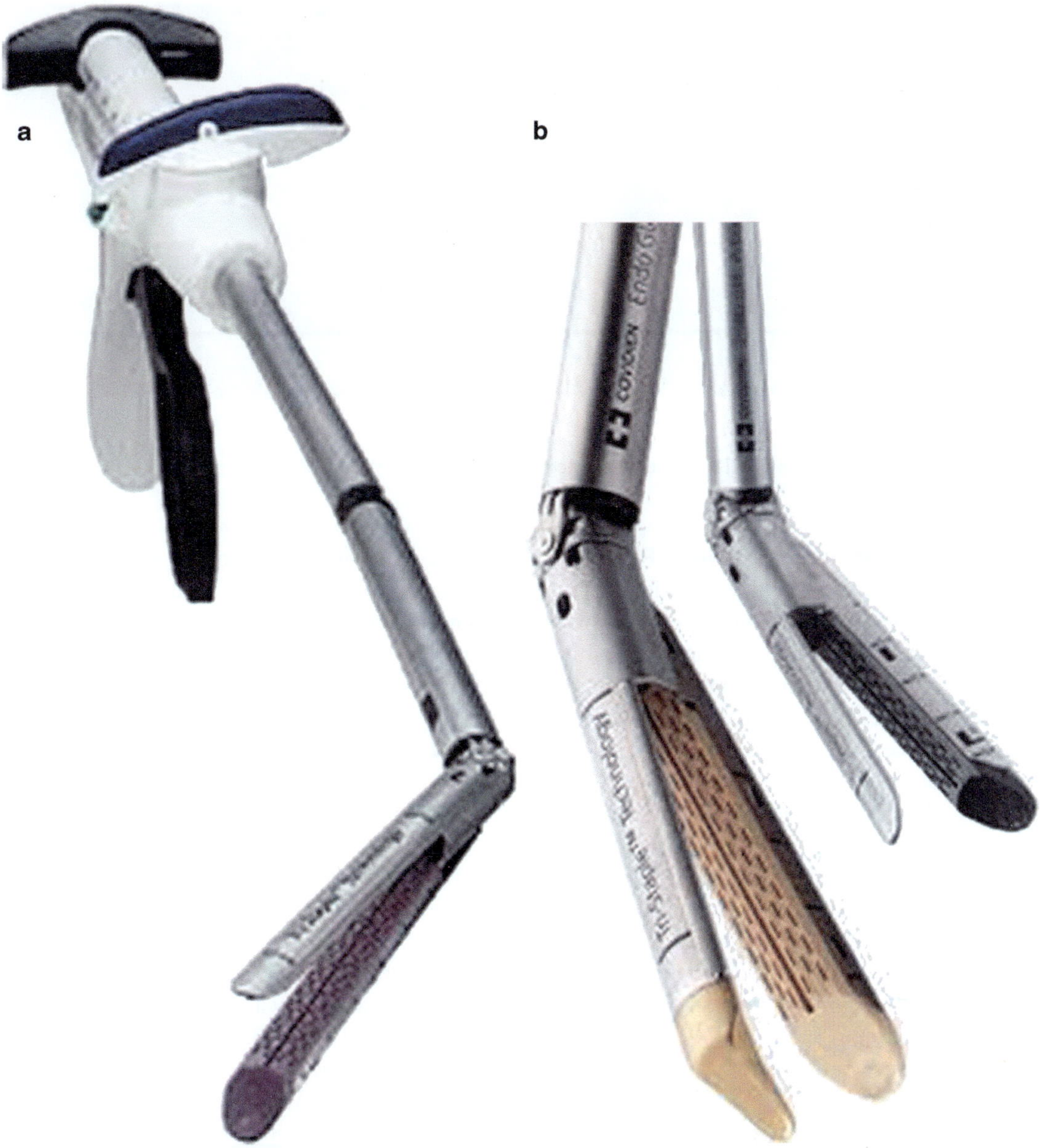

Fig. 19.1a-b Endostaplers used for resection of blebs or bullae during a VATS procedure

VATS, although there is no level A evidence to support this (Fig.19.2a-b). However, Naunheim et al. have demonstrated that the recurrence rate drops from 20% to 1.5% when a resection of bullae is performed [19]. Often endostaplers are used for this; cheaper alternatives include the use of endoloops or endoscopic sutures. Small blebs can be coagulated which is not applicable for large bullae due to frequent recurrences.

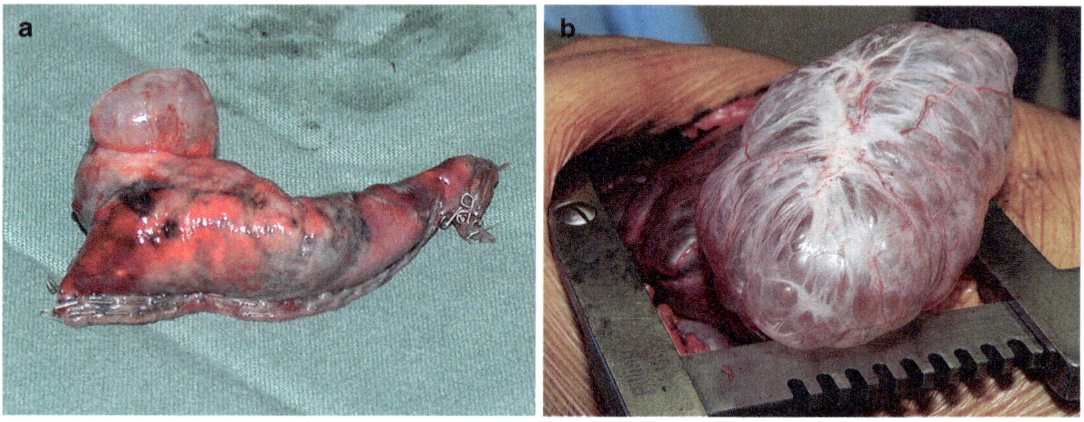

Fig. 19.2 (**a**) Bleb resected by VATS (**b**) Bulla resected by muscle-sparing thoracotomy

19.2.1.2 Treatment of Parietal Pleura

For recurrence prevention, the parietal pleura should be treated to obliterate the pleural space, especially in the apical part where most blebs and bullae occur. In a comparative but nonrandomised study, Horio et al. have shown that the recurrence rate diminished from 16% to 1.9% when a pleurodesis was added to the bullectomy [12]. Many possible techniques have been described, most utilised being pleurectomy and mechanical pleurodesis. There are no prospective randomised studies comparing these techniques or comparing VATS to medical pleuroscopy with talc poudrage. In 1996, a retrospective study was published comparing different techniques in 1,365 VATS procedures [14]. Recurrence rate was 0% after talc instillation, but this technique was only applied in 15 patients, 2.7% after coagulation, 4.4% after pleurectomy, 7.9% after pleural abrasion, 10.2% without pleurodesis and 16.4% after injection of fibrin glue. Due to its retrospective nature, no firm conclusions can be drawn. The studies listed in Table 19.4 show recurrence rates of 0.8–11.7% after pleurectomy, of 2.1–9.4% after abrasion, of 1.9–10.7% after coagulation, and 1.8% after talc injection. As there is mostly no randomization in these studies, level of evidence mainly remains C. Although the best results are obtained after total pleurectomy, this technique makes the hemithorax inaccessible when a new intervention is required later in life. For this reason, most authors advocate an apical, partial pleurectomy and a mechanical pleurodesis down to the diaphragm, technique which is also utilised in our centre (Fig. 19.3).

19.2.2 VATS: Primary Versus Secondary Spontaneous Pneumothorax

Most of the studies on VATS for pneumothorax were performed for primary spontaneous pneumothorax. Reports on secondary spontaneous pneumothorax treated by a VATS approach are less frequent and show a recurrence rate between 0% and 8% [1, 15, 16, 23, 31]. Especially in these patients, a spontaneous pneumothorax may induce severe distress due to a limited pulmonary reserve. Advantages of VATS versus thoracotomy in patients with secondary spontaneous pneumothorax probably include less postoperative pain, a shorter hospitalisation time and less pulmonary dysfunction although this has not been clearly demonstrated. In contrast, the incidence of complications after a VATS procedure for secondary spontaneous pneumothorax varies between 25% and 77%, which is much higher than for primary spontaneous pneumothorax where the percentage of reported complications lies between 3.2% and 25.4% [1, 15, 16, 23, 31]. In patients with a poor pulmonary function who cannot tolerate single lung ventilation, a thoracotomy is indicated.

Table 19.4 Recent studies on treatment of pneumothorax by VATS [4–8, 10–12, 17, 18, 21, 22, 25, 27, 28, 32]

Author	Year	Ref.	Evidence	*n*	Type of procedure	% recurrence
Waller	1999	[32]	C	180	bull, pl	6.6
Liu et al.	1999	[18]	C	757	bull, pl, abr, chem.	2.1
Ohno et al.	2000	[21]	C	424	bull, abr	9.4
Cardillo et al.	2000	[6]	C	153	bull, pl	9.2
				279	bull, talc	1.8
Chan et al.	2001	[8]	C	82	bull, abr	5.7
Horio et al.	2002	[12]	C	50	bull	16.0
				53	bull, coag	1.9
Onuki et al.	2002	[22]	C	59 (SSP)	bull	1.7
Roviaro et al.	2002	[25]	C	171	bull, pl	0.8
Sawabata et al.	2002	[27]	C	99	bull	10.1
Casadio et al.	2002	[7]	C	133	bull, abr	3.8
de Vos et al.	2002	[10]	C	63 (PSP)	bull, pl, abr	4.8
				13 (SSP)	bull, pl, abr	7.7
Lang-Lazdunski et al.	2003	[17]	C	182	bull, abr	3
Freixinet et al.	2004	[11]	B	46	bull, abr	4.3
Sawada et al.	2005	[28]	C	281	bull (apical pl when multiple)	11.7
Ben-Nun et al.	2006	[4]	C	58	bull, abr	3
Bobbio et al.	2006	[5]	C	70	coag Argon	10.7
				67	abr Marlex	3.4

SSP secondary spontaneous pneumothorax, *PSP* primary spontaneous pneumothorax, *Ref.* reference, *bull* bullectomy or resection blebs, *pl* pleurectomy, *abr* abrasion, *chem.* chemical pleurodesis, *coag* coagulation

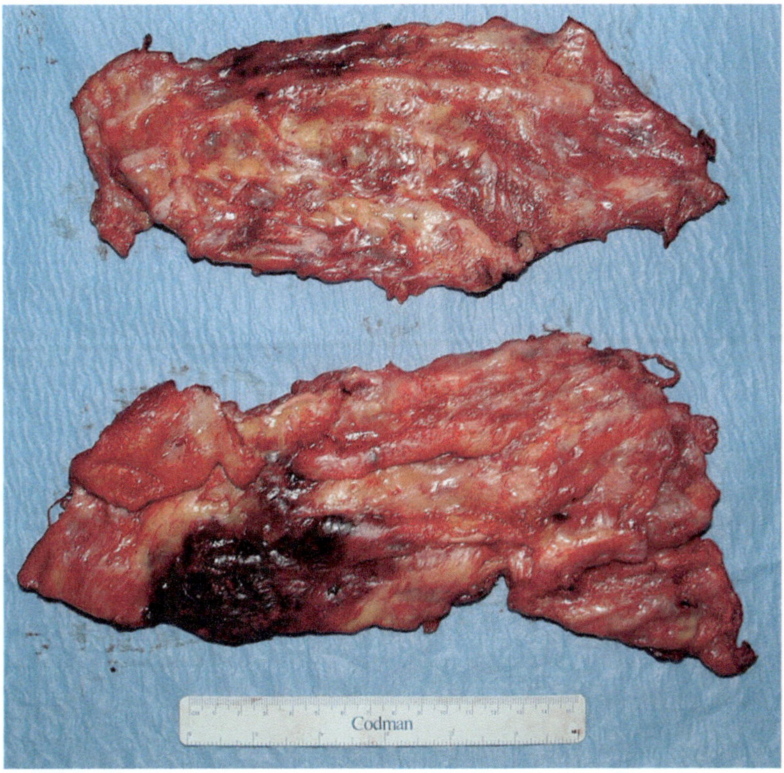

Fig. 19.3 Pleurectomy in a patient with metastatic pleuritis

19.2.3 VATS Versus Thoracotomy

Several prospective studies compare a VATS procedure with a classical thoracotomy (lateral or limited axillary). Waller et al. published a randomised study of 60 patients treated for a pneumothorax by thoracoscopy or lateral thoracotomy [31]. In the VATS group, there was less pulmonary dysfunction, less pain and a shorter hospitalisation time compared to the thoracotomy group.

Kim et al. completed a prospective trial in 66 patients comparing VATS to a limited axillary thoracotomy [16]. This was a nonrandomised trial as the choice of approach was made by the patients themselves. There was no significant difference between both groups regarding the duration of intervention and chest tube drainage, need for analgesics and recurrence rate.

In a prospective and randomised study including 90 patients, VATS was compared to axillary thoracotomy [11]. Specific factors studied were postoperative blood loss, lung function, postoperative pain and use of analgesics, postoperative complications, duration of hospital stay and resumption of normal activity. There were no significant differences for every factor studied, so VATS seems to be equally effective as a limited axillary thoracotomy (level of evidence B). However, with a minimum follow-up of 2 years, the recurrence rate after VATS was 4.3% and after a limited thoracotomy 0% [11].

Two systematic reviews and one best evidence topic evaluated whether VATS was superior to thoracotomy for the treatment of spontaneous pneumothorax [3, 13, 29]. The first systematic review published in 2004 included 670 patients from 12 randomised clinical trials [29]. VATS resulted in a shorter hospital stay, induced less pain and was associated with fewer recurrences compared to pleural drainage. Complication profile was comparable with that of thoracotomy [29]. The second systematic review published in 2007 included 4 randomised and 25 nonrandomised studies. Overall relative risk of recurrent pneumothorax was 4.73 when comparing VATS to open thoracotomy. This result was consistent for both randomised and nonrandomised trials [3]. A best evidence topic published 1 year later compared VATS pleurectomy to open pleurectomy [13]. VATS was associated with a shorter hospital stay and less analgesic requirements. As noted in the previous systematic review, a fourfold increase in recurrent pneumothoraces was noted following VATS pleurectomy [13].

19.2.4 Flowcharts for Treatment of Spontaneous Pneumothorax

Treatment of spontaneous pneumothorax remains controversial due to the lack of level of evidence [9]. Flowcharts for treatment of primary and secondary spontaneous pneumothorax are provided in Figs. 19.4 and 19.5. Level B evidence exists for treatment of a first episode of a primary spontaneous pneumothorax >20% where simple aspiration is preferred as it can be performed in an ambulatory setting. For a secondary spontaneous pneumothorax, a more aggressive approach is warranted as a higher mortality can be anticipated. Regarding recurrence prevention, the optimal technique remains to be determined. VATS provides an attractive surgical method due to its superior visualisation of the thoracic cavity and possible interventions, as well as on the lung parenchyma itself and on the parietal pleura, resulting in an adequate obliteration of the pleural space.

19.3 Recurrent Pleural Effusion in Inflammatory Disorders

In specific cases of inflammatory pleural disorders as, e.g. rheumatoid pleural disease, recurrent large effusions may occur. Treatment by repeated aspiration and nonsteroidal anti-inflammatory agents or steroidal therapy should be attempted [2]. In patients with a refractory recurrent effusion, pleurectomy may be necessary. In some cases, a simultaneous decortication is indicated when the thickened visceral pleura limits lung expansion [2].

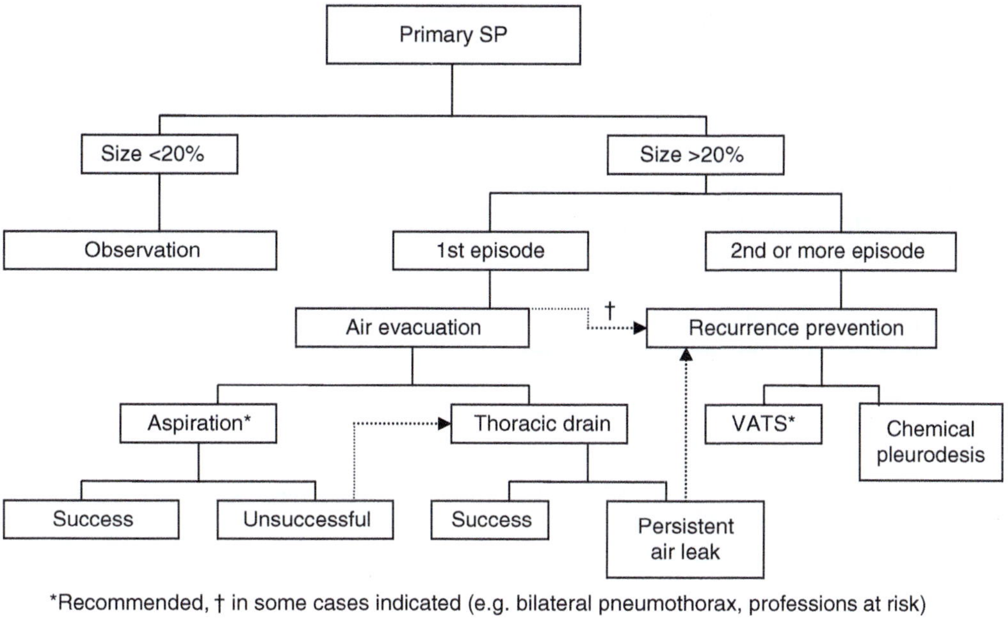

Fig. 19.4 Flowchart for primary spontaneous pneumothorax (*SP*)

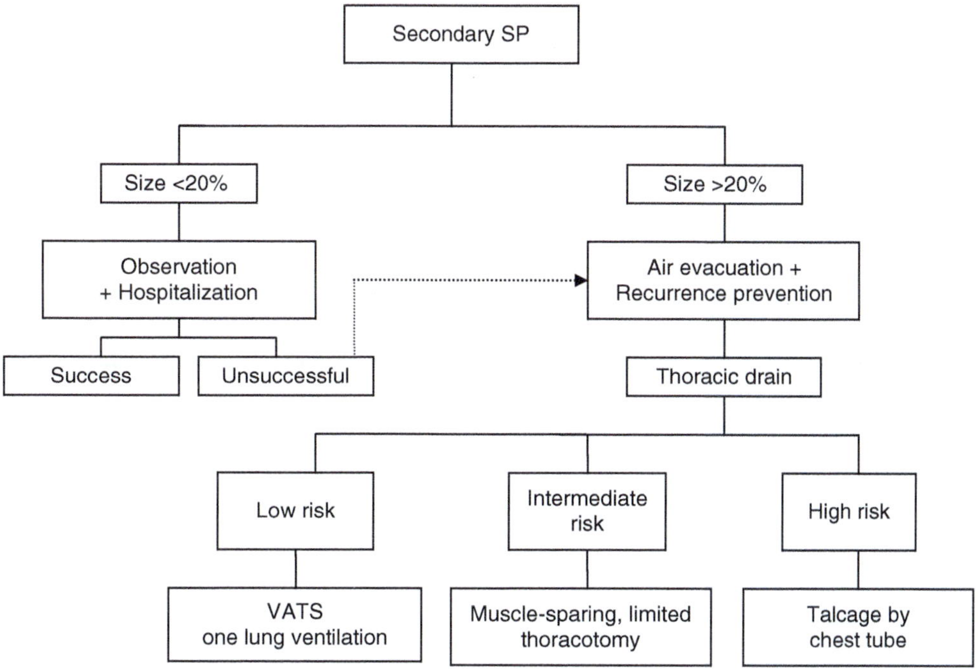

Fig. 19.5 Flowchart for secondary spontaneous pneumothorax (*SP*)

19.4 Metastatic Pleuritis

Metastatic pleuritis may occur with a variety of tumours, as well as intrathoracic and extrathoracic. Most patients with malignant pleural effusion have a poor prognosis. In case of a primary lung cancer, malignant pleural effusion is now considered M1a instead of T4 disease [24]. Other tumours associated with metastatic pleuritis include breast cancer, mesothelioma and gynaecologic malignancies as tumours of the ovary. Treatment is mainly supportive, and in case of worsening dyspnoea, evacuation of the fluid and prevention of recurrent effusion are indicated [20]. Thoracic surgical options include chest tube drainage, VATS associated with chemical or mechanical pleurodesis, external catheter drainage, insertion of a pleuroperitoneal shunt and pleurectomy by VATS or thoracotomy. Talc has been found to be the most successful pleurodesis agent. Complete description of a subtotal pleurectomy for metastatic pleuritis performed by VATS is presented at MMCTS (2012) Vol. 2012 mms008 doi:10.1093/mmcts/mms008. As pleurectomy is associated with a significant morbidity and mortality, it is not justified in patients with a poor prognosis [26]. On the other hand, it may provide symptomatic relief in patients with a reasonable life expectancy.

References

1. Andres B, Lujan J, Robles R, Aguilar J et al (1998) Treatment of primary and secondary spontaneous pneumothorax using videothoracoscopy. Surg Laparosc Endosc 8:108–112
2. Antoniou KM, Bouros D, Wells AU (2010) Immunological diseases of the pleura. In: Bouros D (ed) Pleural disease, 2nd edn. Informa Healthcare, New York
3. Barker A, Maratos EC, Edmonds L et al (2007) Recurrence rates of video-assisted thoracoscopic versus open surgery in the prevention of recurrent pneumothoraces: a systematic review of randomised and non-randomised trials. Lancet 370:329–335
4. Ben-Nun A, Soudack M, Best LA (2006) Video-assisted thoracoscopic surgery for recurrent spontaneous pneumothorax: the long-term benefit. World J Surg 30:285–290
5. Bobbio A, Ampollini L, Internullo E et al (2006) Thoracoscopic parietal pleural argon beam coagulation versus pleural abrasion in the treatment of primary spontaneous pneumothorax. Eur J Cardiothorac Surg 29:6–8
6. Cardillo G, Facciolo F, Giunti R et al (2000) Videothoracoscopic treatment of primary spontaneous pneumothorax; a 6-year experience. Ann Thorac Surg 69:357–362
7. Casadio C, Ottavio R, Giobbe R et al (2001) Primary spontaneous pneumothorax. Is video-assisted thoracoscopy stapler resection with pleural abrasion the gold-standard? Eur J Cardiothorac Surg 20:897–898
8. Chan P, Clarke P, Daniel FJ et al (2001) Efficacy study of video-assisted thoracoscopic surgery for spontaneous pneumothorax. Ann Thorac Surg 71:452–454
9. De Leyn P, Lismonde M, Ninane V et al (2005) Belgian society of pneumology guidelines on the management of spontaneous pneumothorax. Acta Chir Belg 105:265–267
10. de Vos B, Hendriks J, Van Schil P et al (2002) Long-term results after video-assisted thoracic surgery for spontaneous pneumothorax. Acta Chir Belg 102:439–444
11. Freixinet JL, Canalis E, Julia G et al (2004) Axillary thoracotomy versus videothoracoscopy for the treatment of primary spontaneous pneumothorax. Ann Thorac Surg 78:417–420
12. Horio H, Nomori H, Kobayashi R et al (2002) Impact of additional pleurodesis in video-assisted thoracoscopic bullectomy for primary spontaneous pneumothorax. Surg Endosc 16:630–634
13. Hunaid AV, Adamson L, Weeden DF (2008) Does video-assisted thoracoscopic pleurectomy result in better outcomes than open pleurectomy for primary spontaneous pneumothorax? Interact Cardiovasc Thorac Surg 7:673–677
14. Hurtgen M, Linder A, Friedel G et al (1996) Video-assisted thoracoscopic pleurodesis. Thorac Cardiovasc Surg 44:199–203
15. Inderbitzi RGC, Grillet MP (1996) Risk and hazards of video-thoracoscopic surgery: a collective review. Eur J Cardiothorac Surg 10:483–489
16. Kim KH, Kim HK, Han JY et al (1996) Transaxillary minithoracotomy versus video-assisted thoracic surgery for spontaneous pneumothorax. Ann Thorac Surg 61:1510–1512
17. Lang-Lazdunski L, Chapuis O, Bonnet PM et al (2003) Videothoracoscopic bleb excision and pleural abrasion for the treatment of primary spontaneous pneumothorax: long-term results. Ann Thorac Surg 75:960–965
18. Liu HP, Yim AP, Izzat MB et al (1999) Thoracoscopic surgery for spontaneous pneumothorax. World J Surg 23:1133–1136
19. Naunheim KS, Mack MJ, Hazelrigg SR et al (1995) Safety and efficacy of video-assisted thoracic surgical techniques for the treatment of spontaneous pneumothorax. J Thorac Cardiovasc Surg 109:1198–1204
20. Neragi-Miandoab S (2008) Surgical and other invasive approaches to recurrent pleural effusion with malignant etiology. Support Care Cancer 16:1323–1331

21. Ohno K, Myoshi S, Minami M et al (2000) Ipsilateral recurrence frequency after video-assisted thoracic surgery for primary spontaneous pneumothorax. Jpn J Thorac Cardiovasc Surg 48:757–760
22. Onuki T, Murasugi M, Ikeda T et al (2002) Thoracoscopic surgery for pneumothorax in older patients. Surg Endosc 16:355–357
23. Passlick B, Born C, Haussinger K et al (1998) Efficiency of video-assisted thoracic surgery for primary and secondary spontaneous pneumothorax. Ann Thorac Surg 35:324–327
24. Postmus P, Brambilla E, Chansky K et al (2007) The IASLC lung cancer staging project: proposals for revision of the M descriptors in the forthcoming (seventh) edition of the TNM classification of lung cancer. J Thorac Oncol 2:686–693
25. Rovario GC, Varoli F, Vergani C et al (2002) State of the art in thoracoscopic surgery. Surg Endosc 16: 881–892
26. Sahn SA (2010) Malignant pleural effusions. In: Bouros D (ed) Pleural disease, 2nd edn. Informa Healthcare, New York
27. Sawabata N, Ikeda M, Matsumara A et al (2002) New electroablation technique following the first-line stapling method for thoracoscopic treatment of primary spontaneous pneumothorax. Chest 121:251–255
28. Sawada S, Watanabe Y, Moriyama S (2005) Video-assisted thoracoscopic surgery for primary spontaneous pneumothorax: evaluation of indications and long-term outcome compared with conservative treatment and open thoracotomy. Chest 127:2226–2230
29. Sedrakyan A, van der Meulen J, Lewsey J et al (2004) Video-assisted thoracic surgery for treatment of pneumothorax and lung resections: systematic review of randomised clinical trials. BMJ 329:1008
30. Van Schil P, Bellens L, De Maeseneer M et al (2005) Video-assisted thoracic surgery for primary spontaneous pneumothorax: how I do it? Acta Chir Belg 105:397–399
31. Waller DA, Forty G, Morrit GN (1994) Video-assisted thoracoscopic surgery versus thoracotomy for spontaneous pneumothorax. Ann Thorac Surg 58: 372–377
32. Waller DA (1999) Video-assisted thoracic surgery for spontaneous pneumothorax – a 7 year learning experience. Ann R Coll Surg Engl 8:387–392

20 Video-Assisted Thoracoscopic Surgery Techniques in the Treatment of Complicated Parapneumonic Effusions and Empyema

Giovanni L. Carboni

Contents

G.L. Carboni, M.D.
Division of Thoracic Surgery,
University Hospital Berne, Freiburgstrasse,
3010 Zurich, Switzerland
e-mail: giovanni.carboni@triemli.zuerich.ch

20.1 Introduction

Parapneumonic effusions are pleural effusions that occur in the pleural space in association with a bacterial pneumonia. They occur in about 50% of bacterial pneumonias [1]. The usual parapneumonic effusion is small and resolves with appropriate conservative treatment including antibiotic therapy. However, if bacteria invade the pleural space, a complicated parapneumonic effusion or empyema may result, which will necessitate aside of antibiotic therapy additional interventions and frequently surgery. Ten to twenty percent of patients with pneumonia will eventually develop a complicated effusion or pleural empyema [2]. Early adequate therapy is mandatory to avoid unnecessary surgery and complicated courses in patients with pneumonia. The timepoint of drainage and surgery has been object of a considerable amount of debate in the literature. However, the best management remains controversial. In the following chapter, a therapeutic approach with early use of video-assisted thoracoscopic surgery (VATS), and description of current techniques is presented. The focus is placed on decision-making and technical aspects.

20.2 Progression of Infection in the Pleural Space

Uncomplicated parapneumonic effusions are small, less than half of the lung volume and present with no loculation on imaging. The

R.G.C. Inderbitzi et al. (eds.), *Minimally Invasive Thoracic and Cardiac Surgery*,
DOI 10.1007/978-3-642-11861-6_20, © Springer-Verlag Berlin Heidelberg 2012

Table 20.1 Typical laboratory findings in patients with parapneumonic effusions according to the progression of the infection in the pleural space

	Uncomplicated parapneumonic effusion	Complicated parapneumonic effusion	Pleural empyema
Fluid appearance	Clear, thin	Turbid, thick	Frank pus
Bacteria	Sterile	±	+ (−)
pH	>7.30	<7.10	<7.10
Lactate dehydrogenase (LDH)	<500 U/L	>1,000 U/L	>1,000 U/L
Glucose (Glc)	>60 mg/dL	<40 mg/dL	<40 mg/dL
Fluid/serum glucose ratio	>0.5	<0.5	<0.5

Gram stain and culture results are negative, and the fluid is clear in appearance. Uncomplicated parapneumonic effusions will eventually resolve, and usually, diagnostic thoracentesis will reveal an exudate with normal pH and glucose levels (pH > 7.30, Glc > 60 mg/dL, and LDH < 1,000 U/L). The indications for chest tube drainage of parapneumonic effusions are well described elsewhere [3]. Large pleural effusions with low pH (pH < 7.10) need to be drained with a large bored chest tube insertion to avoid further loculation and development of pleural empyema. The American Thoracic Society divides the progression of an empyema into three distinct stages. These are, however, rarely reflected by distinct clinical signs. During the *exudative phase* (stage I), the pleura swells considerably and discharges copious amounts of thin exudate. The fibrin deposits are thin enough to allow the lung for re-expansion. This phase is followed by the *fibrinopurulent stage* (stage II) where heavy fibrin deposits cover the pleural surface and the pleural fluid is turbid and thickened. In this stage loculations develop within about a week. In the following 2 weeks in growth of fibroblasts and formation of collagen fibers on the pleural membrane leading to an entrapment of the lung within the thick peel. This last stage is defined as *organization phase* (stage III). In the chronic stage of the disease, complications such as spontaneous drainage through the skin, contraction of the chest wall, and pulmonary fibrosis are more likely to develop. Typical findings for the progression of the disease are summarized in Table 20.1.

Even with tube drainage of complicated effusion, the treatment may fail, and therefore patients with stage II empyema may need more invasive therapy. Application of fibrinolytics agents through a chest tube has been advocated from several authors with the aim to disrupt fibrin deposits and loculations [4–6]. Although small prospective controlled trial support the early use of fibrinolytic agents and their use is safe [7], a randomized multicenter study did not show any advantage [8] in terms of mortality, morbidity, and hospital stay. Therefore, routinely application of fibrinolytics should be reserved for selected patients until their efficacy is proven. Furthermore, adding additional waiting time prior to proceed to surgical intervention may render a minimal invasive approach less likely to succeed [9].

20.3 Indications for Surgery

Any pleural infection with an undrained infected space and a non-expanded lung will unlikely resolve without surgical intervention. This is undoubtely the case in stage III empyema. Only in selected, mostly inoperable patients a simple drainage procedure should be considered in the knowledge, however, that control of infection might be only last for the time in which the drain is actually draining the infected space. In these cases, computer tomographic-guided drainage placement is preferable because bedside placement of a chest tube will most likely be difficult in view of a thickened and fibrotic parietal pleura.

Considerable differences in the approach of complicated parapneumonic pleural effusion with loculation are described in the literature.

Table 20.2 Simplified algorithm with early surgical treatment in complicated parapneumonic effusions

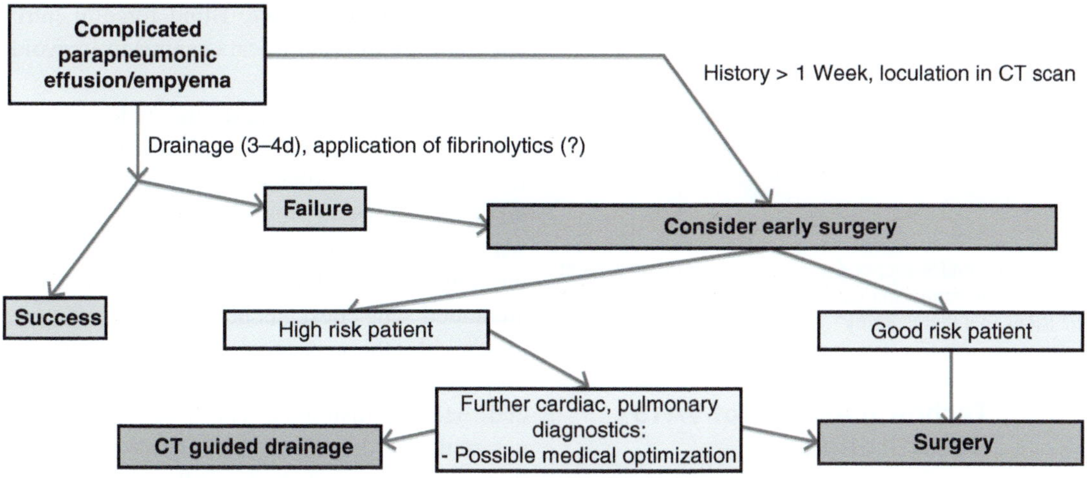

The main goal of surgery is debridement of the infected space, re-expansion of the lung, and adequate drainage. Early intervention is more likely to achieve these goals. The indication for surgery should not be delayed through ineffective conservative measures, such as adjustment of antibiotic therapy or placement of additional drainages. A simplified approach in respect to the natural history of pleural space infection is summarized in the algorithm of Table 20.2. Complicated pleural effusions that do not resolve with drainage as shown by clinical course and CT imaging should undergo early surgery within a week of the diagnosis. Intrapleural instillation of streptokinase (250,000 units in 100 ccm/2 h dwelling time) may be of use; however, it should not delay surgical intervention if needed. In patients with poor surgical risk, care must be taken not to deny adequate surgical treatment in a phase were the patient is operable with acceptable morbidity. Once the patient is septic and intubated, the outcome of surgery is not good [10]. Early VATS deloculation is not associated with the same complications as thoracotomy and should be therefore aggressively used in the management of empyema also in high-risk patients to avoid treatment failure in a later stage and more extensive surgery. VATS or thoracotomy in a more advanced stage empyema is associated with a better outcome [11, 12] compared to conservative treatment.

20.4 Choice of Surgical Technique

Once the decision is taken to proceed with surgery, the choice of the technique depends on time from onset of the disease, patient general conditions, and familiarity of the surgeon with minimal invasive surgery. The axiom that stage III empyema is not amenable to successful VATS decortication has been refuted by recent literature [13]. However, a long history with radiologic evidence of thick-walled multiloculated empyema may warrant the surgeon to proceed directly to open decortication in view of a high likelihood of conversion to achieve the therapeutic goals. As history and radiologic appearance can be deceiving, a rational approach would be to start every case with VATS technique and early convert to open surgery if adequate debridement, expansion of the lung is unlikely to be attained. There are only sparse studies comparing VATS decortication with open decortication for later stage empyema [13, 14]. It is unlikely that further controlled studies will answer all the questions. Therefore, a simplified institutional approach to suppurative pleural disease is advisable. VATS deloculation and decortication is safe, provided the goals of the surgery are achieved. The time from onset of symptoms and the etiology seem to have an influence on feasibility of VATS decortication [9].

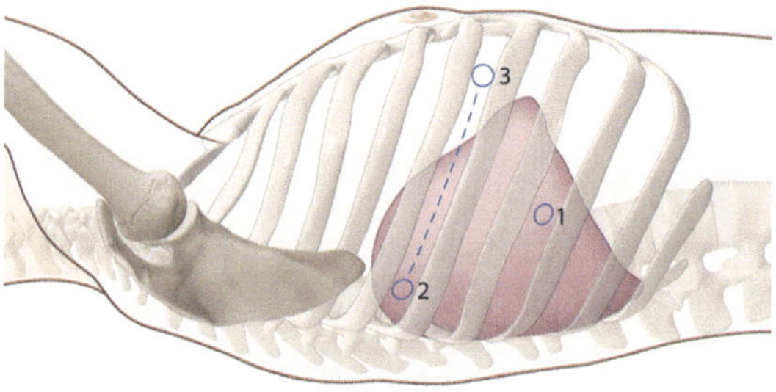

Fig. 20.1 VATS access for empyema. Port placement according to empyema cavity and possible extension of incisions to a thoracotomy

20.5 Technical Aspects of VATS Decortication

To safely perform any decortication, independently of access type, the patient should be adequately prepared and monitored in the perioperative phase. The anesthetist should be able to monitor the patient's urine output and blood pressure continuously, so an arterial line and a Foley catheter are advisable. Intraoperative opening of the infected pleural space with consecutive systemic bacterial load can lead to substantial circulatory instability. Therefore, adequate volume lines are mandatory for intraoperative resuscitation. Unlike in open decortication, the ventilatory isolation of the affected lung is almost uniformly necessary for VATS decortication or deloculation. A bronchial blocker can occasionally be used if double lumen intubation fails.

The patient is placed in lateral decubitus position. It is important to flex the table at the height of the lower back, so that the patient is properly extended, especially in persons with a broad pelvis. An extension of incisions should be possible if needed. The choice of the incision depends on the location of the main collection as depicted in Fig. 20.1. Thus, the incisions are chosen that an extension to a lateral/posterolateral thoracotomy is possible (Fig. 20.1) Therefore, a recent CT imaging should be available, to avoid entering the chest where the lung is adherent to the chest wall. The access should not be too small to allow entering the pleural cavity under direct vision. The parietal pleura is thickened, therefore small S-shaped retractors can be useful to help dissect into the intercostal space. Blind forceful introduction even of blunt trocars can result in avoidable lung laceration.

Once entered the chest, the videothoracoscope is introduced through an adequate trocar. If there are fibrin adhesions, they usually can be disrupted either with the surgeon's finger or with the videothoracoscope by gently dissecting the lung away. At least two additional incisions are added. The chest can be entered at this point under videothoracoscopic control. The pleural fluid as well as the peel is then sent for culture and cytology/histology. The procedure continues with the deloculation of the pleural space that can be accomplished usually with a suction device, a peanut sponge, and a grasper in bimanual technique. In certain situations, the use of curved instruments will facilitate the dissection. Firm adhesions may need sharp dissection with cautery. Every surgeon performing these steps has to have a clear idea how long it should take and have a predefined cutoff point when to convert to open surgery. The next step is the removal of the peel from the lung surface and chest wall. Removing a thick peel from the lung is best achieved by defining the correct plane between lung and peel and dissecting this space (Fig. 20.2a–d). A small amount of positive airway pressure in the ipsilateral lung can facilitate this step initially as it is in open decortication. If this plane cannot be developed, the surgeon may have to decide for a conversion. The chest wall and the diaphragm should be at least thoroughly debrided as this allows a better motility. It is important not to forget an adequate release of the fissures, which will allow a better lung expansion. At the end of the procedure, the lung is reinflated and assessed for parenchyma leaks. Small to moderate leaks are left untouched provided the lung expands adequately. Large lacerations of the parenchyma may present a problem that can lead to prolonged hospital stay. Meticulous control of hemostasis is mandatory and can be achieved either through cautery or thoracoscopic argon beam coagulator, which can also be used to seal small parenchyma leaks.

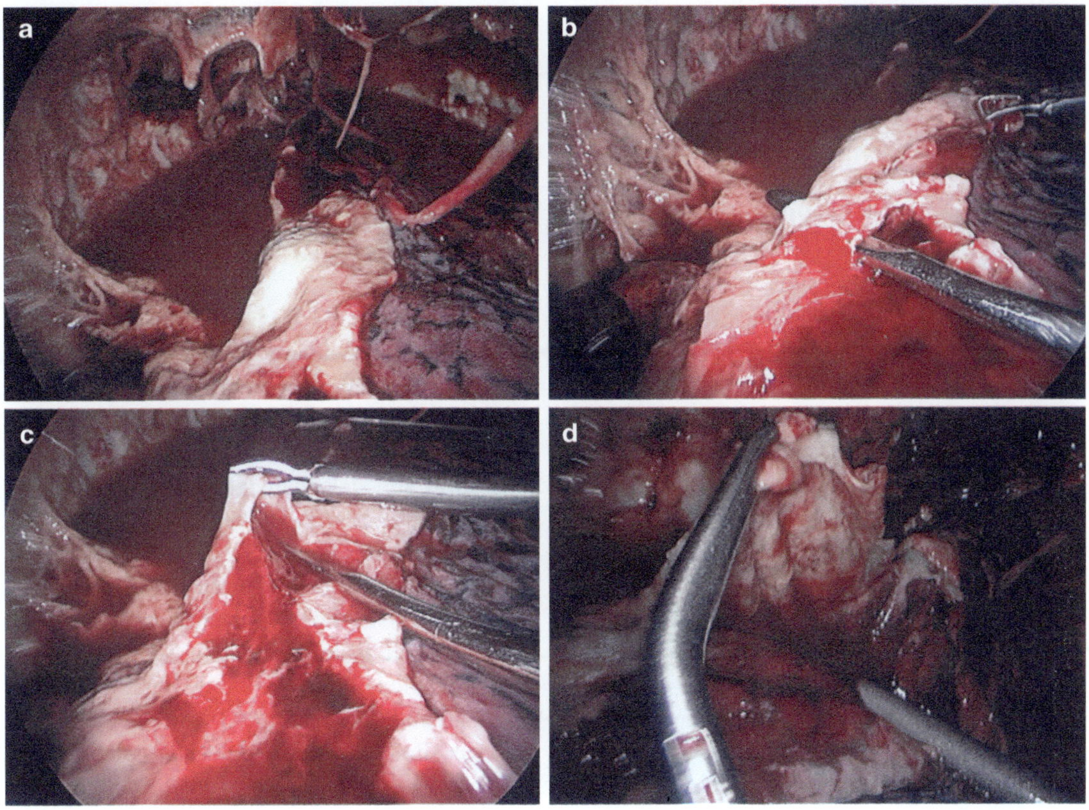

Fig. 20.2 (**a–d**) VATS visceral decortication. Removal of the fibrinous peel after development of correct plane using blunt dissector and suction

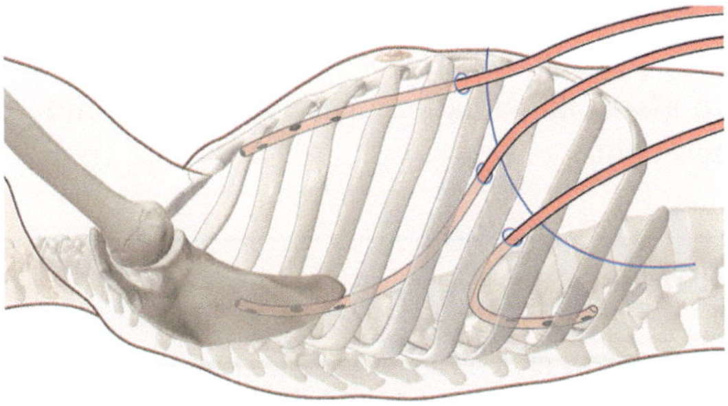

Fig. 20.3 Chest tube placement. Correct placement of three chest tubes for draining of the complete pleural space

The pleural cavity is irrigated and drained with large amount of saline. At our institution, we prefer to generally to insert 2–3 chest drains. One right-angled drain is positioned in the posterior costophrenic space, and the other two drains to the posterior and the anterior part of the chest (Fig. 20.3). Failure of appropriate drainage can result in recurrent empyema. If the lung does not expand sufficiently at the end of the procedure to fill the chest completely, one has to consider open decortication. If the lung is still severely consolidated because of the underlying pneumonia, even an open decortication will not achieve the goal, and a long drainage time or an alternative procedure will be necessary. Flexible bronchoscopy after switching to single lumen intubation should be used generously to clean the airway and resample for culture. To ameliorate the outcome, early extubation, usually in the operating room, is important, and postoperative follow-up should be done in a step down unit or intensive care unit. Respiratory physiotherapy and good pain control are important in the first days after intervention.

20.6 Pitfalls and Dangers

Summarized below are the main dangers that will lead to a failure in the therapy.

20.6.1 Decision-Making

Withhold surgery because of comorbidity
Failure to obtain recent imaging after drainage
Surgery for lung abscess, which is best managed initially without surgery
Rush for surgery in uncomplicated pleural effusion

20.6.2 Technical Problems

Failure to position the patient correctly
Inadequate port-site placement with consecutive lung injury
Failure to release the entire lung including the diaphragm
Insisting in minimal invasive technique when there is no progress in the operation
Failure to develop right surgical dissection plane with consecutive lung injury
Opening of lung abscesses causing large parenchyma leaks and insufficient lung expansion
Large parenchyma leaks in emphysema patients
Incautious parietal pleurectomy with injury to mediastinal structures such as azygos vein
Failure to adequately drain the pleural space at the end of surgery
Skip postoperative bronchoscopy and bronchial cleaning where necessary

20.6.3 Perioperative Occurrences

Inadequate intraoperative monitoring and consecutive hypotension
Inadequate analgesia
Insufficient postoperative respiratory physiotherapy
Missing a postoperative hemothorax
Failure to recognize an air leak and early withdrawal of drainages
Clogging or kinking of drainages

20.7 Special Situations

The management of pleural empyema after lung surgery, in particular after pneumonectomy, is discussed elsewhere. The treatment of an infected pleural space is difficult and may need finally drastic measures such as thoracic window, muscle and/or omental transposition, and thoracoplasty. VATS techniques can be used in the assessment of the infected cavity and for irrigation and debridement in postpneumonectomy empyema without bronchopleural fistula [15–17]. Similar approaches can be used in the management of postlobectomy empyema, provided there is no persistent bronchopleural fistula. As it is for parapneumonic empyema, the avoidance of an infected residual airspace is fundamental.

Occasionally, a lung cancer is detected during surgery for pleural empyema. Resection in a later timepoint can result in formidable technical difficulties. In such cases, individual decision-making depending on size, age of the patient, and likelihood of metastatic disease is necessary. A conversion to an open operation may provide the surgeon with more possibilities to assess the situation and technically facilitate resection.

References

1. Light RW (1985) Parapneumonic effusions and empyema. Clin Chest Med 6(1):55–62
2. Sahn SA (1993) Management of complicated parapneumonic effusions. Am Rev Respir Dis 148(3): 813–817
3. Rahman NM, Chapman SJ, Davies RJ (2006) The approach to the patient with a parapneumonic effusion. Clin Chest Med 27(2):253–266. doi:S0272-5231(05), 00129-2[pii] 10.1016/j.ccm.2005.12.005
4. Diacon AH, Theron J, Schuurmans MM, Van de Wal BW, Bolliger CT (2004) Intrapleural streptokinase for empyema and complicated parapneumonic effusions. Am J Respir Crit Care Med 170(1):49–53. doi:10.1164/rccm.200312-1740OC 200312-1740OC[pii]

5. Bouros D, Schiza S, Tzanakis N, Chalkiadakis G, Drositis J, Siafakas N (1999) Intrapleural urokinase versus normal saline in the treatment of complicated parapneumonic effusions and empyema. A randomized, double-blind study. Am J Respir Crit Care Med 159(1):37–42
6. Tuncozgur B, Ustunsoy H, Sivrikoz MC, Dikensoy O, Topal M, Sanli M, Elbeyli L (2001) Intrapleural urokinase in the management of parapneumonic empyema: a randomised controlled trial. Int J Clin Pract 55(10): 658–660
7. Davies CW, Lok S, Davies RJ (1998) The systemic fibrinolytic activity of intrapleural streptokinase. Am J Respir Crit Care Med 157(1):328–330
8. Maskell NA, Davies CW, Nunn AJ, Hedley EL, Gleeson FV, Miller R, Gabe R, Rees GL, Peto TE, Woodhead MA, Lane DJ, Darbyshire JH, Davies RJ (2005) U.K. controlled trial of intrapleural streptokinase for pleural infection. N Engl J Med 352(9):865–874. doi:352/9/865 [pii]10.1056/NEJMoa042473
9. Lardinois D, Gock M, Pezzetta E, Buchli C, Rousson V, Furrer M, Ris HB (2005) Delayed referral and gram-negative organisms increase the conversion thoracotomy rate in patients undergoing video-assisted thoracoscopic surgery for empyema. Ann Thorac Surg 79(6):1851–1856. doi:S0003-4975(04), 02476-2[pii] 10.1016/j.athoracsur.2004.12.031
10. Hsieh MJ, Liu YH, Chao YK, Lu MS, Liu HP, Wu YC, Lu HI, Chu Y (2008) Risk factors in surgical management of thoracic empyema in elderly patients. ANZ J Surg 78(6):445–448. doi:ANS4532[pii] 10.1111/j.1445-2197.2008.04532.x
11. Wozniak CJ, Paull DE, Moezzi JE, Scott RP, Anstadt MP, York VV, Little AG (2009) Choice of first intervention is related to outcomes in the management of empyema. Ann Thorac Surg 87(5):1525–1530. doi:S0003–4975(09)00123–4[pii] 10.1016/j.athoracsur.2009.01.028; discussion 1530–1521
12. Renner H, Gabor S, Pinter H, Maier A, Friehs G, Smolle-Juettner FM (1998) Is aggressive surgery in pleural empyema justified? Eur J Cardiothorac Surg 14(2):117–122. doi:S1010-7940(98), 00165-1[pii]
13. Cardillo G, Carleo F, Carbone L, Di Martino M, Salvadori L, Petrella L, Martelli M (2009) Chronic postpneumonic pleural empyema: comparative merits of thoracoscopic versus open decortication. Eur J Cardiothorac Surg 36(5):914–918. doi:S1010-7940(09), 00601-0 [pii] 10.1016/j.ejcts.2009.06.017
14. Chan DT, Sihoe AD, Chan S, Tsang DS, Fang B, Lee TW, Cheng LC (2007) Surgical treatment for empyema thoracis: is video-assisted thoracic surgery "better" than thoracotomy? Ann Thorac Surg 84(1):225–231. doi:S0003-4975(07)00598-X[pii] 10.1016/j.athoracsur.2007.03.019
15. Gossot D, Stern JB, Galetta D, Debrosse D, Girard P, Caliandro R, Harper L, Grunenwald D (2004) Thoracoscopic management of postpneumonectomy empyema. Ann Thorac Surg 78(1):273–276. doi:10.1016/j.athoracsur.2004.02.023 S000349750400400X[pii]
16. Hollaus PH, Lax F, Wurnig PN, Janakiev D, Pridun NS (1999) Videothoracoscopic debridement of the postpneumonectomy space in empyema. Eur J Cardiothorac Surg 16(3):283–286. doi:S1010794099002249[pii]
17. Bagan P, Boissier F, Berna P, Badia A, Le Pimpec-Barthes F, Souilamas R, Riquet M (2006) Postpneumonectomy empyema treated with a combination of antibiotic irrigation followed by videothoracoscopic debridement. J Thorac Cardiovasc Surg 132(3):708–710. doi:S0022-5223(06),00886-5[pii]10.1016/j.jtcvs.2006.05.014

Malignant Mesothelioma

21

David A. Waller and Muhammad Javed

Contents

D.A. Waller, M.D., FRCS(CTh) (✉)
M. Javed, M.D., MRCS
Department of Thoracic Surgery, Glenfield Hospital, Groby Road, Leicester LE3 9QP, UK
e-mail: david.waller@uhl-tr.nhs.uk; umair.dr@gmail.com

21.1 VAT Staging

21.1.1 Video-Assisted Thoracoscopy

VAT can be used to confirm the cell type of mesothelioma and assess the T stage of the tumour. Involvement of the parietal and visceral surfaces can be recorded together with involvement of diaphragmatic and pericardial surfaces. When taking a biopsy, full-thickness biopsies including underlying muscle are preferred. VATS pleural biopsy has an accuracy of nearly 100% [1].

21.1.2 Cervical Thoracomediastinoscopy

The nodal stage of the tumour may influence the subsequent choice of surgical therapy. Video-assisted mediastinoscopy can assess at least five mediastinal lymph node stations. It is feasible to enter the pleural cavity via the mediastinal pleura (Fig. 21.1) and perform simultaneous intrathoracic staging, confirm tissue diagnosis and effect pleurodesis with talc insufflation via a single collar incision [2]. This combined approach to diagnosis and staging reduces preoperative delay [3].

21.2 VAT Symptom Control

21.2.1 Talc Pleurodesis

Thoracoscopic talc insufflation has been shown to be superior to instillation of a talc slurry via a

R.G.C. Inderbitzi et al. (eds.), *Minimally Invasive Thoracic and Cardiac Surgery*,
DOI 10.1007/978-3-642-11861-6_21, © Springer-Verlag Berlin Heidelberg 2012

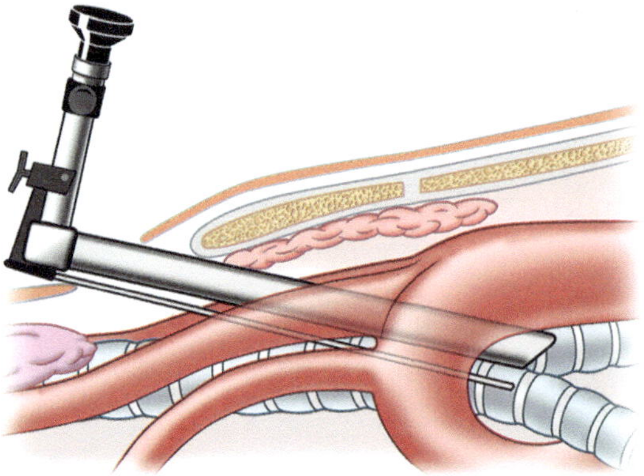

Fig. 21.1 Video-assisted cervical thoraco-mediastinoscopy

chest tube with a 15% greater success rate [4]. A small risk of ARDS is associated with talc insufflations of about 3% [5]. Ideally, 8 g of large particle size talc should be used to avoid the risk of ARDS [6]. VATS talc pleurodesis is over 92% successful in controlling effusion and carries a risk of less than 1% [1].

21.3 VAT Debulking/Cytoreduction

21.3.1 VAT Parietal Pleurectomy

In early stages of mesothelioma, the underlying lung remains expansile. Removal of the parietal tumour mass around the inside of the chest wall may prevent fluid production prolonging symptom control and may delay disease progression. Despite the theoretical risk of bleeding, the feasibility of this technique has been established [7].

21.3.2 Pleurodesis Versus Pleurectomy

The potential benefits of pleurectomy over simple talc pleurodesis include removal of the source of excess fluid production and cytoreduction thus delaying tumour progression. There is nonrandomised evidence that survival may be significantly prolonged by this approach [8]. The comparative benefits are currently under assessment in a multicentre randomised trial in UK: the Meso VATS trial (PI: Dr Robert Rintoul, Papworth Hospital, UK)

21.3.3 VAT Visceral Pleurectomy

In more advanced stages of mesothelioma, tumour involvement of the visceral pleura entraps the lung. Whilst drainage of the pleural effusion will improve symptoms, dyspnoea will not be relieved without releasing the lung. Decortication of the lung may be achieved via thoracotomy, but the consequent morbidity detracts from any symptomatic benefit in the relatively short survival period [9]. VAT has the benefit of faster recovery but is technically more demanding. The technique was initially devised for parapneumonic pleural empyema [10] but has been extended to patients with malignant empyema and thence to those with noninfected trapped lung syndrome secondary to malignant pleural mesothelioma [11]. This technique is associated with relief of dyspnoea in over 80% of cases and has acceptable morbidity and mortality [12]

21.3.4 Surgical Technique

Double lumen endotracheal intubation with single lung ventilation is employed. For most cases, an indwelling thoracic epidural catheter is inserted for postoperative analgesia.

Video-assisted thoracoscopy is performed in the lateral position via three 2-cm incisions. The initial incision is placed just below the tip of the scapula, and two further incisions are placed to complete a triangle based on the intrathoracic anatomy.

The initial phase involves debridement of the thorax using directed suction (Fig. 21.2); specimens of exudate are sent for microbiological analysis. The extent of pleural entrapment can then be assessed.

The thickened visceral pleura is then incised using a fine knife blade (Fig. 21.3) across the surface if the lung just inferior to the oblique fissure. The visceral pleural sheet is then grasped and gently separated from the underlying lung parenchyma using a mounted pledget with attached suction (Fig. 21.4). The raised pleural sheet can then be resected using endoscopic scissors. This process is continued across all lobes until the lung is fully mobilised (Fig. 21.5). The

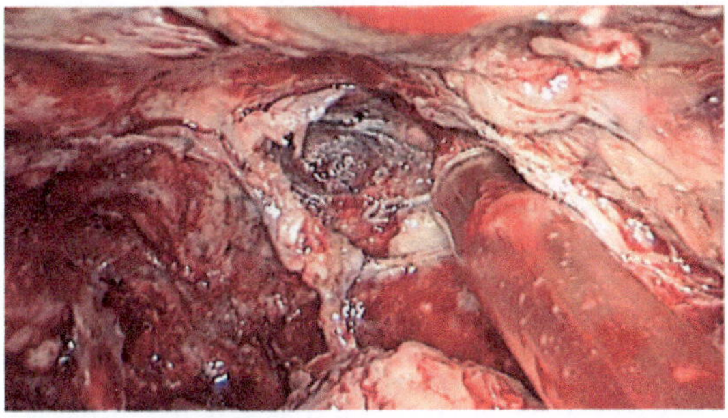

Fig. 21.2 Initial video-assisted pleural debridement

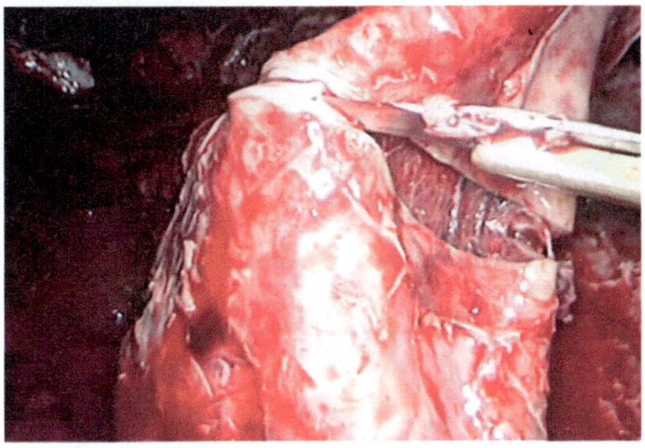

Fig. 21.3 Incision of the visceral pleural tumour

parietal pleural sheet can then be removed by blunt extrapleural dissection. It is not usually possible to remove all of the mediastinal or diaphragmatic pleura. To reduce air leak, the bare parenchymal surface can be covered with a sealant.

Prior to closure, the chest is drained by two large bore tubes connected to suction.

21.3.5 VATS Decortication Versus Pleural Catheter Drainage

There is an increasing trend toward treating a malignant pleural effusion secondary to mesothelioma by insertion of a tunnelled silicone intrapleural catheter connected to a portable suction device [13]. In cases where the lung can re-expand, talc pleurodesis is as effective for less cost [14]. There are reports of spontaneous pleural symphysis, but in the majority of patients, the lung fails to expand [15].

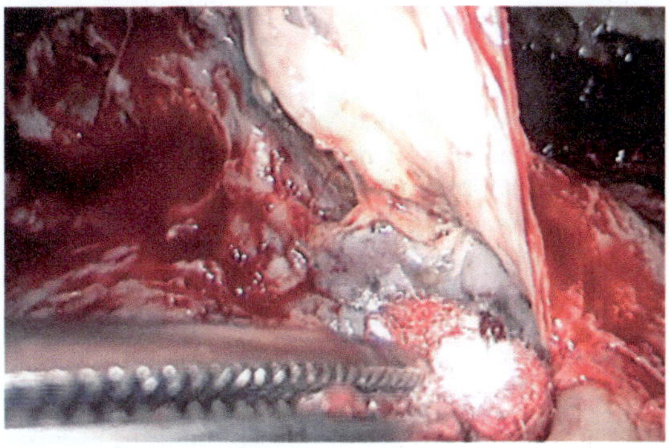

Fig. 21.4 Video-assisted thoracoscopic visceral pleurectomy

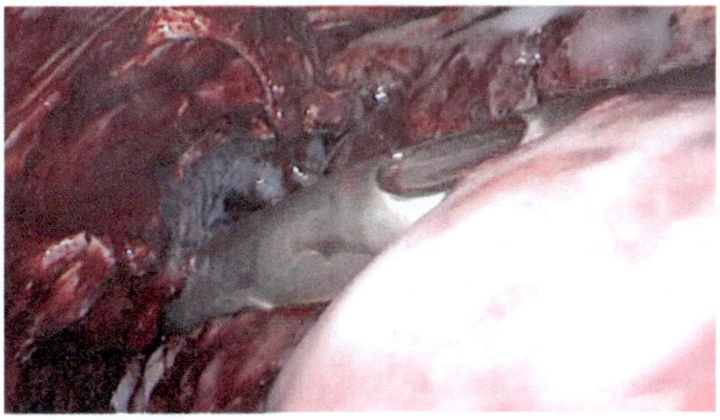

Fig. 21.5 Lung re-expanded by reventilation

The potential advantages of VATS decortication over long-term drainage include: the ability to relieve dyspnoea secondary to the trapped lung. The potential disadvantages of long-term catheter drainage include: catheter blockage or infection necessitating removal and the psychological disadvantage to the patient of wearing a constant reminder of their underlying disease.

Conclusions

The population of patients presenting with malignant pleural mesothelioma is becoming older and therefore of poorer performance status. Fewer patients will be suitable for radical open surgery, thus VATS will become more important. Increasing technical expertise with VATS should broaden the application of cytoreductive techniques, and the completion of ongoing surgical trials may stimulate its use.

References

1. Cardillo G, Facciolo F, Carbone L, Regal M, Corzani F, Ricci A, Di Martino M, Martelli M (2002) Long-term follow-up of video-assisted talc pleurodesis in malignant recurrent pleural effusions. Eur J Cardiothorac Surg 21(2):302–305; discussion 305–6
2. Fowkes L, Lau KK, Shah N, Black E (2009) A cervical approach to investigating pleural disease. Ann Thorac Surg 88(1):315–317
3. Chamberlain MH, Fareed K, Nakas A, Martin-Ucar AE, Waller DA (2008) Video-assisted cervical thoracoscopy: a novel approach for diagnosis, staging and pleurodesis of malignant pleural mesothelioma. Eur J Cardiothorac Surg 34(1):200–203
4. Stefani A, Natali P, Casali C, Morandi U (2006) Talc poudrage versus talc slurry in the treatment of malignant pleural effusion. A prospective comparative study. Eur J Cardiothorac Surg 30(6):827–832
5. Gonzalez AV, Bezwada V, Beamis JF Jr, Villanueva AG (2010) Lung injury following thoracoscopic talc insufflation: experience of a single north American center. Chest 137(6):1375–1381, Epub 2010 Jan 22
6. Ferrer J, Montes JF, Villarino MA, Light RW, García-Valero J (2002) Influence of particle size on extrapleural talc dissemination after talc slurry pleurodesis. Chest 122(3):1018–1027
7. Waller DA, Morritt GN, Forty J (1995) Video-assisted thoracoscopic pleurectomy in the management of malignant pleural effusion. Chest 107(5):1454–1456
8. Halstead JC, Lim E, Venkateswaran RM, Charman SC, Goddard M, Ritchie AJ (2005) Improved survival with VATS pleurectomy-decortication in advanced malignant mesothelioma. Eur J Surg Oncol 31(3):314–320
9. Martin-Ucar AE, Edwards JG, Rengajaran A, Muller S, Waller DA (2001) Palliative surgical debulking in malignant mesothelioma. Predictors of survival and symptom control. Eur J Cardiothorac Surg 20(6): 1117–1121
10. Waller DA, Rengarajan A (2001) Thoracoscopic decortication: a role for video-assisted surgery in chronic postpneumonic pleural empyema. Ann Thorac Surg 71(6):1813–1816
11. Nakas A, Martin Ucar AE, Edwards JG, Waller DA (2008) The role of video assisted thoracoscopic pleurectomy/decortication in the therapeutic management of malignant pleural mesothelioma. Eur J Cardiothorac Surg 33(1):83–88
12. Srivastava V, Dunning J, Au J (2009) Does video-assisted thoracoscopic decortication in advanced malignant mesothelioma improve prognosis? Interact Cardiovasc Thorac Surg 8(4):454–456
13. Efthymiou CA, Masudi T, Thorpe JA, Papagiannopoulos K (2009) Malignant pleural effusion in the presence of trapped lung. Five-year experience of PleurX tunnelled catheters. Interact Cardiovasc Thorac Surg 9(6):961–964, Epub 2009 Jul 28
14. Olden AM, Holloway R (2010) Treatment of malignant pleural effusion: pleuRx catheter or talc pleurodesis? A cost-effectiveness analysis. J Palliat Med 13(1):59–65
15. Sioris T, Sihvo E, Salo J, Räsänen J, Knuuttila A (2009) Long-term indwelling pleural catheter (PleurX) for malignant pleural effusion unsuitable for talc pleurodesis. Eur J Surg Oncol 35(5):546–551

Part IV

Minimally Invasive Thoracic Surgery: The Mediastinum

22 Staging Procedures

Gunda Leschber and Johannes Merk

Contents

Among the several techniques to stage the mediastinum, the most important in the hands of thoracic surgeons remains mediastinoscopy. As a minimal invasive procedure, it allows approach to most parts of the middle compartment of the mediastinum. Besides staging of lung cancer patients, mediastinoscopy is also widely used to diagnose undefined mediastinal masses. In 1959, the Swedish thoracic surgeon Eric Carlens [1] for the first time described mediastinoscopy. With the existing limited radiological options in patients with lung cancer, Carlens wished to obtain information on potential mediastinal tumour spread prior to surgery, since it was not unusual to find inoperable tumours at thoracotomy. Nowadays, the importance of mediastinoscopy in lung cancer lies in the exact determination of the tumour stage. Tumour stage strongly affects survival, especially in stages I to III, since these have far differing prognosis depending on the involvement of mediastinal lymph nodes. In addition, according to current studies, neoadjuvant treatment in stage III increases life expectancy [2]; therefore, mediastinal staging needs to be as accurate as possible even in non-enlarged lymph nodes.

Novel techniques that have emerged over the past 10 years such as EBUS, EUS and PET CT scan are still lacking the prove of reliability in widespread use. There are publications by a handful of specialists indicating excellent results, but the prevalence of lymph node metastasis in these studies is generally much higher than in the daily practice of a thoracic surgeon. Therefore, mediastinoscopy remains the gold standard in mediastinal

G. Leschber, M.D. (✉)
Thoraxchirurgische Klinik, Evangelische Lungenklinik Berlin – Krankenhausbetriebs gGmbH, Lindenberger Weg 27, D-13125, Berlin, Germany
e-mail: gunda.leschber@elk-berlin.de

J. Merk, M.D.
Klinik für Herz-, Thorax- und Gefässchirurgie, Universitätsklinikum Ulm, 9,89075, Ulm Germany

Thoraxchirurgische Klinik, Evangelische Lungenklinik Berlin – Krankenhausbetriebs gGmbH, Lindenberger Weg 27, D-13125, Berlin, Germany
e-mail: johannes.merk@uniklinik-ulum.de; johannes.merk@elk-berlin.de

R.G.C. Inderbitzi et al. (eds.), *Minimally Invasive Thoracic and Cardiac Surgery*,
DOI 10.1007/978-3-642-11861-6_22,

staging of lung cancer although it is a more invasive procedure than the competing techniques.

22.1 Cervical Mediastinoscopy (Conventional Mediastinoscopy)

Cervical mediastinoscopy is performed under general anaesthesia in a supine position. Through a small incision cranial of the jugular notch, dissection is carried down in the midline, and the strap muscles are bluntly separated. The thyroid gland is retracted cranially, and the pretracheal fascia is exposed and opened. By blunt dissection with the index finger (Fig. 22.1), a pretracheal space is created as far down as possible, large enough to introduce a normal mediastinoscope. Under direct vision, further dissection along the anterior surface of the trachea is carried out with a suction device. This metal suction device also allows coagulation of small bleeding sites. In general, the peritracheal as well as the tissues along the main bronchi are dissected with this instrument, and biopsy forceps are used to take small bites of visible subcarinal, tracheobronchial, para-, and pretracheal lymph nodes.

Not accessible by conventional mediastinoscopy are the paraoesophageal (station 8), the left-sided para- and subaortic lymph node stations (station 5 and 6) and lymph nodes of the pulmonary ligament (station 9). The distinction between lymphatic and other tissues (e.g. blood vessels) can be achieved by puncture with a special needle adapted to the use in mediastinoscopy. In case of doubt whether a mediastinal structure might be a vessel, puncture should always be performed prior to taking a bite with the biopsy forceps as this may result in uncontrollable bleeding. Upon completion of the operation, the field is inspected for bleeding before removing the mediastinoscope, and the incision in the jugular fossa is closed with absorbable sutures. Only on rare indications a suction drain is placed for 24 h. An indication and time point for a postoperative X-ray is seen differently in Europe or the USA, especially with an unremarkable course. In the USA as well as in some European hospitals, mediastinoscopy is performed on an outpatient basis, while in most European centres it usually takes place in the course of a hospital stay of a few days.

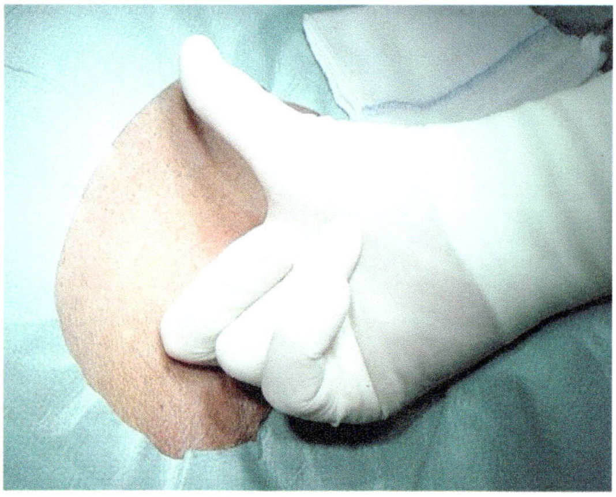

Fig. 22.1 Blunt dissection of a pretracheal space with the index finger

Whether the lymph nodes tissue removed by mediastinoscopy is handled as frozen section allowing only examination of a few nodes at the time of operation or whether removal of several stations such as recommended by the ESTS working group with a thorough workup by the pathologist is performed determines the status of mediastinoscopy in the whole setting of lung cancer treatment.

22.2 Video Mediastinoscopy

In the late 1980s, thoracic surgeons in close cooperation with two German companies, producers of surgical instruments, invented video mediastinoscopy. The technique initially introduced by Lerut showed no major differences to conventional methods. The advantage of integration of a video chip into the mediastinoscope and transmission of the video signal to a monitor was that the surgeon and everyone in the operation room had an unobstructed view into the mediastinum. It remained a one-handed procedure but improved training of young surgeons. The next step in development was a mediastinoscope with spreadable blades: the Linder-Dahan video mediastinoscope (Fig. 22.2). For the first time, it was possible to bluntly enlarge the operating field, creating a

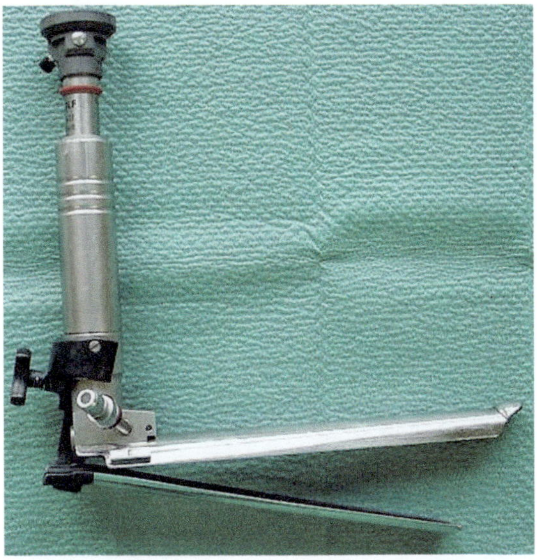

Fig. 22.2 Linder-Dahan video mediastinoscope

space large enough to introduce two instruments for bimanual work. This opened a new dimension in operating in the mediastinum [9] especially when special equipment such as bipolar scissors or clip applicators became available (Fig. 22.3).

The video mediastinoscope is introduced the same way as in the conventional technique through a small skin incision. After insertion of the video mediastinoscope (Fig. 22.4), dissection along the anterior surface of the trachea is performed using two instruments for dissection and retraction of tissue. All anatomical structures are clearly identified: pulmonary artery, vena cava and vena azygos, right and left main bronchus as well as pleura and oesophagus (Figs. 22.5 and 22.6). Visualisation of vulnerable structures such as the recurrent laryngeal nerve is facilitated (Fig. 22.7). By grasping the lymph node with a forceps and holding it under gentle tension, the surrounding tissue are easily dissected from the node. Adjacent blood vessels can be separated and clipped, and eventually the lymph node is completely freed and removed in toto (Fig. 22.8). The alternative in larger nodes or tumours is a biopsy taken by the biopsy forceps without removal of the entire node. Coagulation can be administered by mono- or

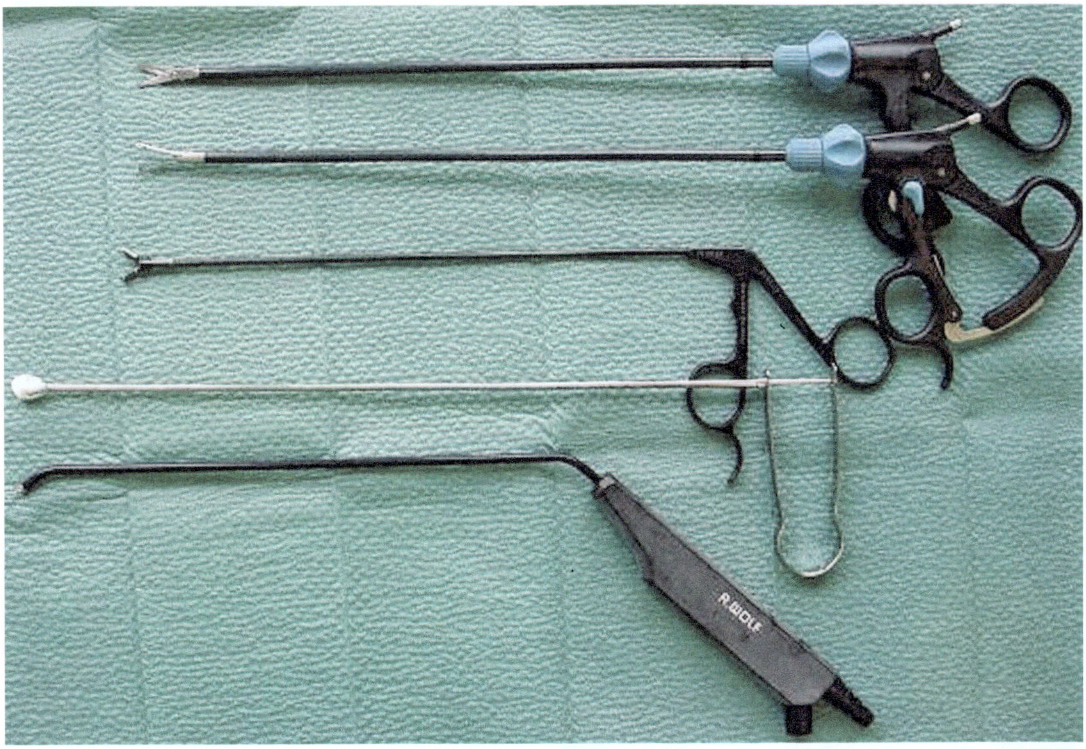

Fig. 22.3 Instruments, usable in video mediastinoscopy

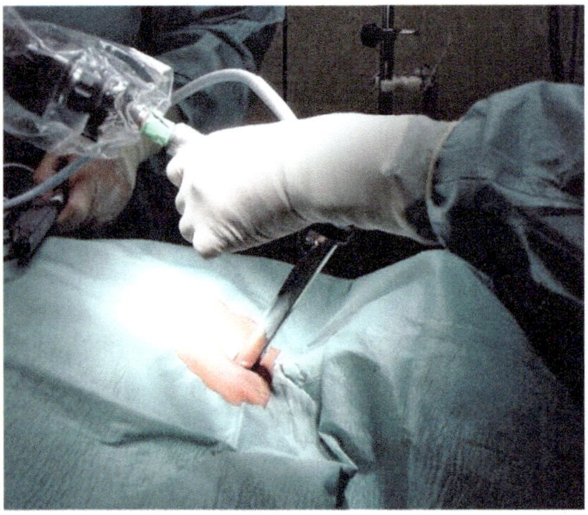

Fig. 22.4 Insertion of the video mediastinoscope

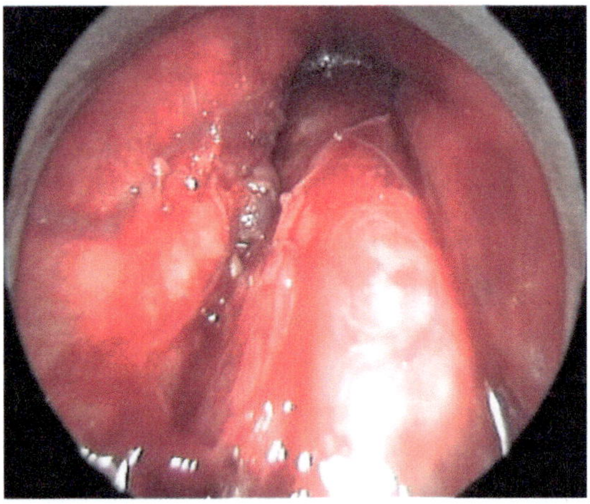

Fig. 22.5 Anterior surface of the trachea after blunt dissection

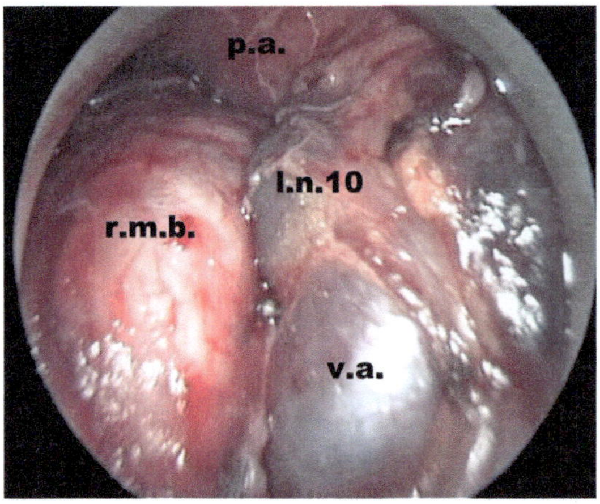

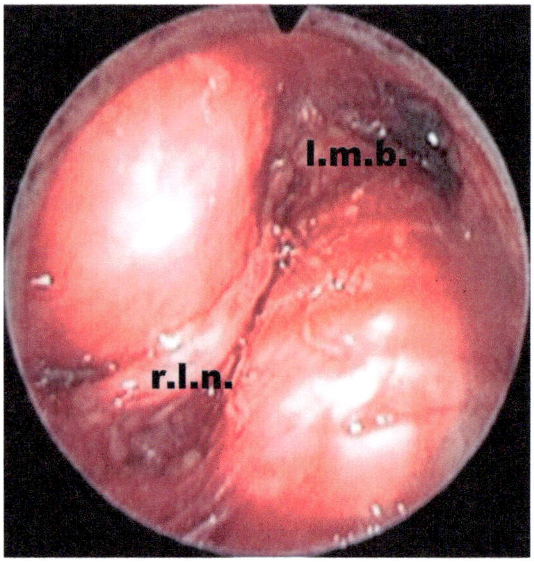

Fig. 22.7 Visualisation of vulnerable structures in video mediastinoscopy (*r.l.n.* recurrent laryngeal nerve, *l.m.b.* left main bronchus)

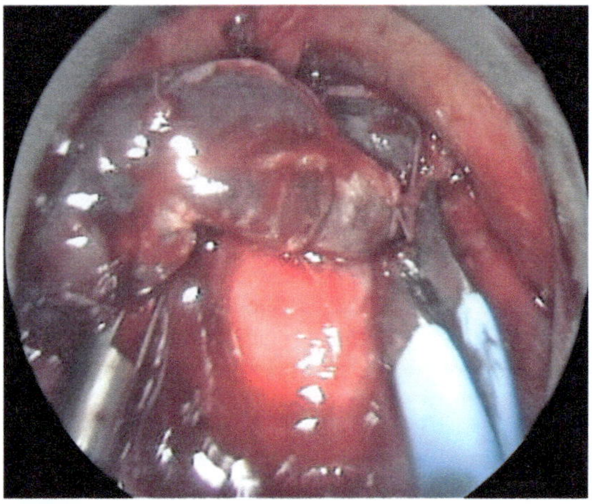

Fig. 22.8 Bimanual technique in dissection of entire lymph nodes

Fig. 22.6 Visualisation of anatomical structures in video mediastinoscopy (*p.a.* pulmonary artery, *v.a.* vena azygos, *r.m.b.* right main bronchus, *l.n.10* lymph node station 10)

bipolar coagulation; the use of a gauze admixed with fibrin is rarely indicated.

Since the videoscopic surgery nowadays is playing a major role in thoracic surgery, video mediastinoscopy has encountered wide spread use. Visualisation of all structures improves the safety of the operation for the patient and even younger surgeons gain an excellent knowledge of the anatomy by merely participating in the procedure. For the experienced thoracic surgeon, new options emerged: VAMLA (video-assisted mediastinal lymphadenectomy).

22.3 VAMLA (Video-Assisted Mediastinal Lymphadenectomy)

First described in 2002 by Hürtgen et al. [6], one of the pioneers in video mediastinoscopy, complete mediastinal lymphadenectomy by mediastinoscopy is the most accurate and complete lymph node staging possible.

Not only single lymph nodes are dissected but also the complete compartment including all nodes and the adjacent fatty tissue are removed [8]. The completeness results in blank anatomical structure such as the pleura, vena cava, vena azygos, and the right main bronchus up to the upper lobe bronchus, the carina and oesophagus. There is no difference in the lymphadenectomy performed in the open fashion. VAMLA is perfect in combination with VATS lobectomy if performed prior to this procedure: Thorough lymph node staging allows inclusion of patients in the early stages only, and at the time of VATS lobectomy, operation time is shortened because most of the lymphadenectomy is already done [11]. In addition, clearance of the subcarinal area is easier by VAMLA than during VATS lobectomy.

22.4 Extended Cervical Mediastinoscopy and TEMLA

Cervical mediastinoscopy does not allow access to the para- and subaortic lymph node stations (stations 5 and 6) which are particularly important for tumours of the left upper lobe. Anterior mediastinotomy was first used to explore these lymph node stations by incision through the second intercostal space and blunt, extrapleural dissection towards the aortopulmonary window. Ginsberg in 1987, however, developed a new method, the extended cervical mediastinoscopy. After performing conventional mediastinoscopy, a space is digitally created anterior to the aortic arch between the innominate and left carotid arter and the mediastinoscope advanced over the aortic arch down to the aortopulmonary window. The same can be done with the video mediastinoscope although care must be taken as due to sheer forces, there is a risk to tear the arteries especially in patients with arteriosclerosis. To reach the lymph nodes in this area under direct vision, Kuzdal et al. [7] described a further extension, the transcervical extended mediastinal lymphadenectomy (TEMLA). The cervical incision is larger to allow insertion of a sternal elevator, and by combination of mediastinoscopy and thoracoscopy, the whole mediastinal space, including the para- and subaortic lymph node stations, is explored and can be dissected. The dissection starts at the level of the upper mediastinal nodes and follows the recurrent laryngeal nerve down under vision until the aortopulmonary window is reached.

22.5 Complications

Major complications of mediastinoscopy and video mediastinoscopy are rare events and consist mostly of bleeding from vessel injuries. These can be life threatening, so that a thoracotomy or sternotomy becomes mandatory to gain control of injured blood vessel.

The pulmonary artery and the azygos vein are mainly at risk. The pulmonary artery is affected when adherent lymph nodes or tumour tissue are removed with excessive traction. The same accounts for calcified lymph nodes encountered at the confluence of vena cava and vena azygos in patients with former tuberculosis. Also, the azygos vein can easily be mistaken for a lymph node if not clearly dissected from the surrounding tissue. If a biopsy is taken this will cause a major bleeding, therefore careful evaluation of the tissue to be biopsied is indicated (i.e. by needle puncture). Still, treatment of bleeding complications consists of initial packing the operating field with a sponge as these vessels belong to the low pressure system and intrinsic coagulation may solve the problem. Bleeding from a bronchial artery can be stopped by clipping or electro coagulation.

Through knowledge of the anatomy should avoid accidental biopsies from the aortic wall or the carotid artery. The implementation of the video technique has resulted in further decrease of these problems.

The most common minor complication is injury of the left recurrent laryngeal nerve with an incidence of up to 5%. The use of a nerve stimulator is not mandatory; instead, application of electric current and intense traction in the left tracheobronchial area should be avoided. One has to keep in mind that the use of the coagulation device can cause severe burns in all tissues that are not "cooled" by blood flow: nerves, trachea and oesophagus.

If the parietal pleura is opened accidentally, a pneumothorax may result, but in general no further action is needed, as the lung is kept inflated by the intubation.

Other rare complications include bradycardia by irritation of the vagus nerve and wound infections.

According to the literature, complication rates vary between 1% and 3%. The mortality rate, stated in all published collectives, is far below 1% [3, 12].

22.6 Alternative Staging Procedures

In addition to classical imaging and computed tomography (CT), magnet resonance imaging (MRI) and positron-emission tomography (PET) are of increasing importance. All three imaging methods, however, suffer from the lack to provide tissue for histopathological examination.

In contrast, endobronchial ultrasound-guided needle aspiration (EBUS) provides specimen for pathologic analysis. Although the samples are very small, due to the ultrasound imaging and the working channel of the bronchoscope, high sensitivity of lymph nodes reached by this technique is described [5]. However, it must be taken into account that the majority of the published studies were performed on patients with enlarged lymph nodes [4]. This reflects the prevalence of lymph node metastases, which is considerably higher than for mediastinoscopy, where all reachable lymph nodes are biopsied in a standard fashion even when of normal size [10].

References

1. Carlens E (1959) Mediastinoscopy: a method for inspection a tissue biopsy in the superior mediastinum. Dis Chest 36:343–352
2. De Leyn P, Lardinois D, Van Schil PE et al (2007) ESTS guidelines for preoperative lymph node staging for non-small cell lung cancer. Eur J Cardiothorac Surg 32(1):1–8
3. Detterbeck FC, Jantz MA, Wallace M et al (2007) Invasive mediastinal staging of lung cancer: ACCP evidence-based clinical practice guidelines (2nd edition). Chest 132(3 Suppl):202S–220S
4. Ernst A, Anantham D, Eberhardt R et al (2008) Diagnosis of mediastinal adenopathy-real-time endobronchial ultrasound guided needle aspiration versus mediastinoscopy. J Thorac Oncol 3(6):577–582
5. Herth FJ, Eberhardt R, Krasnik M et al (2008) Endobronchial ultrasound-guided transbronchial needle aspiration of lymph nodes in the radiologically and positron emission tomography-normal mediastinum in patients with lung cancer. Chest 133(4):887–891
6. Hürtgen M, Friedel G, Toomes H et al (2002) Radical video-assisted mediastinoscopic lymphadenectomy (VAMLA) – technique and first results. Eur J Cardiothorac Surg 21(2):348–351
7. Kuzdzał J, Zieliński M, Papla B et al (2007) The transcervical extended mediastinal lymphadenectomy versus cervical mediastinoscopy in non-small cell lung cancer staging. Eur J Cardiothorac Surg 31(1):88–94
8. Leschber G, Holinka G, Linder A (2003) Video-assisted mediastinoscopic lymphadenectomy (VAMLA) – a method for systematic mediastinal lymph node dissection. Eur J Cardiothorac Surg 24(2):192–195
9. Leschber G, Sperling D, Klemm W et al (2008) Does video-mediastinoscopy improve the results of conventional mediastinoscopy? Eur J Cardiothorac Surg 33(2):289–293
10. Silvestri GA, Gould MK, Margolis ML et al (2007) Noninvasive staging of non-small cell lung cancer: ACCP evidenced-based clinical practice guidelines (2nd edition). Chest 132(3 Suppl):178S–201S
11. Witte B, Hürtgen M (2007) Video-assisted mediastinoscopic lymphadenectomy (VAMLA). J Thorac Oncol 2(4):367–369
12. Yasufuku K, Fujisawa T (2007) Staging and diagnosis of non-small cell lung cancer: invasive modalities. Respirology 12(2):173–183

Video-Assisted Thoracic Lymphadenectomy

23

Godehard Friedel, Stefanie Veit, and Thomas Kyriss

Contents

G. Friedel, M.D. (✉) • S. Veit, M.D. • T. Kyriss, M.D.
Department of Thoracic Surgery,
Robert-Bosch-Hospital, Klinik Schillerhöhe,
Solitudestr. 18, D-70839 Gerlingen-Stuttgart, Germany
e-mail: godehard.friedel@klinik-schillerhoehe.de;
stefanie.veit@klinik-schillerhoehe.de;
thomas.kyriss@klinik-schillerhoehe.de

23.1 Introduction

The role of lymph node dissection is discussed since Borrie, Nohl-Oser, and Cahan first described the intrapulmonary lymphatic anatomy with its interconnecting network and the radical mediastinal lymphadenectomy in the resection of lung cancer in the 1950s [1, 2]. It is still a debate on basic principles whether lymphadenectomy is a part of radical surgery or a just a staging procedure.

23.2 Anatomy

The lung is characterized by an extensive network of lymphatic vessels and nodes. A superficial subpleural lymphatic vessel system is connected to a second large lymphatic network in the interlobar septa. In the parenchyma, the drainage is continued in the perivascular and peribronchial lymphatic pathways, finally leading via the hilar pathways to the mediastinal lymphatic vessels. Direct passages to the mediastinum bypassing the hilar lymphatic vessels have also been described. The pulmonary lymph nodes are divided into the lobar and the hilar ones. Intrapulmonary lymph nodes are rare; at autopsy, Trapnell [3] found direct intrapulmonary lymph nodes in about 18%. On high-resolution computed tomography, these lymph nodes are often visible as peripheral coin lesions and are sometimes interpreted to be metastases. Bronchopulmonary lymph nodes are located close to the origin of the lobar bronchi directly

R.G.C. Inderbitzi et al. (eds.), *Minimally Invasive Thoracic and Cardiac Surgery*,
DOI 10.1007/978-3-642-11861-6_23,

next to bronchus and pulmonary artery. The hilar lymph nodes are defined to reach from the right lateral side of the main bronchus to where the azygos vein crosses the trachea and medially to the lymph nodes bordering on the carina. On the left side, the border is lateral to the midline where the pulmonary artery crosses the main bronchus. Anatomically, the mediastinal lymph nodes are divided into four groups: the anterior, prevascular ones, the tracheobronchial ones, the paratracheal, and the posterior mediastinal lymph nodes. The anterior lymph nodes are located in the anterior mediastinum in front of the large vessels. The tracheobronchial lymph nodes are divided into three groups. The superior right and left groups are located in the angle between trachea and main bronchus outside the pretracheal fascia. The nodes of the inferior tracheobronchial group are commonly called subcarinal lymph nodes and are located inside the pretracheal fascia. The right-sided tracheobronchial lymph nodes are located between the main stem of the pulmonary artery and the azygos vein. The left-sided group is found deep in the aortopulmonary window between the recurrent nerve, the ligamentum arteriosum, and the main stem of the pulmonary artery. The paratracheal lymph nodes are located along the trachea bordered by the cava vein, the aortic arch and the left carotid artery, the brachiocephalic trunk, and the azygos vein. The right paratracheal lymph nodes are commonly larger than the left ones. The posterior mediastinal lymph nodes include the paraesophageal ones and those in the pulmonary ligament either [4].

23.3 Definition

Without a precise staging, a comparison of studies and survival data is impossible, particularly against the background of forthcoming studies of adjuvant and neoadjuvant therapeutic approaches. The different forms of lymph node dissection have mainly been used so far to prove longer survival times. The reports deal with simple and systematic lymph node sampling, complete, radical, or supraradical lymphadenectomy, however, without exactly defining these synonyms. A simple lymph node sampling includes the removal of suspicious lymph nodes; the systematic sampling is intended to describe the routine biopsy of lymph node stations, which had been defined before. Complete lymphadenectomy describes the ipsilateral resection of all lymph nodes including the surrounding tissue. The radical lymphadenectomy additionally removes contralateral and/or supraclavicular lymph nodes [5].

23.4 Lymphadenectomy

VAT lymphadenectomy follows the same steps as it does in open surgery. In case of a carcinoma of the right lung, the lymph nodes were resected en bloc including the mediastinal fat tissue up to the contralateral side. The dissection was performed starting at the pulmonary ligament via the paraesophageal, bifurcational to the tracheobronchial, and paratracheal lymph nodes. In the bifurcational region, the lymph nodes of the left main bronchus were resected additionally. In the paratracheal region, the contralateral lymph nodes were resected as well. On the left side, the procedure was the same up to the tracheobronchial lymph nodes. In addition, the aortopulmonary window was completely dissected with conservation of the recurrent nerve. On the left paratracheal side, only increased and visible lymph nodes were removed. A regular mobilization of the aortic arch was not performed [6].

The first part of VAT lobectomy is the dissection of hilar structures. Thereby, the hilar lymph nodes will be resected. The intrapulmonary lymph nodes will be resected during the dissection of the segmental arteries within the pulmonary fissure. In cases of resection of the lower lobes, the pulmonary ligament will be divided first and the lymph nodes of this region will be resected as well.

After completion of the lobectomy of the right side, the paratracheal lymphadenectomy will be performed first (Figs. 23.1, 23.2, 23.3, 23.4, and 23.5). The azygos vein is dissected and retracted caudally. The mediastinal pleura will be incised along the lateral border of the cava vein, protecting the phrenic nerve. The mediastinal fat is

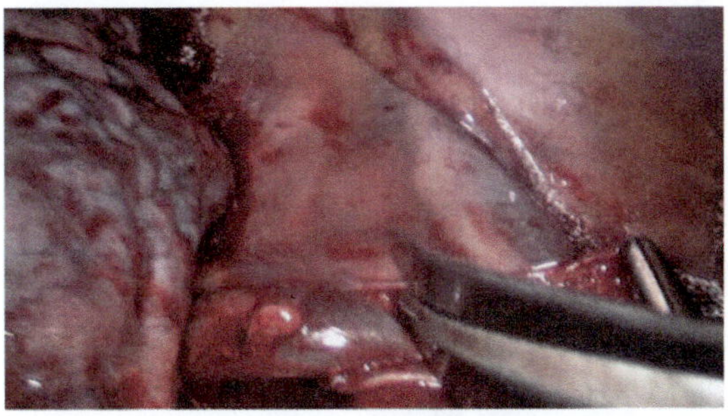

Fig. 23.1 Thoracoscopic separation of azygos vein (starting point to dissection of lymph node stations 4, 2, and 8)

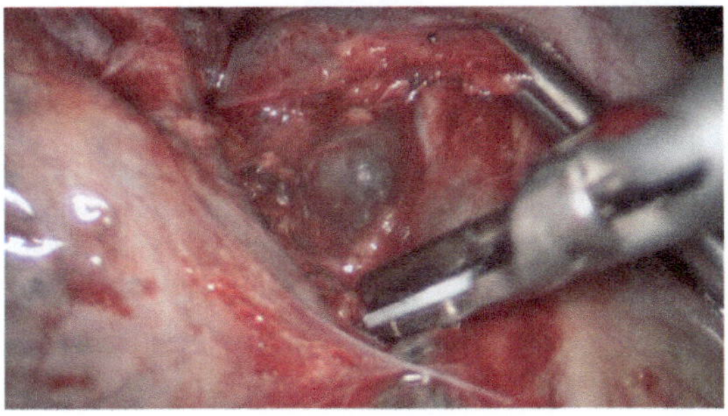

Fig. 23.2 Thoracoscopic preparation of lymph nodes behind and below azygos vein, ATS 4 proceeding to 8

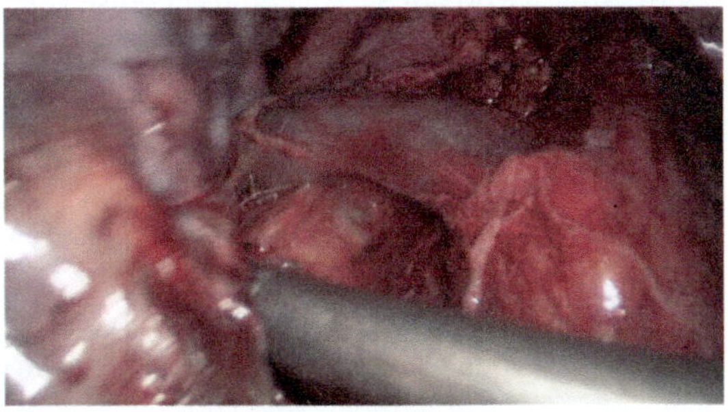

Fig. 23.3 Thoracoscopically removed lymph nodes ATS 4/8. *Above*: azygos vein. *Right*: v. cava

dissected along the cava vein up to the pericardium and the aortic arch below. Attention should be played to small vessels coming off the cava vein which should be closed using clips or ultrasound dissector. The mediastinal fat will be dissected from the trachea under protection of the peritracheal vessels, if possible. The dissection is carried out using ultrasound dissector as well. Now the fat-lymph node packet is grasped by an endoscopic forceps and divided with the ultrasound dissector underneath the brachiocephalic trunk. Hemostasis, especially near brachiocephalic trunk, is performed using bipolar coagulation to protect the recurrent nerve.

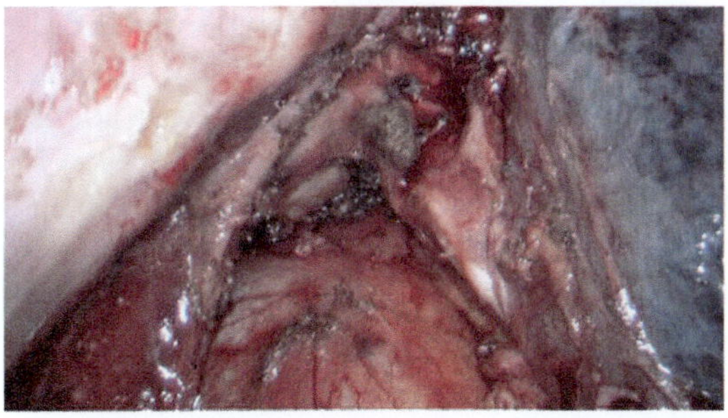

Fig. 23.4 Resected lymph nodes ATS 7. Visible carina

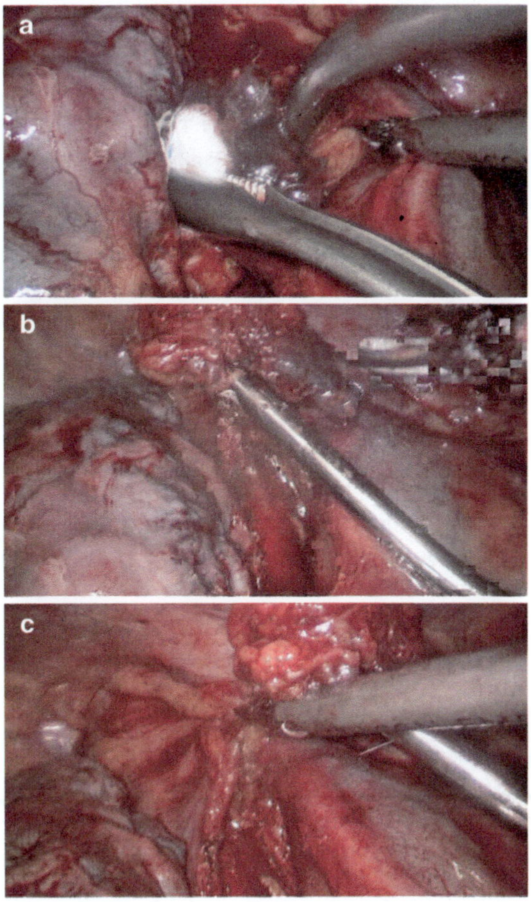

Fig. 23.5 (**a**) Start of removing lymph nodes ATS 4 right. (**b**) Dissection en bloc of lymph node 2/1 right. (**c**) Cutting through of nutritive vessels of en bloc resected lymph nodes ATS 2 /1 right

We do not cut through the azygos vein in order to protect as much tissue as possible. However, it seems to be not problematical and cause no morbidity to divide the vessel.

In left-side lobectomy, the mediastinal pleura around the aortic arch is incised and retracted by a grasp. The vagus nerve is identified, and its branch, the left-side recurrent nerve, should be protected. To assure this, bipolar or ultrasound dissection should be preferred within this region. The medial border is defined by the phrenic nerve which has to be protected also. The complete tissue packet will be dissected in head of the central pulmonary artery, which was freed before.

The subcarinal lymph nodes are included within the tissue between the right main bronchus, the left main bronchus, the pericardium, and the esophagus. The tissue is dissected starting at the right main bronchus and goes up to the pericardium extending to the left main bronchus. The right main bronchus is retracted using a sponge, and the tissue is resected from the esophagus with an ultrasound dissector. Subcarinal lymph node resection at the left side starts with the incision of the mediastinal pleura along the aorta descendens. The aorta is retracted and dissection extends to the right main bronchus. The tissue will be grasped and with the dissection from pericardium and from the border of the left main bronchus resected.

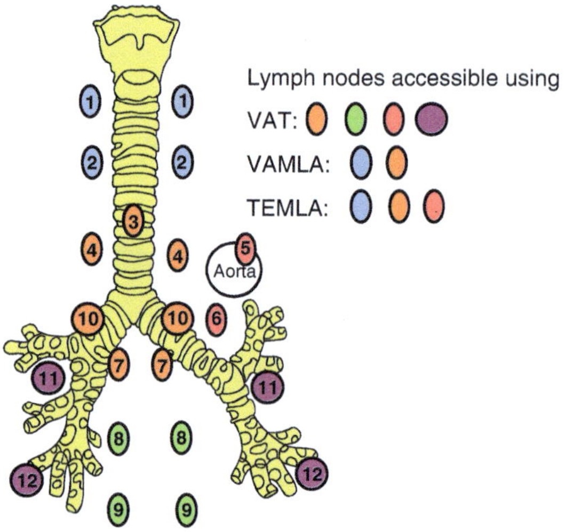

Fig. 23.6 Assessment of mediastinal lymph nodes by minimally invasive techniques in relation to the accessible lymph node stations: video-assisted thoracoscopy, video-assisted mediastinoscopic lymphadenectomy (*VAMLA*), transcervical extended mediastinal lymphadenectomy (*TEMLA*)

23.5 Discussion

The ideal strategy of the assessment of mediastinal lymph nodes is a topic of debate. Other approaches are the video-assisted mediastinoscopic lymphadenectomy (VAMLA) [7] and transcervical extended mediastinal lymphadenectomy (TEMLA) [8] (Fig. 23.6). Both techniques are useful as well for staging as for paratracheal and subcarinal lymphadenectomy. In cases suspected for N2 or hilar N1 disease, VAMLA has to be considered first for staging and in N-negative patients upper lymphadenectomy has to be done only. The disadvantage of both techniques is that an additional approach is necessary; the advantage is that a complete lymphadenectomy of N2 and N3 stages is possible. TEMLA needs a larger incision, and therefore, left-side aortopulmonary window could be reached as well as the hilar lymph nodes. Still, we do not have a common sense what form of lymphadenectomy is the gold standard, the complete ipsilateral lymphadenectomy, the extended lymphadenectomy, the lymph node sampling, or the resection of enlarged lymph nodes only. However, different groups could show that either thoracoscopically or mediastinoscopically all types of lymphadenectomy up to the extended versions are feasible. Purported advantages of complete lymphadenectomy (as compared with systematic sampling) include superior staging as well as improvement in local control and survival [5, 9]. There is evidence to support the concept that radical lymphadenectomy is performed just as effectively using the thoracoscopic approach. Several studies have been performed, comparing thoracoscopic dissection with conventional lymph node dissection [10–13]. Kondo and colleagues performed complete MLND during thoracoscopic lobectomy followed by thoracotomy. In this study, 27–48 lymph nodes were resected thoracoscopically, and subsequent thoracotomy yielded minimal extra lymph node tissue:

mean 1.3 and median zero lymph nodes. In the randomized study by Sugi and colleagues, there was no difference in the number of hilar or mediastinal lymph nodes resected using the open or thoracoscopic approaches [14]. Watanabe and colleagues demonstrated similar lymph node resection rates for the open and thoracoscopic approaches in a lobe-specific study [13].

References

1. Nohl HC (1956) An investigation into the lymphatic and vascular spread of carcinoma of the bronchus. Thorax 11:172–185
2. Cahan WG, Watson WL, Pool JL (1951) Radical pneumonectomy. J Thorac Surg 22:449–473
3. Trapnell DH (1963) The peripheral lymphatics of the lung. Br J Radiol 36:660–672
4. Friedel G, Steger V, Kyriss T et al (2004) Prognosis in N2 NSCLC. Lung Cancer 45(Suppl 2):45–53
5. Keller SM (2002) Complete mediastinal lymph node dissection – does it make a difference? Lung Cancer 36:7–8
6. Friedel G, Linder A, Pfeiffer S et al (1996) Radical lung surgery interventions with special reference to lymphadenectomy. Langenbecks Arch Chir Suppl Kongressbd 113:785–789
7. Hurtgen M, Friedel G, Toomes H et al (2002) Radical video-assisted mediastinoscopic lymphadenectomy (VAMLA)–technique and first results. Eur J Cardiothorac Surg 21:348–351
8. Zielinski M (2007) Transcervical extended mediastinal lymphadenectomy: results of staging in two hundred fifty-six patients with non-small cell lung cancer. J Thorac Oncol 2:370–372
9. Passlick B, Kubuschock B, Sienel W et al (2002) Mediastinal lymphadenectomy in non-small cell lung cancer: effectiveness in patients with or without nodal micrometastases – results of a preliminary study. Eur J Cardiothorac Surg 21:520–526
10. Naruke T, Tsuchiya R, Kondo H et al (1999) Lymph node sampling in lung cancer: how should it be done? Eur J Cardiothorac Surg 16(Suppl 1):S17–S24
11. Asamura H, Nakayama H, Kondo H et al (1999) Lobe-specific extent of systematic lymph node dissection for non-small cell lung carcinomas according to a retrospective study of metastasis and prognosis. J Thorac Cardiovasc Surg 117:1102–1111
12. Kondo T, Sagawa M, Tanita T et al (1998) Is complete systematic nodal dissection by thoracoscopic surgery possible? A prospective trial of video-assisted lobectomy for cancer of the right lung. J Thorac Cardiovasc Surg 116:651–652
13. Watanabe A, Koyanagi T, Ohsawa H et al (2005) Systematic node dissection by VATS is not inferior to that through an open thoracotomy: a comparative clinicopathologic retrospective study. Surgery 138:510–517
14. Sugi K, Kaneda Y, Esato K (2000) Video-assisted thoracoscopic lobectomy achieves a satisfactory long-term prognosis in patients with clinical stage IA lung cancer. World J Surg 24:27–30; discussion 30–1

Minimally Invasive Thymectomy: Introduction

24

Marcin Zieliński and Federico Rea

There are very few issues in thoracic surgery attracting so much interest as thymectomy for myasthenia gravis (MG). This is a rather unique phenomenon if one considers how rare the disease MG is and how few patients need thymectomy. The introduction of surgery for MG was made by Sauerbruch in 1908 and by Blalock in 1936; however, the modern principles of surgical treatment of MG have been established by several later authors, with Masaoka and Jaretzki being the most prominent. The main principle of thymectomy for MG is a complete removal of the whole thymic gland. A subtotal thymectomy is unacceptable and should not be performed. The necessity of removal of the ectopic thymic foci is a matter of controversy.

Generally, there are three types of thymectomies in regard to extensiveness of the procedure. Basic thymectomy includes removal of the thymus gland without any surrounding fatty tissue. Extended thymectomy includes removal of the thymus with the surrounding fatty tissue of the neck and the mediastinum. Maximally extended procedure introduced by Jaretzki includes removal of the thymus with the fatty tissue, from the level of the upper poles of the thyroid gland, down to the diaphragm, with a wide opening of both pleural cavities and radical en bloc exenteration of the anterior mediastinum with the overlying mediastinal pleural sheets; the laryngeal recurrent, vagus, and phrenic nerves are routinely visualized bilaterally. The aim of the extended and maximally extended thymectomies is a complete removal of the whole thymus and all ectopic thymic foci dispersed in the various areas of fatty tissue of the neck and mediastinum.

During the last two decades, there was a shift from standard approach, which was a more or less extended thymectomy performed through a median sternotomy to the less invasive procedures, mainly for the treatment of nonthymomatous MG. The minimally invasive techniques are those, which utilize operative approaches without sternotomy. These techniques include transcervical, videothoracoscopic (VATS), subxiphoid approaches, or combination of these approaches. The advantages of minimally invasive techniques include less pain in the early postoperative period, pulmonary function less compromised, better cosmetic result, and total avoidance of the risk of disruption or infection of the sternotomy wound. The inventors of most of these techniques usually tried to combine the minimally invasive operative approach with preservation of extensiveness of thymectomy.

Even in the largest textbook, it is not possible to describe all types of minimally invasive techniques of thymectomy. In this chapter, three examples of such less invasive procedures are

M. Zieliński, M.D., Ph.D. (✉)
Department of Thoracic Surgery, Pulmonary Hospital,
Ul. Gładkie 1, 34 500 Zakopane, Poland
e-mail: marcinz@mp.pl

F. Rea, M.D.
Division of Thoracic Surgery, University of Padua,
Via Giustiniani 2, 35128 Padua, Italy
e-mail: federico.rea@unipd.it

R.G.C. Inderbitzi et al. (eds.), *Minimally Invasive Thoracic and Cardiac Surgery*,
DOI 10.1007/978-3-642-11861-6_24, © Springer-Verlag Berlin Heidelberg 2012

presented, illustrating different strategy and different technology used by the authors for one of the "hottest" topics in thoracic surgery. The VATS thymectomy with use of the robot da Vinci describes a technique gaining increasing interest due to advantages of the modern robotic technology. The combining transcervical, subxiphoid, and VATS approach with double elevation of the sternum stands for maximally extended thymectomy using minimally invasive techniques. After all, complete thoracoscopic thymectomy indicates that the surgical procedure is carried out entirely by means of endoscopy (closed chest). Taken together, the presented techniques describe almost the whole spectrum of operative approaches and extensiveness of thymectomy available for contemporary thoracic surgeons.

Video-Assisted Thoracoscopic Thymectomy

25

Marcin Zieliński

Contents

25.1 Introduction

Over the period of the last two decades, minimally invasive thymectomy has gained increasing popularity in surgical treatment of myasthenia gravis (MG) [1–3]. The main reason for this phenomenon is an avoidance of sternotomy previously regarded the gold standard approach for thymectomy for MG. Minimally invasive techniques include transcervical thymectomies and videothoracoscopy-assisted (VATS) thymectomies, the last one being the topic of this chapter.

There are several kinds of VATS thymectomies listed in Table 25.1.

There have never been proved that late results of VATS thymectomies were better that transsternal thymectomies in regard to the complete remission rates of MG which is the generally regarded the most important criterion of the effectiveness on thymectomy [11]. There are, however, several advantages of VATS thymectomies in comparison to the transsternal approach which are listed in Table 25.2.

VATS techniques of thymectomy have been criticized for prolonged operative time, long "learning curve" including about 60 patients, inability of complete removal of the upper poles of the thymus, and the ectopic thymic foci found in 39.5–98% of MG patients in the perithymic fatty tissue of the neck and mediastinum [16, 17]. The importance of removal of these ectopic foci has been widely discussed, the same as the problem if the minimally invasive techniques of thymectomy are equally effective as the trans-

M. Zieliński, M.D., Ph.D.
Department of Thoracic Surgery, Pulmonary Hospital, Ul. Gładkie 1, 34 500 Zakopane, Poland
e-mail: marcinz@mp.pl

R.G.C. Inderbitzi et al. (eds.), *Minimally Invasive Thoracic and Cardiac Surgery*, DOI 10.1007/978-3-642-11861-6_25, © Springer-Verlag Berlin Heidelberg 2012

Table 25.1 Types of VATS thymectomies

Technique of thymectomy with the use of a videothoracoscope (VATS)	Author and publication
Unilateral right VATS	Yim et al. *Semin Thorac Cardiovasc Surg* 1999;11:65–73 [1]
Unilateral left VATS	Mineo et al. *Ann Thorac Surg* 2000;69:1537–41 [2]
Bilateral VATS	Roviaro et al. *Chest* 2001;117:1179–83 [3]
Bilateral VTS plus cervical incision	Novellino et al. *Int Surg* 1994;79:378–81 [4]
Bilateral VTS plus cervical and subxiphoid incision	Zielinski et al. *Ann Thorac Surg* 2004;78:404–9 [5]
Subxiphoid incision	Kido et al. *Ann Thorac Surg* 1999;67:263–5 [6]
Subxiphoid incision plus cervical incision	Uchiyama et al. *Ann Thorac Surg* 2001;72:1902–5 [7]
Subxiphoid incision plus bilateral VTS	Hsu et al. *Surg Endosc* 2002;16:1105 [8]
Robotic unilateral VTS	Rea et al. *Ann Thorac Surg* 2006;81:455–9 [9]
Transcervical extended approach with the use of a videothoracoscope inserted into the mediastinum through the neck incision	Cooper. *Chest Surg Clin N Am* 1998;8:827–33 [10]

Table 25.2 Advantages of VATS thymectomies in comparison to the transsternal approach

Advantage of VATS thymectomy	Author and publication
Less pain in the early postoperative period	Ruckert et al. *Ann Thorac Surg* 2000;70:1656–61 [12]
Pulmonary function less compromised	Ruckert et al. *Ann Thorac Surg* 2000;70:1656–61 [12]
Better cosmetic result	Yim et al. *Semin Thorac Cardiovasc Surg* 1999;11:65–73 [1]
Shorter time of hospital stay	Toker et al. *Interact Cardiovasc Thorac Surg* 2009; 9:995–8 [13]
The incidence of the chronic postoperative pain is also probably less frequent after VTS and 27% after sternotomy	Cooper. *Chest Surg Clin N Am* 1998;8:827–33 [10] Kalso et al. *Acta Anaesthesiol Scand* 2001;45:935–9 [14]
Risk of sternotomy wound disruption or infection is avoided	Machens et al. *Jpn J Surg* 1998;28:808–10 [15]

Table 25.3 Disadvantages of VATS thymectomies in comparison to the transsternal approach

Disadvantage of VATS thymectomy	Author and publication
Limited completeness of removal of the upper poles of the thymus with unilateral or bilateral VATS without additional cervical incision	Shigemura et al. *Surg Endosc* 2006;20(10):1614–8 [18]
Limited extent of removal of the adipose tissue of the mediastinum and lower neck containing ectopic foci of thymic tissue	Jaretzki. *Neurology* 1997;48(suppl 5):S52–63 [19] Zielinski et al. *Eur J Cardiothorac Surg* 2010;37:1137–43 [11]
Risk of chronic pain after thoracoscopy in 10–15% of patients	Cooper. *Chest Surg Clin N Am* 1998;8:827–33 [10]
Dissection tedious, technically demanding, may be time consuming	Hiratsuka et al. *Int Surg* 2006;91:44–51 [20]
Learning curve >60 patients	Toker et al. *Eur J Cardiothorac Surg* 2008;34:155–8 [21]
Unproven oncological value in thymomas; no reports >50 patients with >5 years follow-up	

sternal thymectomy [4]. Disadvantages of VATS thymectomies are listed in Table 25.3.

There have been also no larger prospective studies comparing the results of treatment of MG with different types of thymectomies. It must be mentioned, however, that the best results, with the highest complete remission rates reported in the literature, were achieved with use of the most extensive types of thymectomies.

The transcervical-subxiphoid-VATS maximal thymectomy, the technique introduced by the author of this chapter, will be presented in detail [5].

25.2 Operative Technique of the Transcervical-Subxiphoid-VATS Maximal Thymectomy

The patient is positioned supine on the operating table with a roll placed beneath the thoracic spine to elevate the chest and to hyperextend the patient's neck. Under general anesthesia, an endobronchial tube is inserted to conduct selective lung ventilation during the latter part of the procedure. To shorten the operative time and to facilitate performance of the procedure, an operation may be performed by two teams – one called the "cervical team" working from above and the second one called "the subxiphoid team" working from below the sternum with control of the videothoracoscope (VTS) (Figs. 25.1 and 25.2). Alternatively, the whole operation is performed by one surgical team performing "the cervical" and "the subxiphoid" parts of the operation sequentially.

All operative steps are described without specifying if one or two team is involved. In the cervical part of the operation, a transverse 5–8-cm incision is made in the neck above the sternal notch. The whole thyroid gland is visualized, and all foci of the adipose tissue are removed downward from the level of the upper poles of the thyroid gland. The parathyroid glands and both laryngeal recurrent nerves are visualized and carefully preserved (Figs. 25.3 and 25.4). The fatty tissue containing the superior poles of the thymus is separated from the lower poles of the thyroid gland with 1–4 inferior thyroid veins ligated and divided (Fig. 25.5). Alternatively, such devices as a harmonic knife, LigaSure (Valleylab), BiClamp (ERBE), or vascular clips can be used to secure the vessels throughout the procedure. The thymus with the surrounding fat is then separated from the sternohyoid and sternothyroid muscles, the trachea, the internal surface of the sternum, the carotid arteries, the innominate artery, the aorta, and the right innominate vein. At this point, a sternal retractor connected to the firm frame with a traction mechanism is inserted under the manubrium of the sternum to elevate it several centimeters to provide access to the anterior mediastinum. The lower thyroid

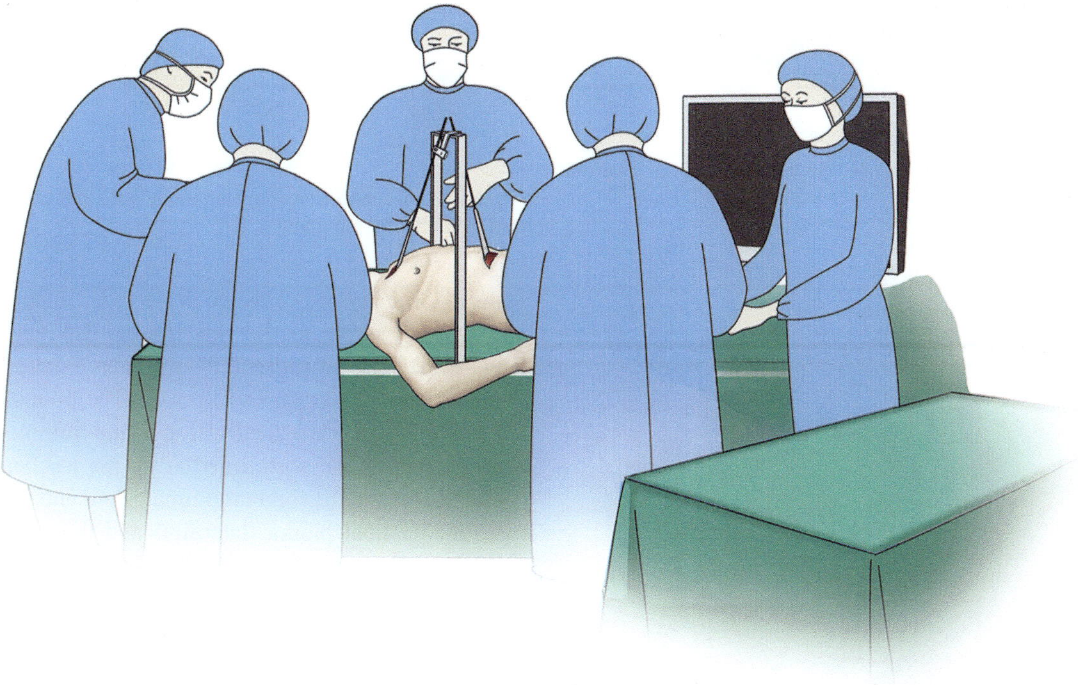

Fig. 25.1 Operating staff for the "two team approach"

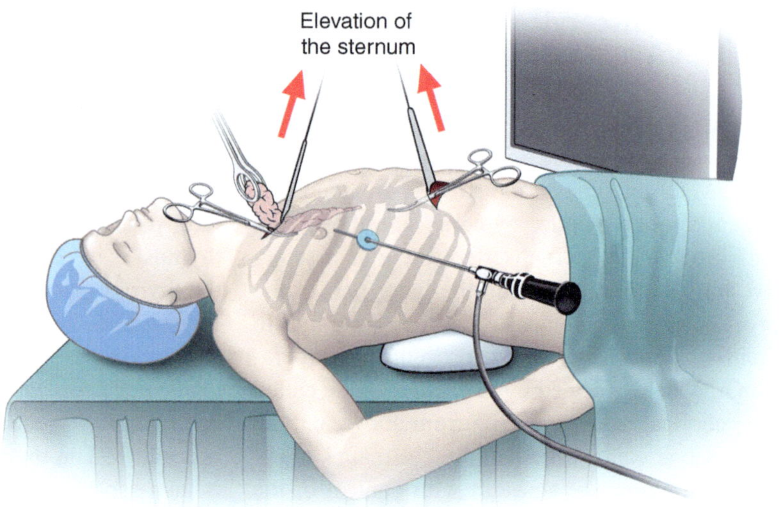

Fig. 25.2 Simultaneous dissection of the thymus performed by the "transcervical" and "subxiphoid" teams. *Arrows* indicate Elevation of the sternum

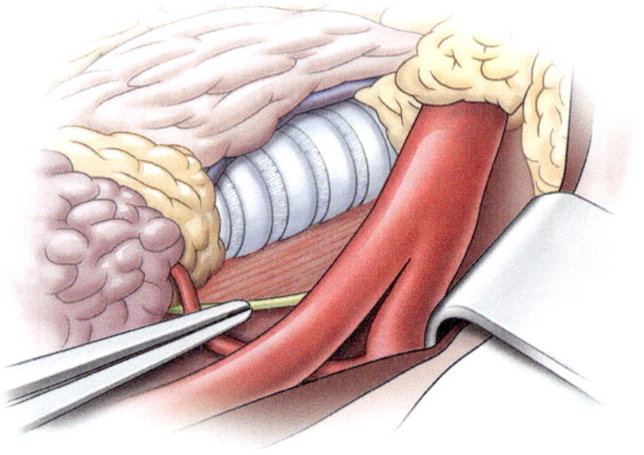

Fig. 25.3 Dissection of the right laryngeal recurrent nerve

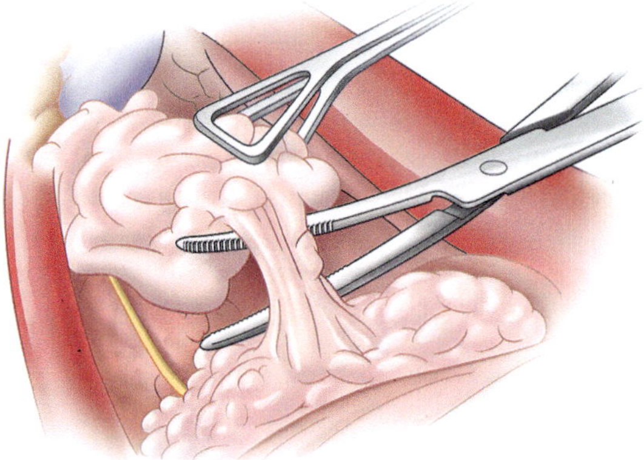

Fig. 25.5 Disconnection of the left upper pole of the thymus from the thyroid gland

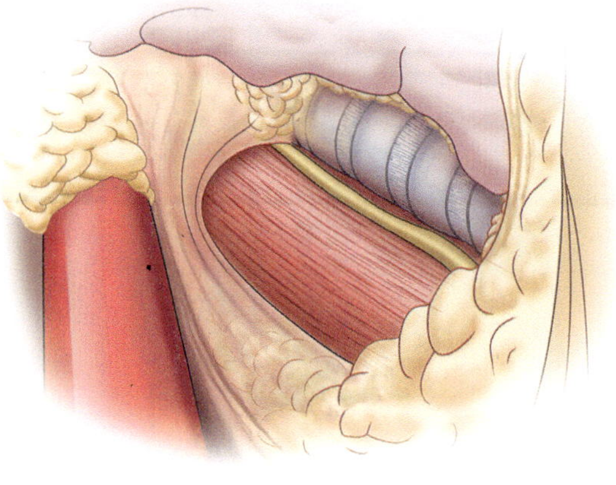

Fig. 25.4 Dissection of the left laryngeal recurrent nerve

veins and the thymic veins are dissected, clipped, and divided close to the left innominate vein (Fig. 25.6). The fatty tissue from the area called "the aorta-caval groove" is removed. The boundaries of this space are the division of the innominate artery and the aorta (medially), the trachea (posteriorly) and the right innominate vein and the right mediastinal pleura (laterally) and the right main bronchus, the azygos vein, and the superior vena cava (inferiorly) (Fig. 25.7). The dissection proceeds caudally, below the left innominate vein, and the specimen is separated from the pericardium at a distance of several centimeters. The most difficult but very important part of this

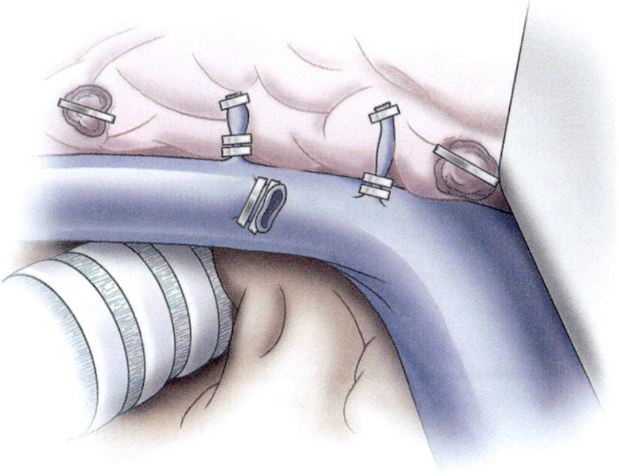

Fig. 25.6 Clipping and division of the inferior thyroid veins and the thymic veins

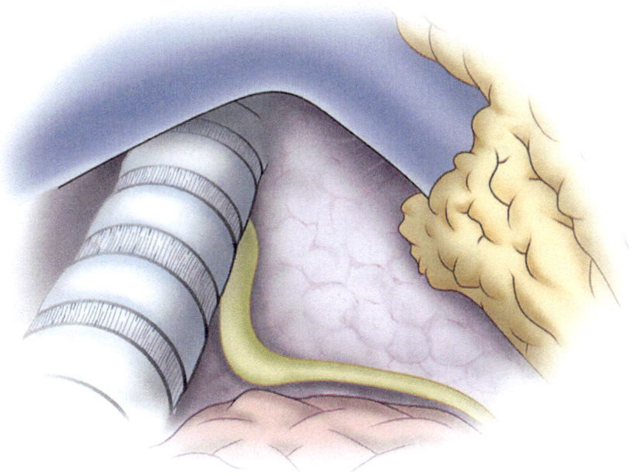

Fig. 25.7 View of the aorta-caval groove

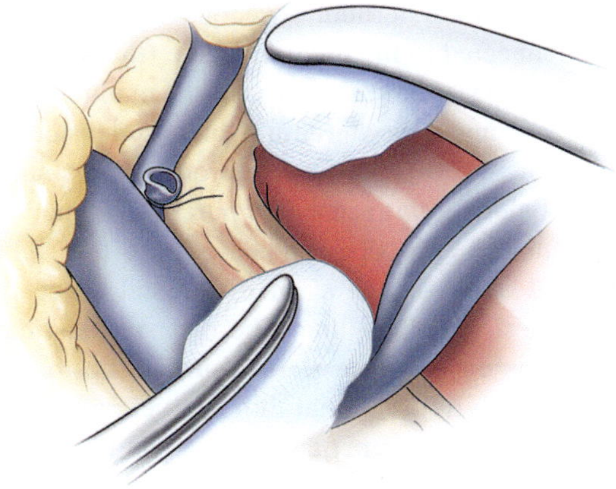

Fig. 25.8 Entrance to the aorta-pulmonary window

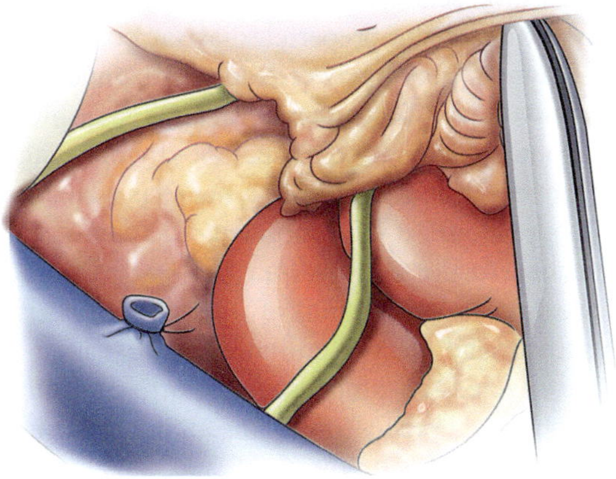

Fig. 25.9 View of the aorta-pulmonary window

operation is the dissection of the adipose tissue from the aorta-pulmonary window. Further dissection of two other branches of the left innominate vein, namely, the left internal thoracic vein and the accessory hemiazygos vein, is mandatory. These two veins are subsequently divided, and their ends are secured with clips or sutures (preferably). The division of these veins provides much better access to the aorta-pulmonary window above the left innominate vein which is retracted toward the aorta (Fig. 25.8). The next step is the visualization of the left phrenic nerve which runs very close to the left internal thoracic vein and the left vagus nerve which runs laterally to the left common carotid artery. With blunt dissection using a peanut sponge, the fatty tissue containing the aorta-pulmonary window is dissected from these nerves, the aorta, and the left mediastinal pleura. At the bottom of the aorta-pulmonary window, the left pulmonary artery is visualized (Fig. 25.9). In difficult cases, the dissection of the aorta-pulmonary window is completed at a later stage of the operation with a videothoracoscopic camera inserted inside the chest.

In the subxiphoid part of the operation, a transverse 4–6 cm-incision is made above the xiphoid process. The subcutaneous tissue is cut and the medial parts of the rectus muscles are cut near the insertions to the costal arches. The xiphoid process is divided transversely and left without removal. The selective left lung ventilation is started resulting in the collapse of the right lung. The anterior mediastinum is opened from below the sternum. A second sternal retractor connected to the traction frame (the same as one which is used for traction of the manubrium) is placed under the sternum, which is elevated to facilitate access to the anterior mediastinum from below. A thoracoscopic port for 5-mm, 30° oblique thoracoscope is inserted into the right pleural cavity in the sixth intercostal space in the anterior axillary line. The right mediastinal pleura is cut near the sternal surface up to the level of the right internal thoracic vein which is left intact. The prepericardial fat and right and left epiphrenic fat pads are dissected from the pericardium and diaphragm with blunt dissection using a peanut sponge and a sharp dissection using scissors or BiClamp (preferably). Dissection of the prepericardial fat containing the thymus gland proceeds upward under the control of the VTS camera with en bloc fashion, without any attempt to dissect the thymus gland separately. The right phrenic nerve is a margin of dissection. At this moment, the thymus is attached to the pericardium only with its left lower pole. Ventilation of the right lung is resumed, and the ventilation of the left lung is disconnected. A thoracoscopic port for 5-mm, 30° oblique thoracoscope is inserted into the left pleural cavity, as on the right side. The operating table is rotated on the right side with elevation of the left side which lowers the mediastinum, improving access to the left pleural cavity. Under the control of the VTS camera, the left mediastinal pleura is divided along the sternum and the left prepericardial fat is dissected from the pericardium above the level of the left internal thoracic vein previously divided. The left lower pole of the thymus is separated from the pericardium, and the specimen is removed. Dissection of the aorta-pulmonary window is completed, if necessary, at this stage of the operation. Hemostasis is checked, the VTS ports are removed, and the chest tubes are inserted into both pleural cavities through the incisions made for insertion of the ports. Ventilation of both lungs is resumed. The cervical and subxiphoid incisions are closed in the standard manner. Generally, a patient is extubated immediately after the operation.

References

1. Yim A, Kay R, Izaat M, Ng S (1999) Video-assisted thoracoscopic thymectomy for myasthenia gravis. Semin Thorac Cardiovasc Surg 11:65–73
2. Mineo T, Pompeo E, Lerut T, Bernardi G, Coosemans W, Nofroni I (2000) Thoracoscopic thymectomy in autoimmune myasthenia: results of left-sided approach. Ann Thorac Surg 69:1537–1541
3. Roviaro G, Varoli F, Nucca O, Vergani C, Maciocco M (2001) Videothoracoscopic approach to primary mediastinal pathology. Chest 117:1179–1183
4. Novellino L, Longoni M, Spinelli L, Andretta M, Cozzi M, Faillace G, Vitellaro M, De Benedetti D, Pezzuoli G (1994) "Extended" thymectomy, without sternotomy performed by cervicotomy and thoracoscopic technique in the treatment of myasthenia gravis. Int Surg 79:378–381
5. Zielinski M, Kuzdzal J, Szlubowski A, Soja J (2004) Transcervical-subxiphoid-videothoracoscopic "maximal" thymectomy—operative technique and early results. Ann Thorac Surg 78:404–409
6. Kido T, Hazama K, Inoue Y, Tanaka Y, Takao T (1999) Resection of anterior mediastinal masses through an infrasternal approach. Ann Thorac Surg 67:263–265
7. Uchiyama A, Shimizu S, Murai H, Kuroki S, Okido M, Tanaka M (2001) Infrasternal mediastinoscopic thymectomy in myasthenia gravis: surgical results in 23 patients. Ann Thorac Surg 72:1902–1905
8. Hsu C (2002) Subxiphoid approach for thoracoscopic thymectomy. Surg Endosc 16:1105
9. Rea F, Marulli G, Bortolotti L, Feltracco P, Zuin A, Sartori F (2006) Experience with the "da Vinci" robotic system for thymectomy in patients with myasthenia gravis: report of 33 cases. Ann Thorac Surg 81: 455–459
10. Cooper J (1998) Video-assisted thoracic surgery for myasthenia gravis: commentary. Chest Surg Clin N Am 8:827–833
11. Zieli ski M, Hauer L, Hauer J, Pankowski J, Nabiałek T, Szlubowski A (2010) Comparison of complete remission rates after 5-years follow-up of three different techniques of thymectomy for myasthenia gravis. Eur J Cardiothorac Surg 37:1137–1143
12. Ruckert J, Walter M, Muller J (2000) Pulmonary function after thoracoscopic thymectomy versus median sternotomy for myasthenia gravis. Ann Thorac Surg 70:1656–1661
13. Toker A, Tanju S, Ziyade S, Ozkan B, Sungur Z, Parman Y, Serdaroglu P, Deymeer F (2009) Early outcomes of video-assisted thoracoscopic resection of thymus in 181 patients with myasthenia gravis: who are the candidates for the next morning discharge? Interact Cardiovasc Thorac Surg 9:995–998
14. Kalso E, Mennander S, Tasmuth T, Nilsson E (2001) Chronic post-sternotomy pain. Acta Anaesthesiol Scand 45:935–939
15. Machens A, Emskotter T, Busch C, Izbicki J (1998) Postoperative infection after transsternal thymectomy

for myasthenia gravis: a retrospective analysis of 125 patients. Jpn J Surg 28:808–810
16. Ashour M (1995) Prevalence of ectopic thymic tissue in myasthenia gravis and its clinical significance. J Thorac Cardiovasc Surg 109:632–635
17. Jaretzki A, Wolff M (1988) "Maximal" thymectomy for myasthenia gravis. Surgical anatomy and operative technique. J Thorac Cardiovasc Surg 96:711–716
18. Shigemura N, Shiono H, Inoue M, Minami M, Ohta M, Okumura M, Matsuda H (2006) Inclusion of the transcervical approach in video-assisted thoracoscopic extended thymectomy (VATET) for myasthenia gravis: a prospective trial. Surg Endosc 20(10):1614–1618
19. Jaretzki A (1997) Thymectomy for myasthenia gravis: analysis of the controversies regarding technique and results. Neurology 48(suppl 5):S52–S63
20. Hiratsuka M, Iwasaki A, Shirakusa T, Yoneda S, Yamamoto S, Shiraishi T, Tsuboi Y (2006) Role of video-assisted thoracic surgery for the treatment of myasthenia gravis: extended thymectomy by median sternotomy versus the thoracoscopic approach with sternal lifting. Int Surg 91:44–51
21. Toker A, Tanju S, Ziyade S, Kaya S, Dilege S (2008) Learning curve in videothoracoscopic thymectomy: how many operations and in which situations? Eur J Cardiothorac Surg 34:155–158

Robotic Thymectomy

26

Federico Rea and Giuseppe Marulli

Contents

F. Rea, M.D. (✉) • G. Marulli, M.D.
Division of Thoracic Surgery, Department
of Cardiologic, Thoracic and Vascular Sciences,
University Hospital of Padua, Via Giustiniani 2,
35128 Padua, Italy
e-mail: federico.rea@unipd.it;
giuseppe.marulli@unipd.it

26.1 Introduction

Since our first experience [1] on a robotic thymectomy in a patient with myasthenia gravis, we adopted this technique in more than 100 cases including patients affected by non-thymomatous myasthenia gravis and, recently, patients with early stage thymoma.

26.1.1 Operative Technique

The patient is under general anaesthesia and has a double-lumen endotracheal tube for selective single lung ventilation during the time of operation. The technique here described is a left-sided robot-aided thoracoscopic approach; we prefer the left-sided approach as it offers a perfect visualization of the aortic window, where often residual thymus can be reached, and it reduces the probability of phrenic nerves injury, with a direct vision of the left phrenic nerve, while the right phrenic nerve is partially protected by the superior vena cava.

26.1.1.1 Patient Position

In the surgical room, the patient is positioned supine with the left side up, 30° upon a bean bag. The right arm is along the body, and the left arm is positioned on a support parallel to the bed; in this way, the axillary region is easily exposed (Fig. 26.1).

R.G.C. Inderbitzi et al. (eds.), *Minimally Invasive Thoracic and Cardiac Surgery*,
DOI 10.1007/978-3-642-11861-6_26, © Springer-Verlag Berlin Heidelberg 2012

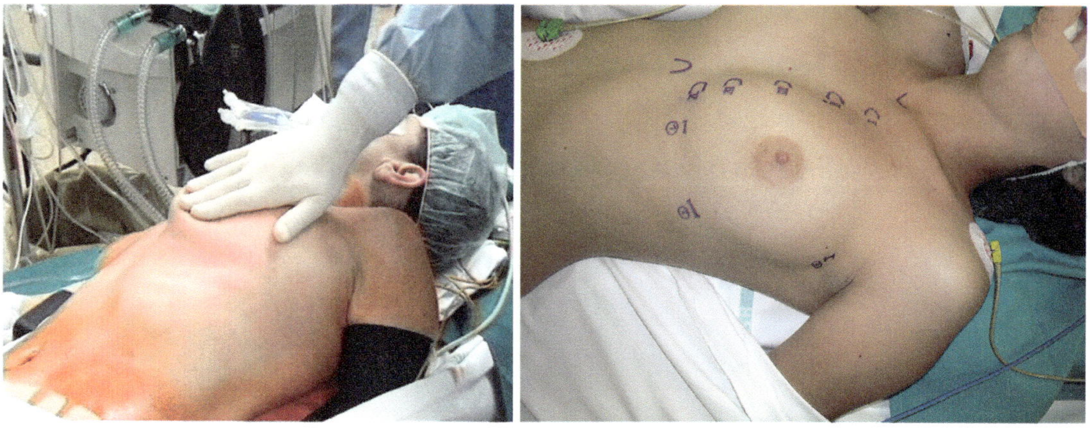

Fig. 26.1 Patient position

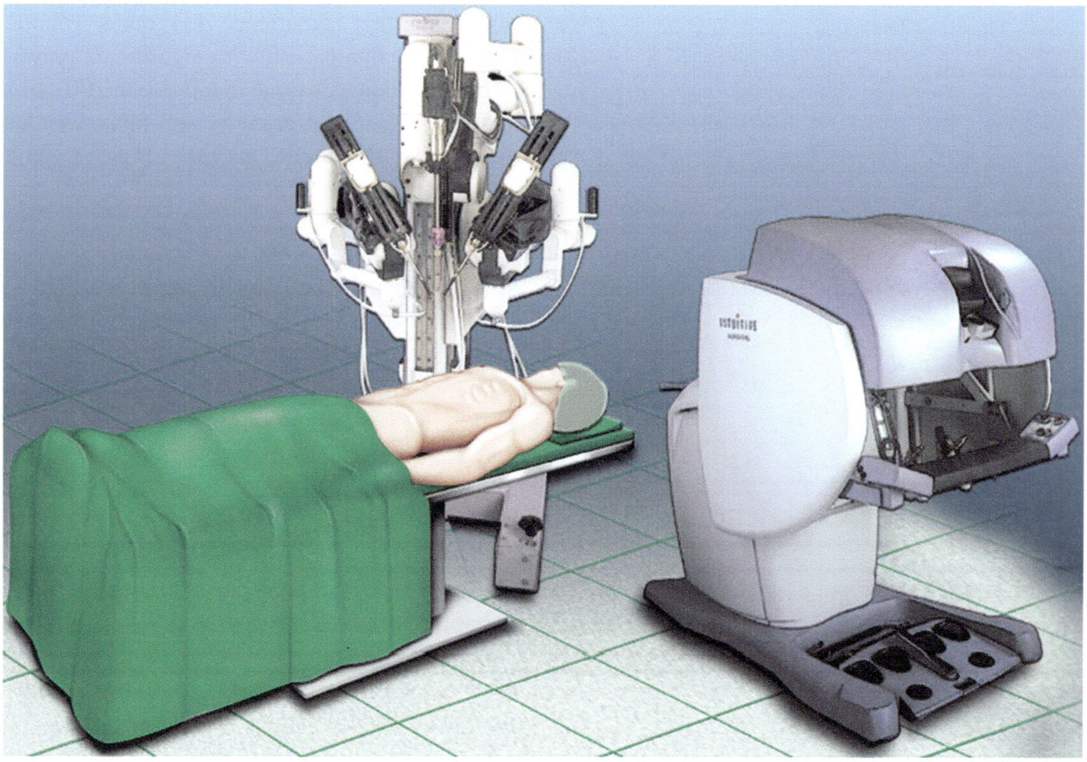

Fig. 26.2 Robotic alignment in relation to patient's position

26.1.1.2 Robot

The surgeon's console is far from the patient in the operating room, and the video tower is at the bottom of the bed. The patient-side cart is positioned on the right of the bed angled of 45° with the longitudinal axis of the patient (Fig. 26.2).

The arms of "da Vinci" surgical system are placed as follows: the 0° camera port for the 3-D videoendoscope is introduced through a 12-mm incision in fifth intercostal space in the anterior axillary line; two additional thoracic ports are inserted through two 5-mm incisions: one in fifth

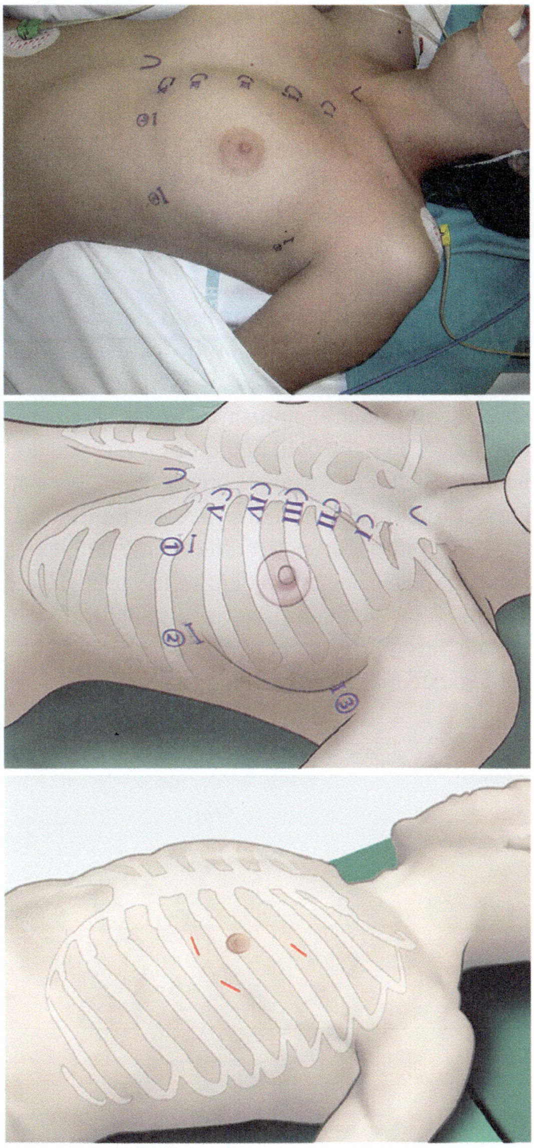

Fig. 26.3 Incisions in relation to ribs and axes of body

intercostal space between the midclavicular line and the parasternal line and another in the third intercostal space on the anterior axillary line (Fig. 26.3).

The arms of the da Vinci system are then attached to the two ports, and another arm is attached to the port-inserted endoscope (Fig. 26.4). The left arm is equipped with an EndoWrist that works by grasping the thymus and the perithymic fat tissue during dissection; the right arm is equipped with an Endo-Dissector device with electric cautery function to perform the dissection (Fig. 26.5). A careful positioning of the ports and the robotic arms with an adequate distance between the accesses is of paramount importance to avoid conflict between arms and instruments outside and inside the chest cavity (Fig. 26.4).

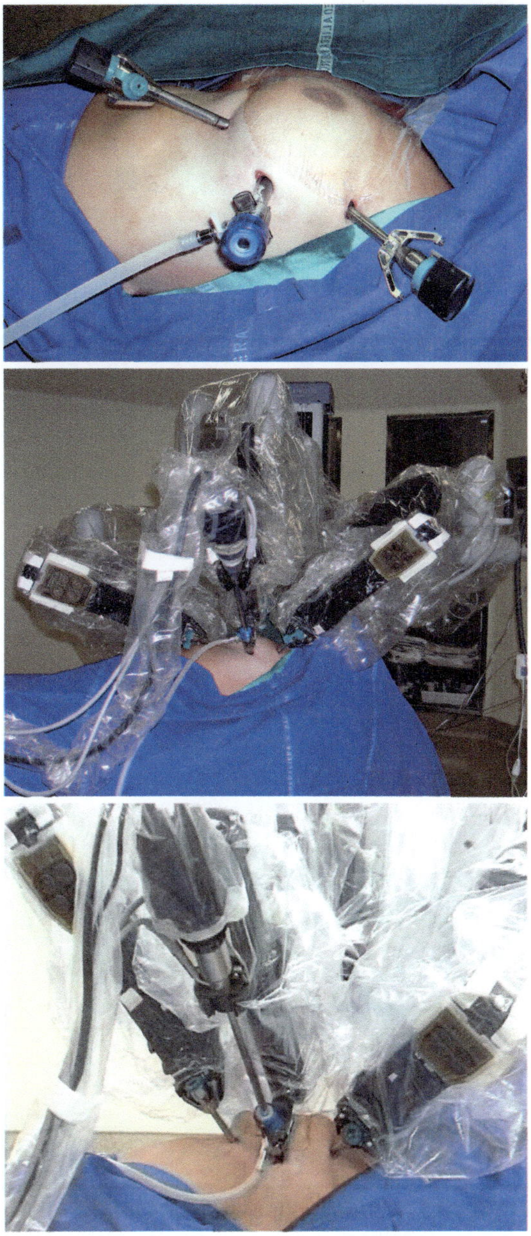

Fig. 26.4 Positioning of the arms of da Vinci

During operation, a continuous inflation of CO_2 maintaining an endocavitary pressure ranging from 8–12 mmHg is delivered in the left hemithorax through a dedicated connection system in the camera port. The CO_2 inflation enlarges the mediastinal space, making easier the dissection, thanks to the wide and clear view within the chest. During CO_2 inflation, a careful attention must be paid by the anaesthesiologist at the possible complication related to this procedure (e.g. hypotension, hypercarbia, contralateral increased ventilatory pressure after opening of the right mediastinal pleura).

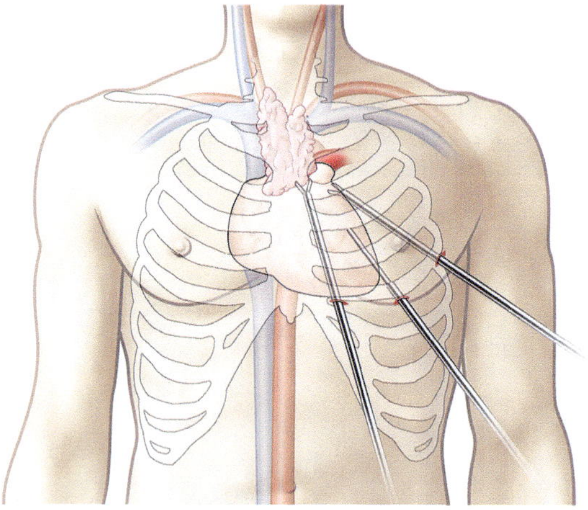

Fig. 26.5 Placement of instruments

26.1.1.3 Surgical Technique

First, a careful exploration of the mediastinal left pleural space is performed to exclude the presence of any pleural implants in case of thymic tumours. Then, the field of the surgical dissection is individuated in a triangle area with the basis at the bottom of pericardium where the fat tissue of the left and right pericardiophrenic angles is localized. The lateral borders of the triangle are delimited by the mammary vessels anteriorly and by the left phrenic nerve posteriorly, with the apex located in the neck (Fig. 26.6).

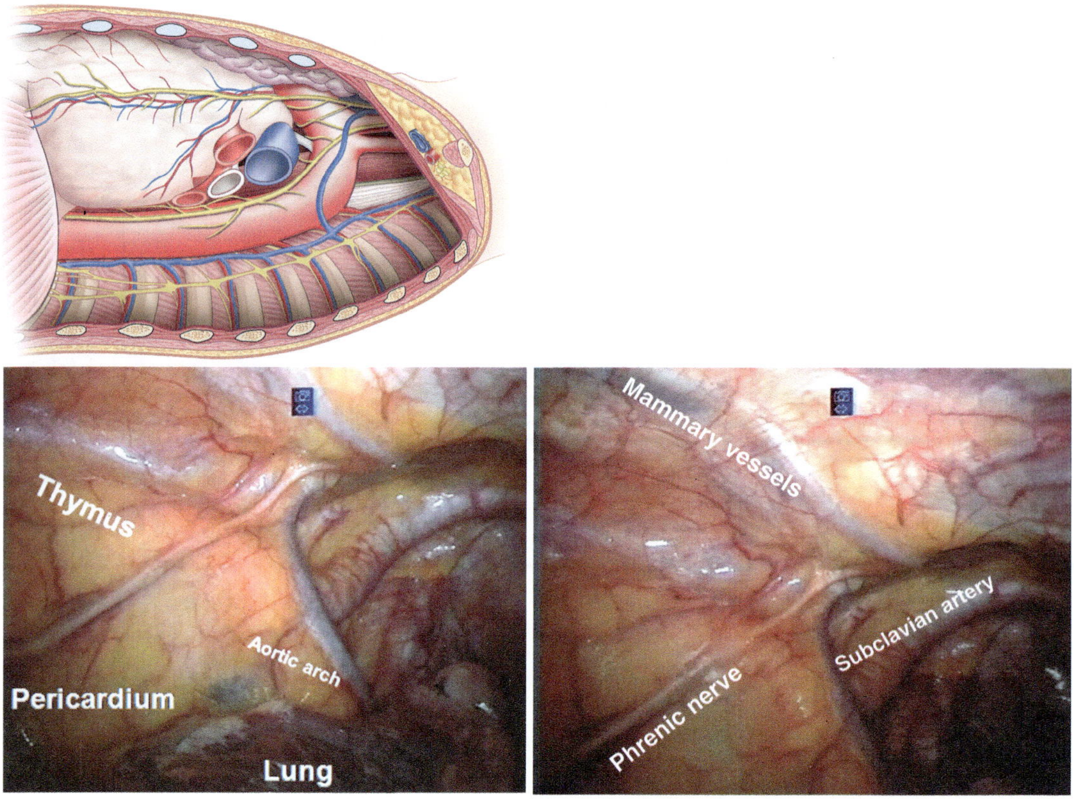

Fig. 26.6 Anatomical landmarks: mammary vessels and phrenic nerve

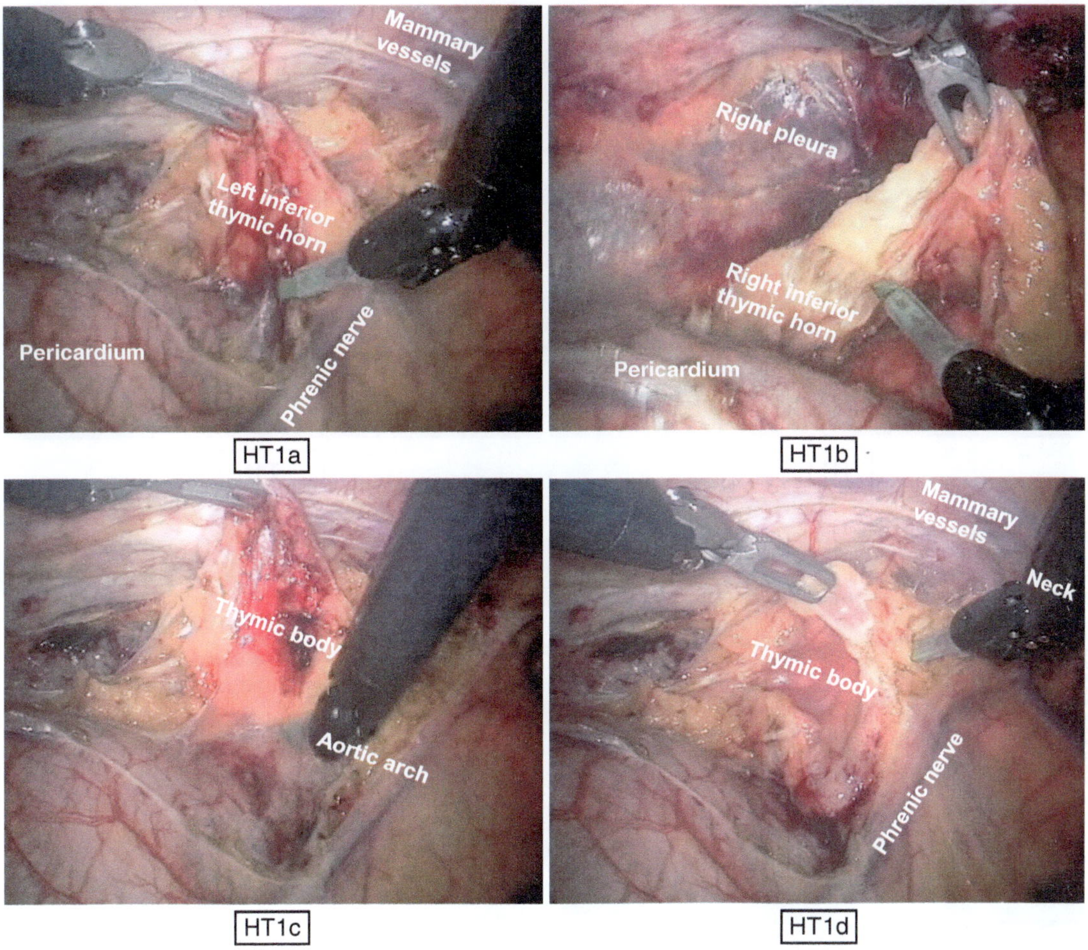

Fig. 26.7 (HT1 **a–d**) Surgical techniques

The dissection starts inferiorly from the fat tissue of the left pericardiophrenic angle and follows the pericardial plane where the left inferior horn and the body of the thymic gland are located (Fig. 26.7 HT1a). On the right side, the dissection involves the retrosternal area starting medially to the left mammary vessels with the visualization of the right mediastinal pleura that may be opened; the retrosternal fat tissue en bloc with the right inferior horn of the thymus is therefore isolated and dissected (Fig. 26.7 HT1b). At this point, the lower part of the thymus is mobilized upwards, and the thymic tissue is dissected from the plane of the pericardium (Fig. 26.7 HT1c).

At the top of the mediastinum, the pleura is incised in the area delimited by the mammary vessels in the anterior limit and by the phrenic nerve in the posterior limit (Fig. 26.7 HT1d).

The isolation proceeds up to into the neck until the superior horns with their fatty tissue are identified and divided from the inferior portion of the thyroid gland by a blunt dissection (Fig. 26.8 HT1e).

Grasping and pulling the superior horns below, the innominate vein is then identified and dissected along its border up to the point where the thymic veins are identified, clipped and divided (Fig. 26.8 HT1f).

The operation ends with the dissection of the tissue laterally and under the left phrenic nerve: by pulling up the nerve with the EndoWrist, paying attention to avoid any nervous damaging, the

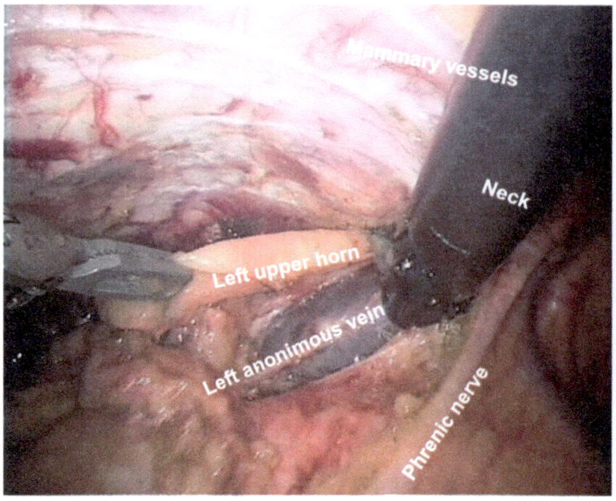

HT1e

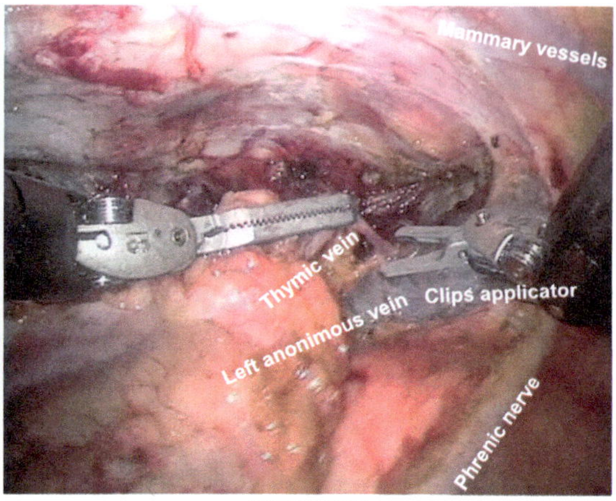

HT1f

Fig. 26.8 (HT1 **e–f**) Surgical techniques

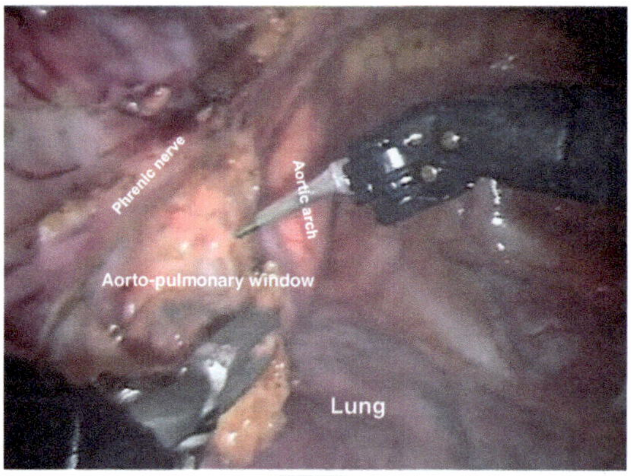

HT2

Fig. 26.9 HT2 Operation field after removing of thymic gland

aorto-pulmonary window area is dissected and cleared up from fatty tissue (Fig. 26.9 HT2). The thymus gland, the mediastinal and the neck's fatty tissue are then radically resected. The specimen is placed in an Endobag so it can be removed by the incision on the fifth intercostal space after removing the left robotic arm and extending the incision up to 15 mm. After the haemostasis, a 28-F drainage tube is inserted through the wound of the fifth intercostal space, the lung is reinflated, and the other wounds are sutured.

The patient is extubated in the operating room and, subsequent to an adequate period of observation, returns to the floor of surgical thoracic ward.

The chest drainage tube is removed 24 h after surgery, and the patient is discharged 48–72 h after surgery.

26.2 Results

Thymectomy may be effectively and safely performed by robotic approach. The surgical technique is sound, but despite no doubt exists on feasibility, the clinical results both on treatment of myasthenia gravis and early stage thymoma need to be confirmed by a long-term follow-up. In Table 26.1, the most important published series on this topic are reported: the morbidity and conversion rate is very low, such as the hospital stay. The operative time is comparable with standard thoracoscopy, but longer than transsternal approach. No randomized studies are available for comparison of different approaches. Most of authors have extended the indication for thymectomy not only to the removal of benign thymus in patients with myasthenia gravis but also to early stage thymoma.

Regarding the most common techniques for thymectomy, the *transsternal approach* is the most popular used surgical approach [9]. The main advantages are: an optimal exposition and

Table 26.1 Recent experiences on robotic thymectomy

Author	Approach	N° patients	Thymoma (%)	Major morbidity (%)	Mean operative time (min)	Conversion rate (%)	Hospital stay (days)
Ruckert et al. [2]	Left-sided	95	12.6	2	186	1	NA
Augustin et al. [3]	Right-sided	32	28.1	6.2	127	3	6
Castle and Kernstine [4]	Right-sided	26	3.8	7.7	90	3.8	1.6
Fleck et al. [5]	Left-sided	18	33.3	12	175	5.5	4
Goldstein and Yang [6]	Right-sided	26	19.2	15.4	127	15.4	NA
Marulli et al. [7]	Left-sided	83	7.2	3.6	120	0	3
Freeman et al. [8]	Left-sided	75	0	4	113	0	2.2

dissection of the thymus and perithymic fat tissue and lower risks of vascular and nervous injuries. Some disadvantages include invasiveness of the approach and a longer hospitalization. The *transcervical thymectomy*, popularized by Cooper [10], is a minimally invasive technique that is easily accepted by young patients and neurologists. The advantages are a short hospitalization, fewer complications and lower costs. The main criticism to this approach related to the small space of access that determines crowding of instruments, thus making surgical manoeuvres difficult, making it impossible to perform a thymectomy that extends to the perithymic fat tissue. *VATS thymectomy* through the left- [11] or right-sided [12] approach is a minimally invasive technique that permits a good visualization of the anterior mediastinum, achieving an extended thymectomy. Disadvantages are the two-dimensional view of the operative field and the limited manoeuvrability of endoscopic instruments. The *robotic approach* combines the advantages of minimally invasive techniques (fewer complications, minimal thoracic trauma, decreased postoperative pain, early improved pulmonary function, shorter recovery period and optimal cosmetic results) and the specific advantages as an intuitive three-dimensional vision, a scale motion with tremor filtering and the EndoWrists with articulated movements permitting a full 7° of freedom. These characteristics allow an accurate dissection, easier than classic VATS, particularly in remote, fixed and difficult to reach areas of the neck and contralateral mediastinum where the dissection is more difficult allowing a safe and comfortable dissection of vascular and nervous structures. We prefer the left-sided approach as it offers a perfect visualization of the aortic window and reduces the probability of phrenic nerves injury, with a direct vision of the left phrenic nerve, while the right phrenic nerve is partially protected by the superior vena cava. Disadvantages of this approach include the initial high cost of the robotic system that may be easily recovered if the robotic instrumentation is used in several different surgical specialties, as in our hospital. Another disadvantage of robotic surgery is its current lack of tactile feedback, but this is compensated by the superior image of the three-dimensional camera. The learning curve associated with robotic technology could be considered a disadvantage, but learning curves are part of any new technology and, in our experience, determined only an initial increased operative time.

References

1. Rea F, Bortolotti L, Girardi R, Sartori F (2003) Thoracoscopic thymectomy with the Da Vinci surgical system in patient with myasthenia gravis. Interact Cardiovasc Thorac Surg 2:70–72
2. Rückert JC, Ismail M, Swierzy M, Sobel H, Rogalla P, Meisel A, Wernecke KD, Rückert RI, Müller JM (2008) Thoracoscopic thymectomy with the da Vinci robotic system for myasthenia gravis. Ann N Y Acad Sci 1132:329–335
3. Augustin F, Schmid T, Sieb M, Lucciarini P, Bodner J (2008) Video-assisted thoracoscopic surgery versus robotic-assisted thoracoscopic surgery thymectomy. Ann Thorac Surg 85:S768–S771
4. Castle SL, Kernstine KH (2008) Robotic-assisted thymectomy. Semin Thorac Cardiovasc Surg 20:326–331
5. Fleck T, Fleck M, Müller M, Hager H, Klepetko W, Wolner E, Wisser W (2009) Extended videoscopic

robotic thymectomy with the da Vinci telemanipulator for the treatment of myasthenia gravis: the Vienna experience. Interact Cardiovasc Thorac Surg 9:784–787
6. Goldstein SD, Yang SC (2010) Assessment of robotic thymectomy using the myasthenia gravis foundation of America guidelines. Ann Thorac Surg 89:1080–1085
7. Marulli G, Schiavon M, Perissinotto E, Zuin A, Di Chiara F, Rebusso A, Battistella L, Rea F (2010) Safety and long-term efficacy of left thoracoscopic robot enhanced thymectomy in patients with myasthenia gravis. Interact Cardiovasc Thorac Surg 11(S1):S49
8. Freeman RK, Ascioti AJ, Van Woerkom JM, Vyverberg A, Robison RJ (2011) Long-term follow-up after robotic thymectomy for nonthymomatous myasthenia gravis. Ann Thorac Surg 92:1018–1022
9. Masaoka A, Yamakawa Y, Niwa H, Fukai I, Kondo S, Kobayashi M, Fujii Y, Monden Y (1996) Extended thymectomy for myasthenia gravis: a 20-year review. Ann Thorac Surg 62:853–859
10. Cooper JD, Al-Jilaihawa AN, Pearson FG, Humphrey JG, Humphrey HE (1988) An improved technique to facilitate transcervical thymectomy for myasthenia gravis. Ann Thorac Surg 45:242–247
11. Mineo TC, Pompeo E, Lerut T, Bernardi G, Coosemans W, Nofroni I (2000) Thoracoscopic thymectomy in autoimmune myasthenia: results of left-sided approach. Ann Thorac Surg 69:1537–1541
12. Mack M, Landreneau R, Yim A, Halzelrigg S, Scruggs G (1996) Results of video-assisted thymectomy in patients with myasthenia gravis. J Thorac Cardiovasc Surg 112:1352–1360

27 Complete Thoracoscopic Thymectomy (cT-Thymectomy)

Rolf G.C. Inderbitzi and Ralph Alexander Schmid

Contents

R.G.C. Inderbitzi, M.D.
Thoraxzentrum Zurich, Hirslanden Clinic,
Witellikerstrasse 40,
CH-8008 Zurich, Switzerland
e-mail: r.inderbitzi@thoraxzentrum.ch

R.A. Schmid, M.D.
Division of General Thoracic Surgery,
University Hospital Berne, Freiburgstrasse,
3010 Berne, Switzerland
e-mail: ralph.schmid@insel.ch

27.1 Introduction

Complete thoracoscopic thymectomy ("cT-Thymectomy") indicates that the operative procedure is completely carried out thoracoscopically claiming comparable results to the open, radical procedures: transsternal extended thymectomy (T-3 according to 3) and transcervical and transsternal thymectomy (T-4 according to 3). cT-Thymectomy is frequently applied. It takes a mid-position between the above depicted "transcervical-subxiphoid-VATS maximal thymectomy" and the "robotic thymectomy". Technically it is less extensive and less expensive than the robotic-assisted resection. Surgically it is less invasive than the VATS resection, but probably less radical than both other techniques.

Over the past two decades, thymectomy has been increasingly carried out thoracoscopically in different techniques [3–5]. Essentially "total thymectomy" is considered the goal of surgery. Standards for the surgical resection in myasthenic patients have been established already in 1997 [1].

In the early years of VATS, an additional cervical incision was routinely performed to remove the upper cervical thymic lobes and the pretracheal fat [6]. In the recent years, the cervical extensions of the thymus are removed from the thoracoscopic approach through the chest [4, 7]. This technique employs a unilateral videoscopic exposure of the mediastinum, from the right or from the left side, with removal of the endoscopic identifiable thymus and radical excision of the anterior mediastinal fat.

R.G.C. Inderbitzi et al. (eds.), *Minimally Invasive Thoracic and Cardiac Surgery*,
DOI 10.1007/978-3-642-11861-6_27, © Springer-Verlag Berlin Heidelberg 2012

Regardless of the different operative techniques, the relationship between the extent of the thymectomy and the rate of complete remission or clinical improvement remains unclear. Hence, the surgeon should clearly describe his operation in as objective terms as possible [2].

27.2 Surgical Technique

The patient lies in the supine position with the thorax disinfected and draped on both sides. The neck is also kept sterile within the field of operation (Fig. 27.1). One-lung ventilation is established on the right side, and the three incisions are placed in a V shape in a sufficient distance from each other (Fig. 27.2). We use a 10-mm 25° lens. Ultrasound scalpels such as the Ultracision® or Harmonic scalpel® are very effective and safe for the dissection alongside the nerves. The surgeon stands on the left side, turned towards the thorax. For the stages of dissection in the upper mediastinum and neck, the assistant holding the camera stands on the left of the surgeon or alternately on the opposite side of the patient. If the thoracoscope and the instruments are directed towards the inferior part of the anterior mediastinum, the assistant moves to the surgeon's right side.

The operation starts with the distal dissection of the mediastinal tissue, approximately 1 cm

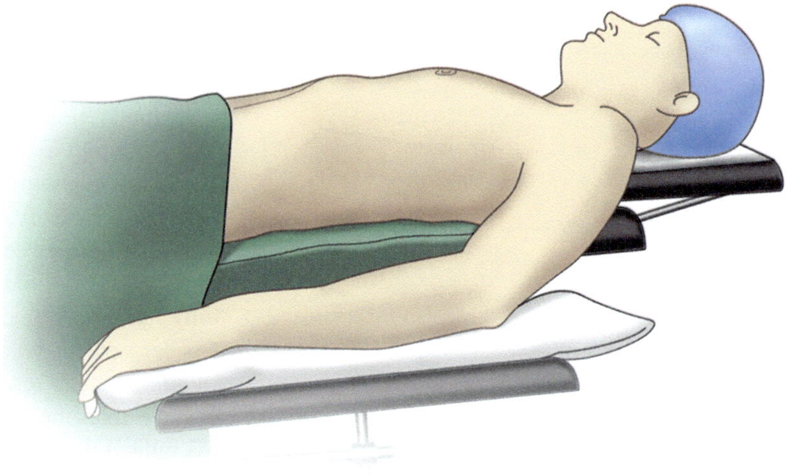

Fig. 27.1 Position on the operating table

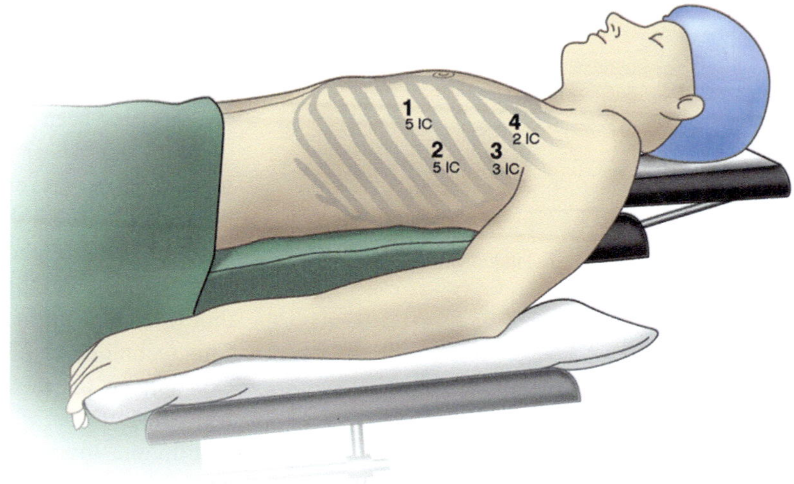

Fig. 27.2 Mini-incisions. Incisions *1* and *3* are used for the instruments and incision *2* for the thoracoscope. Incisions 1 and 2 accept trocar sleeves with a diameter of 10.5 mm, incision 3 a diameter of 7 mm. Depending on the build of the patient, incision *4* may be helpful (7 mm)

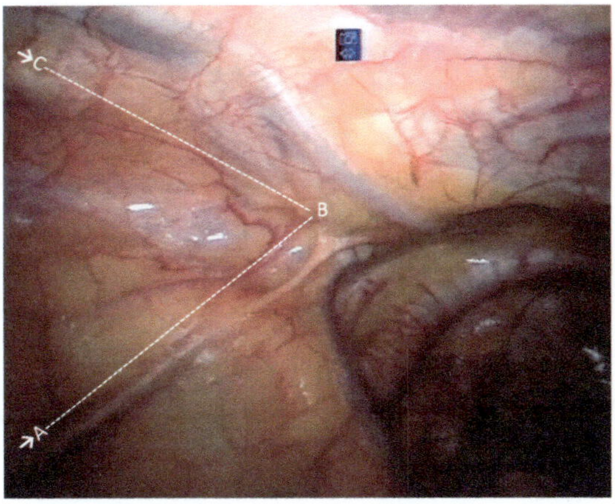

Fig. 27.3 Operation stages *line A–B* followed the phrenic nerve, *line B–C* the mammary vessels (Illustration by Prof. Federico Rea)

anterior to the phrenic nerve (Fig. 27.3, Step A–B). It is essential that the mediastinal tissue is initially dissected around the pericardium, the anterior semi-circumference of the aorta and at the inferior margin of the innominate vein. When the mediastinal tissue retrosternally is dissected in a first step, this tissue will hang like a curtain to the left side, hindering the safe dissection along the phrenic nerve (A–B). The distal mediastinal incision is then extended from caudal to a cranial direction as much as possible to the right side.

In the second step, the mediastinum is opened retrosternally along the mammary artery (Fig. 27.3, Step B–C). The dissection is then performed also distally to cranially as much as possible on the opposite pleural side on the right. Proximal to the level of the origin of the aorta, strict attention must be paid to the anterior wall of the superior vena cava. This structure serves as the guide to lead to the confluence of the brachiocephalic trunk and the innominate vein. Near the confluence, usually a little vein appears in the fat tissue, which has to be clipped.

In the third stage of the operation, the anterior wall of the innominate vein is cautiously visualised over to the confluence with the superior vena cava. An additional incision (4 in Fig. 27.2) may be helpful to lift the vein. The thymic veins, usually two, are dissected from the left to the right and are divided between clips.

When the stages 1–3 of the operation are completed, the whole anterior mediastinal tissue containing the thymus gland hangs at the cranial end of the mediastinum or the entrance to the neck. In the final step, the cervical dissection is performed under gentle tension to free the common bilateral cervical mediastinal body as well as the cervical lobes of the thymus and the adjacent cervical fat which may contain ectopic thymic tissue.

The whole mediastinal tissue is now removed en bloc with the aid of a specimen pouch through incision 1 (Fig. 27.2).

If the right side of the pleura has been opened during the dissection, it is drained by means of the transmediastinal insertion of a thoracic drain into the right thoracic space. A second tube is placed to drain the left side.

References

1. Gronseth GS, Barohn RJ (1997) Practice parameter: thymectomy for autoimmune myasthenia gravis (an evidence-based review report of the quality standards subcommittee of the American academy of neurology). Neurology 48(suppl 5):S52–S63
2. Jaretzki A III, Barohn RJ, Ernstoff RM, Kaminski HJ, Keesey JC, Penn AS, Sanders DB (2000) Myasthenia gravis: recommendations for clinical research standards. Ann Thorac Surg 70:327–334
3. Loscertales J, Ayarra Jarne J, Congregado M, Arroyo Tristán A, Jiménez Merchán R, Girón Arjona JC, Arenas Linares C (2004) Video-assisted thoracoscopic thymectomy for the treatment of myasthenia gravis. Arch Bronconeumol 40:409–413
4. Mack MJ, Landreneau RJ, Yim AP, Hazelrigg SR, Scruggs GR (1996) Results of video-assisted thymectomy in patients with myasthenia gravis. J Thorac Cardiovasc Surg 112:1352–1359, discussion 1359–60
5. Mantegazza R, Baggi F, Bernasconi P, Antozzi C, Confalonieri P, Novellino L, Spinelli L, Ferrò MT, Beghi E, Cornelio F (2003) Video-assisted thoracoscopic extended thymectomy and extended transsternal thymectomy (T-3b) in non-thymomatous myasthenia gravis patients: remission after 6 years of follow-up. J Neurol Sci 212:31–36
6. Scelsi R, Ferrò MT, Scelsi L, Novellino L, Mantegazza R, Cornelio F, Porta M, Longoni C, Pezzuoli G (1996) Detection and morphology of thymic remnants after video-assisted thoracoscopic extended thymectomy (VATET) in patients with myasthenia gravis. Int Surg 81:14–17
7. Yim APC, Kay RLC, Ho JKS (1995) Video-assisted thoracoscopic thymectomy for myasthenia gravis. Chest 108:1440–1443

28 Thoracic Duct Ligation

Rolf G.C. Inderbitzi

Contents

28.1 Introduction

The diagnosis of chylothorax is easy to make using a needle biopsy or drainage of effusion: The milky, often blood-tinged effusion does not clot. However, we must remember that chyle is only milky when it contains fat, but without fat it is clear, i.e. in patients who have been fasting for a long time! If there is any doubt, or for an intra-operative search for a leak or fistula, the administration of 100-ml cream within 60 min has the effect of producing the white coloration of the pleural effusion (Fig. 28.1).

Post-operative chylothorax caused by injury to the thoracic duct is a rare but well-known problem after procedures on the aorta (Fig. 28.2), the oesophagus, heart and – rarely – the lungs [4, 6, 9, 10, 15, 18, 21, 25]. It can also be caused by a blunt injury or more rarely a sharp injury. Besides local injury to the thoracic duct, infection, neoplasia, post-actinic damage or thrombosis of the jugular or subclavian veins can be responsible for the occurrence of a chylothorax (Fig. 28.1) [20, 26].

28.2 Therapy

Conservative therapy options usually comprise drainage treatment and parenteral feeding. However, in spite of supplements, a loss of protein, fat-soluble vitamins, electrolytes and lymphocytes results [3, 21]. Admittedly, in half of all cases, a leak closes spontaneously after several weeks of conservative treatment, although a

R.G.C. Inderbitzi, M.D.
Thoraxzentrum Zurich, Hirslanden Clinic, Witellikerstrasse 40, CH-8008
Zurich, Switzerland
e-mail: r.inderbitzi@thoraxzentrum.ch

R.G.C. Inderbitzi et al. (eds.), *Minimally Invasive Thoracic and Cardiac Surgery*,
DOI 10.1007/978-3-642-11861-6_28, © Springer-Verlag Berlin Heidelberg 2012

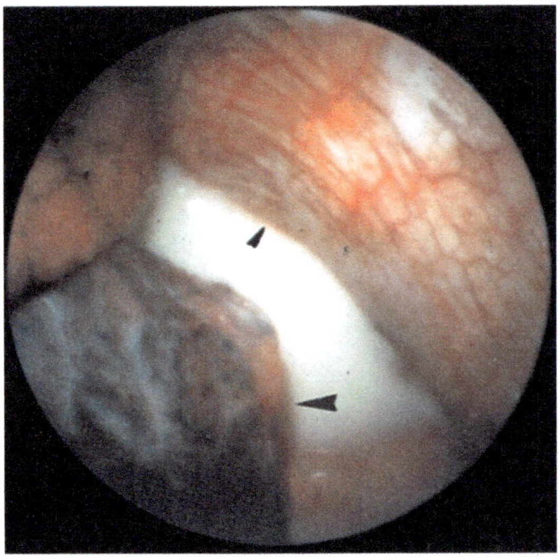

Fig. 28.1 Idiopathic chylothorax of a 56-year-old woman with exertional dyspnoea. Videothoracoscopic view: *small arrow*, parietal pleura with dilation of the pleural capillaries; *large arrow*, atelectatic lung (Illus. 26.23 S 363, Nakhosteen, Inderbitzi)

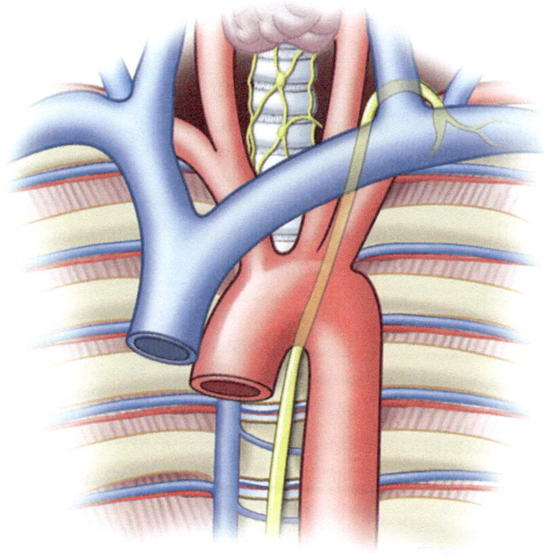

Fig. 28.2 Principal anatomic course of the thoracic duct in the upper part of mediastinum

surgical intervention must be performed on the other half.

The current surgical therapy for post-operative chylothorax consists of ligation of the supradiaphragmatic thoracic duct [14, 16, 19, 22] or bulk ligation on the right side of the thorax of the tissue between the aorta, the pericardium, the oesophagus and the vertebral column [16, 19]. Another therapeutic procedure described is the insertion of a pleuroperitoneal shunt [16, 28].

Since 1989, there have been several case reports describing the successful videothoracoscopic ligation of the thoracic duct [5, 13, 23, 27, 29] or the specific closure of the mediastinal fistula [12]. The thoracoscopic leak closure or the ligation of the thoracic duct represents a minimally invasive procedure which can be used immediately after diagnosis of a chylothorax. This avoids loss of protein, vitamins, electrolytes or immunocompetent lymphocytes. Furthermore, any adhesions to be found inside the thorax as a result of early post-operative thoracoscopic intervention are still easily dividable, [4, 6, 7, 12, 15–17].

28.3 Minimally Invasive Surgical Procedure

In some cases, carrying out a preoperative lymphangio CT (Fig. 28.3) enables the position of the leak in the thoracic duct to be found or a fistula to be visualised. In addition, 100-ml cream is administered to the patient via a gastric tube to colour the chyle white immediately after the commencement of anaesthesia (double-lumen intubation). The surgical procedure basically follows the technique described in Chapter 2. In the left lateral position (or the right lateral position can be selected if the visualisation of the fistula suggests this is appropriate), the level of the three mini-incisions is established, based on the planned level of the ligation. If an escape of contrast medium is found in the CT, the incisions are made according to the level of the fistula. The flow of chyle visible during the operation shows the way to the leak from the duct; this is then visualised and closed both cranially and caudally using clips. If the fistula can be found during the thoracoscopy, this is specifically sealed using an injection of 1-ml fibrin adhesive. If neither the primary leak nor a localised fistula is found, the supradiaphragmatic tissue between the aorta, the pericardium, the vertebral column and the oesophagus is visualised in an open

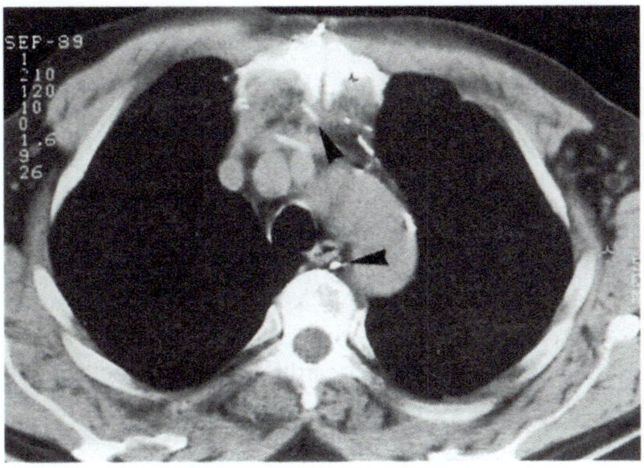

Fig. 28.3 Lymphangio CT section at the level of the exit of the contrast medium from the thoracic duct prevertebrally, retro-aortic (*arrow*), post-operatively after replacement of the aortic valve and aorto-coronary bypass (Illus. 26.35. P 362, Nakhosteen/Inderbitzi)

procedure (cf. Illus. Xy in the Chap. 34) and treated with a bulk ligation. If there is no longer any chyle flow in the subsequent thoracoscopic check, the operation is completed with the insertion of sufficient drainage.

28.4 Diffuse Chylothorax

If a chylothorax occurs as a result of increased capillary permeability (Fig. 28.1), a thoracoscopy is suitable for diagnosis and therapy (cf. Chap. 17). Whether an intrapleural fibrin application [2, 24], a talc pleurodesis [1, 8] or a parietal pleurectomy [11] is used to stop, it depends most likely on the quantity produced and the associated pressure of perfusion in the capillary network. Chapters 17 and 18 will provide you with information on the relevant techniques.

References

1. Adler RH, Levinsky L (1978) Persistent chylothorax. J Thorac Cardiovasc Surg 76:859–864
2. Akaogi E, Kiyohumi M, Sohara Y, Endo S, Ishikawa S, Hori M (1989) Treatment of postoperative chylothorax with intrapleural fibrin glue. Ann Thorac Surg 48:116–118
3. Bessone LN, Ferguson TB, Burford TH (1971) Chylothorax. Ann Thorac Surg 12:527–550
4. Cerfolio RJ, Allen MS, Deschamps C et al (1996) Postoperative chylothorax. J Thorac Cardiovasc Surg 112:1361–1366
5. Christodoulou M, Ris H-B, Pezzetta E (2006) Video-assisted right supradiaphragmatic thoracic duct ligation for non-traumatic recurrent chylothorax. Eur J Cardiothorac Surg 29:810–814
6. Dugue L, Sauvanet A, Farges O, Goharin A, Le Mee J, Belghiti J (1998) Output of chyle as an indicator of treatment for chylothorax complicating esophagectomy. Br J Surg 85:1147–1149
7. Ferguson MK, Little AG, Skinner DB (1985) Current concepts in the management of postoperative chylothorax. Ann Thorac Surg 40:542–545
8. Frey JG, Tschopp JM (1987) Chylothorax: traîtement par pleurodèse au talc. Schweiz Med Wochenschr 117:1624–1627
9. Hillerdal G (1985) Chyliform (cholesterol) pleural effusion. Chest 88:426–428
10. Huwer H, Volkmer I, Feindt P (1991) Tension chylothorax following left-sided surgery. Pneumologie 45:337–339
11. Inderbitzi R, Atay Z, Müller K-M, Karmann U, Furrer M (1994) Einsatz der Thorakoskopie in Diagnostik und Therapie. In: Nakhosteen JA, Inderbitzi R (eds) Atlas und Lehrbuch der thorakalen Endoskopie, 3rd edn. Springer, New York, pp S.341–383
12. Inderbitzi R, Krebs TH, Stirnemann P, Althaus U (1992) Treatment of postoperative chylothorax by fibrin glue under thoracoscopic view using local anesthesia. J Thorac Cardiovasc Surg 104:209–210
13. Kent RB III, Pinson TW (1993) Thoracoscopic ligation of the thoracic duct. Surg Endosc 7:52–53
14. Lampson RS (1948) Traumatic chylothorax. A review of the literature and report of a case treated by mediastinal ligation of the thoracic duct. J Thorac Surg 17:778–791
15. Merigliano S, Molena D, Ruol A, Zaninotto G, Cagol M, Scappin S, Ancona E (2000) Chylothorax complicating esophagectomy for cancer. A plea for early thoracic duct ligation. J Thorac Cardiovasc Surg 119: 453–457
16. Milson JW, Kron IL, Rheuban KS, Rodgers BM (1985) Chylothorax: an assessment of current surgical management. J Thorac Cardiovasc Surg 89: 221–227
17. Orringer MB, Bluett M, Deeb GM (1988) Aggressive treatment of chylothorax complicating transhiatal esophagectomy without thoracotomy. Surgery 104:720–726
18. Orringer MB, Marshall B, Iannettoni MD (1999) Aggressive treatment of chylothorax complicating transhiatal esophagectomy: clinical experience and refinements. Ann Surg 230:392–400
19. Patterson GA, Todd TRJ, Delarue NC, Ilves R, Pearson FG, Cooper JD (1981) Supradiaphragmatic ligation of the thoracic duct in intractable chylous fistula. Ann Thorac Surg 32:44–49
20. Ross JK (1961) A review of surgery of the thoracic duct. Thorax 16:12–21

21. Sarsam MA, Rahman AN, Deiraniya AK (1994) Postpneumonectomy chylothorax. Ann Thorac Surg 57:689–690
22. Selle JG, Snyder WH, Schreiber JT (1973) Chylothorax. Indications for surgery. Ann Surg 177:245–249
23. Shirai T, Amano J, Takabe K (1991) Thoracoscopic diagnosis and treatment of chylothorax after pneumonectomy. Ann Thorac Surg 52:306–307
24. Stenzl W, Rigler B, Tscheliessnigg HK, Beitzke A, Metgler H (1983) Treatment of postsurgical chylothorax with fibrin glue. Thorac Cardiovasc Surg 31:35–36
25. Terzi A, Furlan G, Magnanelli G, Terrini A, Ivic N (1994) Chylothorax after pleuro-pulmonary surgery: a rare but unavoidable complication. Thorac Cardiovasc Surg 42:81–84
26. Valentine VG, Ta R (1992) The management of chylothorax. Chest 102:586–591
27. Watanabe A, Koyanagi T, Nakashima S, Higami T (2007) Supradiaphragmatic thoracic duct clipping for chylothorax through left-sided video-assisted thoracoscopic surgery. Eur J Cardiothorac Surg 31:313–314
28. Weese JL, Schouten JT (1982) Pleural peritoneal shunts for the treatment of malignant pleural effusions. Surg Gynecol Obstet 154:391–392
29. Wurnig PN, Hollaus PH, Ohtsuka T, Flege JB, Wolf RK (2000) Thoracoscopic direct clipping of the thoracic duct for chylopericardium and chylothorax. Ann Thorac Surg 70:1662–1665

Endoscopic Sympathetic Surgery

29

Georg Bischof, Peter Panhofer,
and Christoph Neumayer

Contents

G. Bischof, M.D. (✉)
Department of Surgery, St. Josef Hospital,
Auhofstrasse 189, 1130 Vienna, Austria
e-mail: georg.bischof@sjk-wien.at

P. Panhofer, M.D. • C. Neumayer, M.D.
Department of Surgery,
Medical University of Vienna (MUW),
Währinger Gürtel 18-20, 1090 Vienna, Austria
e-mail: peter.panhofer@meduniwien.ac.at;
christoph.neumayer@meduniwien.ac.at

29.1 Introduction and History

The first article published on upper thoracic sympathetic surgery dates back to 1889, when Alexander aimed to treat a patient with epilepsy [3]. In the following years, toxic goiter, exophthalmos, glaucoma, and angina pectoris were also targeted by resection of the sympathetic trunk at the level of the neck. None of these diseases nowadays are treated by sympathectomy anymore. In 1920, Kotzareff first described partial resection of the cervical sympathetic nerve for treatment of unilateral hyperhidrosis [47, 64, 67, 79]. Only a few years later, Leriche and Royle treated ischemic lesions of the lower extremities by lumbar sympathectomy [87, 138]. This was accepted as treatment of choice for peripheral vasoocclusive diseases for some time.

R.G.C. Inderbitzi et al. (eds.), *Minimally Invasive Thoracic and Cardiac Surgery*,
DOI 10.1007/978-3-642-11861-6_29, © Springer-Verlag Berlin Heidelberg 2012

Several surgical approaches have been used for upper thoracic sympathectomy. The classic posterior thoracotomy [2, 162] required partial rib resection. To ameliorate postoperative pain, Telford [153] introduced a supraclavicular approach, which was technically challenging due to the proximity of the brachial plexus and major vessels. An anterior transthoracic incision was then proposed by Goetz and Marr [51] and a transaxillary method by Atkins [7]. Between 1942 and 1951, Kux and other authors [51, 63, 82] made use of thoracoscopy to access the sympathetic trunk. The low complication rate and less postoperative pain led to the fact that the minimally invasive approach became the gold standard for this type of surgery. For many years, sympathetic surgeons relied on either the resective method or the ablative type of severing the sympathetic chain, the latter using electrocautery to cut or effectively damage the nerve. In a meta-analysis [56], no statistically significant differences were found between the two methods, although a trend toward higher palmar anhidrosis and lower recurrence rates for the resective type of operation was mentioned. Percutaneous methods such as phenol injection [38, 57] and radiofrequency thermal ablation [163] have not gained widespread acceptance.

In 1998, a new method was introduced by Lin et al. [95] named "thoracoscopic or endoscopic sympathetic block." The technique makes use of a 5-mm titanium clip applier to effectively damage the nerve and offers potential reversibility as the clips can again be removed at a later stage. The necessity of reversal operations has originated from a roughly 5% dissatisfaction rate of patients after sympathetic surgery, mainly due to massive compensatory hyperhidrosis in the lower back, inguinal, and abdominal regions. In the same year, Telaranta [151] described a technique of secondary sympathetic chain reconstruction with a free sural nerve graft. Only recently, Korean authors [54] reported clinical results of a small series of patients after reconstruction with a pedicled intercostal nerve graft. Nearly half of their patients had definite or mild resolution of compensatory hyperhidrosis after 22 months.

29.2 Indications

29.2.1 Primary Hyperhidrosis

Primary hyperhidrosis has been reported to occur at an incidence of up to 2.8% [149]. The disease most often affects the palms and soles, the armpits, and the craniofacial area. Typically, symptoms occur bilaterally several times a day/week and are not dependent on outside temperature or physical activity. The onset can be in childhood but most often symptoms start between age 13 and 18. The sweating disorder can lead to severe physical impairment such as recurrent skin infections, mycosis, and sinusitis. Moreover, emotional and psychological distress can limit social interactions of hyperhidrosis patients. A genetic predisposition has been described in a series of patients with positive family history [135] and Kaufmann et al. [72] found an autosomal dominant mode of transmission with incomplete penetration. Secondary hyperhidrosis should be ruled out, which can originate from thyroid disease, obesity, chronic infectious diseases, or others (Table 29.1).

29.2.2 Facial Blushing (Erythrophobia)

This sympathetic disorder can occur in individuals with or without concomitant primary hyperhidrosis and is considered one of the cardinal symptoms of social phobia. Patients exhibit sudden attacks of redness in the face and sometimes also in the neck and upper chest regions. In this situation, they typically experience severe embarrassment and self-consciousness and can hardly refrain from thinking about anything else than the blush in their face. Among others, threats to public identity, scrutiny, and fear of blushing can stimulate the blushing attacks [85]. As a consequence, most of these patients concomitantly suffer from anxiety disorders such as simple phobia (up to 60%) or agoraphobia (up to 45%) [148]. Major depression and alcohol abuse occur at a high percentage in these patients (up to 20% and 30%, respectively) [24]. Dermatological disorders as a result of recurrent blushing include hyperpyrexia, feelings of burning and tingling,

Table 29.1 Causes of secondary hyperhidrosis

Metabolic/endocrine	Diabetes, hyperthyroidism, Cushing disease, carcinoid syndrome
Pharmacologic	Antiemetics, antidepressants, antihypertensive drugs (ACE inhibitors, beta-blockers)
Neoplastic	CNS tumors, Hodgkin disease, pheochromocytoma/paraganglioma
Physiologic/traumatic	Menopause, head/spine injuries
Other	Morbid obesity, chronic infection, alcohol

and acne rosacea caused by increased filling of superficial venous plexus and/or arteriolar dilatation. Blushing or other peripheral circulatory disturbances can be found in up to 50% of hyperhidrosis patients. Conservative treatment includes anticholinergics, beta-blockers, sedatives, MAO inhibitors, and serotonin antagonists [32, 127]. Long-term use cannot be recommended as it may lead to dependency besides severe side effects and early recurrences. Moreover, Davidson et al. showed that the effect of these medication therapies did not differ from placebo [32].

29.2.3 Vascular Disorders

Vasospastic and vasoocclusive diseases have been treated by different technical methods of sympathetic surgery since the early 1920s [2, 13]. Episodical attacks of painful pale fingers becoming cyanotic and followed by reactive hyperthermia characterize primary Raynaud's disease. Low temperatures and/or stress causing acroanesthesia and pain trigger these attacks. Secondary Raynaud's syndrome comprises different systemic diseases such as scleroderma, thromboangiitis, lupus erythematosus, dermatomyositis, or CREST syndrome [11]. Patients with vasoocclusive disorders including thromboangiitis obliterans (Buerger's disease), panarteritis nodosa, thromboembolic disorders, and end-stage atherosclerosis have also been treated by sympathetic surgery [26, 37, 84, 164]. Although primary Raynaud's disease is no longer regarded as an indication for surgery, it has been shown that most of these patients transit to secondary diseases [60, 146]. Patients with systemic sclerosis/scleroderma suffer from recurrent finger tip ulceration (up to 75%), progression to gangrene (up to 30%), and chronic pain (up to 70%) [12]. To date, endothoracic sympathectomy is regarded as "ultima ratio" therapy for selected cases suffering from ulcerations of the finger tips with threatening limb loss and chronic pain [23, 115].

29.2.4 Other Indications

Another indication for sympathetic surgery is social phobia, an anxiety disorder which can be described as a strong, persistent fear of situations in which humiliation or embarrassment occurs [126, 152]. Frequently social phobia is accompanied by erythrophobia, and data for sympathetic surgery in patients with social phobia without erythrophobia are limited.

Congenital long QT syndrome is a cardiac electrophysiological disorder due to genetic mutations. Although beta-blockers can improve clinical symptoms such as ventricular tachycardia and reduce the incidence of sudden cardiac death in approximately 70% of patients, left cardiac sympathetic denervation is an alternative therapy. Candidates are patients who are resistant to beta-blockers or do not want to undergo implantation of a cardioverting/defibrillator device. Recently, it has been recommended as the first-line therapy for long QT syndrome, as microinvasive thoracoscopic sympathectomy was found to be a safe and simple procedure [158].

29.3 Preoperative Evaluation and Conservative Treatment

29.3.1 Preoperative Evaluation

Evaluation of sweat gland activity and extent of hyperhidrosis remains difficult, as it is very subjective and depends on the environment and the physical and emotional situation. First of all, secondary hyperhidrosis has to be excluded (see

Table 29.1). Endocrine or metabolic diseases should be ruled out as well as pharmacologic side effects of medical drugs. Most important is a detailed medical history including the age of the patient at the onset of the sweating disorder. At last, neoplastic and postoperative or posttraumatic sources of sweating may be evaluated. Typically, patients describe their disorder to be independent of the outside temperature, their physical activity, and the time of the year. The degree of sweating can be assessed on a visual analogue scale or severity score using disease-specific questionnaires [118]. A few investigators also evaluate primary hyperhidrosis by using quality of life instruments [125].

The "Minor sweat test," first described in 1928, is frequently used. The affected area is lubricated with iodine liquid followed by the application of starch powder. As a result, the hyperhidrotic area turns from brown into violet and can be visualized on blotting paper [80]. This test is reliable for detection of the hyperhidrotic area in the armpits before minimal invasive suction curettage of the sweat glands. Another modification of this method uses prints with iodine-coated copy paper [8]. These methods can demonstrate the border between hyper- and anhidrotic areas quite precisely but cannot quantify the amount of sweat.

Gravimetric methods were used in former days. Patients were weighed over 24 h with special emphasis on the body fluid secretion, which was rather complicated, time consuming, and still imprecise. A more effective and simple method uses accurate analysis scales assessing the exact weight of sweat-saturated blotting papers.

Hygrometric methods are quantitative and assess the moisture secretion of the skin by using a body box with gas ventilation. The atmospheric humidity is measured at the influx and efflux of the box.

The VapoMeter (Delfin Technologies Inc.) is a small, handheld device, which allows measurement of the evaporation of sweat (TEWL – transepidermal water loss; g/m^2/h), the relative humidity (%), and the ambient temperature (°C) of the affected area. The measurements should be performed in a special testing room under standardized environment: 24°C room temperature and 50% atmospheric humidity. The test is divided in three sections: thermal, emotional, and gustatory provocation. Only recently, the first data have been published [134, 154]. The limitation of these systems is that they can only assess a certain degree of sweat at a specific time point. Therefore, it has been recommended that patients should measure repeatedly at home with the VapoMeter in order to obtain a more realistic reflection of their disorder [36].

29.3.2 Conservative Treatment

Conservative treatment includes topical antitranspirants, iontophoresis, botulinum toxin injections, as well as anticholinergic drugs. In addition, alternative strategies may be recommended such as yoga, autogene training, and traditional Chinese medicine (TCM) including acupuncture or herbal therapy aiming at the vegetative nervous system.

Topical antitranspirants are applied to the skin in order to close the excretory ducts of the sweat glands, mainly aluminum chloride or other tanning agents. The patient lubricates the affected body region in the evening, and the aluminum chloride solution remains on the skin over night. On the next morning, the patient washes off the antitranspirant and creams the skin. The topical agents have to be used daily; otherwise, the effect is likely to fade within days. Nowadays, many deodorants contain antitranspirants such as aluminum chloride.

For tap water iontophoresis, patients put their hands (or feet) in a tray filled with water. A low-voltage direct current is applied, causing ion exchanges on the skin and subcutaneous tissue (sweat glands). Regular usage (2–3 times/week) can improve palmar or plantar hyperhidrosis. Patients suffering from axillary HH use two sponges connected to electrodes. Besides considerable costs of the iontophoretic system, the time-consuming procedure, possible lack of success, dysesthesias, and pain in case of cutaneous fissures are limiting.

Botulinum toxin is a neurotoxic protein of Clostridium botulinum. It blocks signal transduction of neurons at the endplate. As a result, sweat gland secretion and thus sweating stops when the vegetative nervous system is affected. The procedure can be recommended for treatment of axillary hyperhidrosis, as the hyperhidrotic skin region can be clearly visualized by the Minor test and anesthesia can be achieved by local measures. Before treatment, the hyperhidrotic skin is divided into small areas of about 1 cm^2. About 2–4 units of botulinum toxin are injected intracutaneously every centimeter. In total, about 50 units of botulinum toxin are recommended per armpit. Hands and feet arc less effectively treated as local anesthesia is more difficult and painful (usually peripheral nerve blocks are performed) and the hyperhidrotic area is less clearly visible. Ambrogi and colleagues [4] showed that ETS surgery is superior to Botox injections for the hands. Initially, the satisfaction rate was higher in the botox group, but after 6 months, the results significantly reversed. The botox effect lasts for about 3–6 months without much difference between preparations [71]. Possible side effects include dysesthesia, postinterventional cutaneous hematomas and infection, although observed rarely, and the possible risk of neurotoxicity. The major drawback of this therapy is its short-lasting effect and considerable costs for the patient.

Oral medications such as tranquilizers, sedatives, and anticholinergics should not be used over longer time periods due to side effects like nausea, vomiting, glaucoma, dizziness, mouth dryness, and other adverse effects. When patients suffer from severe hyperhidrotic attacks (during exams, presentations, etc.), these drugs may be helpful on demand. Guidelines for a severity-based treatment of focal hyperhidrosis have been presented in 2007 [145].

In order to relax and reduce stress-related sweating, patients may practice yoga or autogene training. Furthermore, traditional Chinese medicine (herbal therapy, acupuncture) can be considered for therapy refractory hyperhidrosis. Nevertheless, the effects of these methods are minor and have not been proven in controlled studies, yet. Consequently, these therapies may provide insufficient results despite high costs.

Local sweat gland excision as performed in former days included resection of the axillary skin. Postoperative sequelae were sometimes strictures and distinct scars, and even impaired arm movement was described. Therefore, this method is no longer used with exception of repeat abscesses of the axillae. Nowadays, minimally invasive sweat gland curettage can be performed in local tumescent anesthesia via two small skin incisions. After dissecting the cutis from the subcutaneous fatty tissue and thus denervating the sweat glands, suction curettage is performed by means of special cannulae. Hematoma and wound infection may occur, and the effect is not everlasting with a high recurrence rate within 3 years [9, 30, 103, 136].

29.4 Anatomy and Physiology of the Sympathetic Trunk

29.4.1 Anatomy

The hypothalamus is the major integrative point of the central autonomic nervous system [106]. The hippocampal formation, the amygdala, the olfactory cortex, and cortical regions have connections to the hypothalamus [114, 128]. In addition, the limbic system plays a major role receiving impulses of the forebrain, the brainstem, and the reticular formation, and vice versa [106, 114]. Some hypothalamic impulses are directly sent to visceral motor nuclei in the brainstem, the reticular formation of the medulla, and the spinal cord [106, 113]. Thus, different visceral reflex activities are regulated and modified by the hypothalamus via these connections. A detailed review has been provided by Marhold et al. recently [107].

The sympathetic chains are situated bilaterally along the vertebral column (Fig. 29.1). The cervical part consists mostly of three ganglia, the superior cervical, the middle cervical, and the inferior cervical ganglion. Sometimes the middle cervical ganglion is absent, whereas the inferior cervical ganglion frequently fuses with the first thoracic ganglion to build the stellate ganglion [44]. In the thoracic, lumbar, and sacral regions, the ganglia are segmentally arranged (up to 12 thoracic, 4 lumbar, and 5 sacral ganglia). At the coccyx, the two trunks fuse in the unpaired coccygeal ganglion. Besides these paravertebral ganglia, there are also prevertebral ganglia surrounding the visceral branches of the aorta.

Preganglionic sympathetic fibers arise from the intermediolateral and intermediomedial

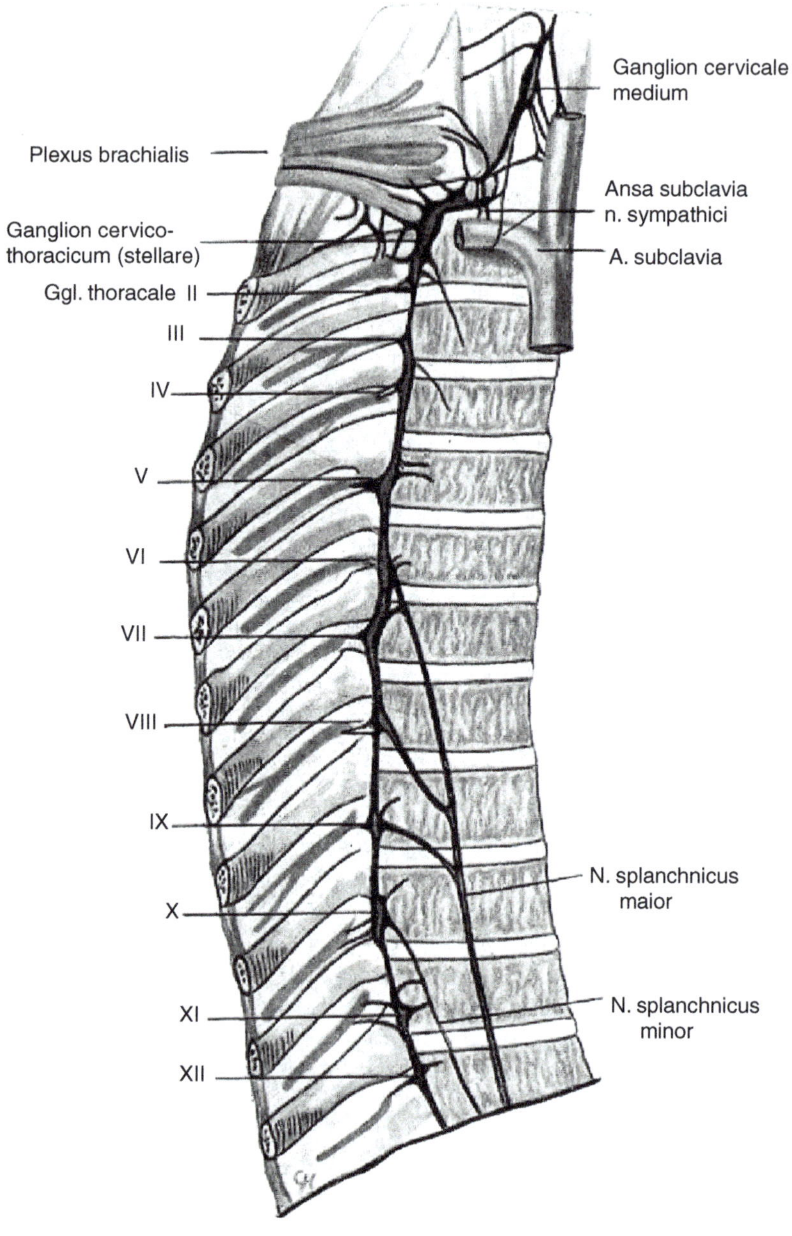

Fig. 29.1 Thoracic sympathetic trunk (Illustration from Sprung [147])

column of the spinal cord from C8 to L2 and emerge via the anterior roots to reach the sympathetic chain via the white communicating rami [106]. After synapsing with cells in the sympathetic ganglia, the unmyelinated postganglionic fibers course through the gray communicating rami and join the somatic nerves. Finally, these cholinergic fibers innervate the sweat glands as sudomotor fibers, the smooth muscles of the peripheral blood vessels as vasoconstrictor fibers, and the erector pili muscles in erectile hairs as pilomotor fibers.

Detailed information of efferent and afferent sympathetic fibers to the sympathetic chain can be derived from Fig. 29.2 [107].

29.4.2 Physiology

Sweating is a physiological condition preventing too rapid raise of the body temperature in hot environments. Secretion of sweat is induced by sympathetic cholinergic nerve impulses. In addition,

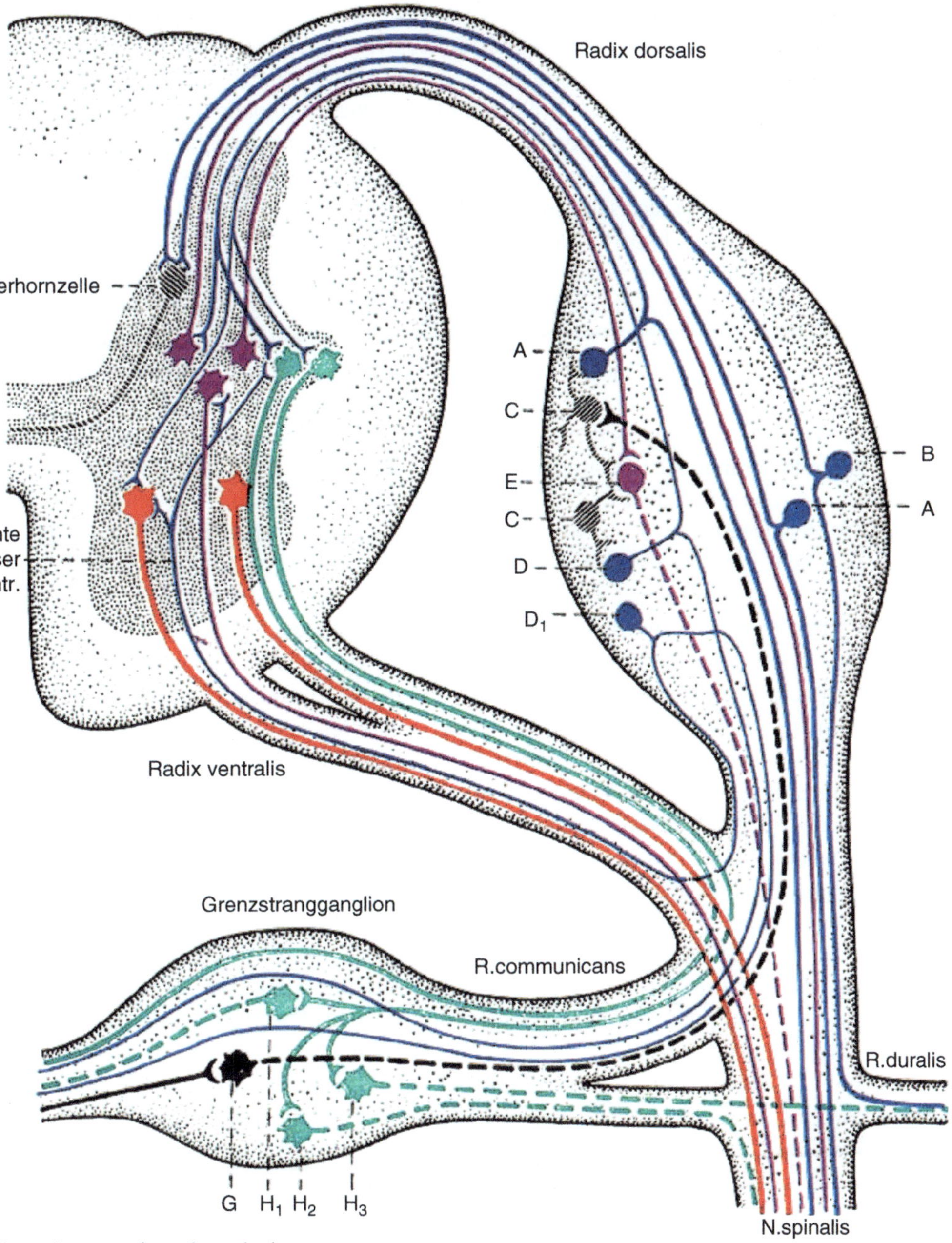

A	cutivisceral neuron from the spinal nerve
B	cutivisceral neuron from the dural branch
C	intraganglionic neuron of the spinal ganglion
D,D1	viscerosensitive neuron of the viscerocutaneous reflex arc
E	alpha-motoneuron
E	interganglionic viscerosensitive neuron
H1	postganglionic visceral neuron to the splanchnic nerve
H2	postganglionic visceral neuron to the spinal nerve
H3	postganglionic visceral neuron to the dural branch

Fig. 29.2 Efferent and afferent sympathetic fibers to the sympathetic chain (Fig. 88 from Max Clara [27])

sweat glands can also be stimulated by circulating hormones that indirectly activate the sympathetic trunk (see Table 29.1). Two kinds of eccrine sweat glands can be distinguished. One is stimulated by emotional and the other by thermoregulatory reasons. Palms and soles contain both forms, whereas the rest of the body surface reacts to thermoregulatory causes. Emotional hyperhidrosis can be detected in other body regions if the environmental temperature rises [122]. Human beings have two to five million sweat glands with the highest density in the palms of the hands (400–1,000 sweat glands per square centimeter skin) compared to about 130 sweat glands per square centimeter skin in the armpits. It is of importance that the rate of sweat secretion does not correspond to the density of sweat glands.

Essential hyperhidrosis is defined as excessive sweating mainly affecting palms, armpits, and feet but also affects other body regions. Although morphology of sweat glands seems to be normal, a theory blames capillary disorders of the sympathetic trunk [14] or dysfunction of cerebral cortical areas including sudomotor fibers [28] for the disorder.

Facial sweating which is frequently found in patients with erythrophobia can be provoked by gustatory stimulation or emotions. Sweat glands in the face have a dual innervation from the 1st and 2nd thoracic ganglia of the sympathetic trunk with connection to both the trigeminal nerve and the external carotid artery. If one pathways fails or is interrupted, the other one can compensate for the missing function [140].

The auriculotemporal branch of the trigeminal nerve contains sympathetic neurons heading toward vessels and sweat glands and parasympathetic secretory fibers to the parotid gland. That cross-link may explain gustatory sweating [49]. Guttmann et al. reported that sympathectomy of the right superior, middle, and stellate sympathetic ganglia led to dryness of the right face, neck, and upper chest during thermoregulatory stimulation, whereas gustatory sweating could not be stopped. Accessory cholinergic fibers originating from the brainstem and innervating facial sweat glands can explain that phenomenon.

Moreover, failure of thermoregulatory sweating due to accidental, disease-specific, or iatrogenic lesions in certain skin areas results in reflex hyperhidrosis in adjacent zones [81].

The Horner syndrome following lesions of the cervical sympathetic trunk including the stellate ganglion consists of miosis, ptosis, and enophthalmus, sometimes amended by vasodilatation of the ipsilateral facial vessels. Sympathetic neurons responsible for that syndrome run through the lateral medullary area. They are accompanied by some fibers from the opposite side resulting very often in partial Horner syndrome with presence of only one or two leading symptoms.

29.5 Surgical Technique

29.5.1 Patient Positioning

Three types of positions have been described for ETS surgery.

The lateral decubitus position used for open thoracotomy can be modified by tilting the patient anteriorly by 30°. The upper arm is fixed in a raised position in order to expose the axillary region (Fig. 29.3). This way, even a ventilated lung can retract to the ventral inferior side, providing ideal working space in the upper posterior thoracic cavity. The major disadvantage is the necessity of patient repositioning for the other side when bilateral operation is performed. There may be some risk for accidental extubation or skin lesions during rearrangement [119]. The great advantage is the possibility of standard single-lumen orotracheal intubation and continuous ventilation of both lungs.

The prone position with 90° abduction of the arms saves rearrangement time. The lungs can collapse to the ventral side, and the posterior thoracic cavity is exposed. When starting with that technique, surgeons have reported orientation problems due to the upside-down view of the sympathetic trunk at the cranial thoracic wall. Another disadvantage could be anesthetic and pulmonary problems in obese patients.

Thirdly, a semi-sitting position with 90° abduction of the arms is commonly used for ETS surgery. Again no rearrangement is necessary for operating bilaterally, but double-lumen intubation

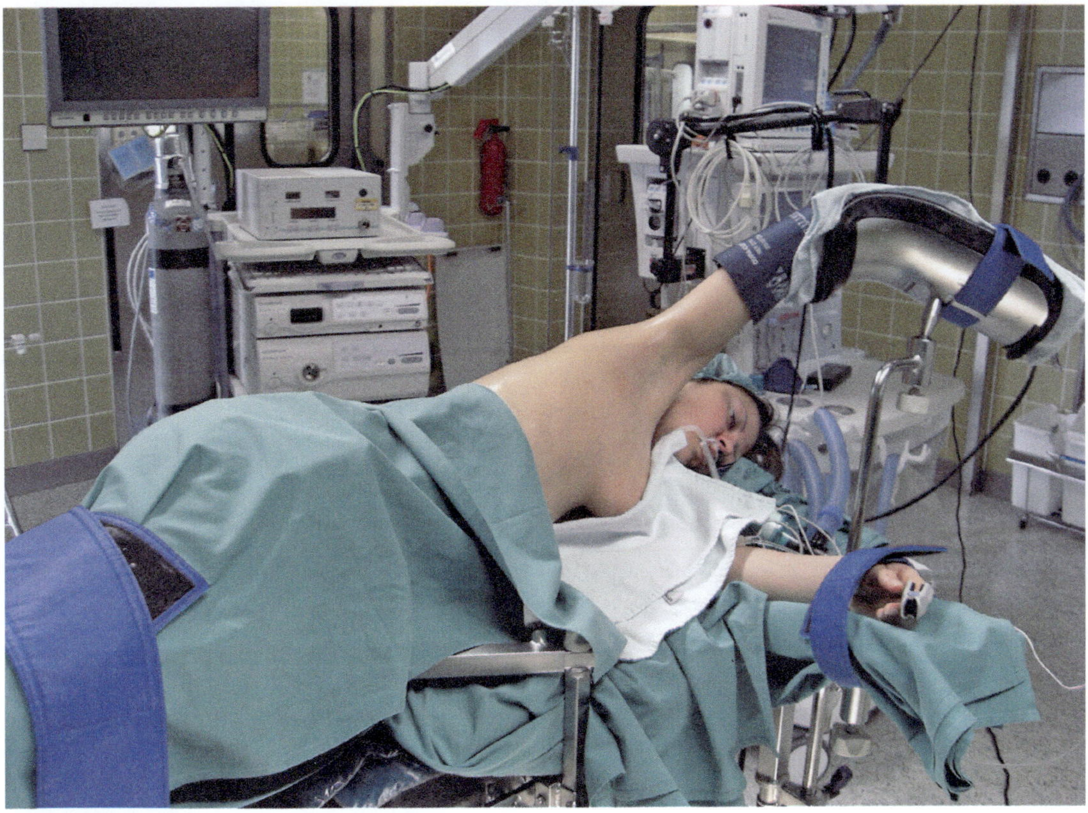

Fig. 29.3 Patient position during endothoracic sympathetic surgery of the right hemithorax (Modified lateral decubitus position)

is usually required. At our department, the modified lateral position is preferred as it has proven to be a very safe method and offers a good intrathoracic overview. Operation time for bilateral surgery currently ranges from 30 to 40 min including the repositioning time.

29.5.2 Surgical Access/Closure

During a short stop of the ventilation, the interpleural space is punctured in the 4th or 5th intercostal space with a Verres needle, and a pneumothorax is achieved by low-pressure insufflation of CO_2 (3 mmHg). A preemptive intercostal block with local anesthetics can be injected [45], and a 5-mm trocar is inserted in the 4th (5th) intercostal space in the midaxillary line. A 5-mm videothoracoscope is inserted and a second 5-mm trocar inserted under direct view in the 2nd (3rd) intercostal space. Other sizes and numbers of trocars (1–3) in different positions have been described by other authors. Even single-access thoracoscopy for a bilateral operation has been achieved. A recent article proclaims uniportal video-assisted thoracoscopic sympathectomy compared to biportal operation. Postoperative results did not differ significantly, whereas operation time and postoperative pain were reduced in the uniportal group [19].

After the preferred ETS operation (cutting, clipping, resection), gas insufflation is stopped. The pneumothorax is aspirated, the skin incisions are closed, and normally no chest drain is used. In the wake-up room, a chest radiogram is taken to rule out hemothorax or pneumothorax. Usually patients are discharged on the first postoperative day. According to the literature, the rate of postoperative pneumothorax drainage ranges from 1% to 3% [116, 118, 119].

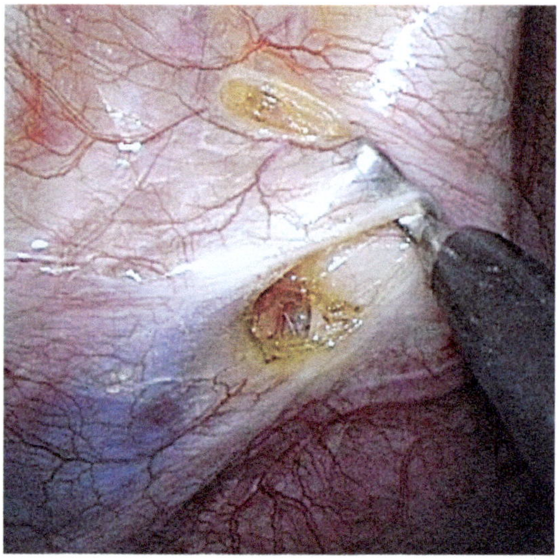

Fig. 29.4 Intrathoracic view: the pleura is incised next to the sympathetic trunk

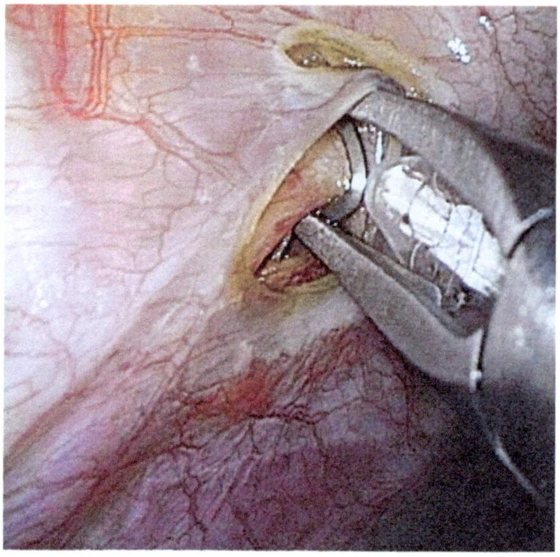

Fig. 29.5 After careful isolation the nerve is blocked by a 5 mm titanium clip

29.5.3 Types of ETS Procedures

Several techniques have been used to accomplish sympathetic surgery over time. During *sympathectomy*, resection of the sympathetic chain and ganglia up to a varying length is carried out [21, 34, 166]. *Sympathicotomy* means dissection of the sympathetic trunk at one or more levels without resection [77, 102, 157]. Diathermic hooks, scissors, laser, and more recently ultrasonic dissection have been used for either technique [10, 34, 160].

In 1998, a new method has been introduced [95], called endoscopic *sympathetic block* (ESB) or *clipping*, using a 5-mm titan clip applier to cause interruption of the sympathetic trunk at the desired level [117–120]. The major advantage is the potential reversibility of the operation by clip removal since few patients suffer from unbearable compensatory sweating postoperatively (see Sect. 29.6.5). Furthermore, total anhidrosis with potential skin fissures is rarely reported in that patient cohort.

As mentioned above, we use two 5-mm trocars in the 2nd and 4th intercostal spaces. Optionally the trocars are placed in the 3rd and 5th intercostal spaces. Trocars that are placed too high can damage axillary vessels and nerve structures. If the trocars are positioned too low, the surgeon might not have ideal access to the upper thoracic sympathetic structures.

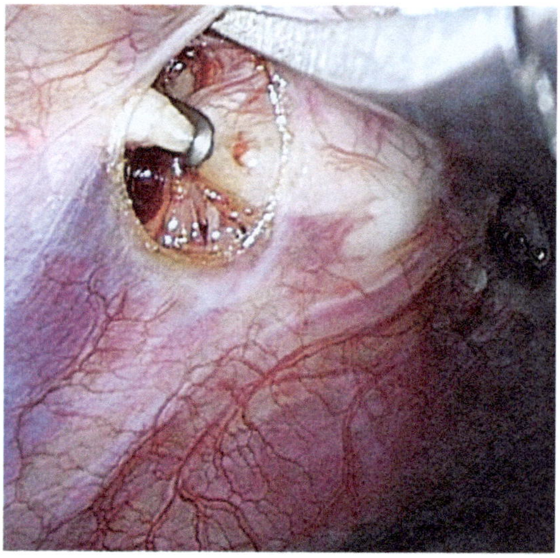

Fig. 29.6 Complete closure of the clip around the sympathetic trunk is achieved

The thoracoscope is inserted into the lower port and a diathermic hook, scissors, or other instrument (ultrasonic shears, etc.) into the other. After identification of the sympathetic trunk at the desired level(s), the pleura is incised and the nerve carefully isolated (see Figs. 29.4, 29.5, 29.6, and 29.7). Any pulling on the nerve

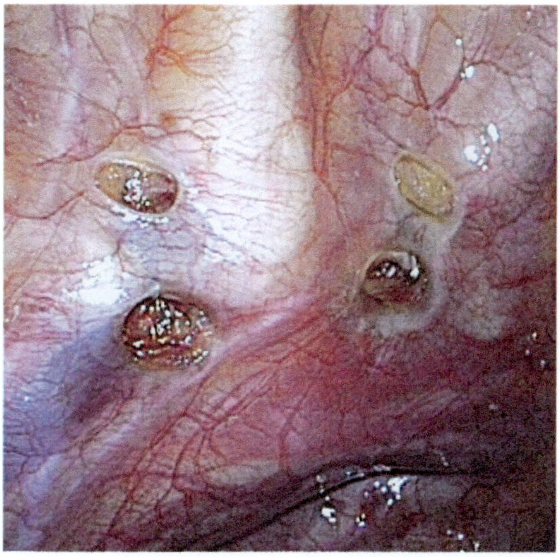

Fig. 29.7 Two clips are applied above and below the fourth thoracic ganglion

structures should be avoided. For sympathetic block (ESB) in patients with palmar hyperhidrosis, we use a 5-mm reusable clip applier (e.g., Aesculap® Challenger) and close one clip above and one below the 4th thoracic (T4) ganglion. After checking the operative field, the pneumothorax is aspirated under endoscopic view. The thoracoscope and the trocars are removed and the incisions closed at the skin level.

29.6 Functional Results and Quality of Life

29.6.1 Results for Palmoaxillary Hyperhidrosis

29.6.1.1 Functional Results

Endoscopic thoracic sympathectomy (ETS) is the method of choice in case of severe palmar hyperhidrosis when conservative treatment measures failed. Short-term results reported cure rates of more than 98% for palmar hyperhidrosis [56, 58, 116, 132]. Recurrence rates are acceptable (about 5%) even in long-term follow-up investigations of more than 10 years [58, 116]. Analysis of the outcome of sympathetic surgery is difficult, as most of the studies report personal series with different surgical methods and different levels of ablation [56]. Moreover, the number of prospective randomized studies is limited [87], and long-term follow-up studies besides that of our own group [58, 116, 118, 171] are rare [17, 55, 96]. The International Society for Sympathetic Surgery defines "long term" by a follow-up period of at least 5 years. Table 29.2 gives an overview of studies with a representative follow-up of at least 20 months.

For isolated excessive axillary hyperhidrosis, the outcome is significantly worse as shown by Herbst and colleagues [58]. Only one third of patients were fully satisfied with the results. Consequently, the ETS procedure is often recommended after failed axillary sweat gland curettage or for recurrences after botulinum toxin A injections. Reisfeld [131] explained the unpredictable results by the two groups of sweat glands in the axillae: the eccrine glands being innervated by sympathetic fibers and the apocrine glands, which respond primarily to epinephrine and are not effectively blocked by sympathectomy. However, Coelho et al. recently reported high success rates for axillary hyperhidrosis after T3–T4 sympathetic block (83.3%) as well as after T3–T4 sympathectomy (92.8%) [29]. This is currently the only study published comparing different operative techniques at the same level. There were no significant differences concerning therapeutic success, satisfaction rate, and incidence and severity of compensatory hyperhidrosis. The study by Herbst and coworkers also showed that satisfaction rates deteriorated with time of follow-up. This finding was explained by compensatory sweating, which became a more prominent problem with time, although the effectiveness of the operation did not deteriorate essentially [58]. As a result, direct comparison of satisfaction rates and rates of dryness is not advisable, as satisfaction rates are usually much lower. In addition, many studies do not differentiate between the outcome of palms and armpits according to the primarily affected body region (isolated palmar, isolated axillary, or combined palmoaxillary hyperhidrosis). Likewise, one cannot read in those reports whether recurrences of upper limb hyperhidrosis include axillary recurrences or not.

Table 29.2 Overview on studies dealing with palmar hyperhidrosis (PH)[a]

Year	Author	Follow-up (months)	Patients	Level	Technique[b]	Results[c]				
						Success rate (%)	Recurrence rate (%)	Satisfaction (%)	CS (%)	GS (%)
2009	Yazbek [167]	20 (Mean)	28	T2	VATS			93	100	
			29	T3	VATS			100	100	
2008	Jeganathan [66]	51 (Mean)	66	T2–T3	VATS	99	5			
2007	Assalia [6]	52 (Mean)	26	T2–T3	VATS	97	4		73	8
2007	Chang [17]	61 (Mean)	86	T2	VATS		26		92	6
		36 (Mean)	78	T3	VATS		8		92	23
		43 (Mean)	70	T4	VATS		23		80	11
2003	Yoon [170]	20 (Mean)	24	T3	VATS	100	0			
2002	Chuang [22]	54 (Max)	35	T2–T3	Sympathectomy	98				
2001	Neumayer [116]	200 (Mean)	221	T2–T4	CTS	98		94	68	50
		23 (Mean)	55	T2–T4	VATS	97		95	56	33
1999	Lin [96]	143 (Mean)	84	T2–T3	UDS		6	55	68	
		43 (Mean)	71	T2–T3	Sympathectomy		3	63	85	
1994	Herbst [58]	197 (Mean)	175	T1–T4	Sympathectomy	98			67	51
1992	Hashmonai [55]	100 (Mean)	62	T2–T3	Sympathectomy	77	13			
1975	Gjerris [50]	94 (Mean)	35	T2–T3/4	Sympathectomy				57	43

CTS conventional thoracoscopic sympathicotomy, *VATS* video-assisted thoracoscopic sympathicotomy, *UDS* upper dorsal sympathetic ganglionectomy, *CS* compensatory sweating, *GS* gustatory sweating

[a]Studies including patients with PH without providing data on their outcome, dealing with a follow-up below 20 months or less than 20 patients, respectively, have been omitted

[b]Sympathectomy: removing of corresponding ganglia

[c]Satisfy: satisfied and satisfaction, respectively

29.6.1.2 Quality of Life

Health is defined by the WHO as follows: "Health is a state of complete physical, mental and social wellbeing and not merely the absence of disease or infirmity." Quality of life is a multidimensional construct comprising physical, psychological, social, and functional domains [68]. In the last 15 years, less than 50 papers dealt with QoL in HH. In comparison, about 1,900 authors used QoL measurement in breast cancer studies [124]. Velanovich reported that 63% of studies used a QoL instrument, whereas only 40% of the studies used a validated QoL instrument [156]. One has to emphasize that SF-36 scores of social functioning and general health status are less applicable for hyperhidrotic patients compared to those suffering from postmastectomy pain or myocardial infarction [76, 105, 125].

In principal, generic QoL instruments have to be differentiated from disease-specific ones. Generic instruments cover all relevant domains of QoL going beyond the specific illness. Specific instruments focus on specific parts of the health state and measure important changes in disease, population functions, and conditions [156]. Three aspects help to identify useful QoL instruments: Validity proves that the developed instrument measures what it intends to measure. Furthermore, the investigator should be able to find conclusions according to the results of the QoL measurements. Reliability guarantees similar data outcomes on a QoL questionnaire in a group of patients, who have gone through it twice. Factors that influence results after patients undergoing a questionnaire repeatedly are neutralized, if the test is reliable. Responsiveness detects study relevant changes, no matter how inconspicuous they are. In generic questionnaires, such as the SF-36, disease-specific changes are mostly not obvious [31, 52, 53].

Two disease-specific QoL instruments have been validated for hyperhidrotic patients. The Keller questionnaire was compared to the SF-36 and showed a high rate of responsiveness, reliability, and variability [73, 118, 120]. The questionnaire, which is easy to handle and to understand, covers important disease-specific areas of hyperhidrosis (e.g., the palms, axillae, or feet). Milanez de Campos presented a disease-specific questionnaire, subdividing 21 questions in 4 domains, summarizing the results in an overall score [33]. Though some questions give place for several interpretations, it fulfills criteria demanded for QoL instruments such as divisions into domains. Unfortunately, no pre- and postoperative results have been included in the paper [33]. We have shown significant improvement of postoperative QoL in most of the 106 patients treated with endothoracic sympathetic block at T4 using both questionnaires [125]. In about 5% of patients, compensatory sweating presented a major postoperative problem and reduced postoperative satisfaction rates and QoL [125].

Lack of literature, different tests with different visual analogue scales, and the absence of a gold standard make it difficult to compare QoL instruments in surgical treatment of hyperhidrosis. Nevertheless, psychological assessment and evaluation of QoL are essential for quality assurance.

29.6.2 Results for Facial Blushing and Craniofacial Hyperhidrosis

29.6.2.1 Results for Facial Blushing

Since the first description by Wittmoser in 1985, numerous reports have been published confirming the effective treatment of facial blushing by sympathetic surgery. Most of these studies included few patients with a short follow-up. All authors operated on the second thoracic ganglion. The largest series were published by Drott [40, 41] and Rex [133] with an efficacy of more than 90%. Patients reported an impressive improvement from VAS 9 preoperatively to 2.5 at follow-up. Satisfaction rates ranged from 85% to 94%. Table 29.3 gives a comprehensive overview on the largest studies with at least 20 patients. One has to keep in mind that the incidence of postoperative Horner syndrome is higher when operating close to the stellate ganglion in this group of patients.

29.6.2.2 Results for Facial Hyperhidrosis

In general, more men than women are operated for facial hyperhidrosis [18, 70, 119, 132].

Table 29.3 Overview on studies dealing with facial blushing (FB)[a]

Year	Author	Follow-up (months)	Patients	Level	Technique[b]	Results[c]				
						Success rate (%)	Recurrence rate (%)	Satisfaction (%)	CS (%)	GS (%)
2008	Rathinam [129]	68 (Mean)	26	T2–T4	VATS	85			18	
2008	Jeganathan [66]	51 (Mean)	25[d]	T2	VATS	84	5			
2006	Chou [20]	35 (Max)	54	T2	ESB	83			43	
2006	Licht [91]	20 (Median)	95	T2	VATS	73			83	
			78	T2–T3	VATS	76			95	
2005	Neumayer [119]	20 (Mean)	26	T2	ESB	96		88	23	54
2005	Adair [1]	20 (Mean)	59	T2–T3	VATS	80			91	32
2004	Callejas [15]	20 (Max)	100	Lower T1–T3	VATS					
2004	Licht [89]	26 (Median)	49[d]	T2	VATS	75			81	
2002	Drott [41]	29 (Mean)	831	T2	Sympathectomy	94		85		
2001	Lin [93]	–	25	T2	ESB				16	
1998	Drott [40]	8 (Mean)	244	Lower T1–T3	Sympathectomy	97		98	75	
1998	Rex [133]	8 (Mean)	244	T2–T3	Sympathicotomy	96		98		
1985	Wittmoser [165]	24 (Max)	70	T2–T3	Sympathicotomy					

ESB endoscopic sympathetic block, clip application at the corresponding ganglia, *VATS* video-assisted thoracoscopic sympathicotomy, *CS* compensatory sweating, *GS* gustatory sweating

[a]Studies including patients with FB without providing data on their outcome and studies with less than 20 patients have been omitted

[b]Sympathectomy: removing of corresponding ganglia; sympathicotomy: severing the corresponding ganglia via diathermy or harmonic scalpel

[c]Satisfy: satisfied and satisfaction, respectively

[d]FB + FH

Whether this fact is related to the male hormonal situation or not remains open for speculation. Different levels of the sympathetic trunk have been treated; most of them included T2 or T3 (either alone or in combination). Table 29.4 summarizes the results with similar success rates as for facial blushing. Patient satisfaction ranges from 76% to 100%. Likewise, visual analogue scores significantly improved from 9 preoperatively to 2 at follow-up [133].

29.6.3 Results for Vascular Disorders

Although immediate success rates of sympathetic surgery are promising, long-term follow-up data are less convincing for patients with vascular disorders compared to those with primary hyperhidrosis. For primary Raynaud's disease, initial success rates ranged from 58% to 100% [5, 24, 25, 144, 155, 161], whereas in the long term only 0–65% of patients reported relief or improvement of primary complaints [24, 25, 48, 110, 142, 144, 161]. To date, primary Raynaud's disease can no longer be recommended for ETS surgery because of these early recurrences. Exceptions are patients with trophic lesions and possible loss of extremities. Better results are obtained in patients with secondary Raynaud's syndrome. Success rates are initially higher than 90% [5, 59, 104, 109, 121, 137] and between 46% and 89% in the long run [48, 59, 109, 121, 137, 139]. Nevertheless, the outcome is hardly predictable as there is a vast variety of underlying diseases with different histories of one and the same disorder. The outcome in patients with scleroderma, dermatomyositis, or CREST syndrome is worst due to the progressive character of the underlying disease [115]. Thromboangiitis obliterans yielded better success rate of more than 50% in the long term [35, 142]. For patients with critical ischemia or arterial occlusion, results were even better, although one has to emphasize that nowadays direct revascularization, either by surgical or interventional methods, is the treatment of choice. A detailed overview of studies dealing with endothoracic surgery for vascular disorders is given in Table 29.5.

In conclusion, sympathectomy can effectively control pain in patients who frequently have a short life expectancy and may additionally attribute to ulcer healing. Therefore, it can prevent or delay amputation in patients in whom other therapies have failed. Whether or not NO donors may represent a less invasive alternative has yet to be demonstrated.

29.6.4 Complications

Endothoracic sympathectomy is considered to be a safe surgical procedure with a low morbidity. A comprehensive review was provided by Hashmonay in 2001 [56]. Our group has shown [116, 171] that the introduction of the videoendoscopic method reduced complication rates (especially Horner syndrome) and the number of unwanted side effects (especially gustatory sweating). In our own series of more than 2,400 operations within the last 15 years, there were no deaths and no conversions to open surgery. Two endothoracic revisions were necessary, one after chest tube drainage and subsequent intercostal arterial bleeding and one for a venous port side bleeding. About 2% of operated hemithoraces had to be treated by chest tube drainage due to a pneumothorax of more than 3 cm. One patient unfortunately required chest tube drainage bilaterally. Horner syndrome, which ranged from 10% to 43% in times of open surgery [116], has not been found in our endothoracic series at all. However, we observed temporary mild miosis in five patients (three after endoscopic sympathetic block at the level of T2 for facial blushing and another two after T3 clipping for facial hyperhidrosis). Three of the patients had their clips removed and the miosis resolved, but it also resolved in the two other patients after about 6 months. Five patients with intercostal neuralgia were treated with nonsteroidal analgesics and infiltration therapy. One wound infection was locally treated and required no antibiotics. Mild subcutaneous emphysemas can be found on the postoperative chest X-rays in about 10% of patients, but none of them required any further treatment.

Table 29.4 Overview on studies dealing with facial hyperhidrosis (FH)[a]

Year	Author	Follow-up (months)	Patients	Level	Technique[b]	Results[c]				
						Success rate (%)	Recurrence rate (%)	Satisfaction (%)	CS (%)	GS (%)
2008	Jeganathan [66]	51 (Mean)	25[d]	T2	VATS	84	5			
2008	Sciuchetti [141]	13 (Mean)	23	T2–T3	VATS	100				
2006	Chou [20]	35 (Max)	33	T3	ESB				28	
2006	Licht [90]	17 (Median)	95[d]	T2	VATS	89			85	27
2005	Neumayer [119]	21 (Mean)	29	T3	ESB	93			28	59
2004	Licht [89]	26 (Median)	49[d]	T2	VATS	85			81	
2004	Doolabh [39]	–	28	T2	VATS	100				
2004	Kim [74]	11 (Mean)	22	T2	VATS	82%			9	9
		20 (Mean)	22	T2	ESB	100		77	23	6
2003	Neumayer [117]	6 (Median)	23	T3	ESB	100		100	25	5
2003	Fischel [46]	42 (Max)	55	T2–T3	VATS	100				
2002	Lin [99]	25 (Mean)	28	Lower T1	ESB	100			86	
2001	Chen [18]	9 (Mean)	25	T2–T3	Sympathicotomy	92			60	
2001	Duarte [43]	47 (Max)	23	T2–T4	Sympathicotomy	100			9%	
2001	Lin [93]	–	55[d]	T3	ESB				6	
2000	Lin [100]	32 (Mean)	46	Lower T1	Sympathicotomy	100	2		80	
1999	Lee [86]	–	190	T1	Sympathectomy			70		
				T2	Sympathicotomy			98		
				T2	ESB			93		
1998	Rex [133]	31 (Mean)	30	T2–T3	Sympathicotomy	97		83		
1998	Duarte [42]	88 (Max)	42	T2–T4	Sympathicotomy	100				
1996	Kao [70]	15 (mean)	30	T2	Sympathicotomy			100		

ESB endoscopic sympathetic block, clip application at the corresponding ganglia, *VATS* video-assisted thoracoscopic sympathicotomy, *CS* compensatory sweating, *GS* gustatory sweating

[a]Studies including patients with FH without providing data on their outcome and studies with less than 20 patients have been omitted

[b]Sympathicotomy: severing the corresponding ganglia via diathermy or harmonic scalpel; sympathectomy: removing of corresponding ganglia

[c]Satisfy: satisfied and satisfaction, respectively

[d]FH + FB

Table 29.5 Overview of studies dealing with endoscopic thoracic sympathectomy for vascular disorders

Year	Author	Key disease	No. of patients	No. of limbs	Level of surgery	Follow-up (months)	Immediate success (%)	Follow-up success (%)
1977	Fritsch [48]	Primary Raynaud	17	n.r.	T2–T5	120 (Max)	n.r.	35
		Secondary Raynaud	28	n.r.	T2–T5	120 (Max)	n.r.	46
		Scleroderma	4	n.r.	T2–T5	120 (Max)	n.r.	0
1978	Rösner [137]	Secondary Raynaud	23	36	T2–T5	72 (Max)	n.r.	35
1978	Sebesteny [142]	Primary Raynaud	62	83	T2–T3	276 (Max)	n.r.	65
		Thromboangiitis obliterans	23	25	T2–T3	276 (Max)	n.r.	48
		Arterial occlusion	31	31	T2–T3	276 (Max)	n.r.	73
1981	Mattassi [110]	Primary Raynaud	47	70	n.r.	132 (Max)	n.r.	52
		Scleroderma	16	27	n.r.	132 (Max)	n.r.	6
		Arterial occlusion	16	18	n.r.	132 (Max)	n.r.	94
1987	Skotnicki [144]	Primary Raynaud	25	35	T1–T4/5	107 (Mean)	89	51
		Arterial occlusion	14	19	T1–T4/5	96 (Mean)	100	53
2002	Matsumoto [109]	Secondary Raynaud	28	54	T2–T4	63 (Mean)	93	89
2004	Andrijevskikh [5]	Primary Raynaud	32	47	n.r.	120 (Max)	100	n.r.
		Secondary Raynaud	248	298	n.r.	120 (Max)	100	n.r.
		Arterial occlusion	393	427	n.r.	120 (Max)	100	n.r.
2006	Thune [155]	Primary Raynaud	19	n.r.	T2–T3/4	36 (Max)	58	n.r.
		Secondary Raynaud	15	n.r.	T2–T3/4	36 (Max)	93	n.r.
		Primary and secondary Reynaud	34	n.r.	T2–T3/4	36 (Max)	83	60

Studies including less than a total of 20 patients with vascular disorders and those providing no essential data on the outcome have been omitted
n.r. not reported

Complication rates in patients with vascular disorders do not differ from that in primary hyperhidrotics and blushers [115]. Careful patient selection, however, is a prerequisite to obtain such results. Moreover, an adequate training in sympathetic surgery as well as in thoracic surgery should be demanded. Drawbacks of ETS surgery include open revisions due to major injury of subclavian vessels and the brachial plexus. Although no deaths have been reported in surgical series, one author described nine anecdotal fatalities from personal communications: five resulted from major bleeding and three from anesthetic mishaps (Cameron A: Specific complications and mortality of endoscopic thoracic sympathectomy [16, 123]).

29.6.5 Side Effects

29.6.5.1 Compensatory Hyperhidrosis

Compensatory sweating (CS) is the most frequent and most impairing side effect after sympathetic surgery. Usually patients suffer from sweating attacks on the trunk, primarily the chest, the back, the abdomen, and the thighs. Less frequently the feet, armpits, or the face are involved. Rates of CS are given from 0% to 100% according to the type of evaluation [56]. Different forms of CS should be evaluated separately: first those with aggravated sweating, meaning an increased sweating under certain circumstances (physical stress including sports or hot environment). This form of CS can be found more or less in all operated patients. Secondly, patients can report increased sweating without any stressors in other body regions than those initially operated for. Finally, there are patients suffering from unbearable, extreme CS causing social stigmatization and retreat from working life due to recurrent illness. These patients usually regret having undergone the operation. In our own series of T2 to T4 sympathicotomies for upper limb hyperhidrosis, we found 55% suffering from CS and 5% being affected by the extreme form [116, 118].

Traditionally, sympathectomy or sympathicotomy comprised the thoracic sympathetic ganglion T2 down to T3/T4 for palmar hyperhidrosis [56, 98, 116], and it was assumed that T4 or even T5 should be included in cases of axillary HH [101, 116]. T2 has been considered as "key ganglion" for the palms. In recent years, "limited sympathectomy" has increasingly gained attention, as it was suggested that the severity of CS is correlated with the number of ablated or resected ganglia [61]. This claim has been recently supported by several papers [82, 110, 117, 159] including a prospective randomized controlled trial, which reported rates of 3% severe CS after T3 versus 10% after T2–T4 ablation [88].

In 2001, Lin and Telaranta [93] presented a new classification. According to their hypothesis, reflex sweating – as they termed compensatory sweating – may be caused by the interruption of afferent sympathetic fibers to the anterior portion of the hypothalamus when the sympathetic trunk is severed at the level of T2 and T3. Consequently, they assumed that CS can be prevented by severing T4 solely [94]. Promising initial results [20, 93] were confirmed by our own group [118, 125]. Although a review published in 2008 concluded that there was no evidence that lowering the level of sympathetic surgery results in less CS [78], further studies support this theory [17, 77].

In our own series including a follow-up of more than 5 years, CS rates were 17% after T4 clamping for upper limb hyperhidrosis, 54% after T3 for facial hyperhidrosis, and 43% after T2 clamping for blushing. Unbearable CS rates were 1% after T4 clamping and 8% after T3 and T2 clamping. There is some evidence that side effects may be worse in patients treated for facial symptoms [65, 83, 130]. Moreover, Reisfeld speculated that the clamping method (clip application) by itself contributes to lower rates of CS, although further studies are needed. Besides multiple-level chain division, greater body mass index and older age have been detected as independent predictors for CS [111].

29.6.5.2 Gustatory Hyperhidrosis

Gustatory sweating (GS) defined as facial sweating after smelling or eating spicy food is another unwanted side effect of sympathetic surgery although less frequently reported. There is no generally accepted pathophysiologic explanation, but the theory explained in the "Physiology" section above seems convincing. Licht reported that 32% of patients were affected by GS and that GS was significantly associated with the extent of sympathectomy [90]. In our series of patients, rates of GS were similar: 33% after T2–T4 sympathicotomy [118] and 32% after limited T4 block [120]. In patients with facial blushing (treated by T3 block), GS rates were 22% and in those with erythrophobia 38% after T2 block. After resection of the lower third of the stellate ganglion and T2 to T5 resection for facial blushing, other authors reported GS in 38% [168]. In summary, the presence of GS is found to be of less importance compared to CS, as patients usually do not feel impaired by this side effect.

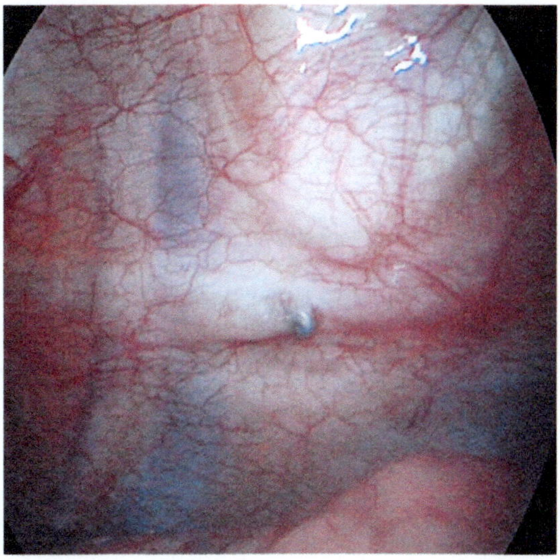

Fig. 29.8 Intrathoracic view during reversal surgery 3 months after primary operation. The clip can well be visualized

29.6.6 Reoperations

29.6.6.1 Reversal Procedures

Operative procedures aiming to reverse the effect of sympathetic surgery have been developed, but are still infrequently needed. Usually they are performed because of severe, unbearable compensatory sweating. Clip removals after endoscopic sympathetic block can be differentiated from surgical techniques aiming to reconstruct the sympathetic chain.

Clip Removals

The introduction of clip application instead of electrocautery for interruption of the sympathetic chain was a further approach to deal with unsatisfied patients due to severe CS [95]. The thoracoscopic procedure of clip removal has been shown to be technically feasible in specialized centers without a higher complication rate than the primary ETS operation [94, 97, 98, 130]. Figure 29.8 depicts the typical thoracoscopic view in a patient 3 months after clip application. Pleural adhesions of the lung are hardly ever seen. The largest series including 34 patients with clip removals after a median of 11 months after clip application was recently published by Sugimura et al. [150]. There was a trend toward fewer subsequent reversal procedures after T3–T4 clip applications compared to T2–T3 and T2 procedures. 48% of patients showed a substantial decrease in CS, and 42% had their initial hyperhidrotic areas well controlled after reversal. There was, however, no significant relationship between the original level of clipping and the interval between clip application and subsequent clip removal and reversibility of symptoms. Others reported improvement of CS in about 60–70% of patients without providing detailed data [130].

Sympathetic Chain Reconstruction

Telaranta first reported in 1998 that reconstruction of the sympathetic chain using a sural nerve graft reduced compensatory sweating in a male patient who underwent sympathicotomy for palmar hyperhidrosis [151]. The intercostal nerve was used as a donor nerve for reinnervation of the sympathetic trunk by Miura et al. [112]. Recently, Haam et al. reported on thoracoscopic sympathetic nerve reconstruction using intercostal nerves in 19 patients with severe compensatory hyperhidrosis after ETS surgery [54]. The median interval between the initial operation and sympathetic nerve reconstruction was 47 months. CS improved in 9 of the 19 patients (47.4%), and 3 out of them (15.8%) had markedly improved symptoms [54].

29.6.6.2 Reoperations and Recurrences

Redo surgery is usually performed because of primary failures or recurrences after sympathetic surgery. For palmar hyperhidrosis, primary failures and early recurrences are reported in 1.9–16% after ETS and in up to 65% for axillary hyperhidrosis [108]. Singh et al. emphasized that the main reason for persisting sympathetic activity is a "misinterpretation" of the sympathetic chain by the surgeon [143]. Other reasons for failed surgery are thought to be nerve regeneration or alternate neural pathways [108, 143]. Most frequently pleural adhesions followed by incorrect identification of the T2 ganglion and vessels overriding the sympathetic trunk have been blamed for technical failures [98]. Pronounced subpleural fatty tissue may be another reason for a low recognizability of the sympathetic trunk [69, 108]. Clip slipping has been reported as the main cause for regeneration after clamping procedures in more than 30% of cases [75]. Nevertheless, resympathectomy can be performed with good results for palmar as well as for axillary hyperhidrosis. Morbidity does not increase compared to primary operations [62, 169]. It is important to inform patients that unilateral technical failures occur and that in such cases CS may worsen after reoperations [92]. Endothoracic redo procedures, however, are technically more demanding and require an adequate experience of the sympathetic surgeon [169].

Conclusions

ETS surgery offers an effective treatment option for patients suffering from primary hyperhidrosis. Also facial blushing and various vascular disorders can be ameliorated. A thorough work-up should rule out secondary causes of hyperhidrosis. When conservative treatments fail, different surgical techniques can be performed by videothoracoscopy with low complication rates. Resection, transsection, or clip application on the upper thoracic sympathetic chain have been shown to be similarly successful in over 90%. The clipping method offers the potential of reversal surgery primarily for patients who suffer from unbearable compensatory sweating. This side effect of ETS surgery is frequently observed, but diminishes quality of life in only 5% of patients. Intra- and postoperative complications are rare, but can be life threatening. Adequate training of surgeons, informed consent of patients, and postoperative follow-up are mandatory.

Acknowledgment The authors want to thank c.m. Catherine Novak for her support in editing the manuscript and providing tables and reference list.

References

1. Adair A, George ML, Camprodon R et al (2005) Endoscopic sympathectomy in the treatment of facial blushing. Ann R Coll Surg Engl 87:358–360
2. Adson AW, Brown GE (1929) Raynaud's disease of the upper extremities; successful treatment by resection of the sympathetic cervicothoracic and second thoracic ganglions and the intervening trunk. JAMA 92:444–449
3. Alexander W (1889) The treatment of epilepsy. Y J Pentland, Edinburgh
4. Ambrogi V, Campione E, Mineo D et al (2009) Bilateral thoracoscopic T2 to T3 sympathectomy versus botulinum injection in palmar hyperhidrosis. Ann Thorac Surg 88:238–245
5. Andrievskikh IA, Fokin AA (2004) Multiyear experience in endoscopic thoracic sympathectomy. Angiol Sosud Khir 10:99–104
6. Assalia A, Bahouth H, Ilivitzki A et al (2007) Thoracoscopic sympathectomy for primary palmar hyperhidrosis: resection versus transaction – a prospective trial. World J Surg 31:1976–1979
7. Atkins HJB (1954) Sympathectomy by the axillary approach. Lancet 1:538–539
8. Bahmer FA (1999) Wound measurement made truly simple by point counting. Arch Dermatol 135:991–992
9. Bechara FG, Sand M, Hoffmann K et al (2008) Aggressive shaving after combined liposuction and curettage for axillary hyperhidrosis leads to more complications without further benefit. Dermatol Surg 34:952–953
10. Black SA, Taylor FG, Russell MH et al (2008) Thorascopic sympathectomy performed using laser. Ann R Coll Surg Engl 90:142–145
11. Block JA, Sequeira W (2001) Raynaud's phenomenon. Lancet 357:2042–2048
12. Bogoch ER, Gross DK (2005) Surgery of the hand in patients with systemic sclerosis: outcomes and considerations. J Rheumatol 32:642–648
13. Brüning F, Stahl O (1923) Über die psychologische Wirkung der Exstirpation des periarteriellen sym-

pathischen Nervengeflechtes. Klin Wochenschr 1:1402–1403
14. Burch GE, Kones RJ (1973) Essential hyperhidrosis – correlation of digital blood flow and capillary ultrastructure after unilateral sympathectomy. Am J Med 54:378–388
15. Callejas MA, Rubio M, Iglesias M et al (2004) Video-assisted thoracoscopic sympathectomy for the treatment of facial blushing: ultrasonic scalpel versus diathermy. Arch Bronconeumol 40:17–19
16. Cameron AE (2003) Specific complications and mortality of endoscopic thoracic sympathectomy. Clin Auton Res 13(Suppl 1):I31–I35
17. Chang YT, Li HP, Lee JY et al (2007) Treatment of palmar hyperhidrosis: T(4) level compared with T(3) and T(2). Ann Surg 246:330–336
18. Chen HJ, Lu K, Liang CL (2001) Transthoracic endoscopic T-2,3 sympathectomy for facial hyperhidrosis. Auton Neurosci 93:91–94
19. Chen YB, Ye W, Yang WT et al (2009) Uniportal versus biportal video-assisted thoracoscopic sympathectomy for palmar hyperhidrosis. Chin Med J 122:1525–1528
20. Chou SH, Kao EL, Lin CC et al (2006) The importance of classification in sympathetic surgery and a proposed mechanism for compensatory hyperhidrosis: experience with 464 cases. Surg Endosc 20:1749–1753
21. Chu D, Chen RC, Lee CH et al (2010) Incidence and frequency of endoscopic sympathectomy for the treatment of hyperhidrosis palmaris in Taiwan. Kaohsiung J Med Sci 26:123–129
22. Chuang KS, Liu JC (2002) Long-term assessment of percutaneous stereotactic thermocoagulation of upper thoracic ganglionectomy and sympathectomy for palmar and craniofacial hyperhidrosis in 1742 cases. Neurosurgery 51:963–969
23. Chung L (2007) Therapeutic options for digital ulcers in patients with systemic sclerosis. J Dtsch Dermatol Ges 5:460–465
24. Claes G (2003) Indications for endoscopic thoracic sympathectomy. Clin Auton Res 13(Suppl 1):I16–I19
25. Claes G, Drott C, Göthberg G (1993) Thoracoscopy for autonomic disorders. Ann Thorac Surg 56:715–716
26. Claes G, Drott C, Göthberg G (1994) Thoracoscopic sympathicotomy for arterial insufficiency. Eur J Surg Suppl 572:63–64
27. Clara M (1959) Das Nervensystem des Menschen: ein Lehrbuch für Studierende und Ärzte, 3rd edn. Barth, Leipzig
28. Cloward RB (1969) Hyperhidrosis. J Neurosurg 30:545–551
29. Coelho Mde S, Silva RF, Mezzalira G et al (2009) T3T4 endoscopic sympathetic blockade versus T3T4 video thoracoscopic sympathectomy in the treatment of axillary hyperhidrosis. Ann Thorac Surg 88:1780–1785
30. Cohen JL, Solish N (2003) Treatment of hyperhidrosis with botulinum toxin. Facial Plast Surg Clin North Am 11:493–502
31. Cohen RD (1999) Validation of health-related quality of life instruments. Hepatology 29(Suppl 6):7S–8S
32. Davidson JRT, Foa EB, Connor KM et al (2002) Hyperhidrosis in social anxiety disorder. Prog Neuro Psychopharm 26:1327–1331
33. De Campos JR, Kauffmann P, Werebe Ede C et al (2003) Quality of life, before and after thoracic sympathectomy: report on 378 operated patients. Ann Thorac Surg 76:886–891
34. De Campos JR, Wolosker N, Yazbek G et al (2010) Comparison of pain severity following video-assisted thoracoscopic sympathectomy: electric versus harmonic scalpels. Interact Cardiovasc Thorac Surg 10:919–922
35. De Giacomo T, Rendina EA, Venuta F et al (2002) Thoracoscopic sympathectomy for symptomatic arterial obstruction of the upper extremities. Ann Thorac Surg 74:885–888
36. De Paepe K, Houben E, Adam R et al (2005) Validation of the VapoMeter, a closed unventilated chamber system to assess transepidermal water loss vs. the open chamber Tewameter. Skin Res Technol 11:61–69
37. Dohn DF, Sava GM (1978) Sympathectomy for vascular syndromes and hyperhidrosis of the upper extremities. Clin Neurosurg 25:637–650
38. Dondelinger RF, Kurdziel JC (1987) Percutaneous phenol block of the upper thoracic sympathetic chain with computed tomography guidance. A new technique. Acta Radiol 28:511–515
39. Doolabh N, Horswell S, Williams M et al (2004) Thoracoscopic sympathectomy for hyperhidrosis: indications and results. Ann Thorac Surg 77:410–414
40. Drott C, Claes G, Olsson-Rex L et al (1998) Successful treatment of facial blushing by endoscopic transthoracic sympathicotomy. Br J Dermatol 138:639–643
41. Drott C, Claes G, Rex L (2002) Facial blushing treated by sympathetic denervation – longlasting benefits in 831 patients. J Cosmet Dermatol 1:115–119
42. Duarte JB, Kux P (1998) Improvements in video-endoscopic sympathicotomy for the treatment of palmar, axillary, facial, and palmar-plantar hyperhidrosis. Eur J Surg Suppl 580:9–11
43. Duarte JB, Kux P (2001) Efficacy of endoscopic thoracic sympathicotomy along with severing the Kuntz nerve in the treatment of chronic non-infectious rhinitis. Ann Chir Gynaecol 90:189–192
44. Eilenberg WH (2010) Topographic anatomy of the upper thoracic sympathetic chain. Thesis, Medical University of Vienna, Vienna
45. Fiorelli A, Vicidomini G, Laperuta P et al (2010) Pre-emptive local analgesia in video-assisted thoracic surgery sympathectomy. Eur J Cardiothorac Surg 37:588–593
46. Fischel R, Cooper M, Kramer D (2003) Microinvasive resectional sympathectomy using the harmonic scalpel. Clin Auton Res 13(Suppl 1):I66–I70

47. Francois-Franck M (1899) Signification physiologique de la resection du sympathique dans la maladie de Basedow, l'epilepsie, l'idiotie et le glaucome. Bull Acad Med Paris 41:565–594
48. Fritsch A, Kokoschka R, Kux M et al (1977) Spätergebnisse der thorakoskopischen Sympathikotomie bei Durchblutungsstörungen der oberen Extremität. Vasa 6:56–58
49. Gardner WJ (1966) Cross talk – the paradoxical transmission of a nerve impulse. Arch Neurol 14:149–156
50. Gjerris F, Olesen HP (1975) Palmar hyperhidrosis. Long-term results following high thoracic sympathectomy. Acta Neurol Scand 51:167–172
51. Goetz RH, Marr JAS (1944) The importance of the second thoracic ganglion for the sympathetic supply of the upper extremities-two new approaches for its removal. Clin Proc 3:102–114
52. Guyatt GH, Feeny DH, Patrick DL (1993) Measuring health-related quality of life. Ann Intern Med 118:622–629
53. Guyatt GH, Naylor DC, Juniper E et al (1997) Users' guides to the medical literature: XII. How to use articles about health-related quality of life. JAMA 277:1232–1237
54. Haam SJ, Park SY, Paik HC et al (2010) Sympathetic nerve reconstruction for compensatory hyperhidrosis after sympathetic surgery for primary hyperhidrosis. J Korean Med Sci 25:597–601
55. Hashmonai M, Kopelman D, Kein O et al (1992) Upper thoracic sympathectomy for primary palmar hyperhidrosis: long-term follow-up. Br J Surg 79:268–271
56. Hashmonai M, Assalia A, Kopelman D (2001) Thoracoscopic sympathectomy for palmar hyperhidrosis. Ablate or resect? Surg Endosc 15:435–441
57. Haxton HA (1949) Chemical sympathectomy. Br Med J 1:1026–1028
58. Herbst F, Plas EG, Függer R et al (1994) Endoscopic thoracic sympathectomy for primary hyperhidrosis of the upper limbs. A critical analysis and long-term results of 480 operations. Ann Surg 220:86–90
59. Heuberger J, Furrer M, Habicht J et al (2000) Indikationen und Ergebnisse der videothorakoskopischen Sympathektomie. Dtsch Med Wochenschr 125:817–821
60. Hirschl M, Hirschl K, Lenz M et al (2006) Transition from primary Raynaud's phenomenon to secondary Raynaud's phenomenon identified by diagnosis of an associated disease: results of ten years of prospective surveillance. Arthritis Rheum 54:1974–1981
61. Hsia JY, Chen CY, Hsu CP et al (1999) Outpatient thoracoscopic limited sympathectomy for hyperhidrosis palmaris. Ann Thorac Surg 67:258–259
62. Hsu CP, Chen CY, Hsia JY et al (1998) Resympathectomy for palmar and axillary hyperhidrosis. Br J Surg 85:1504–1505
63. Hughes J (1942) Endothoracic sympathectomy. Proc R Soc Med 35:585–586
64. Jaboulay M (1900) Chirurgie du grand sympathique et du corps thyroide. A. Storck & Cie, Lyon
65. Jaffer U, Weedon K, Cameron AE (2007) Factors affecting outcome following endoscopic thoracic sympathectomy. Br J Surg 94:1108–1112
66. Jeganathan R, Jordan S, Jones M et al (2008) Bilateral thoracoscopic sympathectomy: results and long-term follow up. Interact Cardiovasc Thorac Surg 7:67–70
67. Jonnesco T (1896) Resectia totala si bilaterala a simpaticuliu cervical in cazuri de epilepsiesi gusa exophtalmica. Rom Med 4:479–496
68. Kamolz T, Pointner R (1998) Quality of life-a factor of medical outcome in surgery. Eur Surg Acta Chir Austriaca 30:355–359
69. Kao MC, Tsai JC, Lai DM et al (1994) Autonomic activities in hyperhidrosis patients before, during, and after endoscopic laser sympathectomy. Neurosurgery 34:262–268
70. Kao MC, Chen YL, Lin JY et al (1996) Endoscopic sympathectomy treatment for craniofacial hyperhidrosis. Arch Surg 131:1091–1096
71. Karsai S, Raulin C (2009) Current evidence on the unit equivalence of different botulinum neurotoxin A formulations and recommendations for clinical practice in dermatology. Dermatol Surg 35:1–8
72. Kaufmann H, Saadia D, Polin C et al (2003) Primary hyperhidrosis: evidence for autosomal dominant inheritance. Clin Auton Res 13:96–98
73. Keller SM, Bello R, Vibert B et al (2009) Diagnosis of palmar hyperhidrosis via questionnaire without physical examination. Clin Auton Res 19:175–181
74. Kim DH, Paik HC, Lee DY (2004) Comparative analysis of T2 selective division of rami-communicantes (ramicotomy) with T2 sympathetic clipping in the treatment of craniofacial hyperhidrosis. Eur J Cardiothorac Surg 26:396–400
75. Kim DH, Paik HC, Lee DY (2005) Video assisted thoracoscopic re-sympathetic surgery in the treatment of re-sweating hyperhidrosis. Eur J Cardiothorac Surg 27:741–744
76. Kim J, Henderson RA, Pocock SJ et al (2005) Health-related quality of life after interventional or conservative strategy in patients with unstable angina or non-ST-segment elevation myocardial infarction. J Am Coll Cardiol 45:221–228
77. Kim WO, Kil HK, Yoon KB et al (2010) Influence of T3 or T4 sympathicotomy for palmar hyperhidrosis. Am J Surg 199:166–169
78. Kopelman D, Hashmonai M (2008) The correlation between the method of sympathetic ablation for palmar hyperhidrosis and the occurrence of compensatory hyperhidrosis: a review. World J Surg 32:2343–2356
79. Kotzareff A (1920) Resection partielle du tronc sympathique cervical droit pour hyperhidrose unilaterale. Rev Med Suisse Romande 40:111–113
80. Kreyden OP, Scheidegger EP (2004) Anatomy of the sweat glands, pharmacology of botulinum toxin, and

distinctive syndromes associated with hyperhidrosis. Clin Dermatol 22:40–44
81. Kuntz A (1953) The autonomic nervous system. Lea & Febiger, Philadelphia
82. Kux E (1951) The endoscopic approach to the vegetative nervous system and its therapeutic possibilities. Dis Chest 20:139–147
83. Kwong KF, Hobbs JL, Cooper LB et al (2008) Stratified analysis of clinical outcomes in thoracoscopic sympathicotomy for hyperhidrosis. Ann Thorac Surg 85:390–393
84. Lazarides MK, Georgiadis GS, Papas TT et al (2006) Diagnostic criteria and treatment of Buerger's disease: a review. Int J Low Extrem Wounds 5:89–95
85. Leary MR, Britt TW, Cutlip WD II et al (1992) Social blushing. Psychol Bull 112:446–460
86. Lee DY, Hong YJ, Shin HK (1999) Thoracoscopic sympathetic surgery for hyperhidrosis. Yonsei Med J 40:589–595
87. Leriche R (1939) The surgery of pain. Bailliere, Tindall & Cox, London
88. Li X, Tu YR, Lin M et al (2008) Endoscopic thoracic sympathectomy for palmar hyperhidrosis: a randomized control trial comparing T3 and T2–4 ablation. Ann Thorac Surg 85:1747–1751
89. Licht PB, Pilegaard HK (2004) Severity of compensatory sweating after thoracoscopic sympathectomy. Ann Thorac Surg 78:427–431
90. Licht PB, Pilegaard HK (2006) Gustatory side effects after thoracoscopic sympathectomy. Ann Thorac Surg 81:1043–1047
91. Licht PB, Ladegaard L, Pilegaard HK (2006) Thoracoscopic sympathectomy for isolated facial blushing. Ann Thorac Surg 81:1863–1866
92. Licht PB, Clausen A, Ladegaard L (2010) Resympathicotomy. Ann Thorac Surg 89:1087–1090
93. Lin CC, Telaranta T (2001) Lin-Telaranta classification: the importance of different procedures for different indications in sympathetic surgery. Ann Chir Gynaecol 90:161–166
94. Lin CC, Wu HH (2001) Kuntz's fiber: the scapegoat of surgical failure in sympathetic surgery. Ann Chir Gynaecol 90:170–171
95. Lin CC, Mo LR, Lee LS et al (1998) Thoracoscopic T2-sympathetic block by clipping – a better and reversible operation for treatment of hyperhidrosis palmaris: experience with 326 cases. Eur J Surg Suppl 580:13–16
96. Lin CL, Yen CP, Howng SL (1999) The long-term results of upper dorsal sympathetic ganglionectomy and endoscopic thoracic sympathectomy for palmar hyperhidrosis. Surg Today 29:209–213
97. Lin TS (2001) Endoscopic clipping in video-assisted thoracoscopic sympathetic blockade for axillary hyperhidrosis. An analysis of 26 cases. Surg Endosc 15:126–128
98. Lin TS (2001) Video-assisted thoracoscopic "resympathicotomy" for palmar hyperhidrosis: analysis of 42 cases. Ann Thorac Surg 72:895–898
99. Lin TS, Chou MC (2002) Needlescopic thoracic sympathetic block by clipping for craniofacial hyperhidrosis: an analysis of 28 cases. Surg Endosc 16:1055–1058
100. Lin TS, Fang HY (2000) Transthoracic endoscopic sympathectomy for craniofacial hyperhidrosis: analysis of 46 cases. J Laparoendosc Adv Surg Tech A 10:243–247
101. Lin TS, Kuo SJ, Chou MC (2002) Uniportal endoscopic thoracic sympathectomy for treatment of palmar and axillary hyperhidrosis: analysis of 2000 cases. Neurosurgery 51(Suppl 5):S84–S87
102. Liu Y, Yang J, Liu J et al (2009) Surgical treatment of primary palmar hyperhidrosis: a prospective randomized study comparing T3 and T4 sympathicotomy. Eur J Cardiothorac Surg 35:398–402
103. Lowe N, Campanati A, Bodokh I et al (2004) The place of botulinum toxin type A in the treatment of focal hyperhidrosis. Br J Dermatol 151:1115–1122
104. Lowell RC, Gloviczki P, Cherry KJ Jr et al (1993) Cervicothoracic sympathectomy for Raynaud's syndrome. Int Angiol 12:168–172
105. Macdonald L, Bruce J, Scott NW et al (2005) Long-term follow-up of breast cancer survivors with post-mastectomy pain syndrome. Br J Cancer 92:225–230
106. Malcolm B, Carpenter JS (1983) The autonomic nervous system. In: Malcolm B, Carpenter JS (eds) Human neuroanatomy. Williams and Wilkins, Baltimore/London
107. Marhold F, Neumayer C, Tschabitscher M (2005) The sympathetic trunk and its neural pathway to the upper limb: review of the literature. Eur Surg 37:114–120
108. Marhold F, Izay B, Zacherl J et al (2008) Thoracoscopic and anatomic landmarks of Kuntz's nerve: implications for sympathetic surgery. Ann Thorac Surg 86:1653–1658
109. Matsumoto Y, Ueyama T, Endo M et al (2002) Endoscopic thoracic sympathicotomy for Raynaud's phenomenon. J Vasc Surg 36:57–61
110. Mattassi R, Miele F, D'Angelo F (1981) Thoracic sympathectomy. Review of indications, results and surgical techniques. J Cardiovasc Surg 22:336–339
111. Miller DL, Bryant AS, Force SD et al (2009) Effect of sympathectomy level on the incidence of compensatory hyperhidrosis after sympathectomy for palmar hyperhidrosis. J Thorac Cardiovasc Surg 138:581–585
112. Miura J, Doita M, Miyata K et al (2003) Horner's syndrome caused by a thoracic dumbbell-shaped schwannoma: sympathetic chain reconstruction after a one-stage removal of the tumor. Spine 28:33–36
113. Nauta WJH (1958) Hippocampal projections and related neural pathways to the midbrain in the cat. Brain 81:319–340
114. Nauta WJH (1972) The central visceromotor system: a general survey. In: Hockman CH (ed) Limbic system mechanisms and autonomic functions. Charles C Thomas, Springfield, pp 21–33

115. Neumayer C (2010) Effect of endoscopic thoracic sympathectomy on vascular disorders. In: Frezza EE, Gagner M, Li MKW (eds) International principles of laparoscopic surgery. Ciné-Med, Woodbury
116. Neumayer C, Bischof G, Függer R et al (2001) Efficacy and safety of thoracoscopic sympathicotomy for hyperhidrosis of the upper limb. Results of 734 sympathicotomies. Ann Chir Gynaecol 90:195–199
117. Neumayer C, Zacherl J, Holak G et al (2003) Experience with limited endoscopic thoracic sympathetic block for hyperhidrosis and facial blushing. Clin Auton Res 13(Suppl 1):I52–I57
118. Neumayer C, Zacherl J, Holak G et al (2004) Limited endoscopic thoracic sympathetic block for hyperhidrosis of the upper limb: reduction of compensatory sweating by clipping T4. Surg Endosc 18:152–156
119. Neumayer C, Panhofer P, Jakesz R et al (2005) Surgical treatment of facial hyperhidrosis and blushing: mid-term results after endoscopic sympathetic block and review of the literature. Eur Surg 37:127–136
120. Neumayer C, Panhofer P, Zacherl J et al (2005) Effect of endoscopic thoracic sympathetic block on plantar hyperhidrosis. Arch Surg 140:676–680
121. Nicholson ML, Dennis MJ, Hopkinson BR (1994) Endoscopic transthoracic sympathectomy: successful in hyperhidrosis but can the indications be extended? Ann R Coll Surg Engl 76:311–314
122. Ogawa T (1975) Thermal influence on palmar sweating and mental influence on generalized sweating in man. Jpn J Physiol 25:525–536
123. Ojimba TA, Cameron AE (2004) Drawbacks of endoscopic thoracic sympathectomy. Br J Surg 91:264–269
124. Panhofer P, Neumayer C, Zacherl J et al (2005) A survey and validation guide for health-related quality-of-life status in surgical treatment of hyperhidrosis. Eur Surg 37:143–152
125. Panhofer P, Zacherl J, Jakesz R et al (2006) Improved quality of life after sympathetic block for upper limb hyperhidrosis. Br J Surg 93:582–586
126. Pohjavaara P, Telaranta T (2005) Endoscopic sympathetic block as treatment of social phobia. Eur Surg 37:137–142
127. Pohjavaara P, Telaranta T, Väisänen E (2003) The role of the sympathetic nervous system in anxiety: is it possible to relieve anxiety with endoscopic sympathetic block? Nord J Psychiatry 57:55–60
128. Raisman G (1966) Neural connexions of hypothalamus. Br Med Bull 22:197–201
129. Rathinam S, Nanjaiah P, Sivalingam S et al (2008) Excision of sympathetic ganglia and the rami communicantes with histological confirmation offers better early and late outcomes in video assisted thoracoscopic sympathectomy. J Cardiothorac Surg 3:50
130. Reisfeld R (2006) Sympathectomy for hyperhidrosis: should we place the clamps at T2-T3 or T3-T4? Clin Auton Res 16:384–389
131. Reisfeld R, Nguyen R, Pnini A (2000) Endoscopic thoracic sympathectomy for treatment of essential hyperhidrosis syndrome: experience with 650 patients. Surg Laparosc Endosc Percutan Tech 10:5–10
132. Reisfeld R, Nguyen R, Pnini A (2002) Endoscopic thoracic sympathectomy for hyperhidrosis: experience with both cauterization and clamping methods. Surg Laparosc Endosc Percutan Tech 12:255–267
133. Rex LO, Drott C, Claes G et al (1998) The Boras experience of endoscopic thoracic sympathicotomy for palmar, axillary, facial hyperhidrosis and facial blushing. Eur J Surg Suppl 580:23–26
134. Rieger R, Pedevilla S (2007) Retroperitoneoscopic lumbar sympathectomy for the treatment of plantar hyperhidrosis: technique and preliminary findings. Surg Endosc 21:129–135
135. Ro KM, Cantor KM, Lange KL et al (2002) Palmar hyperhidrosis: evidence of genetic transmission. J Vasc Surg 35:382–386
136. Rompel R, Scholz S (2001) Subcutaneous curettage vs. injection of botulinum toxin A for treatment of axillary hyperhidrosis. J Eur Acad Dermatol Venereol 15:207–211
137. Rösner K, Goldberg S (1978) Der Stellenwert der thorakoskopischen Sympathikotomie bei der Behandlung des Raynaud-Syndromes. Z Gesamte Inn Med 34:127–128
138. Royle ND (1924) The treatment of spastic paralysis by sympathetic rami-section. Surg Gynecol Obstet 39:701–720
139. Sayers RD, Jenner RE, Barrie WW (1994) Transthoracic endoscopic sympathectomy for hyperhidrosis and Raynaud's phenomenon. Eur J Vasc Surg 8:627–631
140. Schliack H, Schiffter R, Goebel HH et al (1972) Untersuchungen zur Frage der Schweissdrüseninnervation im Bereich des Gesichts. Acta Anat 81:421–438
141. Sciuchetti JF, Corti F, Ballabio D et al (2008) Results, side effects and complications after thoracoscopic sympathetic block by clamping. The monza clinical experience. Clin Auton Res 18:80–83
142. Sebesteny M, Morgan I, Papp S et al (1978) Spätergebnisse der thorakalen Sympathektomie bei verschiedenen Krankheitsbildern. Acta Chir Acad Sci Hung 19:69–74
143. Singh B, Moodley J, Ramdial PK et al (2001) Pitfalls in thoracoscopic sympathectomy: mechanisms for failure. Surg Laparosc Endosc Percutan Tech 11:364–367
144. Skotnicki SH, Van de Wal HJ, Lacquet LK et al (1987) Treatment of patients with Raynaud's phenomenon by thoracic sympathectomy. Vasa Suppl 18:42–47
145. Solish N, Bertucci V, Dansereau A et al (2007) A comprehensive approach to the recognition, diagnosis, and severity-based treatment of focal hyperhidrosis: recommendations of the Canadian

Hyperhidrosis Advisory Committee. Dermatol Surg 33:908–923
146. Spencer-Green G (1998) Outcomes in primary Raynaud phenomenon: a meta-analysis of the frequency, rates, and predictors of transition to secondary diseases. Arch Intern Med 158:595–600
147. Sprung HB (1951) Grundlagen der Sympathikus-Chirurgie, vol Band 35, Medizinische Praxis. Steinkopff Verlag, Dresden/Leipzig
148. Stravynski A, Greenberg D (1998) The treatment of social phobia: a critical assessment. Acta Psychiatr Scand 98:171–181
149. Strutton DR, Kowalski JW, Glaser DA et al (2004) US prevalence of hyperhidrosis and impact on individuals with axillary hyperhidrosis: results from a national survey. J Am Acad Dermatol 51:241–248
150. Sugimura H, Spratt EH, Compeau CG et al (2009) Thoracoscopic sympathetic clipping for hyperhidrosis: long-term results and reversibility. J Thorac Cardiovasc Surg 137:1370–1376
151. Telaranta T (1998) Secondary sympathetic chain reconstruction after endoscopic thoracic sympathectomy. Eur J Surg Suppl 580:17–18
152. Telaranta T (1998) Treatment of social phobia by endoscopic thoracic sympathicotomy. Eur J Surg Suppl 580:27–32
153. Telford ED (1935) The technique of sympathectomy. Br J Surg 23:448–450
154. Tetteh HA, Groth SS, Kast T et al (2009) Primary palmoplantar hyperhidrosis and thoracoscopic sympathectomy: a new objective assessment method. Ann Thorac Surg 87:267–274
155. Thune TH, Ladegaard L, Licht PB (2006) Thoracoscopic sympathectomy for Raynaud's phenomenon – a long term follow-up study. Eur J Vasc Endovasc Surg 32:198–202
156. Velanovich V (2001) The quality of quality of life studies in general surgical journals. J Am Coll Surg 193:288–296
157. Walles T, Somuncuoglu G, Steger V et al (2009) Long-term efficiency of endoscopic thoracic sympathicotomy: survey 10 years after surgery. Interact Cardiovasc Thorac Surg 8:54–57
158. Wang L, Feng G (2004) Left cardiac sympathetic denervation as the first-line therapy for congenital long QT syndrome. Med Hypotheses 63:438–441
159. Weksler B, Blaine G, Souza ZB et al (2009) Transection of more than one sympathetic chain ganglion for hyperhidrosis increases the severity of compensatory hyperhidrosis and decreases patient satisfaction. J Surg Res 156:110–115
160. Weksler B, Pollice M, Souza ZB et al (2009) Comparison of ultrasonic scalpel to electrocautery in patients undergoing endoscopic thoracic sympathectomy. Ann Thorac Surg 88:1138–1141
161. Welch E, Geary J (1984) Current status of thoracic dorsal sympathectomy. J Vasc Surg 1:202–214
162. White JC, Smithwick RH, Allen AW et al (1933) A new muscle splitting incision for resection of the upper thoracic sympathetic ganglia. Surg Gynecol Obstet 56:651–657
163. Wilkinson HA (1984) Radiofrequency percutaneous upper-thoracic sympathectomy. Technique and review of indications. N Engl J Med 311:34–38
164. Williams SJ 2nd (1986) Chronic upper extremity ischemia: current concepts in management. Surg Clin North Am 66:355–375
165. Wittmoser R (1985) Treatment of sweating and blushing by endoscopic surgery. Acta Neurochir 74:153–154
166. Wolosker N, Yazbek G, de Campos JR et al (2010) Quality of life before surgery is a predictive factor for satisfaction among patients undergoing sympathectomy to treat hyperhidrosis. J Vasc Surg 51:1190–1194
167. Yazbek G, Wolosker N, Kauffmann P et al (2009) Twenty months of evolution following sympathectomy on patients with palmar hyperhidrosis: sympathectomy at the T3 level is better than at the T2 level. Clinics 64:743–749
168. Yilmaz EN, Dur AH, Cuesta MA et al (1996) Endoscopic versus transaxillary thoracic sympathectomy for primary axillary and palmar hyperhidrosis and/or facial blushing: 5-year-experience. Eur J Cardiothorac Surg 10:168–172
169. Yim AP, Liu HP, Hazelrigg SR et al (1998) Thoracoscopic operations on reoperated chests. Ann Thorac Surg 65:328–330
170. Yoon DH, Ha Y, Park YG et al (2003) Thoracoscopic limited T-3 sympathicotomy for primary hyperhidrosis: prevention for compensatory hyperhidrosis. J Neurosurg 99(Suppl 1):39–43
171. Zacherl J, Huber ER, Imhof M et al (1998) Long-term results of 630 thoracoscopic sympathicotomies for primary hyperhidrosis: the Vienna experience. Eur J Surg Suppl 580:43–46

Video-Assisted Thoracoscopic Pericardial Window

30

Rolf G.C. Inderbitzi

Contents

30.1 Introduction

The treatment of chronic pericardial effusion depends on the underlying disease and the symptoms caused by the effusion. The latter frequently ranges from dyspnoea to orthopnoea, cough and chest pain, as well as tachycardia, tachypnoea, paradoxical pulse, hypertension and leg oedema [4, 7, 12, 15]. Making sure of the characteristics of the process is of crucial significance for choosing the therapy. If the patient does not respond to an initially administered anti-inflammatory therapy with steroids or nonsteroidal medication with close clinical checks, the next diagnostic step after non-invasive diagnostic methods have been exhausted (electrocardiography or echocardiography) is the echocardiographically guided needle biopsy, followed, if the results are unclear, by a surgical biopsy.

The diagnostic and therapeutic range of procedures for the treatment of effusion is large. It ranges from conservative concepts to pericardiocentesis [2], balloon pericardiotomy [20], subxiphoidal pericardiotomy [1, 13], thoracoscopic pericardial fenestration [6, 11, 19] to radical pericardiectomy [9].

Thoracoscopic pericardial fenestration represents a comprehensive option for simultaneous diagnosis and treatment of chronic pericardial effusion [14]; very often, pericardial effusion also occurs together with pleural effusions [16, 18].

R.G.C. Inderbitzi, M.D.
Thoraxzentrum Zurich, Hirslanden Clinic,
Witellikerstrasse 40, CH-8008
Zurich, Switzerland
e-mail: r.inderbitzi@thoraxzentrum.ch

R.G.C. Inderbitzi et al. (eds.), *Minimally Invasive Thoracic and Cardiac Surgery*,
DOI 10.1007/978-3-642-11861-6_30, © Springer-Verlag Berlin Heidelberg 2012

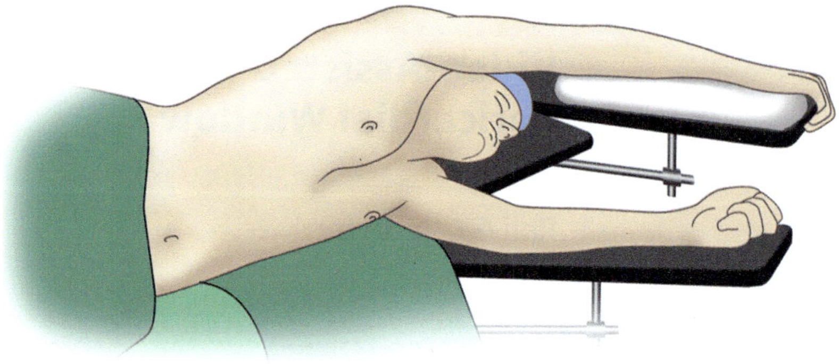

Fig. 30.1 Typical lateral decubitus of the patient for thoracoscopy

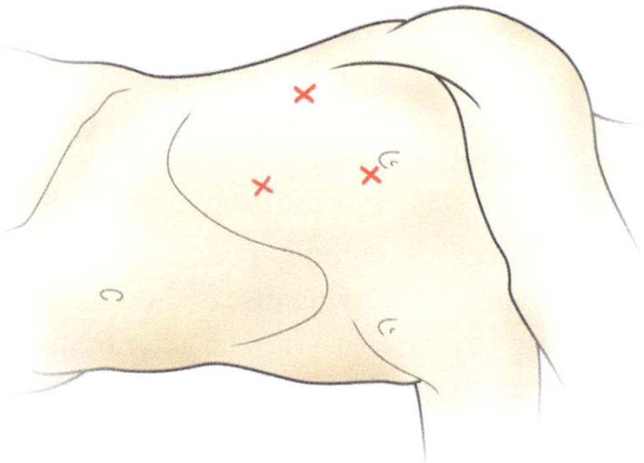

Fig. 30.2 Incisions for pericardial fenestration. Endoscope is inserted through the median. Surgeon is standing behind the patients back, screen ventrally

30.2 Surgical Technique [6]

The patient lies in the lateral decubitus position (Fig. 30.1) with tracheal intubation using a double-lumen tube. Positioning on the right or left is chosen depending on the position of the effusion; if there is no loculation in the echosonography, the preference is for the left side for the thoracoscopic approach. It is easy to identify the phrenic nerve here and the protruding heart muscle is strong. In contrast, the right side of the pericardium presents as flat, with a small diameter, and the underlying right atrium has a thin wall and is more susceptible to injury. The surgeon stands behind the patient with a view of the screen, which is positioned on the other side. The three incisions are chosen as an inverse triangle in the lower third of the thorax (cf. Fig. 30.2).

After diagnostic visual exploration of the thoracic space, the outer side of the pericardium is inspected and the phrenic nerve is defined as the lead structure. Depending on its course, the fenestration is planned to the front or back of this. The pericardium is raised using forceps and then cautiously incised. Depending on the intrapericardial pressure, fluid now trickles or flows out. This is preserved for microbiological, cytological and chemical examination, and the pericardial cavity is suctioned until it as empty as possible. The surgeon should avoid suctioning the epicardium to avoid the risk of provoking heart rhythm disorders; nevertheless, it is hard to prevent occasional supraventricular extrasystoles. A flap of the required size is then shaped (Fig. 30.3), and this is made ready for when the histological examination has been completed. The fenestration, which is of at least 3 cm^2 in size, is concluded with a thorough check on haemostasis.

The relevant half of the pericardium can be cautiously palpated through the pericardial opening with a curved palpation probe and under endoscopic guidance with rigid and flexible endoscopes to look for any adhesions. Any pathological findings are biopsied.

The procedure is completed with the placement of up to two thoracic drains and the reinflation of the lung under endoscopic guidance.

30.3 Discussion

The time for therapeutic intervention is dictated primarily by the clinical symptoms. The quantity of effusion is not the main consideration; it is the speed of its development which is of greatest importance, as a rapid increase in effusion can

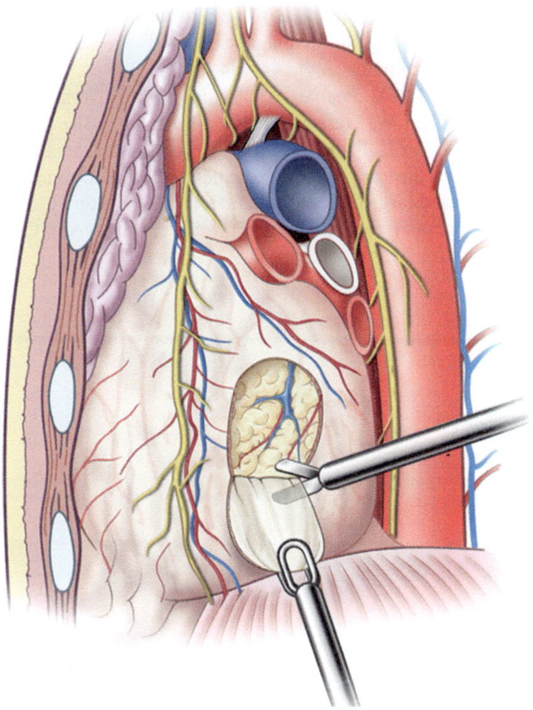

Fig. 30.3 Shaping of a flap with monopolar electric scissors, Ultracision® or by means of ordinary scissors

lead to acute tamponade [3, 4, 17]. The decision to move to an active procedure is supported by the echocardiography findings, which, based on the location and volume of the effusion, help to determine the choice of surgical technique.

With the aid of the thoracoscopy, recurrent pericardial effusions cannot only be drained under visualisation, the endoscopy also allows comprehensive diagnosis, thanks to the extensive inspection options and the targeted biopsy of pathological processes [10, 14], with an accuracy of greater than 90% for malignant effusions [8]. Without unreasonable stress, thoracoscopic pericardial fenestration is also capable of providing rapid and effective relief of symptoms for malignoma patients at an advanced stage of the disease and in severely reduced general condition, as was evidenced by the first studies of this in 1994 [5].

Technically, effusive constrictive pericarditis can make thoracoscopic opening and fenestration impossible, in spite of free access to the pericardium, as pericardial scars mean the pericardium cannot be grasped and lifted safely. In this situation, the endoscopic method does not represent a safe alternative to open pericardial fenestration, in spite of suspected effusion and information on the location from the echocardiogram.

References

1. Allen KB, Faber LP, Warren WH et al (1999) Pericardial effusion: subxiphoid pericardiostomy versus percutaneous catheter drainage. Ann Thorac Surg 67:437–440
2. Callahan JA, Seward JB, Tajik AJ, Dr H, Smith HC, Reeder GS, Milles FA (1983) Pericardiocentesis assisted by two-dimensional echocardiography. J Thorac Cardiovasc Surg 85:877–879
3. Fraser RS, Viloria JB, Wang NS (1980) Cardiac tamponade as a presentation of extracardiac malignancy. Cancer 45:1697–1704
4. Haskell RJ, French WJ (1985) Cardiac tamponade as the initial presentation of malignancy. Chest 88:70–73
5. Inderbitzi R, Grillet MP (1996) Risks and hazards of video assisted thoracic surgery (VATS): a 4 year review. Eur J Cardiothorac Surg 10:483–489
6. Inderbitzi R, Leupi F, Furrer M, Althaus U (1991) Die thorakoskopische Perikardfenestration – eine neue MethodezurBehandlungrezidivierenderPerikardergüsse. Schweiz Med Wochenschr 21(Suppl 36):27
7. Klatt EC, Heitz DR (1990) Cardiac metastases. Chest 65:1456–1459
8. Kralstein J, Frishman W (1987) Malignant pericardial diseases: diagnosis and treatment. Am Heart J 113:785–790
9. Little AG, Kremser PC, Wade JL, Levett JM, De Meester TR, Skinner DB (1984) Operation for diagnosis and treatment of pericardial effusion. Surgery 96:738–744
10. Loddenkemper R (1983) Diagnostik des Pleuraergusses. Internist Welt 10:293–301
11. Mack MJ, Landreneau RJ, Hazelrigg SR, Acuff TE (1993) Video thoracoscopic management of benign and malignant pericardial effusions. Chest 103(4 Suppl):390S–393S
12. Mather EA, Shepherd FA, Todd TJ (1996) Pericardial sclerosis as the primary management of malignant pericardial effusion and cardiac tamponade. J Thorac Cardiovasc Surg 112:637–643
13. McDonald JM, Meyers BF, Guthrie TJ, Battafarano RJ, Cooper JD, Patterson GA (2003) Comparison of open subxiphoidal pericardial drainage with percutaneous catheter drainage for symptomatic pericardial effusion. Ann Thorac Surg 76:811–815; discussion 816
14. Meyers DG, Bouska DJ (1989) Diagnostic usefulness of pericardial fluid cytology. Chest 95:1142–1143
15. Moores DW, Allen KB, Faber LP, Dziuban SW, Gillman DJ, Warren WH, Ilves R, Lininger L (1995) Subxiphoid pericardial drainage for pericardial

tamponade. J Thorac Cardiovasc Surg 109:546–551; discussion 551–552
16. Okamoto H, Shinkai T, Yamakido M, Saijo N (1993) Cardiac tamponade caused by primary lung cancer and the management of pericardial effusion. Cancer 71:93–98
17. Spodick DH (2003) Acute cardiac tamponade. N Engl J Med 349:684–690
18. Swanepoel E, Apffelstaedt JP (1997) Pericardial effusion in breast cancer: terminal event or treatable complication? J Surg Oncol 64:308–311
19. Vogel B, Mall W (1990) Thorakoskopische perikardfenestrierung – diagnostische und therapeutische aspekte. Pneumologie 44:184–185
20. Ziskind AA, Pearce AC, Lemmon CC, Burstein S, Gimple LW, Herrmann HC, McKay R, Block PC, Waldman H, Palacios IF (1993) Percutaneous balloon pericardiotomy for the treatment of cardiac tamponade and large pericardial effusion: description of technique and report of the first 50 cases. J Am Coll Cardiol 21:1–5

Part V

Minimally Invasive Thoracic Surgery: Chest Wall

Minimal-Invasive Repair of Pectus Excavatum

31

Beatrix Hoksch, Jan Siebenga, and Ralph Alexander Schmid

Contents

B. Hoksch, M.D.
Division of Thoracic Surgery, Inselspital Berne, Berne, Switzerland
e-mail: beatrix.hoksch@insel.ch

J. Siebenga, M.D. (✉)
Division of Thoracic Surgery, Department of General Surgery, Atrium Medical Centre, Henri Dunantstraat 5, Heerlen 6401 CX, The Netherlands
e-mail: j.siebenga@atriummc.nl

R.A. Schmid, M.D.
Division of General Thoracic Surgery, University Hospital Berne, Freiburgstrasse, Berne 3010, Switzerland
e-mail: ralph.schmid@insel.ch

31.1 Introduction

31.1.1 Definition

Pectus excavatum (PE) is defined as the sinking of the lower or medium portion of the sternal region in the direction of the spinal column. Pectus excavatum is also known as sunken or funnel chest (Fig. 31.1).

31.1.2 History

Since the sixteenth century, the congenital deformities of the thoracic wall have been described. Johannes Bauhinus and Johannes Schenk von Grafenberg provided the first recognized description of pectus excavatum in 1594 [20].

R.G.C. Inderbitzi et al. (eds.), *Minimally Invasive Thoracic and Cardiac Surgery*,
DOI 10.1007/978-3-642-11861-6_31, © Springer-Verlag Berlin Heidelberg 2012

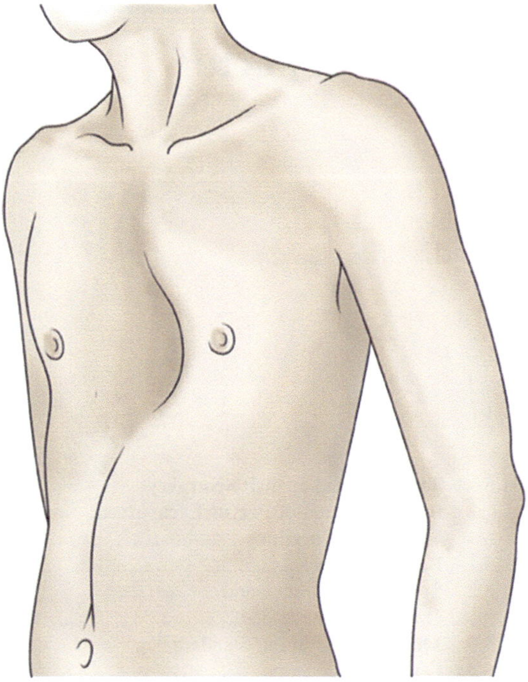

Fig. 31.1 Pectus excavatum

The term "pectus excavatum" was coined by Erich Ebstein in 1882 [12]. Mark M. Ravitch wrote in his book *Congenital Deformities of the Chest Wall and Their Operative Correction*: "We owe to the scholarship of Erich Ebstein of Leipzig the exhumation of Johannes Schenk's 1594 publication of a letter of Bauhinus concerning a case of funnel chest" [56]. First operative correction of pectus excavatum was done by Alexander Tietze in 1899. The history of pectus excavatum repair can be traced through several phases: early attempts at correction from 1911 through 1920 included complete resection of the deformed ribs and sternum (chondrosternal resection; Ludwig Meyer in Vienna 1911 and Ferdinand Sauerbruch in Berlin 1911). External traction in combination with cartilage incision/resection and sternal osteotomy was the dominating surgical method from 1921 through 1939. Mark M. Ravitch published a new operative treatment in 1949 [55]. His method, modified by Friedrich Rehbein in 1957, was the method of choice until the mid-1990s. The Ravitch technique and further modifications included: transection of or resection of distorted rib cartilages, transverse sternotomy, and adequate lifting and stabilization of the anterior chest wall. Since the end of the 1990s, the management of pectus excavatum has undergone major changes [48].

31.1.3 Epidemiology of Pectus Excavatum

Pectus excavatum accounts for 90% of congenital chest wall deformities. It affects 1 in 400 to 1 in 1,000 live births. The deformity is four times more frequent among males than females [8, 9].

In most cases, the deformity is discovered within the first year of life. The deformity appears initially or becomes more prominent during growth spurts [59]. Deterioration of the chest's appearance is usually reported during the rapid growth in the early teenage years [16].

31.1.4 Etiology of Pectus Excavatum

The malformations of the anterior chest wall can be classified as deformities caused by the abnormal skeletal structure growth that is secondary to the incomplete fusion of the sternal blades, Poland's syndrome, and mixed or complex lesions of the dorsal column and costal arches. Within the defects related to abnormal cartilage growth, pectus excavatum is the most frequent deformity [57].

The widely accepted hypothesis is that the underlying pathology is an overgrowth of the costal cartilage that displaces the sternum dorsally [63]. In recent studies, this hypothesis has been challenged. Reconstructed three-dimensional computed tomogram images show that costal cartilage of the fifth and sixth costae is significantly shorter [43]. The relative costal cartilage length can be calculated by the C/R ratio, defined as the quotient of the costal cartilage length divided by the adjacent rib length. In pectus patients, the C/R ratio on the left sixth rib is significantly smaller, indicating that costal cartilage overgrowth is not the cause for pectus excavatum [44]. The biomechanical stability of the cartilage is decreased in PE patients. This is possibly might be caused by the disorderly arrangement and distribution of the collagen in the cartilage [14]. These facts suggest that PE is a systemic disease.

There is a positive family history in up to 37% of the cases [60]. Two-thirds of patients with Marfan's syndrome have a pectus excavatum [53]. However, up to now, a genetic link has not been established [9].

31.2 Clinical Features of Pectus Excavatum

In patients, pectus excavatum characteristics range from asymptomatic to exercise intolerance and chest pain. In severe cases, there is a dislocation of the heart, mostly to the left hemithorax, and a reduction of thoracic volume.

31.2.1 Pain

Sometimes patients experience chest and back pain. The pain is usually musculoskeletal in origin, and the cause is poorly understood [64]. Pectus excavatum is often associated with changes of the spinal column. Scoliosis is an excellent example of this type of change [16]. Patients with pectus excavatum frequently develop poor posture which may be one cause of the pain. However, it is unknown whether the posture is the cause for the pain or the pain is the cause for the posture [24].

31.2.2 Pulmonary Function

Trials of pulmonary function in patients with pectus excavatum described improvement of pulmonary reserve, maximal voluntary ventilation, and exercise tolerance after operative correction [54]. Other studies showed in adolescents a significantly lower forced vital capacity in the pectus excavatum group compared to an age-matched control group. The inverse relationship between vital capacity and the degree of sternal compression led to the suggestion that the patients would benefit from surgery for pectus excavatum [4, 65].

31.2.3 Cardiac Function

Limitation of cardiac stroke volume in patients with pectus excavatum has been described in several trials [4]. Surgery for pectus excavatum gives improvement in cardiac function [50].

However, as in the case of pulmonary function, the role of conditioning and subjective response to surgery is difficult to assess and may play an important role.

31.2.4 Psychological Factors

Among the most important consequences of the deformity are the psychological issues. Several psychological alterations have been described, among which are anxiety, difficulty in participating in social relationships, depression, and reduction in tolerance to frustration [13].

The psychological factors are highly relevant because they lead to social retraction, especially during adolescence. Patients avoid sports activities with physical deconditioning.

31.2.5 Pectus Excavatum in Female Patients

In female patients, the repair of pectus excavatum deformities has often been deferred since breast development commonly conceals the severity of the deformity [15].

As respiration in pectus excavatum patients utilized wider phrenic excursions than the normal chest, most conditions that cause abdominal distention will limit the depth of respiratory movements. In pregnancy, patients may experience progressive dyspnea with activity and tachypnea during the last trimester, which may improve dramatically within a few days of postpartum [15].

Female patients with pectus excavatum typically develop asymmetry of the breasts. This can be an additional cause of psychological problems [15].

31.3 Morphology and Classification of Pectus Excavatum

31.3.1 Morphology

There is a wide but distinguishable variety of morphologic characteristics presenting pectus excavatum. The marked depression of the sternum is frequently close to the xiphoid.

Many different distinctions in pectus excavatum exist: localized depressions vs. diffuse depressions, short and long length, symmetry, sternal torsion, slope/position of absolute depth, and unique patterns such as the horns of steer depression [5]. Few studies have objectively classified the degree of anatomic distortion to enable the quantification of the depression of the anterior chest wall and to aid in corrective surgery. In general, the assessment of these patients was carried out only subjectively during a clinical inspection [21]. Later indices were created to quantify the deformity and/or to enable the comparison between the preoperative and postoperative periods more objectively [2, 11, 28, 66]. Most of the indices are obtained with measurements that relate the approximation of the sternum to the thoracic spine column and not with the unevenness of the sternal region in relation to the costal cartilage in the direction of the column.

31.3.2 Classification

The internationally accepted Haller index is undoubtedly the predominate assessment parameter among surgeons who operate on patients with pectus excavatum (Fig. 31.2). In Haller's original study with 33 patients with pectus excavatum and 19 normal individuals, the cut point of the index was 3.25. Above this point, patients were classified as having moderate or severe pectus excavatum and were referred to surgery. Haller et al. did not identify differences in the index regarding the age [22]. In contrast, Daunt et al. showed important differences regarding age and gender: Children under 2 years have a lower Haller index than older ones, and females have a higher Haller index than males from 0 to 6 and from 12 to 18 years [10].

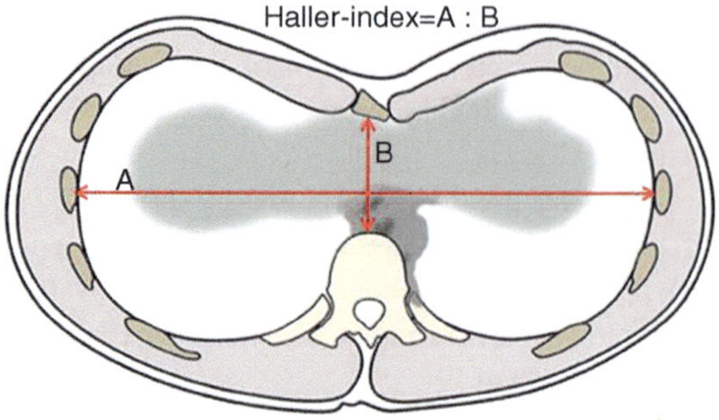

Fig. 31.2 Calculation of the Haller index

The Haller index is evaluated by radiologic methods (X-ray of the chest, CT).

Rebeis et al. developed an anthropometric index for pectus excavatum as a method for diagnosis and for pre- and postoperative assessment by comparing it to the Haller index and the lower vertebral index [57].

31.4 Indication to Surgery

The treatment of choice for pectus excavatum is surgery. Indications for surgery are mixed and can be for physiological and cosmetic reasons [32]. A Haller index >3.2 can be an objective indication for correction and is mentioned by a number of authors [31]. A Haller index <3.2 does not necessarily exclude patients for correction because in a barrel chest deformation, the Haller index can be normal despite a pectus excavatum. Other indications are symptoms; history of progression of the deformity; paradoxical movement of the chest wall with deep inspiration; cardiac compression, displacement, or pulmonary compression identified on echocardiogram or CT; abnormal pulmonary function studies showing significant restrictive disease; mitral valve prolapse, bundle branch block, or other cardiac pathology secondary compression of the heart; history of failed previous repair(s); and significant body image disturbance [33].

Many aspects of the repair of pectus excavatum remain controversial. Because evidence is conflicting concerning the pathophysiology of the deformity, consensus has never been reached about the indications for surgery. This fact has led to difficulty in scientifically evaluating the outcomes after surgery.

The scope of this book is minimal-invasive thoracic surgery; therefore, only the minimal-invasive techniques for the treatment of pectus excavatum will be discussed.

31.5 The Minimal-Invasive Surgery for Correction of Pectus Excavatum: The Nuss Procedure

31.5.1 Basic Principles

Observations about the correction of skeletal abnormalities in orthopedic surgery (scoliosis, club foot) and the possible chest remodeling in emphysema patients aided in the development of a minimal-invasive surgical procedure for pectus excavatum by Donald Nuss in the 1990s [46].

The basis of this "Nuss procedure" is the placement of a convex stainless steel bar under the sternum through two small lateral thoracic incisions. This bar position allows the anterior displacement of sternum and ribs. There is no need for bone or cartilage resection.

31.5.2 Standard Technique and Operating Course

31.5.2.1 Patient Position

The patient is placed in the supine position with both arms folded and polstered in front of the head without traction (Fig. 31.3). The arms may also be abducted, but attention must be paid to avoid injuries of the brachial plexus (Fig. 31.4) [17].

31.5.2.2 Antibiotic and Anesthesia

A first-generation cephalosporin antibiotic should be given 1 h prior to surgery. Some authors recommend the continuation of antibiotics for 48 h [24].

A general endotracheal anesthesia (double-lumen tube) in combination with a thoracic epidural one should be obligate. Central venous or arterial lines are not necessary.

As patients experience significant pain after Nuss procedure, the epidural catheter has to remain in place for up to 1 week following the operation. The surgeon must give information to the patient

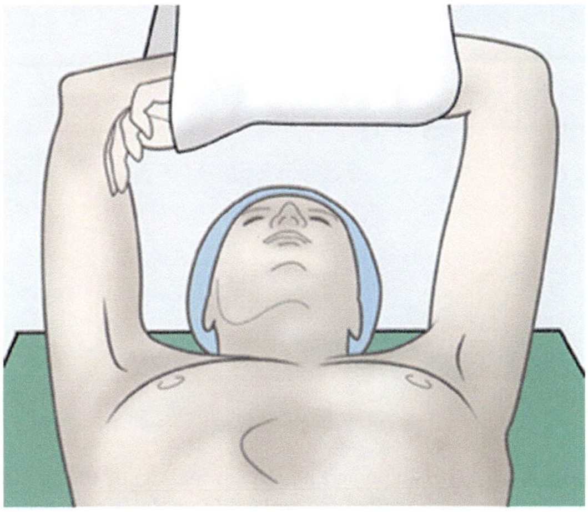

Fig. 31.3 Patient with both arms folded and polstered in front of the head

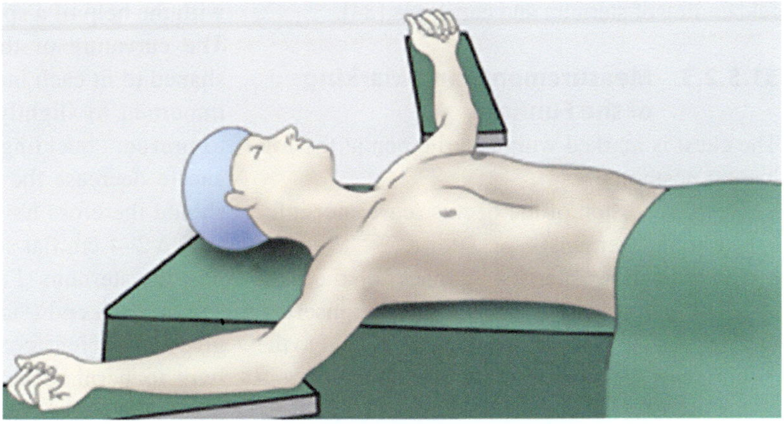

Fig. 31.4 Patient with abducted arms

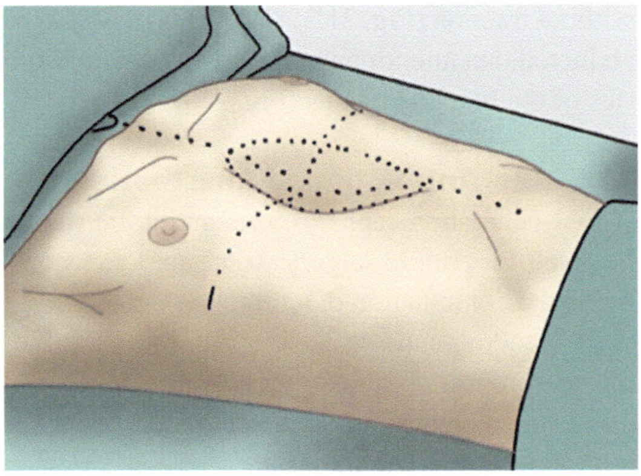

Fig. 31.5 Marking of the deepest portion of the pectus, the corresponding intercostals spaces on both sides, and the points of the pectus ridge that correspond to the horizontal plane from the deepest point of pectus to the lateral chest wall incisions

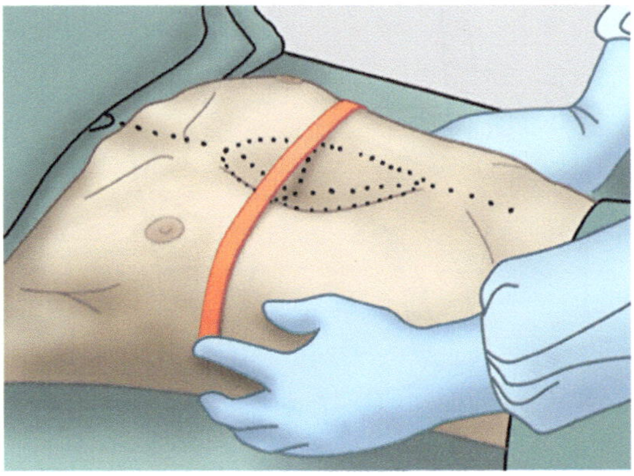

Fig. 31.6 The shape and length (in inches) of the bar is determined with the help of a plastic template (*orange*)

about the postoperative pain because of the forceful bending of sternum and cartilages [24].

31.5.2.3 Measurements and Marking of the Funnel

The chest is marked with a sterile pen at the following positions:

- Deepest portion of the pectus (cave: not inferior to the sternum)
- Corresponding intercostals spaces on the right and left sides where the bar has to be inserted
- Points of the pectus ridge that correspond to the horizontal plane from the deepest point of pectus to the lateral chest wall incisions (Fig. 31.5)

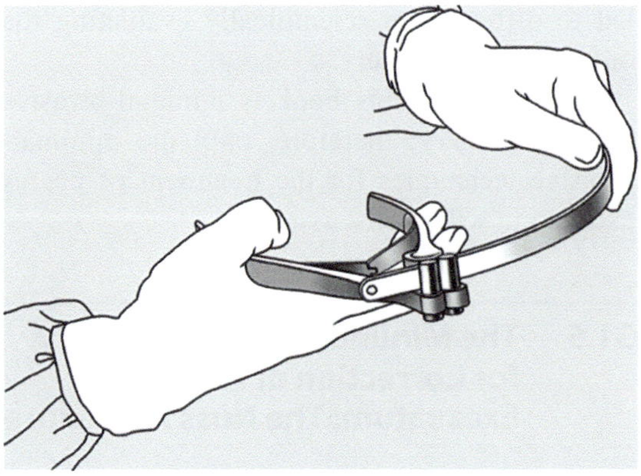

Fig. 31.7 Bending of the bar with the help of the special bar bender

The final length of the bar (in inches) has to be measured from the midaxillary line in one side to the opposite midaxillary line and is typically obtained by substracting 1–2.5 cm from this measurement [48]. A plastic template is used to determine length and shape of the bar (Fig. 31.6). However, some characteristics may interfere with this estimate, including age, thickness of subcutaneous fat, and breasts in females. Computed tomography measurement is assumed to be more precise for determining the length and shape of the bar [36]. In contrast, other studies showed that clinical methods are more sensitive or precise than radiological ones by measuring the deformity in a direct manner external to the chest [3].

31.5.2.4 Preparation of the Bar

The bar is bent from the center out to both ends with the help of a special bar bender (Fig. 31.7). The curvature of the bar (convexity) must be shaped to fit each individual patient's chest. It is important to slightly overcorrect the deformity to prevent "buckling" of the anterior chest wall and to decrease the risk of recurrence. The bar should therefore have a semicircular shape with only a 2–4-cm flat section in the middle to support the sternum (Fig. 31.8). A bar that is only bent at each end ("table top configuration") will give insufficient correction and may allow the lung to herniate between the bar and anterior chest wall [45].

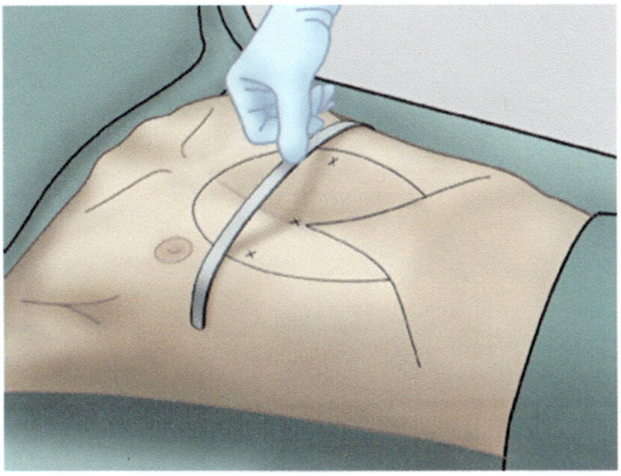

Fig. 31.8 The prepared final bar

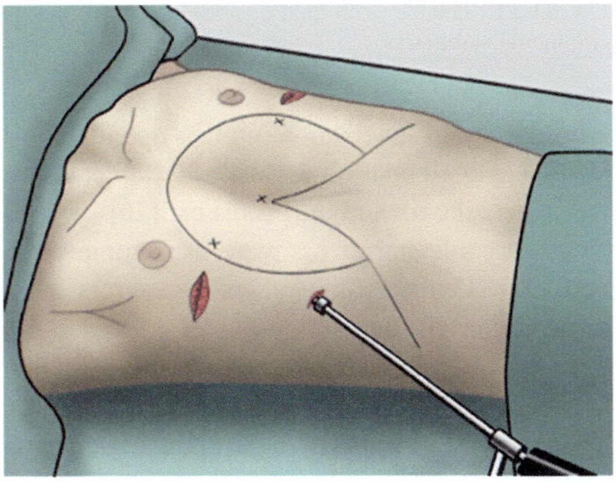

Fig. 31.9 Skin incisions and preparing of the tunnel for the bar

31.5.2.5 Skin Incisions and Skin Tunnel

Two 2-cm transverse incisions are made on the midaxillary line at the levels of the skin marks in line with the deepest point of depression on each side (Fig. 31.9).

The skin tunnel is raised anteriorly from both incisions in direction to the top of the pectus ridge at the previously selected intercostal space.

A skin pocket is extended posteriorly to give space for the distal end of the bar.

31.5.2.6 Videothoracoscopy

A 30° thoracoscope is inserted by a small blunt trocar just inferior to the axilla on the right side or two intercostal spaces below the transverse incisions and the place for the bar on the right side. A 30° thoracoscope gives good visualization of the

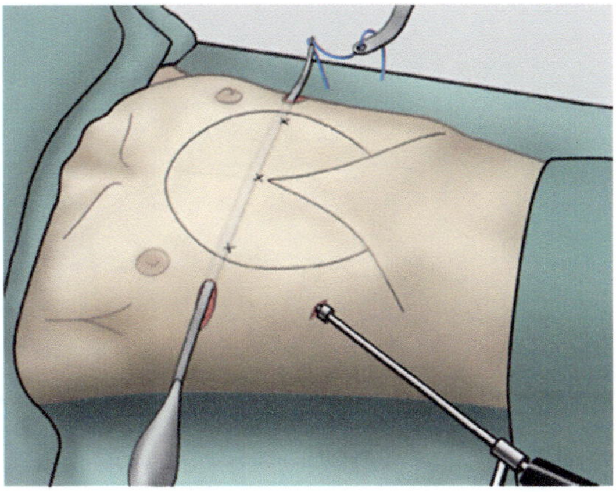

Fig. 31.10 The Pectus Schwert is inserted, and a strong strand is fixed to the anterior tip of the introducer

pleural cavity and mediastinal structures. To reduce pressure on the ribs and for the best cosmetic result, a 5-mm scope can be used. The thoracoscope is usually used only on the right side, but in case of extreme pectus defect, bilateral thoracoscopy may be also helpful (Fig. 31.9).

31.5.2.7 Pectus Introducer

The S-shaped Lorenz pectus introducer (Pectus Schwert, two different sizes) is inserted through the appropriate right intercostals space at top of the pectus ridge, in line with the point that corresponds to the deepest depression of the sternum.

With careful thoracoscopic guidance, the introducer is advanced across the anterior mediastinum immediately under the sternum. This step must be completed with extreme caution to avoid any injury to mediastinal structures including the heart.

With passing the introducer to the contralateral side, the sternum is forcefully lifted.

The tip of the introducer is pushed through the intercostals space at the top of the pectus ridge on the left side and brought out through the left skin incision (Fig. 31.10).

A strong strand (e.g., Mersilene strand or umbilical cloth tape) is fixed to the anterior tip of the introducer. Under thoracoscopic guidance, the introducer has to be pulled backwards. The prepared bar is attached at the other end of the strand at the right side. By using traction on

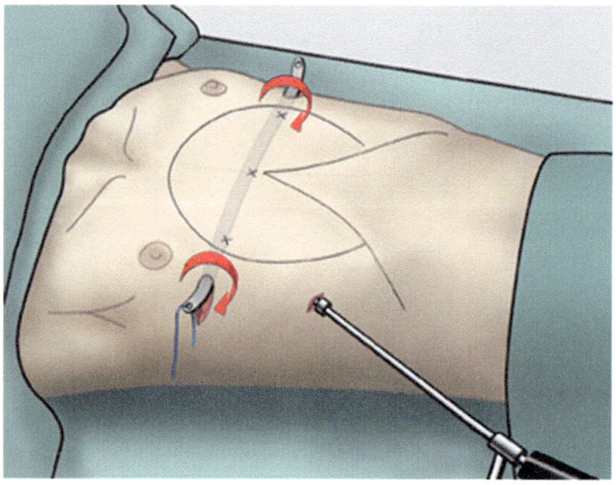

Fig. 31.11 The ends of the bar are brought out on each side through the skin incisions, and the bar is turned over (*red arrows*)

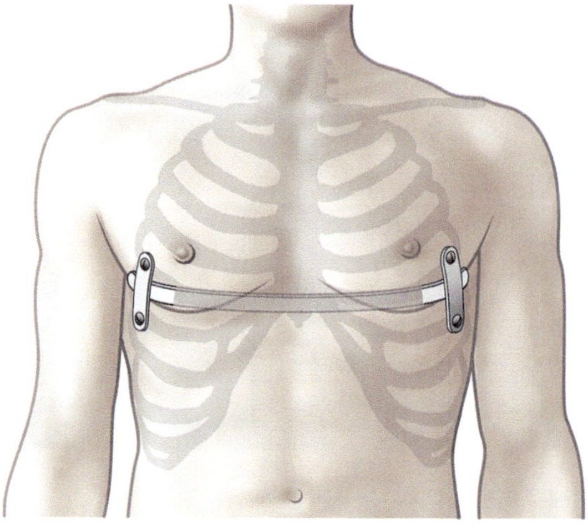

Fig. 31.12 The bar is in final position and is fixed with two lateral stabilizers

the strand, the bar is inserted with convexity facing posteriorly between sternum and mediastinum. In this way, every movement through the thoracic cavity is from right to left (Fig. 31.10).

31.5.2.8 Placement of the Bar

The ends of the bar are brought out on each side through the skin incisions. The strand and the introducer are removed. With the help of a special rotational instrument (Lorenz pectus bar rotational instrument/"bar flipper"), the bar is turned over: Now the convex part faces anteriorly (to the sternum) (Fig. 31.11). The ends of the bars are placed in the subcutaneous tissue under the skin pocket, anterior to the muscles of the chest wall. The ends should hug the chest, and they should not protrude under the skin pocket.

31.5.2.9 Fixation of the Bar

Once the correction of the pectus excavatum has proved satisfactory and no under- or overcorrection has been done, the bar must be fixed by lateral stabilizer bars (Fig. 31.12). Stainless steel stabilizer bars are placed at one or both sides of the pectus bar. Figure-of-8 sutures (stainless steel wire or Ethibond/Prolene number 0 or 1) are placed to secure the bar and the stabilizer(s) to the lateral chest wall (sutures should go around the ribs). Another technique is to fix a cerclage behind the stabilizer(s) to avoid sliding of the stabilizer. In this case, no further suture is necessary.

A third point-of-fixation suture is optional. This suture is placed on the anterior chest wall parasternal around the rib and the pectus bar [26].

Absorbable stabilizers were used some years ago [52]. Unfortunately, these stabilizers were more vulnerable and are no longer utilized.

31.5.2.10 Chest Tube

The insertion of a chest tube is optional. By placing the patient in the Trendelenburg position and using of large tidal volumes with positive-end expiratory pressure, a residual pneumothorax can be eliminated. A chest tube can be inserted in the thoracic cavity, and the end is held under water. This way, a water seal is made. Residual air can be removed in this manner.

31.5.3 Modifications of the Standard Operative Procedure

31.5.3.1 Length of Bar

Pilegaard routinely uses bars that are 5 cm shorter than the ones originally described by Nuss because this facilitates placement of the stabilizer close to the entry of the pectus bar into the thoracic cavity [51]. The stabilizer is placed on the left side of the bar as close as possible to the entry into the thoracic cavity. This gives additional stability because the stabilization plate is more anterior and closer to the turning point of the bar [51].

31.5.3.2 Bar Fixation

Various types of bar fixation are used to prevent bar dislocation [26]. In some patients – mild symmetric pectus excavatum – a submuscular bar fixation would be sufficient [35, 58].

31.5.3.3 Reducing Postoperative Chest Wall Tension

To facilitate retrosternal dissection and to reduce the chest wall tension, relaxing or "kerf" incisions along the cartilaginous ribs at point of maximal chest wall concavity were performed by Al-Assiri et al. [1].

31.5.3.4 Extrapleural Approach

Han et al. evaluated the safety and efficiency of an extrapleural approach to perform the Nuss procedure. The benefit of an extrapleural approach is avoiding irritations of the pleura and the lungs by the bar. Han et al. used this method especially in cases of mild symmetric pectus excavatum. In severe cases, the use of a thoracoscope aids in visualizing the structures inside the thorax to ensure that vascular structures are not injured during insertion of the introducer or the bar [23].

31.5.3.5 Insertion of the Introducer

The introducer can be inserted into the pleura between sternum and thymus instead of the thoracic depression [49].

31.5.4 Postoperative Management

31.5.4.1 Pain

A pain management program is mandatory. Therefore, epidural catheter and nonsteroidal anti-inflammatory drugs are used. The epidural catheter should not be removed before the pain is adequately controlled with oral medications.

31.5.4.2 Mobilization

Mobilization is permitted immediately after the operation. Effective instruction by a physiotherapist helps to avoid trunk rotation or stretching of the chest.

31.5.4.3 Sports

For the first 3 months, physical activities of the chest including heavy lifting, stretching, trunk rotation, and push-ups should be avoided. After that time, regular activity is permitted. Additionally, all contact sports (e.g., karate) are not permitted for at least 3 months.

31.5.5 Impacts of the Pectus Excavatum Repair to the Chest Wall

31.5.5.1 Stress Distribution on the Chest Wall

Adults are more likely than children to complain of pain after Nuss surgery. In children, the costal cartilages are more flexible. However, in adults, they are rigid because of age-related ossification. In the adult group, the Nuss procedure leads to greater stress on all 12 ribs than in those of a child patient. There is also a wider stress distribution on a wider range of the thorax in adults [42].

In ultrasonographic examinations, 29% of the patients showed localized, self-limited costochondral changes after a Nuss procedure [67]. These changes include acute angulation of the costochondral junction and rib fractures near the pectus bar.

31.5.5.2 Changes to the Anterior Chest Wall

Chang et al. reported about a method to record the deviation of the anterior chest wall in patients before and after Nuss repair and after removal of the metal bar. The bar leads to a significant increase in the height and width of the anterior chest wall. After removal of the bar, a reduction of the corrective effects was registered with significant decrease in the height and an increase in the width. These facts are of importance for planning the correction in case of severe pectus excavatum and for understanding the restriction of chest wall growth by mechanical constraints [6, 7].

31.5.5.3 Intrathoracic Volume

After a Nuss procedure, the intrathoracic volume is increased by approximately 2.72–8.88%, providing indirect evidence that repair of the pectus excavatum could have a positive effect on pulmonary function [7].

31.5.6 Outcomes

31.5.6.1 Satisfaction/Quality of Life

Various extensive studies have examined the outcomes after the Nuss procedure. In these studies, patient satisfaction was found to be very good, with excellent and good results reported in over 90% of cases [25, 32, 37].

Jacobsen et al. were able to show that the repair of pectus excavatum led to a positive effect on self-confidence. Children and adolescents perceived their health-related quality of life as significantly better after the Nuss procedure compared with the preoperative status [29].

The positive impact of Nuss repair on the well-being in children and adolescents persists also after bar removal. Thus, Metzelder et al. consider a Nuss procedure to be justified for cosmetic reasons [40].

31.5.6.2 Cardiopulmonary Outcome

Objective measures of pulmonary function such as FEV1 or total lung capacity offered significant improvement (after bar removal) in comparison to the preoperative values [30, 34, 38, 39]. The biggest improvement is measured in the cardiovascular function. Surgical repair of the pectus excavatum significantly improves cardiovascular function and contradicts arguments that surgical repair is primarily cosmetic yielding minimal physiologic improvement [38].

31.5.6.3 Recurrences

The reported mean incidence of recurrence in larger studies is as low as 1% (0–3.3%). Most frequently reported cases are in patients with Marfan's syndrome and in case of early bar removal [31].

31.5.7 Bar Removal

The bar(s) should remain in the chest for 2–4 years after pectus repair. Most patients tolerate the bar well for 3 years and are able to participate in competitive sports. There have been a few patients who have kept their bar in situ for 4 or more years without any problems. If a patient grows more than 6 in. (13 cm) after bar insertion and becomes symptomatic with lateral chest pain, then he needs to be evaluated to see whether early bar removal is required [45].

Bar removal can be an outpatient procedure. The scars on both sides have to be reopened. Bar, stabilizer(s), and sutures must be freed from the surrounding tissues. After removal of the lateral stabilizer(s), the bar is bent into its original straight shape. The bar is then pulled out of the thorax.

An extensive description of the technique for bar removal is published by St. Peter et al.: Two operating tables are abutted perpendicular to each other forming a T. The patient's arms are extended 90° on the transverse table, and by shifting the other table, an open space around the chest is created. The lateral chest incision(s) are incised simultaneously to remove the lateral stabilizers that are routinely used on each side. After removal of the stabilizers, the end of the bar is grasped on one side with vice grip pliers and removed with a single pull taking advantage of the open space to rotate the bar around the torso and under the patient's back [62]. Thoracoscopy is not necessary unless extensive adhesions between bar and pericardium are expected. This would be in case of postcardiotomy syndrome or pericarditis after Nuss procedure [19].

31.5.8 Complications

An overall rate of complications of almost 20% was reported by Hebra et al. [25]. Many centers have reported marked improvement in their complication rate after the learning curve [45].

31.5.8.1 Bar Dislocation

In the initial time of Nuss repair, the most common complication requiring a second operation was the displacement of the retrosternal bar (initially up to 9.5%). The displacement can include different rotations (90° or 180°) and lateral migration. The risk for a displacement is increased in teenagers and young adults. The experience of the last years shows that stabilization of the bar is absolutely essential. The introduction of a lateral stabilizer and the third point of fixation led to a decrease of bar displacement of less than 2% [25].

31.5.8.2 Pneumothorax and Pleural Effusion

Pneumothorax is one of the most common complications after a Nuss procedure. The incidence is between 3.6% and 4.2%, but an invasive treatment (chest tube) is seldom required [34, 45]. Pleural effusion occurs in about 0.3% [45, 47].

31.5.8.3 Wound Infection

Risk of an infection is increased with the implantation of a surgical device. These infections can range from a simple postoperative wound complication to deep infections including hematogenous spread (bacteremia). Infectious complications after Nuss procedure are uncommon (0.42–6.8%) [24, 27, 45–47, 61]. Protocol for the Nuss procedure includes: sterile technique, perioperative antibiotic prophylaxes, and gentle preparation of the pocket for the stabilizer to prevent seroma [61].

Superficial infections can be treated with surgical debridement and antibiotics. Occasionally a long-term antibiotic treatment is helpful in allowing the bar to remain in place until the correction of the pectus excavatum is finished.

Deep infections usually require the removal of the implant. Moss et al. describe one case with a thorax empyema [41]. A bar removal should be reserved only for complicated or recurrent multiple infections. If possible, the removal should be prolonged until the bar was in place for 18 months. In literature, early bar removal due to infections was described with an incidence of 0.34% [61].

31.5.8.4 Life-Threatening Complications

Only a few cases of cardiac perforation are mentioned in the literature, only one of them with lethal consequence [18, 25, 41].

Surgeons should be aware of possible severe complications including the need for converting to open procedure and emergency sternotomy. The use of videothoracoscopy for correct guidance of the bar is highly recommended.

31.5.8.5 Pericarditis/Pericardial Effusion

In about 0.5–1% of the patients, pericarditis or pericardial effusion can be observed [24].

References

1. Al-Assiri A, Kravarusic D, Wong V et al (2009) Operative innovation to the "Nuss" procedure for pectus excavatum: operative and functional effects. J Pediatr Surg 44:888–892
2. Backer OG, Brunner S, Larsen V (1961) The surgical treatment of funnel chest. Initial and follow-up results. Acta Chir Scand 1961(121):253–261
3. Brigato RR, Campos JRM, Jatene FB et al (2008) Pectus excavatum: evaluation of Nuss technique by objective methods. Interact Cardiovasc Thorac Surg 7:1084–1088
4. Cahill JL, Lees GM, Thomas RH (1984) A summary of preoperative and postoperative cardiorespiratory performance in patients undergoing pectus excavatum and carinatum repair. J Pediatr Surg 19:430–433
5. Cartoski MJ, Nuss D, Goretsky MJ et al (2006) Classification of the dysmorphology of pectus excavatum. J Pediatr Surg 41:1573–1581
6. Chang PY, Chang CH, Lai JY et al (2009) Analysis of changes to the anterior chest wall after the Nuss procedure-an objective measurement of pectus excavatum. J Pediatr Surg 44:2291–2295
7. Chang PY, Hsu ZY, Lai JY et al (2010) Increase in intrathoracic volume in pectus excavatum patients after the Nuss procedure. Med Biol Eng Comput 48:133–137
8. Chung CS, Myrianthopoulus NC (1975) Factors affecting risks of congenital malformations. I. Analysis of epidemiologic factors in congenital malformations. Report from the collaborative perinatal project. Birth Defects Orig Artic Ser 11:1–22
9. Creswick HA, Stacey MW, Kelly J et al (2006) Family study of the inheritance of pectus excavatum. J Pediatr Surg 41:1699–1703
10. Daunt S, Cohen J, Miller S (2004) Age-related normal ranges for the Haller index in children. Pediatr Radiol 34:326–330
11. Derveaux L, Clarysse I, Ivanoff I et al (1989) Preoperative and postoperative abnormalities in chest x-ray indices and in lung function in pectus deformities. Chest 95:850–856
12. Ebstein E (1901) Über die angeborene und die erworbene Trichterbrust. In: Sammlung klinischer Vorträge 1–42. Breitkopf und Härtel, Leipzig, pp 541–542
13. Einsiedel E, Clausner A (1999) Funnel chest. Psychological and psychosomatic aspects in children,

youngsters, and young adults. J Cardiovasc Surg 40:733–736
14. Feng J, Hu T, Liu W et al (2001) The biomechanical, morphologic, and histochemical properties of the costal cartilages in children with pectus excavatum. J Pediatr Surg 36:1770–1776
15. Fonkalsrud EW (2004) Management of pectus chest deformities in female patients. Am J Surg 187:192–197
16. Frick SL (2000) Scoliosis in children with anterior chest wall deformities. Chest Surg Clin N Am 10:427–436
17. Fox ME, Bensard DD, Roaten JB et al (2005) Positioning for the Nuss procedure: avoiding brachial plexus injury. Paediatr Anaesth 15:1067–1071
18. Gips H, Zaitsev K, Hiss J (2009) Cardiac perforation by a pectus bar after surgical correction of pectus excavatum: case report and review of the literature. Pediatr Surg Int 24:617–620
19. Haecker FM, Berberich T, Mayr J et al (2009) Near-fatal bleeding after transmyocardial ventricle lesion during removal of the pectus bar after the Nuss procedure. J Thorac Cardiovasc Surg 138:1240–1241
20. Haller JA (2000) History of the operative management of pectus deformities. Chest Surg Clin N Am 10:227–235
21. Haller JA Jr, Shermate DW, Tepas JJ et al (1978) Correction of pectus excavatum without prostheses or splints: objective measurement of severity and management of asymmetrical deformities. Ann Thorac Surg 26:73–79
22. Haller JA Jr, Kramer SS, Lietman SA (1987) Use of CT scans in selection of patients for pectus excavatum surgery: a preliminary report. J Pediatr Surg 22:904–906
23. Han Y, Wang J, Li W et al (2010) Non-thoracoscopic extrapleural Nuss procedure for the correction of pectus excavatum in children. Eur J Cardiothorac Surg 37:312–315
24. Hebra A (2009) Minimally invasive repair of pectus excavatum. Semin Thorac Cardiovasc Surg 21:76–84
25. Hebra A, Swoveland B, Egbert M et al (2000) Outcome analysis of minimally invasive repair of pectus excavatum: review of 251 cases. J Pediatr Surg 35:252–258
26. Hebra A, Gauderer MWL, Tagge EP et al (2001) A simple technique for preventing bar displacement with the Nuss repair of pectus excavatum. J Pediatr Surg 36:1266–1268
27. Hosie S, Sitkiewicz T, Petersen C et al (2001) Minimally invasive repair of pectus excavatum-the Nuss procedure. A European multicentre experience. Eur J Pediatr Surg 12:235–308
28. Hümmer HP, Willital GH (1984) Morphologic findings of chest deformities in children corresponding to the Willital-Hümmer classification. J Pediatr Surg 19:562–566
29. Jacobsen EB, Thastum M, Jeppesen JH et al (2010) Health-related quality of life in children and adolescents undergoing surgery for pectus excavatum. Eur J Pediatr Surg 20:85–91
30. Johnson JN, Hartman TK, Pianosi PT et al (2008) Cardiorespiratory function after operation for pectus excavatum. J Pediatr 153:359–364
31. Krasopoulos G, Goldstraw P (2011) Minimally invasive repair of pectus excavatum deformity. Eur J Cardiothorac Surg 39:149–158
32. Krasopoulos G, Dusmet M, Ladas G et al (2006) Nuss procedure improves the quality of life in young male adults with pectus excavatum deformity. Eur J Cardiothorac Surg 29:1–5
33. Kelly RE Jr (2008) Pectus excavatum: historical background, clinical picture, preoperative evaluation and criteria for operation. Semin Pediatr Surg 17:181–193
34. Kelly RE Jr, Shamberger RC, Mellins RB et al (2007) Prospective multicenter study of surgical correction of pectus excavatum: design, perioperative complications, pain, and baseline pulmonary function facilitated by internet-based data collection. J Am Coll Surg 205:205–216
35. Kim HK, Choi YH, Cho YH et al (2007) A comparative study of pericostal and submuscular bar fixation technique in the Nuss procedure. J Korean Med Sci 22:254–257
36. Lai JY, Wang CJ, Chang PY (2009) The measurement and designation of the pectus bar by computed tomography. J Pediatr Surg 44:2287–2290
37. Lawson ML, Cash TF, Akers R et al (2003) A pilot study of the impact of surgical repair on disease-specific quality of life among patients with pectus excavatum. J Pediatr Surg 38:916–918
38. Malek MH, Berger DE, Housh TJ et al (2006) Cardiovascular function following surgical repair of pectus excavatum. Chest 130:506–516
39. Malek MH, Berger DE, Marelich WD et al (2006) Pulmonary function following surgical repair of pectus excavatum: a meta-analysis. Eur J Cardiothorac Surg 30:637–643
40. Metzelder ML, Kuebler JF, Leonhardt J et al (2007) Self and parental assessment after minimally invasive repair of pectus excavatum: lasting satisfaction after bar removal. Ann Thorac Surg 83:1844–1849
41. Moss RL, Albanese CT, Reynolds M (2001) Major complications after minimally invasive repair of pectus excavatum: case reports. J Pediatr Surg 36:155–158
42. Nagasao T, Miyamoto J, Tamaki T et al (2007) Stress distribution on the thorax after the Nuss procedure for pectus excavatum results in different patterns between adult and child patients. J Thorac Cardiovasc Surg 134:1502–1507
43. Nakaoka T, Uemura S, Yano T et al (2009) Does overgrowth of costal cartilage cause pectus excavatum? A study on the lengths of ribs and costal cartilages in asymmetric patients. J Pediatr Surg 44:1333–1336
44. Nakaoka T, Uemura S, Yoshida T et al (2010) Overgrowth of costal cartilage is not the etiology of pectus excavatum. J Pediatr Surg 45:2015–2018
45. Nuss D (2008) Minimally invasive surgical repair of pectus excavatum. Semin Pediatr Surg 17:209–217
46. Nuss D, Kelly RE Jr, Croitoru DP et al (1998) A 10-year review of a minimally invasive technique for

the correction of pectus excavatum. J Pediatr Surg 33:545–552
47. Nuss D, Croitoru DP, Kelly RE et al (2002) Review and discussion of the complications of minimally invasive pectus excavatum repair. Eur J Pediatr Surg 12:230–234
48. Nuss D, Croitoru DP, Kelly RE Jr (2005) Congenital chest wall deformities. In: Ashcraft KW, Holocomb GW, Murphy JP (eds) Pediatric surgery, 4th edn. Elsevier, Philadelphia
49. Ohno K, Nakamura T, Azuma T et al (2009) Modification of the Nuss procedure for pectus excavatum to prevent cardiac perforation. J Pediatr Surg 44:2426–2430
50. Peterson RJ, Young WG Jr, Godwin JD et al (1985) Noninvasive assessment of exercise cardiac function before and after pectus excavatum repair. J Thorac Cardiovasc Surg 90:251–260
51. Pilegaard HK, Licht PB (2008) Early results following the Nuss operation for pectus excavatum – a single-institution experience of 383 patients. Interact Cardiovasc Thorac Surg 7:54–57
52. Pilegaard HK, Licht PB (2009) Can absorbable stabilizers be used routinely in the Nuss procedure? Eur J Cardiothorac Surg 35:561–564
53. Pyeritz RE, McKusick VA (1979) The Marfan syndrome: diagnosis and management. N Engl J Med 300:772–777
54. Quigley PM, Haller J, Jelus KL et al (1996) Cardiorespiratory function before and after corrective surgery in pectus excavatum. J Pediatr 128:638–643
55. Ravitch MM (1949) The operative treatment of pectus excavatum. Ann Surg 129:429–444
56. Ravitch MM (1997) Congenital deformities of the chest wall and their operative correction. W.B. Saunders Company, Philadelphia
57. Rebeis EB, Campos JR, Fernandez A et al (2007) Anthropometric index for Pectus excavatum. Clinics 62:599–606
58. Schaarschmidt K, Kolberg-Schwerdt A, Dimitrov G et al (2002) Submuscular bar, multiple pericostal bar fixation, bilateral thoracoscopy: a modified nuss repair in adolescents. J Pediatr Surg 37:1276–1280
59. Serafin J, Swiatkowski J, Majkusiak RNP (2003) 40-Year experience in surgical treatment of congenital chest deformations – ethiopathogenesis, operative techniques and clinical results. Acta Chir Orthop Traumatol Cech 70:207–213
60. Shamberger RC, Welch KJ (1988) Surgical repair of pectus excavatum. J Pediatr Surg 23:615–622
61. Shin S, Goretsky MJ, Kelly J et al (2007) Infectious complications after the Nuss repair in a series of 863 patients. J Pediatr Surg 42:87–92
62. St Peter SD, Sharp RJ, Upadhyaya P (2007) A straightforward technique for removal of the substernal bar after the Nuss operation. J Pediatr Surg 42:1789–1791
63. Sweet RH (1944) Pectus excavatum: report of two cases successfully operated upon. Ann Surg 119:922–934
64. Tsirikos AI, McMaster MJ (2005) Congenital anomalies of the ribs and chest wall associated with congenital deformities of the spine. J Bone Joint Surg Am 87:2523–2536
65. Weg JG, Krumholz RA, Harkleroad LE (1967) Pulmonary dysfunction in pectus excavatum. Am Rev Respir Dis 96:936–945
66. Welch KJ (1958) Satisfactory surgical correction of pectus excavatum deformity in childhood; a limited opportunity. J Thorac Surg 36:697–713
67. Zeng Q, Lai JY, Wang XM et al (2008) Costochondral changes in the chest wall after the Nuss procedure: ultrasonographic findings. J Pediatr Surg 43:2147–2150

Part VI

Minimally Invasive Thoracic Surgery: The Oesophagus

Resection of Mid and Distal Esophageal Diverticulum

32

Sebastian F. Schoppmann and Johannes Zacherl

Contents

S.F. Schoppmann, M.D. (✉) • J. Zacherl, M.D.
Department of General Surgery, Medical University of Vienna, Waehringer Guertel 18-20, Vienna A-1020, Austria
e-mail: sebastian.schoppmann@meduniwien.ac.at; johannes.zacherl@meduniwien.ac.at

32.1 Introduction

Mid and distal diverticula of the esophagus are very rare entities with a prevalence of approximately 0.015% [1]. Traditionally, patients with symptomatic mid and distal esophageal diverticula have been treated surgically via laparotomy or thoracotomy including resection of the diverticulum, myotomy, and anti-reflux procedure. The amount of myotomy and the need of additional anti-reflux procedure are continuously discussed in this topic [2].

Aim of this chapter is to describe and discuss minimally invasive approaches to the surgical treatment of mid and distal diverticula of the esophagus.

32.2 Aetiology and Pathophysiology

Diverticula of the esophageal body (95% occur in the middle and distal esophagus) are relatively rare with published prevalence data of about 0.015%. When occurring in the distal esophagus, in the lower 6–10 cm, diverticula are termed epiphrenic diverticula. Most esophageal diverticula occur in middle-aged adults and elderly people and presentation in infants and children is rarely seen [3, 4].

Diverticula of the mid and distal esophagus may have various aetiologies. They can be divided in congenital (mostly seen in the middle esophagus) or acquired diverticula caused by traction or pulsion.

R.G.C. Inderbitzi et al. (eds.), *Minimally Invasive Thoracic and Cardiac Surgery*,
DOI 10.1007/978-3-642-11861-6_32, © Springer-Verlag Berlin Heidelberg 2012

Epiphrenic diverticula typically occur from increased pressure during esophageal propulsive contractions against the lower esophageal sphincter. In contrast, traction diverticula occur as a consequence of pulling forces on the outside of the esophagus (ligament like structure between left bronchus and esophagus) from an adjacent inflammatory process (e.g. involvement of inflamed mediastinal lymph nodes in tuberculosis or histoplasmosis).

The most common causes of mid esophageal and epiphrenic diverticula are motility disorders of the esophageal body, including achalasia, diffuse esophageal spasm and hypertensive lower esophageal sphincter. Other, rather rare causes of diverticula of the mid and distal esophagus include iatrogenic surgical impairment of the esophageal wall and the Ehlers-Danlos syndrome [5]. Epiphrenic pseudodiverticula – to be distinguished from true diverticula – occur in the setting of long-standing peptic esophagitis and strictures.

32.3 Clinical Presentation

Findings on physical examination often are normal in patients with esophageal diverticula, and around 60% of patients with mid and distal esophageal diverticula have minimal or no symptoms. Dysphagia presents the most common symptom associated with mid esophageal and epiphrenic diverticula, particularly if it is very large and filled with food or a bezoar. However, the dysphagia usually is closely related to the underlying motility disorder (e.g. hypertensive lower esophageal sphincter that fails to relax, absence of esophageal body peristalsis) than to the diverticulum by itself. Retention of undigested food in large diverticula results in regurgitation, nocturnal cough and/or aspiration pneumonia in up to half of the patients. Halitosis also may be present and is secondary to accumulated food debris or medicines within the diverticulum.

32.4 Diagnostics

Barium radiography is the diagnostic procedure of choice defining the structure of the diverticula on the one side and additionally providing information about underlying motility disturbances (Fig. 32.1). Especially, if the patient has dysphagia or odynophagia, flexible endoscopy is indicated to rule out structural conditions (strictures, neoplasm). Esophageal manometry is indicated in symptomatic patients if achalasia or another esophageal motility disorder is suspected or if surgery is being considered (Fig. 32.2) [4, 6].

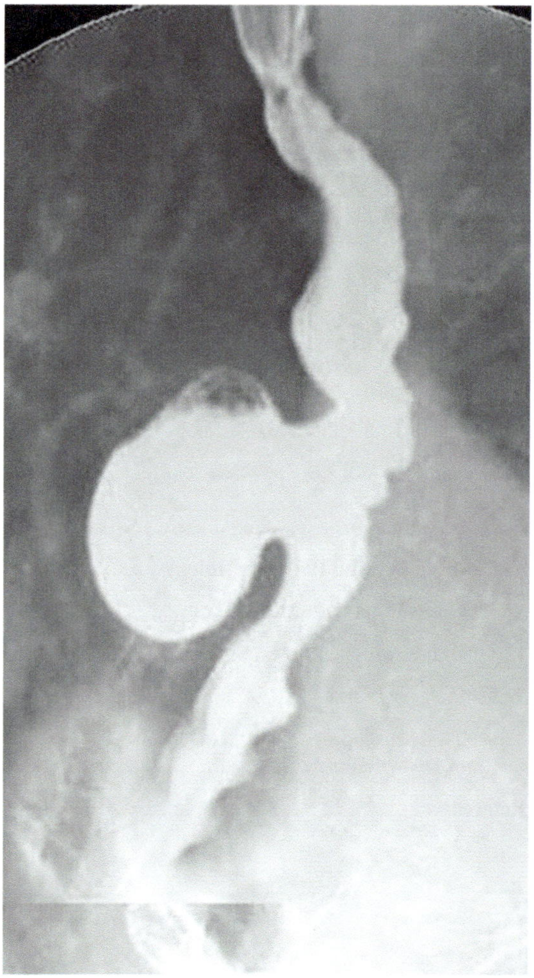

Fig. 32.1 Barium upper gastrointestinal study demonstrating an epiphrenic diverticulum

32.5 Surgery

Asymptomatic and oligosymptomatic esophageal body diverticula do not require treatment. As in most patients with mid and epiphrenic diverticula, dysphagia is related to the under lying

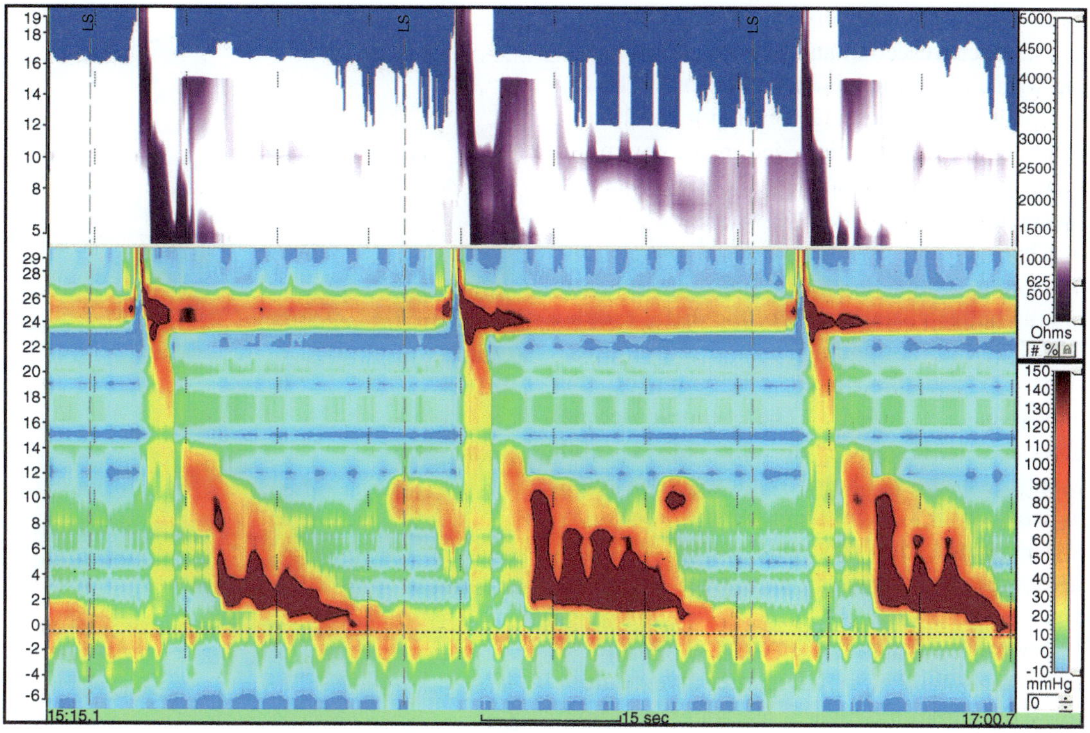

Fig. 32.2 High-resolution manometry from a patient with achalasia and a small epiphrenic diverticulum. Note the repetitive pressure amplitudes (up to 40 mmHg) and the bolus retention in the distal esophagus.

dysmotility, and the treatment should be directed to the underlying cause with botulinum toxin injection in the lower esophageal sphincter, dilatation (pneumatic or mechanic), or myotomy. If esophageal body diverticula are believed to be responsible for the symptoms (dysphagia, aspiration), surgical diverticulectomy should be considered to be added to myotomy (+ anti-reflux procedure). The surgical therapy of large and symptomatic diverticula has traditionally been performed via thoracotomy or laparotomy. However, there is growing evidence for the feasibility and benefits of minimally invasive approaches to mid and epiphrenic esophageal diverticula by laparoscopic or thoracoscopic access, respectively. [4] To date, there is very limited data about the outcome of minimally invasive approaches to mid esophageal and epiphrenic diverticula (see Table 32.1) [7–10]. The topics discussed are if complication rates and success rates are comparable to the open procedures on the one side (Table 32.1) and the benefits of adding myotomy and/or fundoplication to the diverticulectomy. Depending on the location but also on the surgeon's preference, the operation can be performed via laparoscopy or thoracoscopy.

Table 32.1 Comparison of open versus minimally invasive Surgery

	Minimally invasive (21 VATS, 78 laparoscopic)	Open
Studies (*n*)[a]	10	7
Published patients (*n*)	99	165
Mortality (%)	1.8	5
Complication (%)	25	20
Leak (%)	12	9
Conversion (%)	1	
Re-operation (%)	8	4
Hospital stay (days)	5	10
Treatment success (%)	98	96

VATS video-assisted thoracoscopic surgery, *MI* minimally invasive

Values are means, [a]only studies included with more than five patients reported

In epibronchial diverticula (traction caused), transthoracic resection and in some cases covering with a pleural flap is the treatment of choice. In epiphrenic diverticula (pulsion caused), the combination of resection and myotomy plus/minus anti-reflux procedure is the preferred procedure.

The reported benefits of the laparoscopic compared to the thoracoscopic approach are (1) the better visualization of the distal esophagus, (2) easier myotomy and/ or fundoplication, (3) and the better alignment of the endoscopic stapler. The thoracoscopic approach is favorable in cases of (1) mid esophageal and (2) large, inflamed diverticula as well as if (3) significant pleural adhesions are expected. In very rare cases of giant diverticula, a combination of both might be appropriate [11].

There is an ongoing discussion whether a myotomy should be included after diverticulectomy of epiphrenic diverticula, and if yes how long this should be. However, data on the recurrence and leak rates after diverticulectomy dependent on the performance of myotomy are controversial. Most series have described higher rates of recurrences and leakages after diverticulectomy without myotomy. Generally, a length of myotomy extending from the upper limit of the diverticular neck to the proximal 3 cm of the stomach is reported to be sufficient. Some centers also adjust the length of myotomy to the extent of motility disorder after manometry. In our experience, performing a myotomy is essential for avoiding recurrence and treating the problem at its origin (epiphrenic diverticula) as well as to avoid staple line rupture [8].

The necessity and type of accompanying anti-reflux surgery is a further area of debate within the field of epiphrenic esophageal diverticula treatment. Most centres perform a fundoplication after myotomy, but there is great controversy regarding the type of fundoplication. In general, all types of wraps (Nissen, Toupet, Dor) have been described, and some kind of tailoring due to preconditions might be appropriate [12, 13].

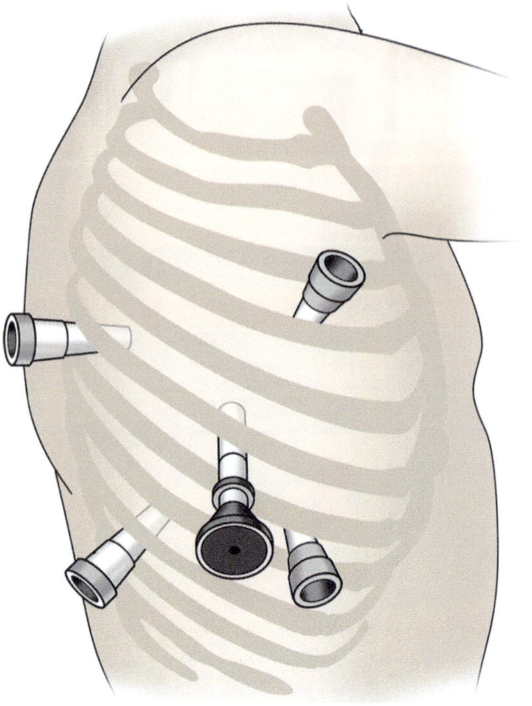

Fig. 32.3 Patient in a right lateral position, with five trocar sleeves

32.6 Thoracoscopic Steps of Resection of Diverticulum

The patient is positioned in a right lateral decubitus position, and single lung ventilation is conducted. For port position, see Fig. 32.3. The lung is mobilized by dividing the pulmonary ligament. After dividing the pleura over the esophagus, the esophagus is mobilized orally and aborally of the diverticulum, and a flexible drain is used to encircle the mobilized esophagus. Now the neck of the diverticulum is visualized. The vagus nerves are identified and preserved (Fig. 32.4). A 40-Fr bougie is carefully inserted and introduced across the gastresophageal junction. Diverticulum is relieved from surrounding tissue (Fig. 32.4). Both corner angles of diverticulum now are tagged (Fig. 32.5). Then the diverticulum is resected using an Endo GIA parallel to the longitudinal axis of the esophagus. We usually not reinforce the staple line with buttress material.

If Endo GIA scarcely can be positioned, alternatively one may carefully excise the diverticulum

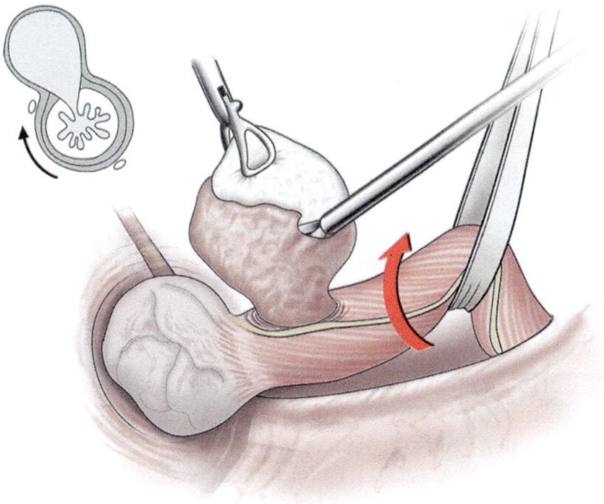

Fig. 32.4 Thoracoscopic dissection of diverticulum

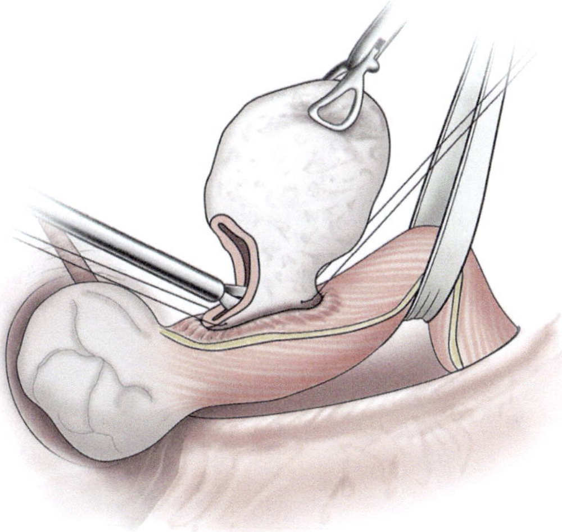

Fig. 32.5 Resection of diverticulum

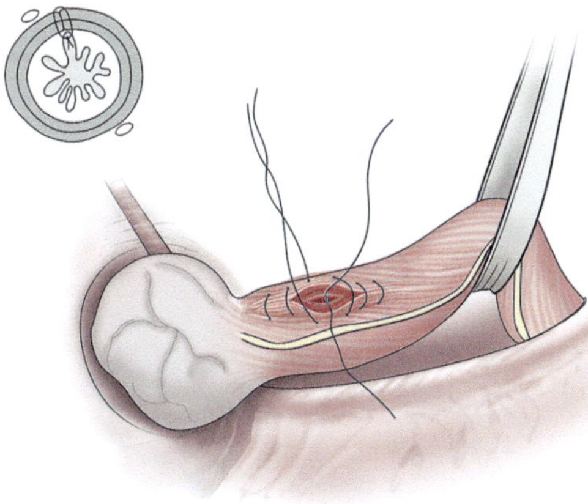

Fig. 32.6 Suture of esophageal lesion

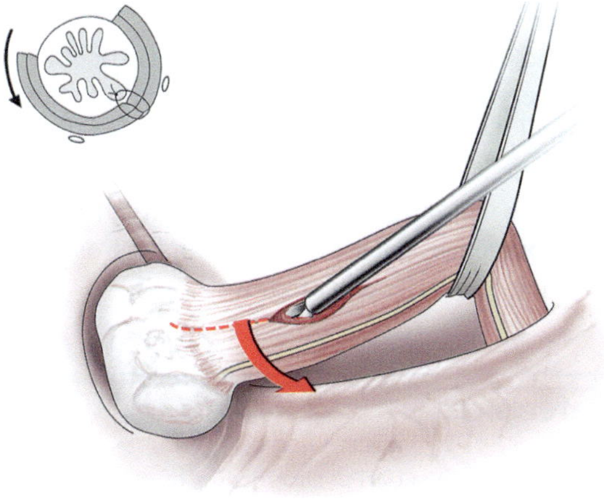

Fig. 32.7 Performing esophageal myotomy proximal of the diverticulum

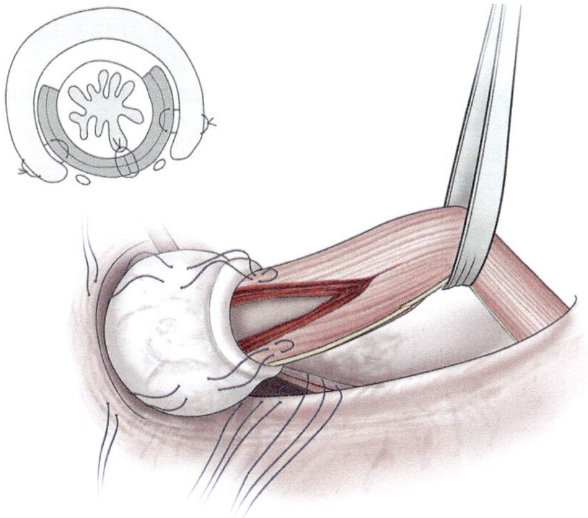

Fig. 32.8 Ending the operation with performing a fundoplication

by scissors (Fig. 32.5). Subsequently it is of particular importance closing all layers of esophagus with accurate stitches (Fig. 32.6).

In epiphrenic diverticula (not in epibronchial), an opposite myotomy utilizing scissors and/or a diathermy hook, accurately referred to the underlying motility disorder, completes intervention (Fig. 32.7). Esophagomyotomy has to be performed preventing suture-line leaks as well as relieving symptoms from the underlying motility disorder. The incision has to be clearly carried onto the stomach (Fig. 32.7), followed by the antireflux procedure illustrated in Fig. 32.8. Finally, the air-bubble test is used to exclude leakage.

Conclusions

Mid esophageal and epiphrenic diverticula are a very rare entity and for sure should be handled in a multidisciplinary and specialized centre. The treatment of symptomatic diverticula is surgery, and minimally invasive approaches (thoracoscopy and laparoscopy) seem to be safe and effective.

References

1. Wheeler D (1947) Diverticula of the foregut. Radiology 49(4):476–482
2. Benacci JC, Deschamps C, Trastek VF et al (1993) Epiphrenic diverticulum: results of surgical treatment. Ann Thorac Surg 55(5):1109–1113; discussion 1114
3. Jordan PH Jr, Kinner BM (1999) New look at epiphrenic diverticula. World J Surg 23(2):147–152
4. Melman L, Quinlan JA, Hall BL et al (2009) Clinical utility of routine barium esophagram after laparoscopic anterior esophageal myotomy for achalasia. Surg Endosc 23(3):606–610
5. Tedesco P, Fisichella PM, Way LW, Patti MG (2005) Cause and treatment of epiphrenic diverticula. Am J Surg 190(6):891–894
6. Melman L, Quinlan J, Robertson B et al (2009) Esophageal manometric characteristics and outcomes for laparoscopic esophageal diverticulectomy, myotomy, and partial fundoplication for epiphrenic diverticula. Surg Endosc 23(6):1337–1341
7. Fernando HC, Luketich JD, Samphire J et al (2005) Minimally invasive operation for esophageal diverticula. Ann Thorac Surg 80(6):2076–2080
8. Melman L, Azar R, Beddow K et al (2009) Primary and overall success rates for clinical outcomes after laparoscopic, endoscopic, and open pancreatic cystgastrostomy for pancreatic pseudocysts. Surg Endosc 23(2):267–271
9. Palanivelu C, Rangarajan M, John SJ et al (2008) Laparoscopic transhiatal approach for benign supradiaphragmatic lesions of the esophagus: a replacement for thoracoscopy? Dis Esophagus 21(2):176–180
10. van der Peet DL, Klinkenberg-Knol EC, Berends FJ, Cuesta MA (2001) Epiphrenic diverticula: minimal invasive approach and repair in five patients. Dis Esophagus 14(1):60–62
11. Varghese TK Jr, Marshall B, Chang AC et al (2007) Surgical treatment of epiphrenic diverticula: a 30-year experience. Ann Thorac Surg 84(6):1801–1809; discussion 1801–1809
12. Richards WO, Torquati A, Holzman MD et al (2004) Heller myotomy versus Heller myotomy with Dor fundoplication for achalasia: a prospective randomized double-blind clinical trial. Ann Surg 240(3): 405–412
13. Rebecchi F, Giaccone C, Farinella E et al (2008) Randomized controlled trial of laparoscopic Heller myotomy plus Dor fundoplication versus nissen fundoplication for achalasia: long-term results. Ann Surg 248(6):1023–1030

Resection of Benign Tumours

33

Yelena Devyatko, Sebastian F. Schoppmann, and Johannes Zacherl

Contents

Y. Devyatko, M.D. • S.F. Schoppmann, M.D. •
J. Zacherl, M.D. (✉)
Department of General Surgery,
Medical University of Vienna,
Waehringer Guertel 18-20, Vienna, A-1020, Austria
e-mail: yelena.devyatko@meduniwien.ac.at;
sebastian.schoppmann@meduniwien.ac.at;
johannes.zacherl@meduniwien.ac.at

33.1 Introduction

Benign oesophageal tumours (BOTs) are rare clinical conditions are asymptomatic in the majority of cases. Rapid improvement of diagnostic imaging techniques and increasing availability of diagnostic imaging techniques during the recent decades led to an increased number of incidentally diagnosed benign tumours of the oesophagus. The determination of the incidence is very difficult because of the asymptomatic clinical presentation in many cases. In three autopsy series, only 172 BOTs were reported from 42.985 autopsies, with estimated prevalence of benign oesophageal tumours of 400/100,000 [1–3]. The BOTs account for about 1% of all oesophageal tumours [4, 5, 34].

The most useful classification for BOTs was offered by Avezzano et al. [6] and is dependent on the distribution of the tumour to the oesophageal wall layers (Table 33.1). The majority of BOTs are located in the middle and lower third of the oesophagus [5, 7] and may originate from different extramucosal layers of the oesophageal wall.

Among these tumour types, leiomyomas are the most common and represent about 80% of all benign neoplasms [8, 9], followed by congenital cysts and duplications, although these are not true neoplasms and will not be discussed here. A review of 1,679 cases with oesophageal leiomyoma reported between 1875 and 1996 revealed an age incidence peak for men and women between 30 and 59 years [7]. In the recently published series of BOTs [10–17], the median patients' ages

R.G.C. Inderbitzi et al. (eds.), *Minimally Invasive Thoracic and Cardiac Surgery*,
DOI 10.1007/978-3-642-11861-6_33, © Springer-Verlag Berlin Heidelberg 2012

Table 33.1 Classification of benign oesophageal tumours

Intraluminal	
	Fibrovascular polyp
	Adenoma
	Lipoma
	Inflammatory polyp
	Squamous cell papilloma
	Inflammatory pseudotumor
Submucosal	
	Haemangioma
	Granular cell tumour
	Neurofibroma, neurinoma
	Paraganglioma
Intramural	
	Leiomyoma
	Rhabdomyoma
	Lipoma
	Hamartoma
	Haemangioma
	Granular cell tumour
	Neurofibroma
	Inclusion cysts
	Schwannoma
Extraoesophageal	
	Cysts and duplications

were 44.5 (range 19–76) years. The male/female ratio for cumulative data amounts to about 2:1 [7, 11–17]. Leiomyomas are characterised by very slow growth and measured less than 5 cm in maximum diameter in about 50% of cases, 5–9 cm in 31% and 10 cm or more in 19% [7]. However, cases with huge tumours (giant leiomyoma) measuring up to 29 cm have been reported [7].

The next most common type of BOTs are intraluminal benign oesophageal polyps of different histologic origin.

More than 85% of benign oesophageal tumours remain asymptomatic [1], incidentally found by endoscopic or radiologic investigation. They are generally characterised by very slow growth and may coexist with other oesophageal disorders, such as GERD, achalasia, diverticula or malignant neoplasms [7, 18]. If symptomatic, the most common complains are dysphagia, chest pain and regurgitation [5, 7, 10, 13, 18]. However, gastrointestinal bleeding due to ulceration or respiratory symptoms because of tracheobronchial compression may occur. Regurgitation of a pedicled intraluminal tumour, mostly fibrovascular polyps, is extremely rare, but a pathognomonic sign. In giant leiomyomas, central necrosis has been observed, which may cause accelerated pseudogrowth due to fluid shift into the tumour centre.

Diagnosis: Contrast swallow frequently is the initial diagnostic test for evaluation of symptomatic patients [2]. The quality of this examination is quite higher, if performed as a cinematographic study. The CT scan offers important topographic and size information [2], it proved to be of utmost value in distinguishing tumours originating in the oesophageal wall from extrinsic compression (Fig. 33.1). Endoscopy depicts the intraluminal aspect and mucosal condition and may be very helpful in the assessment of the degree of obstruction (Fig. 33.2) [7, 19, 20]. Furthermore, coexisting oesophageal diseases may be discovered. It is not recommended to obtain standard endoscopic forceps biopsies in cases of extramucosal tumours with intact mucosal surface because it is not to be expected to offer representative samples, but may complicate surgical enucleation. Endoscopic ultrasonography (EUS) may be used for determination of the tumour localisation within the oesophageal wall layers, for the measurement of the tumour size and for the description of the homogeneity and echogenicity of the respective lesion [19, 20].

33.2 Indications for Surgery

While mucosal and submucosal benign oesophageal neoplasm may be accessible by interventional endoscopic techniques (endoscopic mucosal resection, endoscopic submucosal dissection), intramural BOTs are removed surgically once the path of observation has been left.

The general consensus is that a benign intramural oesophageal tumour should be removed, if (1) it is symptomatic, (2) it is growing or (3) if clinical diagnosis is not clear and histologic examination is a indicated to exclude a malignant process.

As a self-explaining precondition, the individual patient's risk of surgery should be counterbalanced with the benefit of the operative procedure.

The most common benign tumours of the oesophagus – leiomyomas – are located intramu-

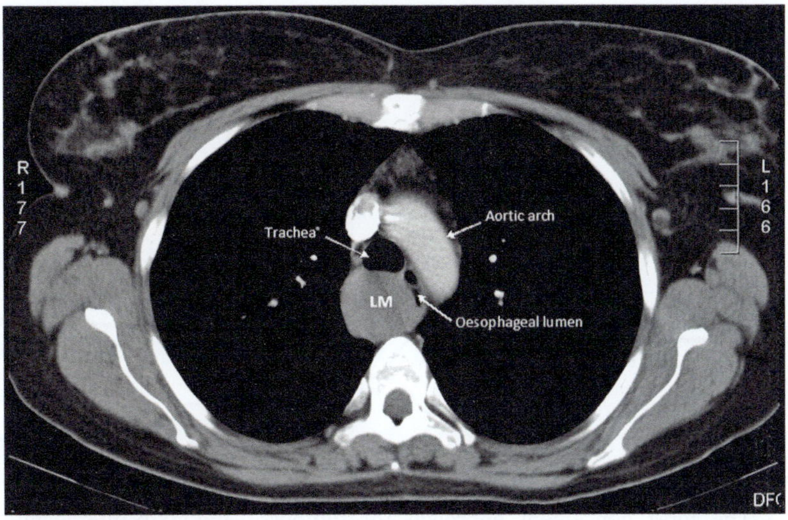

Fig. 33.1 CT scan: leiomyoma (*LM*) is located in middle third of the oesophagus and narrows the lumen

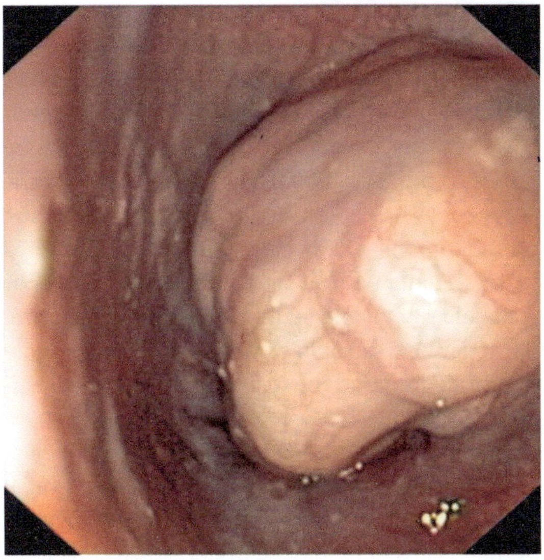

Fig. 33.2 Endoscopic view: leiomyoma of the lower third of the oesophagus: intact mucosal layer, large multilobular intramural tumour protrudes into the lumen of the oesophagus

rally in 72% of cases [7] and in the lower two-thirds of the oesophagus in over 80% [5, 7, 21]. It is important for the treatment concept to distinguish leiomyoma from potentially malignant (GISTs) or definitely malignant (leiomyosarcomas) neoplasms. The malignant potential of a lesion may be estimated non-invasively by the ultrasonic criteria of Yamada et al. [22]: (1) tumour size ≥3 cm, (2) nodular shape, (3) ulceration depth of ≥5 mm, 4 heterogeneous internal echo and (5) the presence of anechoic areas. If an intramural oesophageal tumour shows less than three of these features, it may be interpreted as a rather benign neoplasm. Under certain circumstances, a higher level of diagnostic evidence may be reached by US-guided fine-needle aspiration and histologic examination.

Generally, if oesophagus-preserving tumourectomy is aimed, transmucosal biopsies' sampling should be considered very carefully. Mucosal damage and scar formation following biopsy may increase the risk of intraoperative mucosal injury during enucleation.

33.3 Minimally Invasive Surgical Treatment

Since minimally invasive techniques have been established in oesophageal surgery, benign oesophageal tumours became a classical indication for this surgical approach. The first cases of thoracoscopic or laparoscopic enucleation of BOTs were published in the 1990s [8, 9, 18, 23–27].

The surgeon has to choose the most suitable access among the following three approaches in dependence of tumour localisation: (1) laparoscopic transhiatal, (2) video-assisted thoracoscopic surgery (VATS) in the right hemithorax and (3) VATS in the left hemithorax.

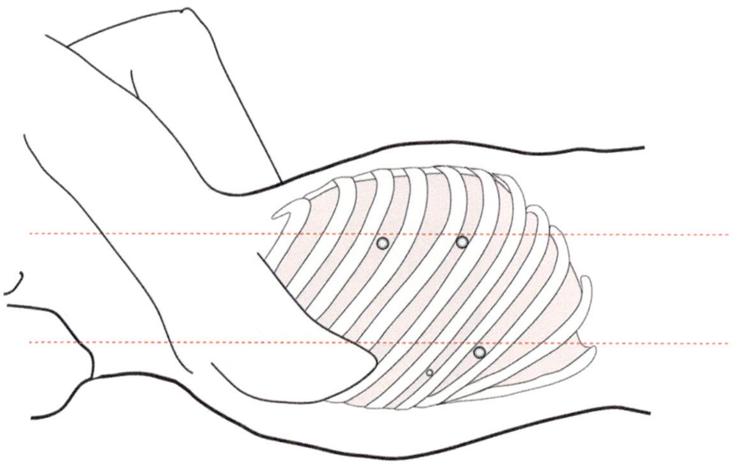

Fig. 33.3 Port positions at the right hemithorax for VATS approach. *AAL* anterior axillary line, *PAL* posterior axillary line

The most convenient approach for tumours located in the upper and middle third of oesophagus is right-sided VATS. Tumours of the distal and abdominal oesophagus as well as tumours located at the gastroesophageal junction (GEJ) could be reached more suitable through a laparoscopic access. Tumours in the lower third of the oesophagus with some distance to the diaphragm may be more comfortable accessible by left-sided VATS.

The operative technique for endoscopic enucleation of leiomyoma will be described in detail Section 33.3.1.

The principles of the minimally invasive enucleation of BOTs include the removal of the entire lesion with an intact tumour capsula. The injury of the mucosal layer is to be avoided. Re-approximation of muscle layers may prevent the development of a pseudodiverticulum and should be intended. In cases of a resulting muscular defect, a pleural flap may be raised to augment the oesophageal wall.

33.3.1 Right-Sided VATS Approach (Fig. 33.4)

The patient is placed in a left lateral decubitus position. The surgical procedure is performed with the patient in general anaesthesia with contralateral single-lung ventilation.

We use four endoscopic ports: three 12-mm and one 5-mm port. Exact port position is given in Fig. 33.3. The camera port (12 mm) is placed in the sixth intercostal space near the anterior axillary line. The 12-mm port for the lung retractor is placed at the forth intercostal space also at the level of anterior axillary line. The 5-mm working port is placed near the scapular angle, and another 12-mm working port is located one or two intercostal spaces lower than the camera port at the posterior axillary line. The exact position of the ports could be chosen higher or lower depending on the tumour localisation. The lung is retracted to the sternum with an endoretractor. If the tumour is not clearly visible by thoracoscopy, we perform intraoperative oesophagoscopy. After exact location of the tumour, the dissection of the mediastinal pleura is performed over the tumour using a cautery hook or endoscissors (Fig. 33.4a). Special care should be taken for the azygos vein and vagal trunks. If required, the oesophagus-crossing part of the azygos vein may be divided using an endoscopic vascular stapler (Fig. 33.4b). After adequate mobilisation, the external longitudinal muscle layer of the oesophagus is dissected directly over the tumour with a hook or endoscopic scissors to expose the tumour (Fig. 33.4c). Mobilisation of the tumour-bearing segment of the oesophagus over sufficient length above and below the tumour performed with a hook, endoscissors or ultrasonic scalpel may be facilitated by the placement of a silicon tube around the oesophagus enabling gentle traction. Especially for tumours located at the left side of thoracic oesophagus, the complete circumferential mobilisation is necessary.

We recommend enucleating the tumour by blunt dissection with a Maryland dissector or endoscopic peanut swabs (Fig. 33.4d). If sharp dissection is needed at certainy points, it may be done by endoscopic scissors or cauter hook. Caution should be kept for using of electrocautery near the mucosa. Bipolar cautery forceps might be helpful in juxtamucosal preparation. Once a mucosal injury occurs, the efect usually can be closed thoracoscopically with monofilament

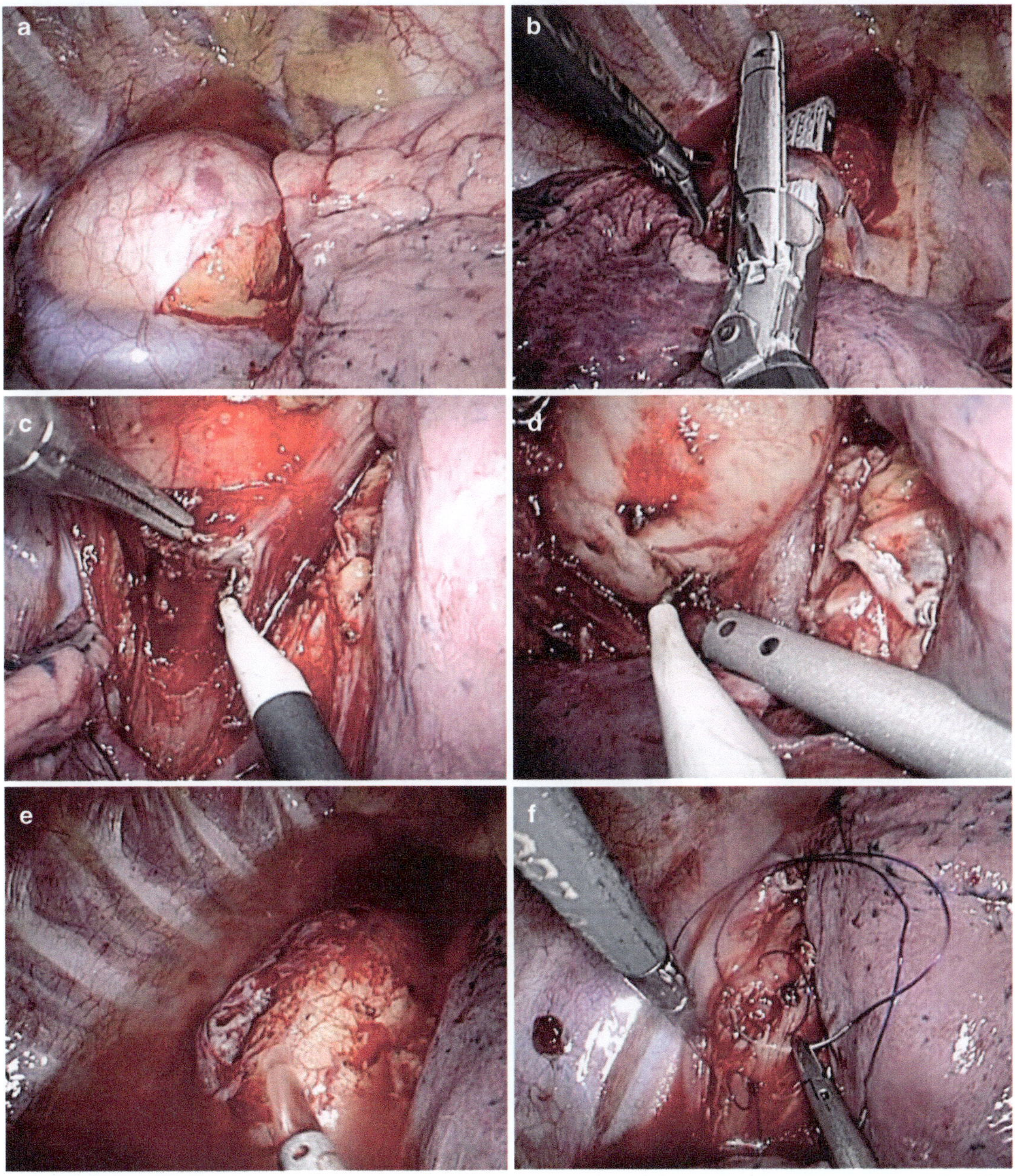

Fig. 33.4 VATS enucleation of a leiomyoma of the thoracic oesophagus. (**a**) Leiomyoma is well visible; mediastinal pleura is dissected. (**b**) Dividing of azygos vein. (**c**) Longitudinal myotomy over the leiomyoma. (**d**) Submucosal enucleation of the leiomyoma. (**e**) Intraoperative gastroscopy with air leak test after tumour enucleation. (**f**) Closure of longitudinal myotomy. (**g**) Closure of mediastinal pleura covers the myotomy suture. (**h**) Specimen

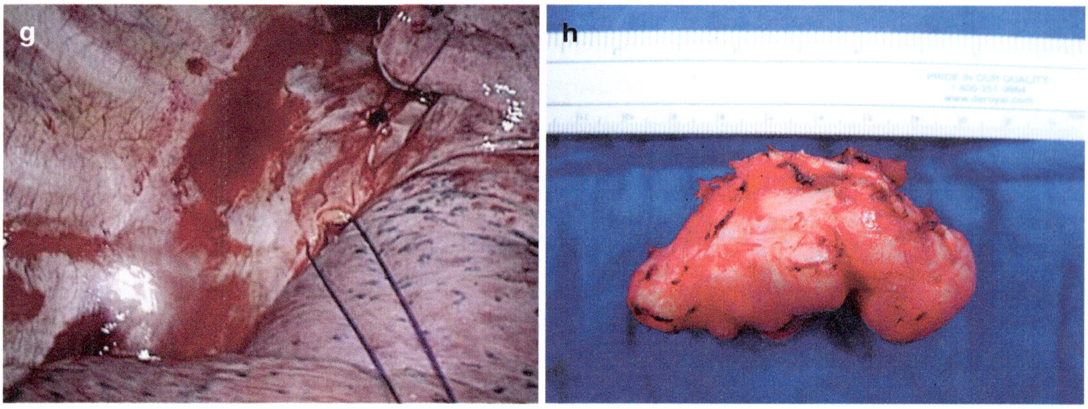

Fig. 33.4 (continued)

absorbable sutures (recommended strength 4.0 USP). After complete removal of the tumour, it should be harvested through a mini-thoracotomy of adequate length with a retrieval bag to avoid intrathoracic spillage. The incision should be protected to prevent any contamination of the chest wall with tumour material. Intraoperative air leak test should be performed to prove the mucosa integrity (Fig. 33.4e).

The resulting defect of the oesophageal muscular layer is closed by a running suture (Fig. 33.4f) with monofilament absorbable material 2.0 USP. Alternatively a pleural patch may be used to cover the defect. If possible, the mediastinal pleura should be closed over the oesophagus (Fig. 33.4g). The right lung will be reinflated after removal of all instruments and insertion of chest tubes. Closing of port sites follows.

fluid oral nutrition may be started at the following day, if a routinely performed swallow study (we recommend a water-soluble contrast medium) is without pathological findings. Alternatively a dye test may prove wall integrity, if a drainage is in adequate position.

If the tumour is located in the lower third of the oesophagus, a similar VATS procedure may be performed at the left side.

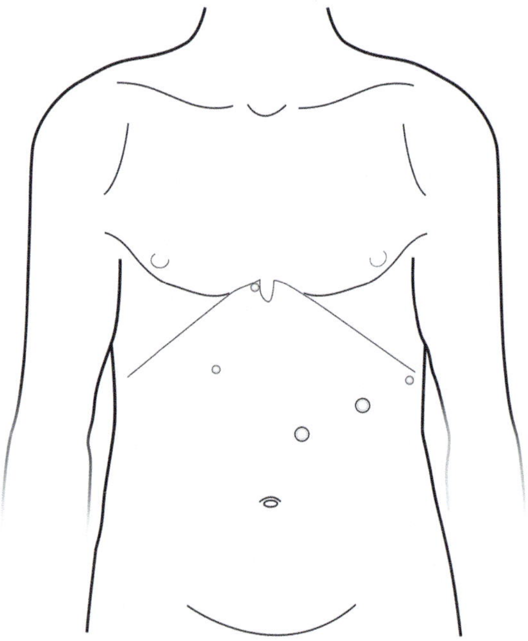

Fig. 33.5 Port positions at the abdominal wall for the laparoscopic transhiatal approach

33.3.2 Laparoscopic (Transhiatal) Approach (Fig. 33.6)

The patient is placed in the supine Lloyd-Davis-like position. The port positions are similar to other procedures at the GEJ. Our standard port positions are exposed on the Fig. 33.5. Shortly, we use five ports (two 12 mm, three 5 mm). After adequate circumferential transhiatal mobilisation of the oesophagus (Fig. 33.6a) and longitudinal myotomy over the tumour (Fig. 33.6b), blunt and sharp enucleation is performed using a cauter hook, endoscissors or ultrasonic shears (Fig. 33.6c), as described earlier (see above: VATS approach). The muscle layer defect should also be re-approximated by

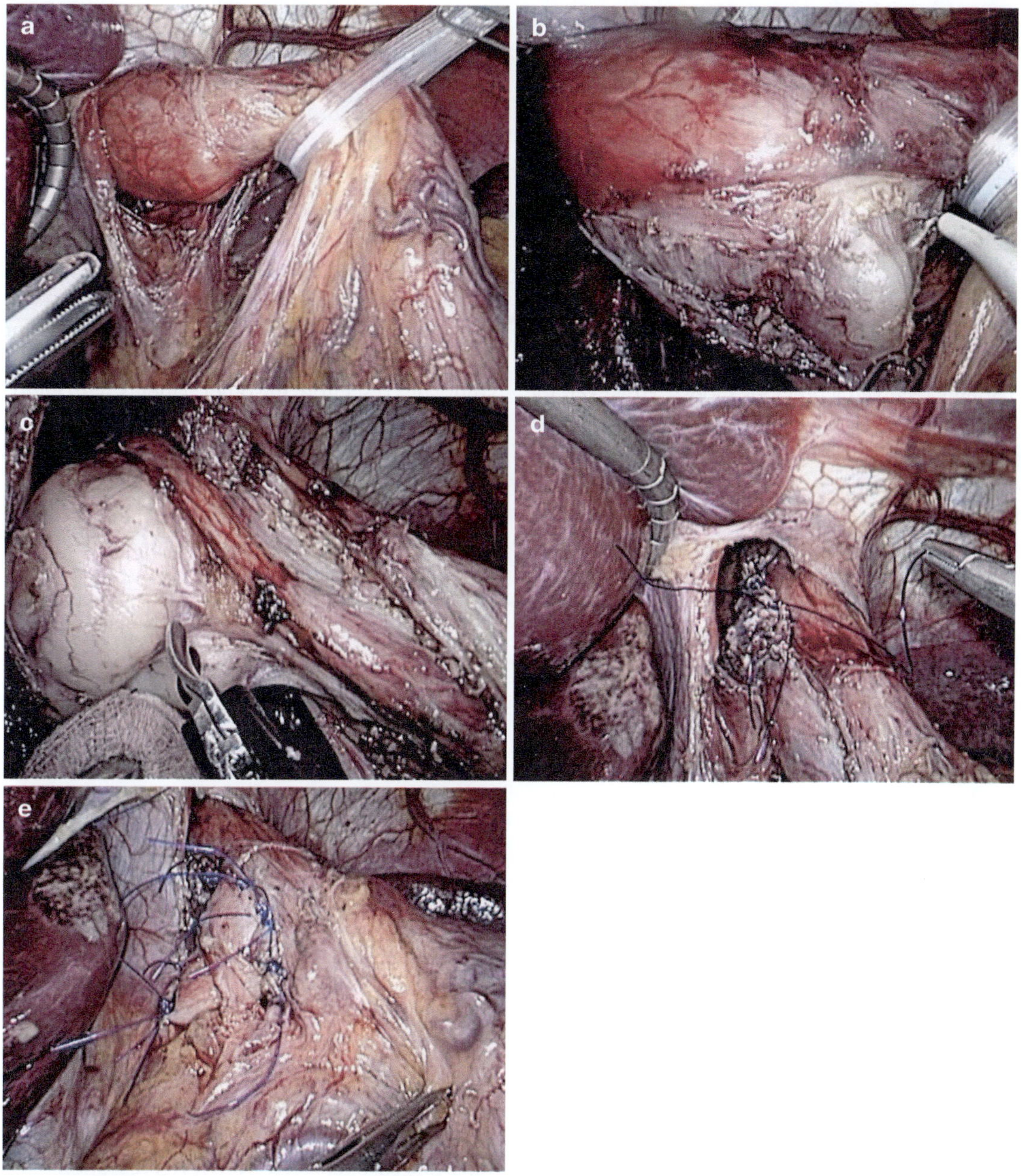

Fig. 33.6 Laparoscopic enucleation of an oesophageal leiomyoma, localised in the lower third at the posterior wall. (**a**) Oesophagus is transhiatally mobilised, leiomyoma at the posterior wall is well visible. (**b**) Longitudinal myotomy over the leiomyoma. (**c**) Oesophageal leiomyoma is mobilised. (**d**) Closure of longitudinal myotomy after completed enucleation of leiomyoma. (**e**) Posterior hemiplication

absorbable sutures (Fig. 33.6d). Furthermore, a hemi- or fundoplication may be added to cover the suture or any resulting defect (Fig. 33.6e). This procedure has also an anti-reflux effect.

Endoscopic enucleation of oesophageal leiomyoma is a safe and effective method. Over 90% of symptomatic patients experienced complete resolution of symptoms lasting over long follow-up period [21]. Since considerable experience with minimally invasive surgical approach has been gained in the last two decades, no study reported any mortality so far [7, 10, 11, 13–18,

21, 23, 24, 26, 28]. There was also no operative mortality for open procedure in the largest series about leiomyoma enucleation [5, 18]. The cumulative rate of conversion to an open access in 200 minimally invasive endoscopic procedures is 8.5% [13–17]. The causes for conversion are too large tumour size, too small non-visible tumour with difficult localisation and the presence of pleural adhesions. Two intraoperative perforations were reported by Kent M. et al. in a series of 20 patients [13] and one by Zaninotto G. et al. in a series comprising 11 patients [12]. All of these patients received a previous biopsy. However, the mucosal injury was recognised intraoperatively and could be successfully managed by a suture. Cardiac arrhythmia in the early postoperative period was described in 3/17 patients [15] and 1/16 [13]. One patient was readmitted to the hospital at the fifth postoperative day because of pneumonia [13]. No leakage or other severe complications were reported after minimally invasive approaches so far [8–17, 21, 23, 26, 27].

Pseudodiverticula have been reported in three cases after VATS enucleation [12, 18, 23]. In two of these cases, the muscle defect of oesophageal wall was not closed. Only two cases of recurrence are documented in the literature for open surgery [7], none after minimally invasive approach. Five out of 20 patients with BOTs, described by Kent M. et al., required an anti-reflux procedure after primary enucleation for development or worsening of GERD after a median follow-up of 6 (1–45) months. Except this report, only in one more series of 14 cases with a follow-up of 19 (1–50) months [17], the development of GERD-like symptoms was reported (one patient). The same authors described two cases with mild pain on the incision sites persisting for 3 months after surgery and required medication.

Oesophagectomy may be the adequate surgical option for about 10% of patients with extended, circular or multiple benign oesophageal tumours [5]. In such a situation, the careful review of technical feasibility and indication with active involvement of the patient should be aimed keeping in mind the risky nature of oesophagectomy and possible impairment in quality of life. Minimally invasive techniques for oesophagectomy are described lower (see Chap. 9, Sect. 4). Lymphadenectomy is not required if the dignity of the tumour is clearly benign.

Other intramural benign oesophageal tumours, such as granular cell tumours, haemangiomas, schwannomas, neurofibromas and paragangliomas, are much more uncommon than leiomyomas. Very few case reports are available regarding oesophageal fibrovascular polyps [29]. Accompanying literature review identified 75 patients with this pathology. Fifty-seven percent were treated with surgical (transcervical or transthoracic) resection, the other patients with endoscopic removal, which include electrocautery loop resection or laser ablation. Squamous papilloma [35] and submucosal paraganglioma [31] have also been removed endoscopically with forceps or endoscopic snares. The literature review regarding schwannoma revealed 30 cases [30, 32]. In 24 patients, an enucleation was performed, including one case with minimally invasive (thoracoscopic) approach, one tumour required oesophagectomy, and in five cases, endoscopic treatment was successful.

Special attention should be paid for haemangiomas, which are more often located in the submucosal layer of middle oesophagus and may present primary with the upper gastrointestinal bleeding. If a lesion suspect for haemangioma is diagnosed during oesophagoscopy, the biopsy is strictly contraindicated; CT scan and EUS may be helpful for further diagnosis. Recently, haemangiomas are usually treated by endoscopic procedures (sclerotherapy, laser ablation, endoscopic resection) [28]. Cases with persisting tumour bleeding needed emergent surgical treatment typically by an open approach. There is only one case reported with VATS resection of an oesophageal haemangioma [25].

Gastrointestinal stromal tumour (GIST) is a rare mesenchymal malignancy of the oesophagus, which must be distinguished from the BOTs. In many cases, only histologic examination reveals the diagnosis GIST. Therapeutic management of GISTs depends on size, tumour localisation and count of mitotic cells. c-kit mutation analysis may help to predict response to treatment with tyrosine-kinase inhibitors [33].

33.4 Summary

Benign oesophageal tumours are rare conditions, represented by leiomyomas in about 80% of cases. Most of the patients are asymptomatic. If symptomatic, the leading clinical features are dysphagia and chest discomfort. Frequently the diagnosis occurs incidentally by endoscopic or radiologic investigation due to other reasons. Contrast swallow, CT scan, endoscopy and EUS contribute to further diagnosis. Therapy concept must be developed for every individual patient and may include observation alone or tumour extirpation. Usually, organ-preserving resection is the preferred method which is followed by low morbidity, excellent long-term results and quality of life. As established in almost every gastrointestinal surgical procedure, minimally invasive approaches have successfully been adopted for the treatment of BOTs with a benefit by reduction of surgical trauma.

References

1. Plachta A (1962) Benign tumors of the esophagus: review of literature and report of 99 cases. Am J Gastroenterol 38:639–52
2. Levine MS (2003) Benign tumors of the esophagus: radiologic evaluation. Semin Thorac Cardiovasc Surg 15:9–19, Review
3. Attah EB, Hajdu SI (1968) Benign and malignant tumors of the esophagus at autopsy. J Thorac Cardiovasc Surg 55:396–404
4. Schmidt HW, Clagett OT, Harrison EG Jr (1961) Benign tumors and cysts of the esophagus. Ann Otol Rhinol Laryngol 70:1148–57
5. Seremetis M, Lyons W, DeGuzman V (1976) Leiomyomata of the esophagus: an analysis of 838 cases. Cancer 38:2166–77
6. Avezzano EA, Fleischer DE, Merida MA et al (1990) Giant fibrovascular polyps of the esophagus. Am J Gastroenterol 85:299–302
7. Hatch GF 3rd, Wertheimer-Hatch L, Hatch KF et al (2000) Tumors of the esophagus. World J Surg 24:401–11
8. Gossot D, Fourquier P, el Meteini M et al (1993) Technical aspects of endoscopic removal of benign tumors of the esophagus. Surg Endosc 7:102–3
9. Peracchia A, Rosati R, Bardini R (1996) Thoracoscopic removal of tumors of the esophagus. In: Gossot D, Hunter JG, Toouli J (eds) Endosurgery. Churchill Livingston, Edinburgh
10. Samphire J, Nafteux P, Luketich J (2003) Minimally invasive techniques for resection of benign esophageal tumors. Semin Thorac Cardiovasc Surg 15:35–43
11. von Rahden BH, Stein HJ, Feussner H et al (2004) Enucleation of submucosal tumors of the esophagus: minimally invasive versus open approach. Surg Endosc 18:924–30
12. Zaninotto G, Portale G, Costantini M et al (2006) Minimally invasive enucleation of esophageal leiomyoma. Surg Endosc 20:1904–8
13. Kent M, d'Amato T, Nordman C et al (2007) Minimally invasive resection of benign esophageal tumors. J Thorac Cardiovasc Surg 134:176–81
14. Vallböhmer D, Hölscher AH, Brabender J et al (2007) Thoracoscopic enucleation of esophageal leiomyomas: a feasible and safe procedure. Endoscopy 39:1097–9
15. Palanivelu C, Rangarajan M, Madankumar MV et al (2008) Minimally invasive therapy for benign tumors of the distal third of the esophagus – a single institute's experience. J Laparoendosc Adv Surg Tech A 18:20–6
16. Jiang G, Zhao H, Yang F et al (2009) Thoracoscopic enucleation of esophageal leiomyoma: a retrospective study on 40 cases. Dis Esophagus 22:279–83
17. Li ZG, Chen HZ, Jin H et al (2009) Surgical treatment of esophageal leiomyoma located near or at the esophagogastric junction via a thoracoscopic approach. Dis Esophagus 22:185–9
18. Bonavina L, Segalin A, Rosati R et al (1995) Surgical therapy of esophageal leiomyoma. J Am Coll Surg 181:257–62
19. Rice TW (2003) Benign esophageal tumors: esophagoscopy and endoscopic esophageal ultrasound. Semin Thorac Cardiovasc Surg 15:20–6, Review
20. Kinney T, Waxman I (2003) Treatment of benign esophageal tumors by endoscopic techniques. Semin Thorac Cardiovasc Surg 15:27–34, Review
21. Mutrie CJ, Donahue DM, Wain JC et al (2005) Esophageal leiomyoma: a 40-year experience. Ann Thorac Surg 79:1122–5
22. Yamada Y, Kida M, Sakaguchi T (1992) A study of myogenic tumors of the upper gastrointestinal tract by endoscopic ultrasonography with special reference to the differential diagnosis of benign and malignant lesions. Dig Endosc 4:396–408
23. Bardini R, Segalin A, Ruol A et al (1992) Videothoracoscopic enucleation of esophageal leiomyoma. Ann Thorac Surg 54:576–7
24. Izumi Y, Inoue H, Endo M (1996) Combined endoluminal-intracavitary thoracoscopic enucleation of leiomyoma of the esophagus. A new method. Surg Endosc 10:457–8
25. Rämö OJ, Salo JA, Bardini R et al (1997) Treatment of a submucosal hemangioma of the esophagus using simultaneous video-assisted thoracoscopy and esophagoscopy: description of a new minimally invasive technique. Endoscopy 29:S27–8
26. Roviaro GC, Maciocco M, Varoli F et al (1998) Videothoracoscopic treatment of oesophageal leiomyoma. Thorax 53:190–2

27. Tamura K, Takamori S, Tayama K et al (1998) Thoracoscopic resection of a giant leiomyoma of the esophagus with a mediastinal outgrowth. Ann Thorac Cardiovasc Surg 4(6):351–3, Review
28. Sogabe M, Taniki T, Fukui Y et al (2006) A patient with esophageal hemangioma treated by endoscopic mucosal resection: a case report and review of the literature. J Med Invest 53:177–82, Review
29. Drenth J, Wobbes T, Bonenkamp JJ et al (2002) Recurrent esophageal fibrovascular polyps: case history and review of the literature. Dig Dis Sci 47:2598–604, Review
30. Murase K, Hino A, Ozeki Y et al (2001) Malignant schwannoma of the esophagus with lymph node metastasis: literature review of schwannoma of the esophagus. J Gastroenterol 36:772–7
31. Harries K, Nunn T, Shah V et al (2004) First reported case of esophageal paraganglioma. A review of the literature of gastrointestinal tract paraganglioma including gangliocytic paraganglioma. Dis Esophagus 17:191–5
32. Park BJ, Carrasquillo J, Bains MS et al (2006) Giant benign esophageal schwannoma requiring esophagectomy. Ann Thorac Surg 82:340–2
33. Ploner F, Zacherl J, Wrba F et al (2009) Gastrointestinal stromal tumors: recommendations on diagnosis, therapy and follow-up care in Austria. Wien Klin Wochenschr 121:780–90
34. Moersch HJ, Harrington SW (1944) Benign tumors of the esophagus. Ann Otol Rhinol Laryngol 53:800–17
35. Mosca S, Manes G, Monaco R et al (2001) Squamous papilloma of the esophagus: long-term follow up. J Gastroenterol Hepatol 16:857–61

Minimally Invasive Esophagectomy

34

Philippe Nafteux, Georges Decker,
and Toni E.M.R. Lerut

Contents

P. Nafteux, M.D. (✉) • G. Decker, M.D.
T.E.M.R. Lerut, M.D., Ph.D.
Department of Thoracic Surgery, UZ Gasthuisberg,
Herestraat 49, Leuven 3000, Belgium
e-mail: philippe.nafteux@uzleuven.be;
georges.decker@uzleuven.be;
toni.lerut@uz.kuleuven.ac.be

34.1 Introduction

Radical surgery currently offers the most realistic chance of cure for cancer of the esophagus or gastroesophageal junction (GEJ) when spread beyond the most superficial epithelial layers, but not extending beyond locoregional lymph nodes [1, 2]. Nowadays experienced centers can consistently perform such an aggressive "conventional" surgery with mortality rates of 3–5% and consistently obtain overall 5-year survival rates of at least 35–40% [1–3]. Few other oncological operations however are as heavily influenced by experience than esophagectomy for cancer, and experienced centers not only achieve lower mortality rates but also much higher cure rates than low-volume centers [4, 5]. However, despite considerable improvements in outcome due to better cancer staging, patient selection, and surgical techniques during the last decade, overall and pulmonary complication rates have remain sufficiently high to encourage the search for alternative operative techniques that could potentially achieve similar cure rates but with less morbidity and probably a better post-operative quality of life.

R.G.C. Inderbitzi et al. (eds.), *Minimally Invasive Thoracic and Cardiac Surgery*,
DOI 10.1007/978-3-642-11861-6_34, © Springer-Verlag Berlin Heidelberg 2012

With this objective in mind, less invasive surgical approaches have been introduced since the 1980s under the form of transhiatal resection (e.g., without any opening of the chest), either with or without the use of (video) mediastinoscope [6–8]. Benefits over transthoracic resection particularly in terms of reduced pulmonary were recently be formally proven by a large randomized study [3, 9]. However, transhiatal esophagectomy (THE) did not reduce mortality compared to transthoracic approaches, and its drawback is clearly the inability to perform a radical lymph node dissection of the mediastinum, thus compromising the chance for long-term survival in any patient with cancer of the thoracic esophagus, including those of the distal third [3, 10].

The use of thoracoscopy and/or laparoscopy for esophageal resection was introduced in 1992 by Cushieri et al., hoping it would further reduce pulmonary morbidity while potentially improving the oncological quality of the resection by enhancing visual control during the mediastinal dissection [11]. Several small series subsequently demonstrated the feasibility of this new approach, but again, pulmonary morbidity was substantial and the early enthusiasm quickly faded [12–14]. Despite the considerable morbidity, the term minimally invasive esophagectomy (MIE) was born and would continue to be applied [7]. During the late 1990s, general advances in laparoscopic skills and equipment encouraged many centers to reintroduce the minimally invasive technology using laparoscopy, thoracoscopy, video-assisted minilaparotomy, or minithoracotomy (VATS) as well as various forms of hand-assisted, robot-assisted, or hybrid techniques for esophageal resection. A few large series have since reported reasonable outcome with some of these approaches, leading to a more frequent use of MIE [15–17]. However, 15 years after the introduction of MIE, evidence from randomized controlled trials is still lacking to confirm neither any benefit of MIE in terms of surgical outcome and safety nor its oncological adequacy as compared to standard open resection.

In this chapter, we will present several minimally invasive esophagectomy techniques as well as review the available evidence in the literature and our own results in an attempt to define a place for minimally invasive esophagectomy in the armamentarium of the surgeon dealing with esophageal cancer.

34.2 Preoperative Evaluation

The preoperative work-up done before MIE is comparable to the one performed before open esophagectomy. Upper GI endoscopy with biopsy is mandatory for diagnosis. Classically, an endo-ultrasound will be performed as to define the “T” and “N” stage of the tumor. For early tumors, an endomucosal resection can be performed as a staging procedure (proving T1b) or as a definitive treatment in case of T1a lesion. Barium swallow, CT chest/abdomen, and PET scan are routinely performed in our department to rule out metastasis (M) and to further refine T and N assessment. A bronchoscopy can be performed in selected cases (to rule out T4 stage or second primary cancer in the lung especially in case of squamous cell carcinoma).

Thorough physiologic evaluation will be performed and involves routine biochemistry, pulmonary function tests, and electrocardiogram and cardiac stress testing. Echo-Doppler of the carotids can be performed in vascular high-risk patients.

34.3 Techniques

The most frequently used technique is the totally thoracoscopic and laparoscopic esophagectomy performed in three stages. During our early experience, we noted that when performing the laparoscopic part after the thoracic part, esophageal dissection in the hiatus and lower mediastinum creates an open communication with the chest which can lead to important CO_2 leak into the chest cavity due to the broad open pleura. This can cause an important drop in intra-abdominal pressure, leading to impaired visualization during this important dissection step. This is less of a problem when the abdominal part is performed first even when a complete periesophageal lymph node clearance is performed in the hiatus. On the other hand, starting with the abdominal part necessitates the patient to be turned twice (when performing the cervical anastomosis) instead of once, making the operation longer. We will describe this technique in detail as this is our preferred approach.

Elements specific for other techniques will be highlighted later.

34.3.1 Laparoscopic and Thoracoscopic Esophagectomy

34.3.1.1 Anesthesia

General anesthesia in combination with thoracic epidural is used.

As single-lung ventilation is mandatory for the thoracic part, a left-sided double-lumen endotracheal tube is placed and will be replaced by the regular endotracheal tube once the thoracic part is over and the patient is again turned in supine position for the cervical part of the procedure.

Arterial catheter for pressure monitoring, a central venous line, and a bladder catheter for urine output monitoring are placed *lege artis*.

34.3.1.2 Surgical Technique: Laparoscopic and Thoracoscopic Esophagectomy

Thoracoscopic and laparoscopic esophagectomy is classically performed in three stages.

1. In the first stage, the patient is positioned in the supine position for laparoscopic mobilization of the stomach, gastric tubulization, and lymphadenectomy.
2. In the second stage, the patient is placed in the left lateral decubitus for thoracic esophageal dissection and lymphadenectomy.
3. The third stage is performed through a left cervical incision anterior to the sternocleidomastoid muscle. The cervical esophagus is mobilized, and the gastric conduit is under direct laparoscopic vision brought through the hiatus and mediastinum into the neck. The esophageal anastomosis is then performed in the neck in an end-to-side fashion.

Stage 1 Laparoscopic Gastric Mobilization and Tubulization

The patient is placed in supine position, and the legs are placed in the leg support. The patient is prepped and draped. The surgeon takes place in between the legs, the first assistant on the right side of the patient, the second assistant on the left side of the patient. Typically five abdominal ports are placed in a similar fashion to the approach used for a laparoscopic Nissen fundoplication (Fig. 34.1a–b). The first port (12 mm) is placed in a supra-umbilical position after insufflation of a pneumoperitoneum to a pressure of 15 mmHg. Subsequently a 12-mm port is placed in the right upper quadrant for

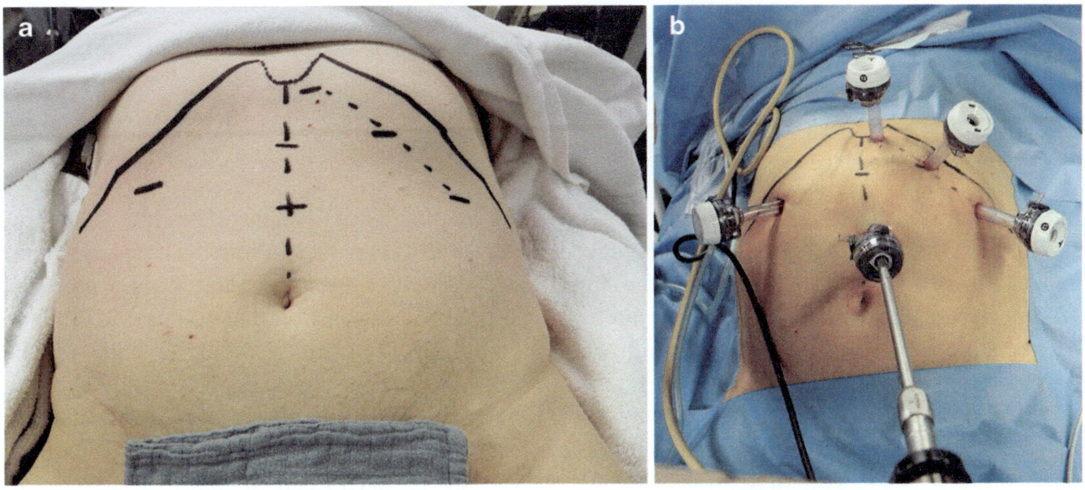

Fig. 34.1 (**a**, **b**) Typical installation showing the positions of the five ports and their relations to the surface anatomy of the abdomen

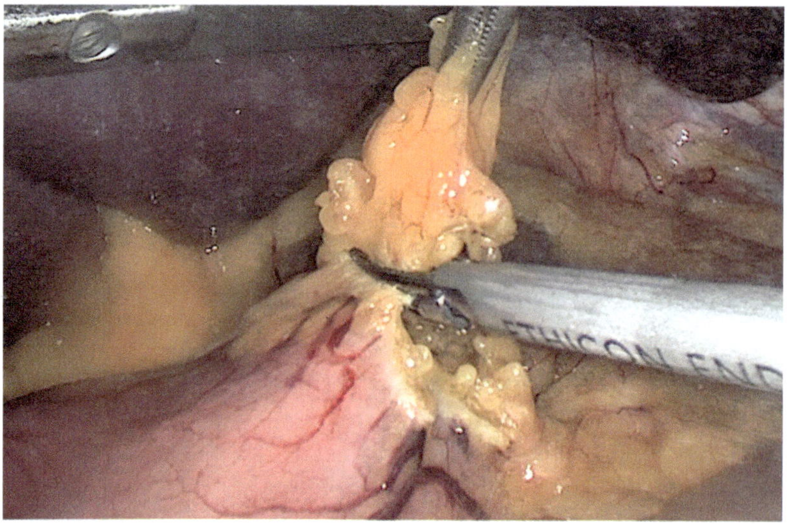

Fig. 34.2 A small incision in the gastrohepatic ligament is performed alongside the lesser curve a few cm proximally from the pylorus. The right gastric artery and the gastrohepatic ligament are subsequently transected using the harmonic scalpel

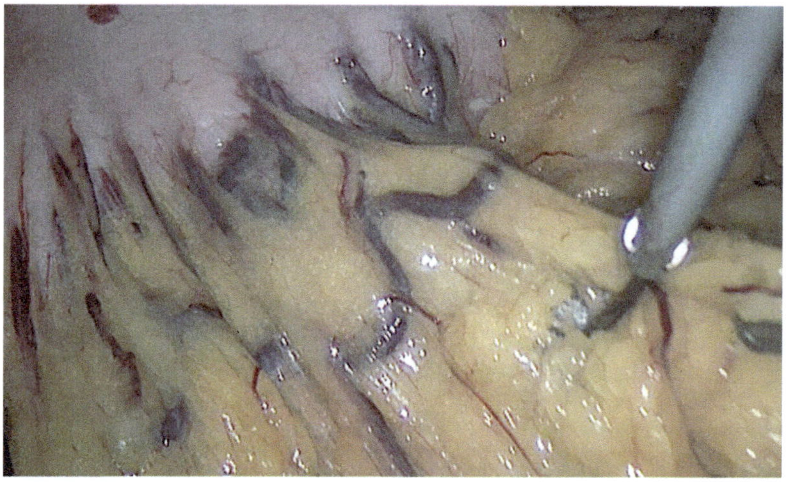

Fig. 34.3 During mobilization of the greater curve, great care has to be taken not to damage the right gastroepiploic artery and vein. It is not always possible to visualize those structures, especially in obese patients, but most of the time, a bulging at the level of the arteriovenous gastroepiploic axis can be seen alongside the greater curve. Dissecting away from this bulge assures the integrity of both vessels

liver retraction. One 5-mm port is placed on a subxiphoidal position, a 12-mm port is placed under the left upper quadrant, and the final 10-mm port is placed below the costal arch in between ports 3 and 4. The liver is retracted medially, and the dissection starts with transection of the gastrohepatic ligament and transection of the right gastric artery using the harmonic scalpel (Fig. 34.2). The dissection continues along the greater curvature of the stomach, taking great care not to damage the right gastroepiploic artery (Fig. 34.3). From the lesser curvature side, the left gastric artery and vein are prepared and clipped at their base as to ensure complete lymph node clearance in along both vessels (Fig. 34.4). The esophagus is then dissected in the hiatus with en bloc resection of the periesophageal tissue (Fig. 34.5). The gastric tubulization is performed using endostaplers to achieve a gastric tube of 4–5 cm width

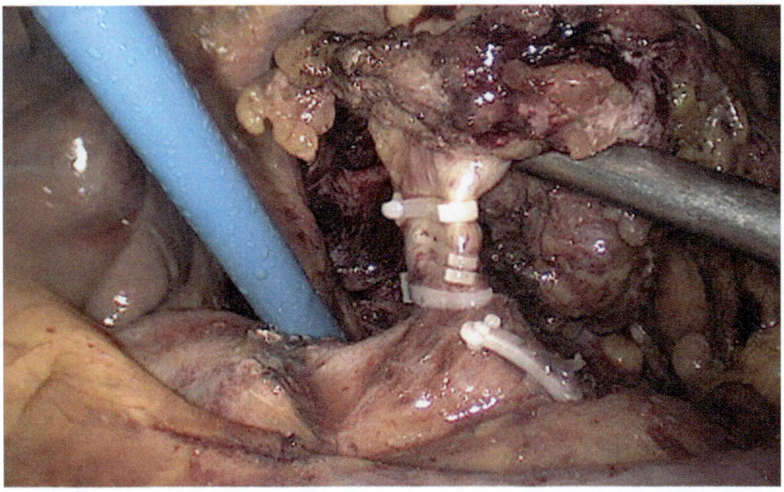

Fig. 34.4 From the lesser curvature side, the left gastric vein and artery are dissected. The vein is first encountered more anteriorly and to the left; the artery lies behind the vein and more to the right. The vein has in this patient already been clipped, and the periarterial lymph nodes have been completely removed

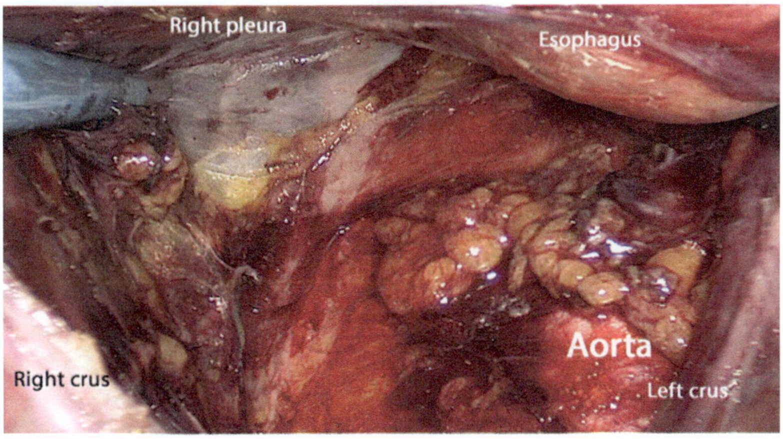

Fig. 34.5 Before performing gastric tubulization, it is important to free the esophagus in the hiatus, especially in case of hiatal hernia. It will enhance mobilization of the stomach and in that way greatly facilitate gastric tubulization

(Fig. 34.6). This tube is most of the times 30 cm long. We do not perform a pyloric drainage procedure.

Once the tubulization has been performed, a lymph node dissection alongside the hepatic artery, the splenic artery and celiac trunk is routinely performed. During this abdominal part, great care is taken not to grasp the gastric conduit to avoid trauma and serosal tears. The gastric tube is then fixed to the proximal gastrectomy specimen using two temporary stitches. Trocars are removed under visual control, pneumoperitoneum is deflated, and incisions are closed. We do not routinely perform a pyloric drainage procedure nor leave a drain in the abdominal cavity.

Stage 2 Thoracoscopic Mobilization of the Esophagus

The patient is now placed in left lateral decubitus and stabilized using a beanbag and taped to the table on the level of the iliac crest top. The surgeon is positioned at the back of the patient, the

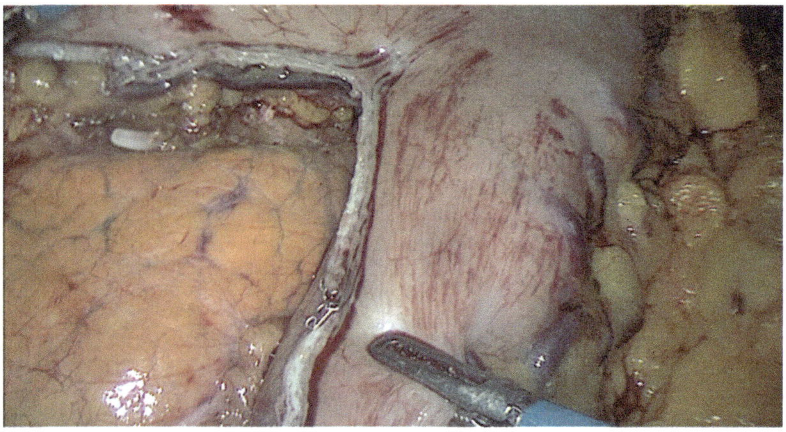

Fig. 34.6 The gastric tubulization is performed using endostaplers to achieve a gastric tube of 4–5-cm width, starting a few centimeters away from the pylorus

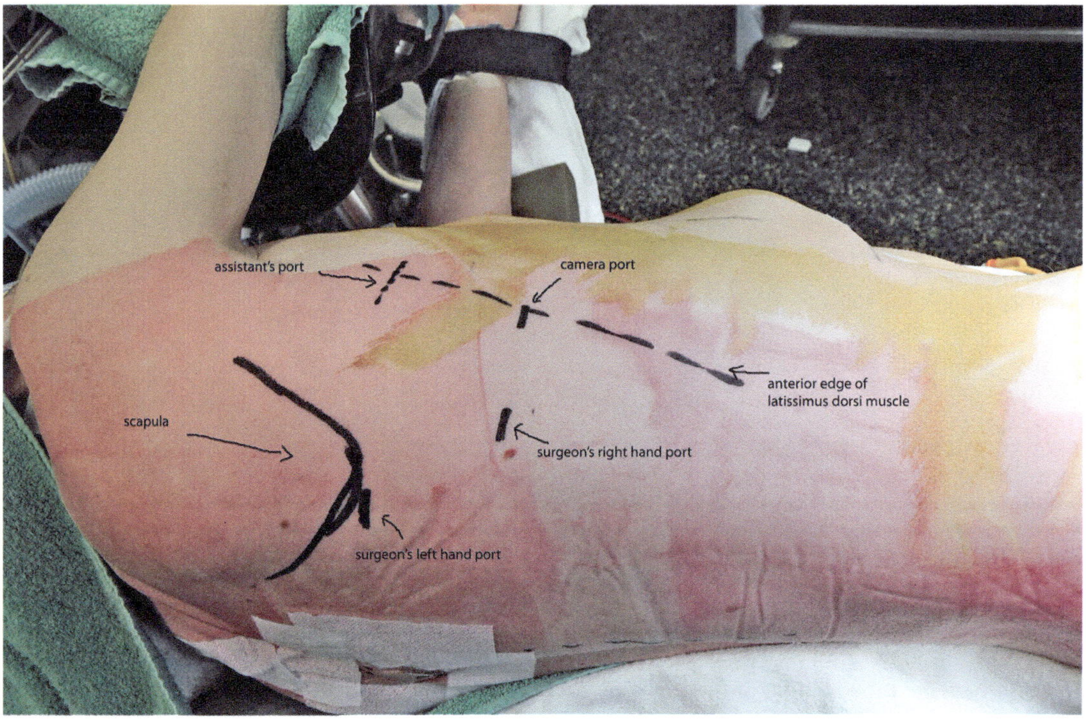

Fig. 34.7 Classical installation for right thoracoscopy showing the locations of the ports and their relation with the thoracic anatomy

first assistant in front of the patient. The patient is prepped and draped. Four thoracoscopy ports are introduced (Fig. 34.7). The 10-mm camera port is placed anteriorly to the latissimus dorsi muscle in the 6th or 7th intercostal space. Another 10-mm port is placed in the 7th intercostal space at the level of the scapula tip for the surgeon's right hand. Two additional ports are placed: one for the

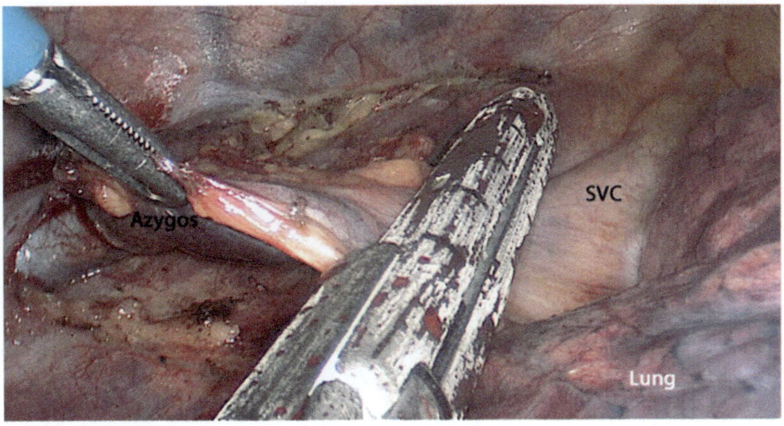

Fig. 34.8 After opening of the mediastinal pleura overlying the azygos, this vein is transected using endostaplers. This will greatly facilitate removal of the periesophageal tissue; SVC: superior vena cava

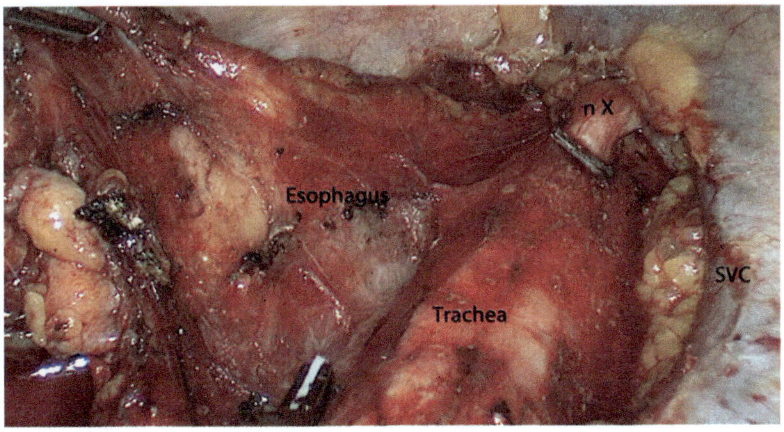

Fig. 34.9 During circumferential mobilization of the esophagus in the upper chest, great care is taken not to damage the membranous part of the trachea which lies just anteriorly to the dissection; SVC: superior vena cava; n X: vagus nerve

surgeon's second hand just posterior from the tip of the scapula and one at the third intercostal space at the anterior axillary line for lung retraction by the first assistant during esophageal dissection.

The mediastinal pleura overlying the esophagus is divided, and the entire thoracic esophagus is exposed. The azygos vein is dissected free and dividing using endostaplers (Fig. 34.8). Circumferential mobilization of the esophagus with all periesophageal tissue and lymph nodes is performed starting routinely from the azygos vein towards the top of the chest (Fig. 34.9). When the esophagus has been completely mobilized in the top of the chest, a Penrose drain is placed around the esophagus to facilitate traction and exposure. Further dissection up into the neck is performed which will facilitate the third step (cervical) of the procedure. During this part of the esophageal dissection, great care is taken not to damage the recurrent nerves while performing a lymph node dissection alongside both nerves (Fig. 34.10). Further dissection towards the subcarinal region is performed; subcarinal lymph node clearance can be performed either en bloc or in an independent step. Further mobilization of the esophagus is performed towards the diaphragm removing completely at the same time the surrounding esophageal tissues and finishing on top of the diaphragm. During the esophageal mobilization, great care is also taken not to

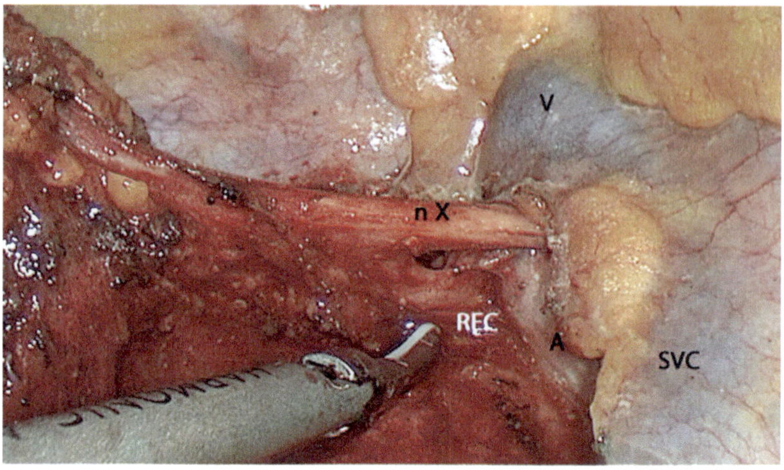

Fig. 34.10 Visualization of both recurrent nerves is critical during MIE and lymph node dissection. Traction on the vagus nerve helps during location of the right recurrent nerve n X: vagus nerve; SVC: superior vena cava; REC: recurrent nerve; A: subclavian artery; V: subclavia vein

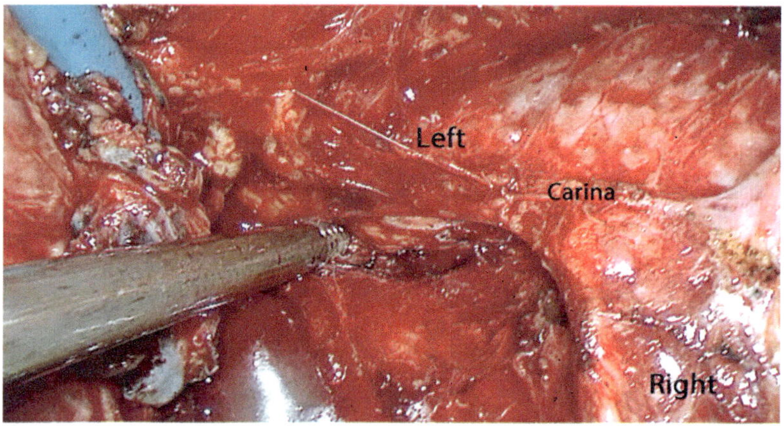

Fig. 34.11 Following the lower edge of the right main bronchus, a complete subcarinal lymph node clearance can be easily performed

damage the membranous part of the trachea or left main bronchus.

Lymph node dissection is also performed at the level of the right tracheal gutter and subcarinal region (Fig. 34.11). The thoracic duct is clipped on the top of the chest and in a retrograde manner is dissected with all its surrounding tissues downwards the chest (Fig. 34.12). It is clipped just above the diaphragm and extracted. When this has been achieved, careful hemostasis is performed and classically two chest drains are placed using therefore the two most anterior ports. The right lung is reinflated and the ports are closed.

Part 3 Mobilization of the Esophagus in the Neck and Anastomosis

An 8-cm-long left cervical incision anterior to the sternocleidomastoid muscle and finishing in the suprasternal notch is performed. Omohyoid and strapped muscles are transected. Dissection is performed medially from the great vessels and laterally from the thyroid gland clipping and transecting eventually its feeding arteries. During this procedure, again great care is taken not to damage the left recurrent nerve. The cervical esophagus is then mobilized till the thoracic part of the dissection is reached. The esophagus with the proximal gastrectomy specimen can be exteriorized through the neck incision, thus pulling

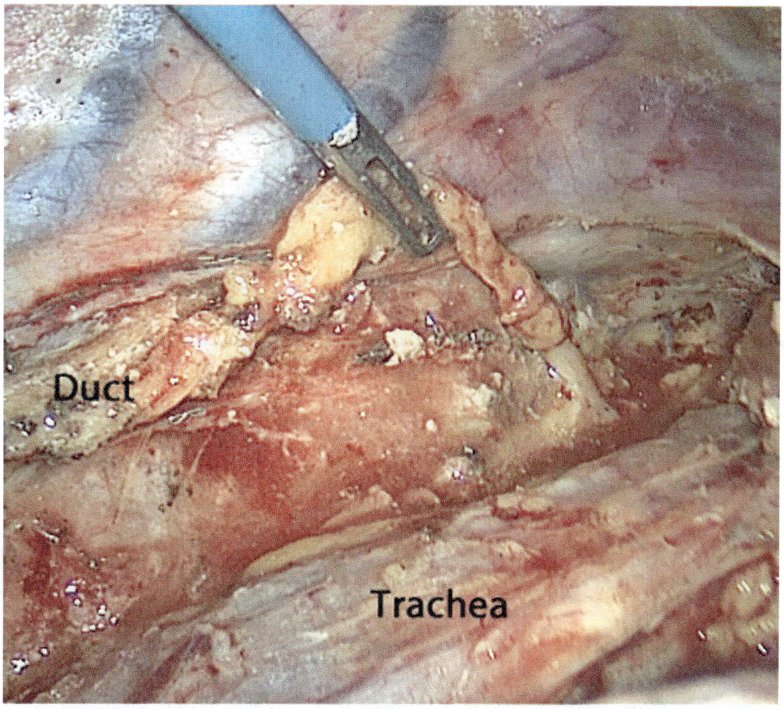

Fig. 34.12 Using the magnifying effect of the scope, the thoracic duct can be visualized in the top of the chest as a light gray shinny structure. It is then clipped on the top of the chest and in a retrograde manner is dissected with all its surrounding tissues downwards the chest

up the gastric conduit. At this point, a classic end-to-side anastomosis is performed: we prefer a semi-mechanical anastomosis, using an endostapler for the posterior esophagogastric anastomosis and finishing the anterior part of the anastomosis using continuous stitches after transection and resection of the esophagus. The nasogastric tube is then under visual control placed again into the stomach tube before finishing the anterior part of the anastomosis. The anastomosis is then reduced in the chest behind the trachea. The neck incision is then closed after placement of a closed suction drain system.

34.4 Other Operative Techniques

34.4.1 Thoracoscopic Esophageal Resection in Prone Decubitus Position

The claimed advantages of this approach in comparison with the standard lateral decubitus position are:

1. The attainable range of thoracic cage and diaphragmatic excursion is greater than in the side position.
2. The extent of mediastinal swing or displacement is less.
3. Exposure of the posterior aspect of the hilum and the esophageal area is facilitated.
4. The weight of the lung itself allows it to fall forward, alleviating the need for lung retraction during surgery.
5. In the event of hemorrhage, the blood flows away from its source, thus permitting its control with greater ease.

However, the major drawback of this procedure is the difficulty to open the chest sufficiently if an urgent thoracotomy is needed.

The patient is positioned in prone decubitus position on a standard device (Fig. 34.13) in order to support on the head, chest, and pelvis. Abdomen is maintained free for breathing excursions. Position of the arms is very important in order to get abduction of the scapula. The arms are positioned on the support device in flexion of the shoulder and elbow. In this way, the area between

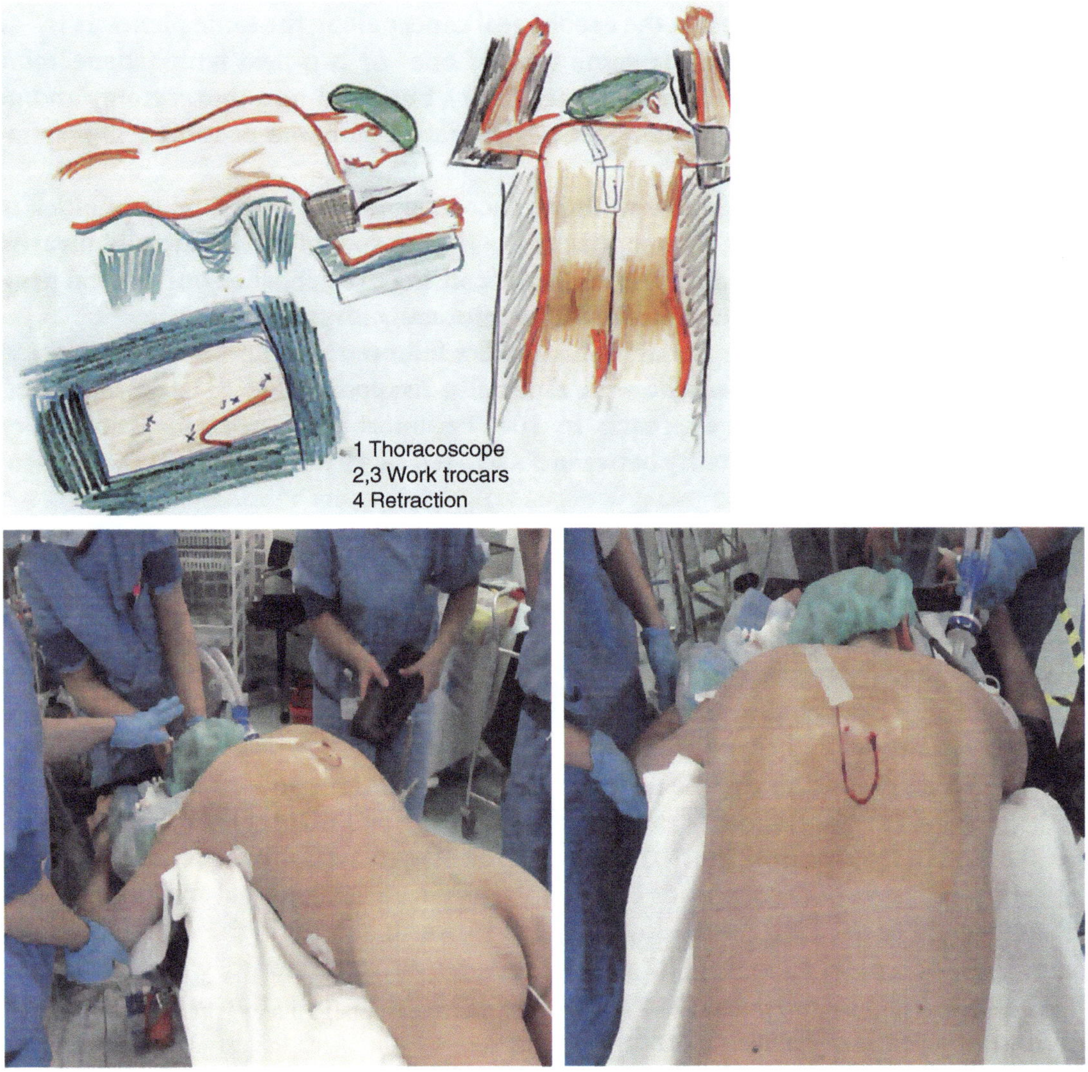

Fig. 34.13 Classical prone position installation. The patient is positioned on a standard device in order to support on the head, chest and pelvis. Abdomen is maintained free for breathing excursions. Position of the arms is very important in order to get abduction of the scapula. The arms are positioned on the support device in flexion of the shoulder and elbow. In this way, the area between the spine and the inner edge of the scapula is broadened

the spine and the inner edge of the scapula is broadened. The surgeon stands on the right side of the patient with the first assistant on his or her right side looking to the monitor in front of them. Four trocars are placed along the inner edge of the right scapula: the first at the level of the lowest point of the scapula for the thoracoscope (usually at 10 mm), the second at the level of the 4th intercostal space (5 mm), the third at the level of the 8th intercostal space (12 mm) and the last at the level of the 2nd intercostal space, as work trocar for the assistant (suction, eventually lung retraction) (Fig. 34.14). After introduction of the first trocar, a positive insufflation of 5–8 mmHg is initiated in order to compress enough the right lung for an adequate visualization of the posterior mediastinum. A 30° thoracoscope is used. The operation steps during this thoracic part are

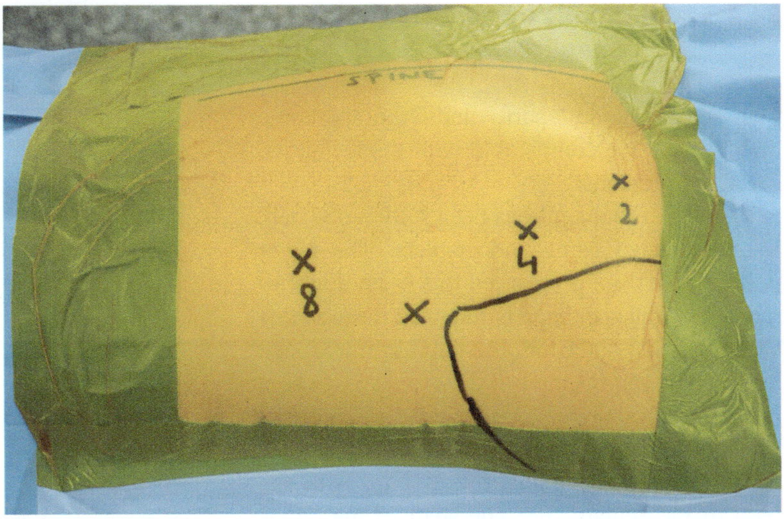

Fig. 34.14 Classical trocar position for thoracoscopy in prone position

then comparable to the one described previously. Further laparoscopic and cervical parts of the procedure are comparable to the ones described previously.

34.4.2 Laparoscopic Transhiatal Esophagectomy

The conventional operative technique described by Akijama and popularized in the Western World by Orringer is performed laparoscopically.

In supine position, the abdominal dissection is performed, as described during the classical thoracoscopic and laparoscopic minimally invasive esophagectomy. To facilitate traction on the esophagus caudally, a sling is placed around the esophagus. The hiatus is enlarged by dividing the anterior part of the hiatus after ligating and dividing the overrunning vein at this level. Anteriorly the dissection is performed in the anterior mediastinal avascular plane with visualization of the pericardium and pulmonary veins. Dissection is continued anteriorly up to the level of the carina below which it is claimed the lymph nodes can be visualized. The aorta is approached at the level of the hiatus, and in an avascular plane, the esophagus is dissected away from the aorta as high as possible in the posterior mediastinum. Lateral dissection is performed on both sides of the level of the pleura. If required, the pleura can be opened on both sides with resection of some part of it. The esophagus is dissected laparoscopically in this way together with paraesophageal tissue and lymph node up to the level of the carina if possible. Gastric mobilization and cervical incision are comparable to the ones previously described. At the same time, another surgeon introduces the HandPort system (Smith & Nephew, Inc., Andover, MA) through a 7-cm longitudinal periumbilical incision. Through the lateral left trocar, a venous stripper is introduced into the gastric lumen by a small incision in the lesser gastric curvature and after performing a left cervicotomy is identified at the level of the cervical esophagus. The cervical esophagus is divided, after which its distal part is tied with an umbilical tape around the stripper. A nasogastric tube is attached to it. This can be used afterwards to lead the gastric tube upwards to the cervical incision. In this way, with the hand of the surgeon in the abdomen, the controlled stripping can be safely performed. Once the specimen is retrieved outside the abdomen, the gastric conduit is created. It is then oversewn and attached to the nasogastric tube and replaced in the abdomen. The pneumoperitoneum is then re-established, and the gastric tube is pulled up under vision into the neck. An anastomosis as previously described is then performed.

34.4.3 Minimally Invasive Ivor-Lewis Esophagectomy

The laparoscopic part and thoracoscopic mobilization are comparable with the technique described previously.

Once the esophagus has been fully mobilized, it is transected using endostaplers. The lower posterior port site is enlarged to a 4-cm minithoracotomy. The specimen is removed through this site. Using this incision, the anvil is introduced in the chest and inserted in the esophagus where it is secured using purse string sutures. The anvil of the circular stapler can also be introduced transorally and perforates the esophagus at the level of the stapler line. The shaft of the circular endostapler is introduced through an anterior incision in the gastric conduit and is connected to the anvil to perform a stapled esophagogastric anastomosis (Fig. 34.15). This anastomosis can be reinforced using interrupted 2/0 sutures.

A Gastrografin contrast study is performed on day 5 to check the integrity of the anastomosis before reinstitution of oral feeding.

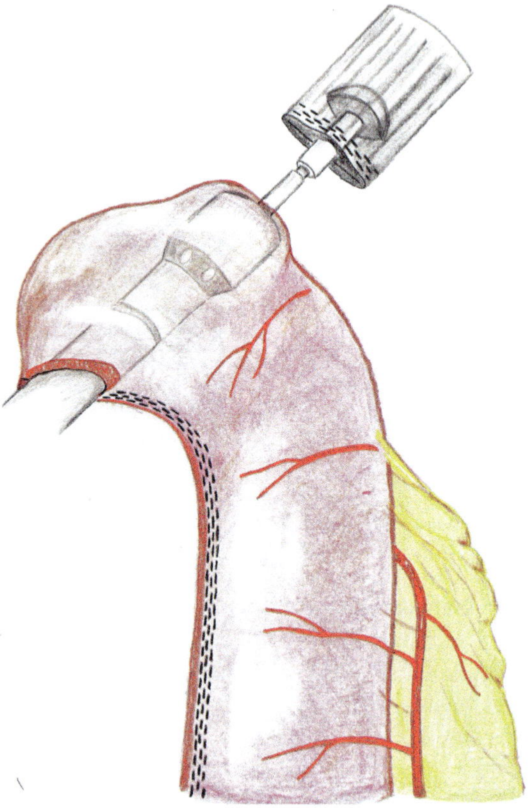

Fig. 34.15 Intrathoracic esophagogastric anastomosis using a circular endostapler

34.5 Post-operative Management

To optimize the results of surgery, this type of procedure should be performed in an appropriately equipped center that is familiar with the meticulous management of the post-operative course. A chest radiography is obtained in the OR to confirm complete lung expansion and appropriate placement of the chest drains. Most patients can be extubated on the table immediately after surgery. An adequately placed epidural anesthesia enables patient to sit upright in bed, breathe deeply, and cooperate fully with physiotherapists. If necessary, bronchoscopy or eventually a minitracheostomy placed either at the time of surgery or sometimes thereafter can be used to ensure adequate bronchial toilet.

Fluid balance and oxygen saturation should be closely monitored, and oxygen supplementation is mandatory. Fluid restriction is essential to avoid cardiac and respiratory complications. It is also vital to maintain adequate and balanced nutrition during the whole post-operative period, and therefore, total parenteral nutrition is preferred. A number of authors prefer to place a feeding jejunostomy at the time of surgery.

Thrombosis prophylaxis is continued by subcutaneous injection of fractionated heparin, and prophylactic antibiotics are given for 2 days.

Since it is essential to avoid intragastric stasis in the stomach tube and subsequent respiratory complications secondary to aspiration, the nasogastric tube is kept in place and prokinetic drugs (domperidone and erythromycin) are administered.

In case these preventive measures are of no avail and gastric stasis and subsequent gastric dilation occur, endoscopic balloon dilation of the pylorus will be performed.

We do not routinely perform a contrast study to check the integrity of the anastomosis in case of cervical location. At day 5, if there is no clinical signs of anastomotic leak, oral fluids are started. In case of intrathoracic anastomosis, a Gastrografin swallow will be performed at day 5, and oral fluid and soft diet are started if no leak is visualized. On the same day, the epidural catheter is removed and the patient is encouraged to mobilize fully. Oral analgetics are administered lege artis. The chest drain will be removed when the effluent amounts to less than 300 ml of fluids. Patients are discharged when they are able to tolerate the soft diet and the pain is sufficiently controlled to permit normal mobilization. The patient is then seen in the outpatient clinic 1 month after discharge.

34.6 Complications

34.6.1 Atelectasis and Respiratory Complications

Atelectasis and other respiratory problems can be minimized using adequate analgesia, physiotherapy, fluid balance (i.e. avoiding over hydration of the lungs) and early mobilization. If necessary, bronchoscopy or eventually a minitracheostomy placed either at the time of surgery or sometimes thereafter can be used to ensure adequate bronchial cleansing.

34.6.2 Anastomotic Leak

Anastomotic leaks may occur in the early postoperative period (2–3 days) when due to a technical failure. Leaks also can occur later (3–7 days) and are thought to be due to ischemic changes in the stomach, usually at the suture line and rather exceptionally as a result of necrosis of the proximal end of the gastric tube. Minor leak needs conservative treatment (i.e. nothing by mouth, antibiotics, total parenteral nutrition, proton pomp inhibitors, nasogastric tube, and eventually octreotide). Early endoscopy is useful for determining the viability of the gastric tube and for evaluating a leak. Early dilation, if needed, is mandatory to allow free passage of saliva. Occasionally the leaks will require a debridement through the neck incision. These leaks will heal spontaneously.

In case of an intrathoracic leak, it is of the utmost importance to adequately drain all collections using pigtail catheters or chest tubes, preferably placed under CT scan guidance for optimal positioning. Re-intervention is necessary occasionally to control sepsis, especially in the event of uncontained leaks, in particular in the presence of disseminated intrathoracic collections. In the event of endoscopically documented gastric tube necrosis, immediate re-intervention with resection of the necrotic stomach and diverting esophagostomy is the safest option. Placement of a jejunostomy tube for feeding is in these cases mandatory. Reconstruction can be made after 3–6 months, usually using a retrosternal colon.

34.6.3 Anastomotic Stricture

In many reports, at least a third of patients develop a stricture at the anastomosis. Dilation of the stricture can be accomplished by several means. The preferred method is endoscopic dilation with Savary dilators. The success rate, eventually after several dilations, is high (more than 90%). When dealing with the more resistant stricture, balloon dilation and local steroid injection usually resolve the problems. Re-intervention is extremely rare. Since the introduction of the semi-mechanical anastomosis, the incidence of anastomotic strictures has fallen dramatically.

34.6.4 Delayed Gastric Emptying

Causes of impaired gastric emptying include lack of a pyloric drainage procedure when the whole stomach or wide gastric tubes are used, obstruction at the severely narrow passage through the hiatus and a redundant intrathoracic stomach resulting in kinking, axial twisting, or both. Those infrequent but sometimes bothersome complications are best tackled by endoscopic balloon dilation of the pylorus along with prokinetic agents (e.g., domperidone, erythromycin) in case of pyloric outlet obstruction. If conservative management fails, reoperation with an adequate drainage procedure or repositioning of the gastric tube may become necessary.

34.6.5 Reflux

Reflux is a common problem after gastric pull-up because the residual antrum resumes its autonomic acid production over time. Small frequent meals, avoidance mixing liquids with meals, avoidance of the supine position after meals and elevation of the head of the bed at night can help symptoms of regurgitation. Acid reflux is best treated with chronic proton pump inhibitors to avoid the higher risk of anastomotic stricture formation, owing to continuous acid damage to the anastomosis. Intestinal metaplasia may develop eventually in the remaining proximal esophagus as a result of mixed acid and biliary reflux. Therefore, regular endoscopic surveillance during follow-up is mandatory.

34.7 Results

Although almost two decades have passed since its introduction, minimally invasive esophagectomy (MIE) has not become widespread (unlike other minimally invasive procedures). It is still considered one of the most complex gastrointestinal surgical procedures and its learning curve is steep. Furthermore, to be acceptable as an alternative to open procedure, MIE must be at least as good as the open counterparts in relation to the post-operative characteristics, oncologic results, and quality of life.

Although the number of published series has increased over the last years, most of them are case series. No randomized controlled trials comparing MIE to open esophagectomy have been published, and the few retrospective comparative cohort studies are limited by small number of patients[18–20] or major selection biases, making both MIE and open group incomparable [16]. Comparing results is thus difficult the more because of the various techniques available, the use of hybrid techniques combining partially open and partially videoscopic approaches, the possible selection bias, etc.

Therefore, many questions remain unanswered as to the real advantages of this technique, and even published systematic reviews and meta-analysis failed to report consistent results [21–24].

34.7.1 Post-operative Characteristics

In our experience between January 2005 and January 2010, comparing 2 matched group of open esophagectomy (OO) ($n=101$) and MIE patients ($n=65$) presenting with early esophageal or GEJ cancer, hospital stay was comparable between both groups, although a trend was seen in favor of the MIE group (19.2 vs. 14.4 days; $p=0.1$). Intra-operative characteristics were comparable although blood loss was less (290 vs. 491 ml; $p=0.01$) and duration of operation longer (322 vs. 375 min; $p=0.001$) in the MIE group.

As esophagectomy for cancer is a formidable undertaking, its inherent risks for morbidity and mortality remain reliable criteria for outcome assessment. Hospital mortality (OO 1.98% vs. MIE 3.08%; $p=0.66$) and post-operative complications (OO 40% vs. MIE 32%; $p=0.34$) were comparable. However, respiratory complications (64.5% vs. 26.2%; $p=0.008$) and ICU admission (20.8% vs. 7.7%; $p=0.02$) were higher in the OO group. Gastrointestinal complications (5.9% vs. 20.0%; $p=0.005$) in particular gastroparesis were more frequent in the MIE group.

We have also performed a systematic review of the literature [21], and the results are summarized in Tables 34.1 and 34.2.

Mortality after MIE varies between 2% and 4.6% and does not seem improved compared to the accepted 3–5% mortality in high-volume centers after open esophagectomy.

As pulmonary complications are the most frequent source of complications and mortality [1, 2], their reduction should be the primary aim of MIE. But considerable variations are seen in those series (0–76% of patients, median 20%), related to the variations in definition and way of reporting pulmonary complications (all versus only major complications). These numbers remain high and not obviously inferior to open surgery [1, 3–9]. Reported rates of vocal cord palsy causing an increased risk for aspiration seem high after MIE (9%), seemingly higher than in open surgery [9, 25, 26]. Impairment of swallowing with subsequent inhalation may play a major role in the development of respiratory infections after MIE [25, 27].

Table 34.1 Overall results of the different techniques for MIE

	N series	*N* patients	Induction treatment (%)	Conversion rates (%)	Operative time (min)	Hospital stay[a] (days)	Lymph node retrieval[a]	Duration of follow-up[a] (months)
1. Transhiatal esophagectomy	16	433 (10–68)	17	7	294 (200–448)	10 (5.5–17)	10.5 (5–15)	17 (11–39)
2. Laparoscopy + VATS	10	609 (12–222)	36	4.7	350 (220–550)	9 (6.5–16)	16.5 (9–48)	23 (3–32)
3. Laparotomy + VATS	14	743 (10–319)	27	6.3	330 (240–476)	18 (10–28)	20 (7–62)	15.5 (10–23)
4. Laparoscopy + thoracotomy	4	147 (13–82)	44	5.4	368 (260–484)	18 (11–29)	27 (12–28)	10.6 (7.2–14)
All transthoracic (TTE) (=Sum 2+3+4)	28	1,499 (10–319)	33	5.6	340 (220–550)	12 (6.5–29)	17 (7–62)	17 (3–32)
Robotic MIE	3	54	7	5.5	274 (267–450)	14 (10–18)	17 (14–20)	No data

[a]Median of all series

Table 34.2 Surgical outcome of the different techniques for MIE

	N series	*N* patients	Mortality	Overall morbidity (%)	Respiratory complications (%)	Reoperation rate (%)	Vocal cord palsy (%)	Anastomotic leaks (%)
1. Transhiatal esophagectomy	15	433 (10–68)	20 (4.6%)	46.1	22	3	9.7	13
2. Laparoscopy + VATS	11	609 (12–222)	14 (2.4%)	43	16.7	8.3	3.1	9
3. Laparotomy + VATS	14	743 (10–319)	18 (2.4%)	51.6	23	5.3	8.9	6.5
4. Laparoscopy + thoracotomy	4	147 (13–82)	3 (2%)	47.6	30.6	4.8	5	7
All transthoracic (TTE) (=Sum 2 + 3 + 4)	29	1,499 (10–319)	35 (2.4%)	47.7	21.7	6.8	6.4	7.6
Robotic MIE	3	54	2.6%	77	30.7	5.1	10	23

With an overall median stay of 11.5 days in this review, MIE does not seem to reduce length of hospital stay as compared to what can be expected today after conventional open esophagectomy in high-volume centers [28, 29].

On the other hand, some studies suggest that at least post-operative ventilation times, blood loss, transfusion rates, length of ICU stay, and hospital stay could be favorably influenced by MIE [17, 30–34]. Those results were confirmed by a recent meta-analysis showing also reduced total morbidity and respiratory complications after MIE [22].

Those results are in some way conflicting, and therefore further studies are necessary to clarify the exact impact of MIE on the direct post-operative evolution. However, our results indicate lower rate of respiratory complications and need for ICU admission.

34.7.2 Oncologic Results

Literature reviews on conventional esophagectomy in the 1980s and 1990s reported overall 5-year survival rates of 22–26% [9, 26]. Nowadays, most high-volume centers report overall 5-year survivals of 40% or more. Even in the setting of controlled trials and national databases, 40% 5-year survival appears to be an adequate benchmark for esophageal cancer surgery [1–3, 35].

Available literature on oncological outcome is limited. In our extensive review [21], we noted that 56% of the papers did not report oncological outcome or follow-up whatsoever. Rate of incomplete resection was only reported in 33% of series (0–24%; median 12%). Only six papers reported removal of any regional abdominal lymph node, and 65% of the studies reported a less than standard mediastinal lymph node dissection. Median of lymph node retrieval in all series was very variable and reached 14 nodes (range 5–62). In our own experience, between 2005 and 2009, a median of 15 lymph nodes were retrieved, but we most certainly noted an effect of the learning curve on the number of lymph node retrieved (Fig. 34.16). From 10 in 2005, the numbers gradually increased till 20 in 2009. For 2010, we have so far reached the level of 25 lymph nodes resected per single patient. This underlines again the importance of experience and high volume when performing this kind of procedures.

Overall 4–5-year survival rates of 22–52% have been reported for transthoracic MIE [16,

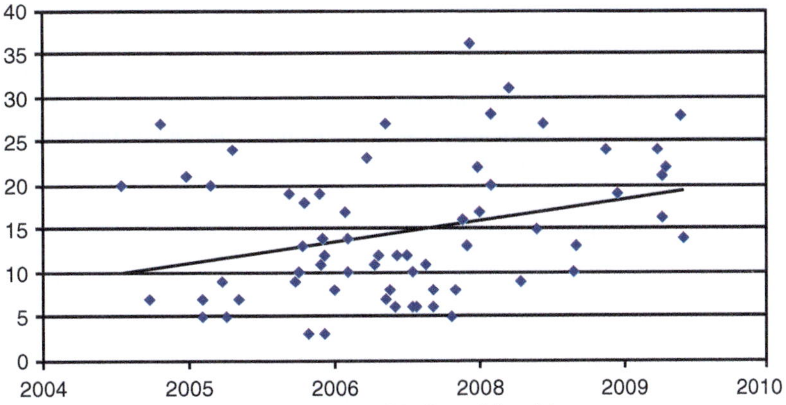

	Mean	Median	Min	Max
2005	13.8	9	5	27
2006	12.0	12	3	19
2007	10.8	9	5	27
2008	21.8	21	9	36
2009	19.3	21	10	28

Fig. 34.16 Cox regression analysis graph showing the improvement of lymph node clearance with growing experience

36–38]. In our extensive review on MIE [21], 5-year survival was available in some studies. Five-year survival rate for stage I was 86% (62–100%; median of five studies), stage II 45% (35–69%), and stage III 16% (0–27%; median of five papers). The survival rate for stage I patients seems similar to the results of conventional esophagectomy. On the other hand, an increasing body of evidence also suggests that many tumors confined to the mucosa (T1a) or very superficial submucosa might be adequately treated by non-resectional endoluminal techniques, which are by definition less invasive than MIE [2, 39]. For tumors extending into the submucosa (T1b), lymph node involvement is encountered in at least 30% of patients, and radical lymph node dissection seems to be most beneficial for such patients [40, 41].MIE with adequate lymph node dissection could be an attractive option in these early cancers.

But so far, except for early cancers, the body of evidence in the literature does not allow us to make any statement on the oncologic usefulness of MIE in treating esophageal cancer. Its use should therefore be limited to high-volume centers and in well-designed study protocols. This is the reason for which, for the time being in our center, the indication for MIE is limited to early cancers as we consider that oncologic safety is of paramount importance.

34.7.3 Quality of Life

Open esophagectomy results in substantial tissue trauma necessary for surgical access, and this has a detrimental impact on the health-related quality of life (HRQL) with long-term residual deficits [42]. Following surgery, it takes up to 1 year for patients to recover their baseline HRQL, and these baseline levels are never achieved in case of recurrence within 2 years [43].

Minimally invasive techniques aim to achieve the same clinical outcomes as open surgery but with significantly less tissue trauma related to the surgical incisions, aiming in this way to improve quality of life outcomes.

Using Short-Form 36 to assess general quality of life, it was shown that there was no significant difference between pre- and post-operative scores, indicating preservation of the HRQL after MIE [15]. In addition, using the gastresophageal reflux disease-health-related quality of life score (ranging from 0 for no symptoms to 45 for most severe symptoms), the same group showed a mean score of 4.6 overall (normal score) and a score of 3 for another group of only early carcinoma at a mean follow-up of 48.2 months [44]. Dysphagia scores were also excellent with a mean score of 1.4 (scale of 1 for no dysphagia to 5 for severe dysphagia) [15]. A more recent report, using the EORTC-approved QLQ-C30 and QLQ-OES18 questionnaires in 62 MIE patients, showed that at 6 weeks after surgery, most patients reported deterioration in functional aspects of HRQL and more symptoms than at baseline. However, most improved at 3 months and had returned to baseline levels by 6 months. These levels were maintained 1 year after surgery, with 85% of patients recovering in more than 50% of the HRQL domains [45].

34.8 Conclusion

This overview has shown the feasibility of this type of surgery in selected patients.

In experienced hands, MIE could be an attractive approach for patients with both benign conditions requiring esophageal resection and for early cancers.

However, the mortality and morbidity of MIE do not seem to be inferior to open esophagectomy when performed by experienced surgeons.

From an oncologic point of view, there appears to be insufficient evidence in the literature to support MIE as an oncologic safe treatment option for the more advanced invasive esophageal carcinoma. Quality of life seems improved after MIE, although the evidence so far is not strong enough to permit definite conclusions.

Use of this procedure should be therefore limited to high-volume centers and within the context of study protocols and/or randomized controlled trials.

References

1. Lerut T, Coosemans W, De Leyn P, Van Raemdonck D, Nafteux P, Moons J (2001) Optimizing treatment of carcinoma of the esophagus and gastroesophageal junction. Surg Clin N Am 10:863–884
2. Vrouenraets BC, van Lanschot JJB (2006) Extent of surgical resection for esophageal and gastroesophageal junction adenocarcinomas. Surg Oncol Clin N Am 15:781–791
3. Hulscher JBF, van Sandick JW, de Boer AG, Wijnhoven BPL, Tijssen JGP, Fockens P, Stalmeier PFM, Ten Kate FJW, van Dekken H, Obertop H, Tilanus HW, van Lanschot JJB (2002) Extended transthoracic resection compared with limited transhiatal resection for adenocarcinoma of the esophagus. N Engl J Med 347:1662–1669
4. Birkmeyer JD, Siewers AE, Finlayson EVA, Stukel TA, Lucas FL, Batista I, Welch HG, Wennberg DE (2002) Hospital volume and surgical mortality in the United States. N Engl J Med 346:1128–1137
5. Birkmeyer JD, Sun Y, Wong SL, Stukel TA (2007) Hospital volume and late survival after cancer surgery. Ann Surg 245:777–783
6. Orringer MB (1984) Transhiatal esophagectomy without thoracotomy for carcinoma of the thoracic esophagus. Ann Surg 200:282–288
7. Perrachia A, Bonavina L, Segalin A, Ruol A, Fumagalli U (1994) Minimally invasive esophageal surgery. Esophagectomy without thoracotomy or transmediastinal endodissection for esophageal carcinoma. Dis Esophagus 7:36–38
8. Buess G, Kayser J, Manncke K, Walter DJ, Bessell JR, Becker HD (1997) Endoscopic microsurgical dissection of the esophagus. Int Surg 82:109–112
9. Hulscher JBF, Tijssen JGP, Obertop H, van Lanschot JJB (2001) Transthoracic versus transhiatal resection for carcinoma of the esophagus: a meta-analysis. Ann Thorac Surg 72:306–313
10. Hulscher JBF, van Lanschot JJB (2005) Individualised surgical treatment of patients with an adenocarcinoma of the distal oesophagus or gastro-oesophageal junction. Dig Surg 22:130–134
11. Cushieri A, Shimi S, Banting S (1992) Endoscopic oesophagectomy through a right thoracoscopic approach. J R Coll Surg Edinb 37:7–11
12. Mc Anena OJ, Rogers J, Williams NS (1994) Right thoracoscopically assisted oesophagectomy for cancer. Br J Surg 81:236–238
13. Robertson GSM, Lloyd DM, Wicks ACB, Veitch PS (1996) No obvious advantages for thoracoscopic two-stage oesophagectomy. Br J Surg 83:675–678
14. Dexter SPL, Martin IG, McMahon MJ (1996) Radical thoracoscopic esophagectomy for cancer. Surg Endosc 10:147–151
15. Luketich JD, Alvelo-Rivera M, Buenaventura PO, Christie NA, McCaughan JS, Litle VR, Schauer PR, Close JM, Fernando HC (2003) Minimally invasive esophagectomy. Outcomes in 222 patients. Ann Surg 238:486–495
16. Smithers BM, Gotley DC, Martin I, Thomas JM (2007) Comparison of the outcomes between open and minimally invasive esophagectomy. Ann Surg 245:232–240
17. Palanivelu C, Prakash A, Senthilkumar R, Senthilnathan P, Parthasarathi R, Rajan PS, Ventkatachlam S (2006) Minimally invasive esophagectomy: thoracoscopic mobilization of the esophagus and mediastinal lymphadenectomy in prone position-experience in 130 patients. J Am Coll Surg 203:7–16
18. Bernabe KQ, Bolton JS, Richardson WS (2005) Laparoscopic hand-assisted vs open transhiatal esophagectomy. A case-control study. Surg Endosc 19: 334–337
19. Bresadola V, Terrosu G, Cojutti A, Benzoni E, Baracchini E, Bresadola F (2006) Laparoscopic versus open gastroplasty in esophagectomy for esophageal cancer: a comparative study. Surg Laparosc Endosc Percutan Tech 16:63–67
20. Nguyen NT, Follette DM, Wolfe BM, Schneider PD, Roberts P, Goodnight JE (2000) Comparison of minimally invasive esophagectomy with transthoracic and transhiatal esophagectomy. Arch Surg 135:920–925
21. Decker G, Coosemans W, De Leyn P, Decaluwé H, Nafteux P, Van Raemdonck D, Lerut T (2009) Minimally invasive esophagectomy for cancer. Eur J Cardiothorac Surg 35:13–21
22. Nagpal K, Ahmed K, Vats A, Yakoub D, James D, Ashrafian H, Darzi A, Moorthy K, Athanasiou T (2010) Is minimally invasive surgery beneficial in the management of esophageal cancer? A meta-analysis. Surg Endosc 24:1621–1629
23. Verhage R, Hazebroek E, Boone J, Van Hillegersberg R (2009) Minimally invasive surgery compared to open procedures in esophagectomy for cancer: a systematic review of the literature. Minerva Chir 64:135–146
24. Biere S, Cuesta M, Van Der Peet D (2009) Minimally invasive versus open esophagectomy for cancer: a systematic review and meta-analysis. Minerva Chir 64:121–133
25. Lerut TE, van Lanschot JJB (2004) Chronic symptoms after subtotal or partial oesophagectomy: diagnosis and treatment. Best Pract Res Clin Gastroenterol 18:901–915
26. Rindani R, Martin CJ, Cox MR (1999) Transhiatal versus Ivor-Lewis oesophagectomy: is there a difference? Aust N Z J Surg 69:187–194
27. Atkins BZ, Fortes DL, Watkins KT (2007) Analysis of respiratory complications after minimally invasive esophagectomy: preliminary observation of persistent aspiration risk. Dysphagia 22:49–54
28. Lanuti M, de Delva PE, Maher A, Wright CD, Gaissert HA, Wain JC, Donahue DM, Mathisen DJ (2006) Feasibility and outcomes of an early extubation policy after esophagectomy. Ann Thorac Surg 82: 2037–2041
29. Cerfolio RJ, Bryant AS, Bass CS, Alexander JR, Bartolucci AA (2004) Fast-tracking after Ivor Lewis esogastrectomy. Chest 126:1187–1194

30. Bonavina L, Bona D, Binyom PR, Peracchia A (2004) A laparoscopy-assisted approach to esophageal carcinoma. J Surg Res 117:52–57
31. Akaishi T, Kaneda I, Higuchi N, Kuriya Y, Kuramoto J, Toyoda T, Wakabayashi A (1996) Thoracoscopic en bloc total esophagectomy with radical mediastinal lymphadenectomy. J Thorac Cardiovasc Surg 112:1533–1541
32. Swanstrom LL (2002) Minimally invasive surgical approaches to esophageal cancer. J Gastrointest Surg 6:522–526
33. Law S, Fok M, Chu KM, Wong J (1997) Thoracoscopic esophagectomy for esophageal cancer. Surgery 122:8–14
34. Puntambekar S, Agarwal G, Joshi S, Rayate N, Sathe R, Patil A (2010) Thoracolaparoscopy in the lateral position for esophageal cancer: the experience of a single institution with 112 consecutive patients. Surg Endosc 24:2407–2414
35. Thompson AM, Rapson T, Gilbert FJ, Park KGM, The Scottish Audit of Gastric and Oesophageal Cancer (2007) Hospital volume does not influence long-term survival of patients undergoing surgery for oesophageal or gastric cancer. Br J Surg 94:578–584
36. Martin DJ, Bessell JR, Chew A, Watson DI (2005) Thoracoscopic and laparoscopic esophagectomy. Initial experiences and outcome. Surg Endosc 19:1597–1601
37. Yamamoto S, Kawahara K, Maekawa T, Shiraishi T, Shirakusa T (2005) Minimally invasive esophagectomy for stage I and II esophageal cancer. Ann Thorac Surg 80:2070–2075
38. Leibman S, Smithers BM, Gotley DC, Martin I, Thomas J (2006) Minimally invasive esophagectomy. Initial experiences and outcome. Surg Endosc 20: 428–433
39. Ell C, May A, Pech O, Gossner L, Guenter E, Behrens A, Nachbar L, Huijsmans J, Vieth M, Stolte M (2007) Curative endoscopic resection of early esophageal adenocarcinomas (Barrett's cancer). Gastrointest Endosc 65:3–10
40. Peyre CG, DeMeester SR, Rizzetto C, Bansal N, Tang AL, Ayazi S, Leers JM, Lipham JC, Hagen JA, DeMeester TR (2007) Vagal sparing esophagectomy. The ideal operation for intra-mucosal adenocarcinoma and Barrett with high-grade dysplasia. Ann Surg 246:665–674
41. Wijnhoven BPL, Tran KTC, Esterman A, Watson DI, Tilanus HW (2007) An evaluation of prognostic factors and tumor staging of resected carcinoma of the esophagus. Ann Surg 245:717–725
42. Lagergren P, Avery K, Hughes R, Barham C, Alderson D, Falk S (2007) Health-related quality of life among patients cured by surgery for esophageal cancer. Cancer 110:686–693
43. Zieren H, Jacobi C, Zieren J, Müller J (1996) Quality of life following resection of oesophageal carcinoma. Br J Surg 83:1772–1775
44. Pennathur A, Awais O, Luketich J (2010) Minimally invasive esophagectomy for Barrett's with high-grade dysplasia and early adenocarcinoma of the esophagus. J Gastrointest Surg 14:948–950
45. Parameswaran R, Blazeby J, Hughes R, Mitchell K, Berrisford R, Wajed S (2010) Health-related quality of life after minimally invasive oesophagectomy. Br J Surg 97:525–531

Part VII

Minimally Invasive Thoracic Surgery: The Diaphragm

The Diaphragm: Introduction and Basics

35

Willem Nicolaas Welvaart and Marinus A. Paul

Contents

W.N. Welvaart, M.D. (✉)
Department of Surgery, Rivierland Ziekenhuis Tiel, Pres. Kennedylaan 1, Tiel 4002 WP, The Netherlands
e-mail: w.welvaart@rzt.nl

M.A. Paul, M.D., Ph.D.
Department of Surgery, VU University Hospital, Boelelaan 1117, Amsterdam 1081 HV, The Netherlands
e-mail: ma.paul@vumc.nl

35.1 Introduction

The diaphragm (Greek: dia = between; phragma = fence) is a musculoaponeurotic structure that separates the thoracic and abdominal cavities [1]. It is, however, not just "the thoracic floor" but the most important muscle of respiration [2] and also plays an important role in preventing gastroesophageal reflux. Impairment of diaphragmatic function can have major physiological consequences. Many of these impairments are amenable for surgical correction, but correct diagnosis and treatment require thorough understanding of form and function. The old maxim: "Let them never forget that without anatomy there is no physiology, no surgery, no medicine" holds true also for the diaphragm [3].

There is, however, more to be gained by increasing knowledge. Pulmonary complications after surgery are common, and they may be, in part, be related to inspiratory muscle weakness. Anesthetics and neuromuscular blockers play a role and a systemic inflammatory response secondary to inflammation, or trauma may also affect diaphragmatic function. Ways to prevent these adverse effects are presently being studied.

35.2 Embryology

The diaphragm arises from four morphological elements: (1) the transverse septum, (2) the pleura-parietal membranes, (3) the body wall

R.G.C. Inderbitzi et al. (eds.), *Minimally Invasive Thoracic and Cardiac Surgery*,
DOI 10.1007/978-3-642-11861-6_35, © Springer-Verlag Berlin Heidelberg 2012

Fig. 35.1 Undersurface of the diaphragm, showing the three foramina (*e* esophageal, *a* aortic, *c* caval), the sites of possible congenital hernias (*m* Morgagni's hernia, *b* Bochdalek's hernia), the distribution of the phrenic nerves (*yellow lines*), and safe areas for incision (*red lines*)

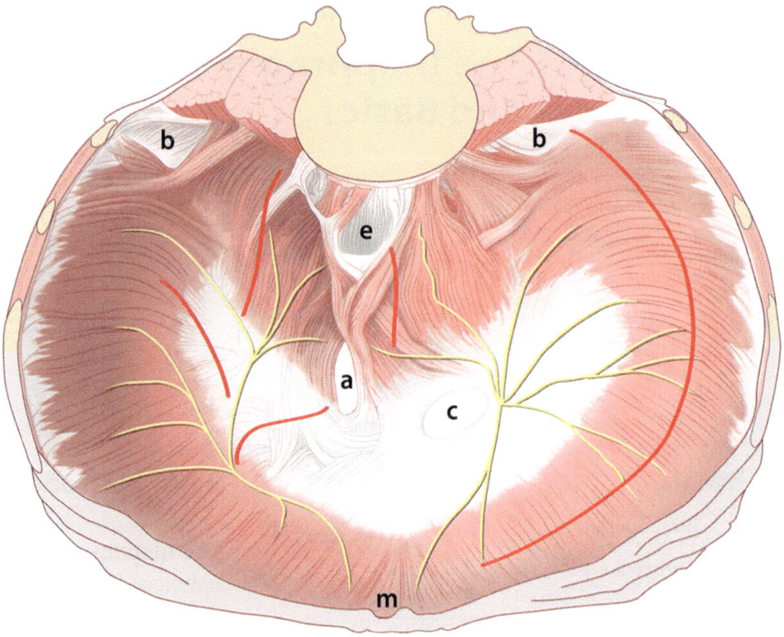

muscles, and (4) the dorsal mesentery of the esophagus [4].

The transverse septum, which becomes the central tendon of the diaphragm, starts in the cervical region as a tissue layer between the heart and the liver. During development it migrates downward.

The pleura-peritoneal membranes develop ventrolaterally on both sides and become attached to the transverse septum. This fusion closes the pleura-parietal canals, thereby separating the thoracic and abdominal cavities. Early in this process, myoblasts appear in these membranes, which later on will form the costal part of the diaphragmatic muscle. Initially this fusion process is incomplete, leaving pleura-peritoneal foramina on both sites. If these foramina persist, herniation occurs.

The third part of the diaphragm is derived from the body wall. The body wall muscles split into an inner and outer layer: The inner layer becomes the posterolateral portion of the diaphragm; the outer layer forms the thoracic wall. The fourth part, which will develop in the crural part of the diaphragm muscle, is derived from the dorsal mesentery of the esophagus.

Thus, the diaphragm is functionally characterized by two separate functional parts: the costal diaphragm which is innervated by the phrenic nerves and the crural diaphragm innervated by the vagal nerve.

During development, there is an extensive caudal migration of the diaphragm, due to the heart and the expanding lungs. The diaphragm's origin, development, and the migration explain its innervation from the cervical plexus, its function, and why fusion defects, closed by peritoneum, fascia, and pleura only, lead to herniation. It also explains why large fusion defects are associated with abnormal development of the lung.

The most well-known fusion defects are in the area between the costal and crural muscles, called the lumbocostal triangle, and, anteriorly, between the sternal adhesion of the central tendon and the border of the costal muscle. Herniation at the lumbocostal angle is named after Bochdalek, an eighteenth century Polish anatomist, and hernias at the sternocostal gaps are named after Morgagni, a sixteenth century Italian anatomist (Fig. 35.1).

35.3 Anatomy

The diaphragm consists of a tendinous central portion from which striated muscle fibers radiate downward and outward. The fibers of the costal part attach to the xiphoid and lower ribs, those of the crural muscles to the upper lumbar segments. The right crus splits to form the esophageal hiatus, thereby creating a sphincter-like opening. These split fibers meet again to form the anterior margin of the aortic opening, which therefore lies also in the muscular part of the diaphragm. The opening for the caval vein, in contrast, lies in the tendinous part [5]. In contrast to man, whales have a strong sphincter around the caval vein, which diverts the blood to collateral systems, e.g., around the spine, before it can reach the heart. It is thought that in this way, heat generated by metabolic processes in the liver is used to preserve body temperature before the blood reaches the lungs and cools down by inhaled air [6].

The central tendon is an aponeurotic structure with a clover-leave-like shape: a single anterior leaflet, inserting in the sternum and two lateral leaflets. The right leaflet is somewhat larger than the left one. The middle part of the central tendon is firmly attached to the undersurface of the pericardium and has a fixed position. The lateral leaflets are free and their position depends on ventilation. Because the posterior crural fibers are longer than the anterior costal fibers, the lateral leaflets are situated more anteriorly. This can clearly be seen by the position of the domes on lateral chest X-rays.

35.4 Blood Supply

The diaphragm is well vascularized to cope with a high demand on maximum exercise. This large blood supply is provided by (1) the pericardiophrenic arteries, which accompany the phrenic nerves; (2) the musculophrenic arteries, branches of the internal thoracic arteries; (3) the superior phrenic arteries, branches from the thoracic aorta; and (4) the inferior phrenic arteries, branches of the abdominal aorta or the celiac trunk. These last named arteries are the largest suppliers. The peripheral parts of the diaphragm muscles also get blood supply from the intercostals muscles.

In general, the veins in the diaphragm follow the arteries. The thoracic side drains into the azygos and hemiazygos system, the abdominal side in the inferior phrenic veins, which in turn empty into the caval vein. The peripheral parts drain into the intercostals veins, the sternal portion into the internal thoracic veins.

35.5 Lymphatic Flow

The diaphragm has a rich lymphatic network that accompanies the blood vessels. The anterior part drains to the parasternal nodes, the lateral systems follow the phrenic nerve toward higher mediastinal nodes, and the posterior part of the diaphragm drains to the posterior mediastinal lymph nodes. The diaphragmatic drainage system is thought to play a major role in the absorption of material from the peritoneal cavity. The extensive network may also explain why locally advanced NSCLC growing into the diaphragm carries a worse prognosis than tumors invading the pericardium of thoracic wall [7].

35.6 Innervation

The diaphragm is mainly innervated by the phrenic nerves, which originate in the cervical plexus. The costal muscle also receives branches of the sixth and seventh thoracic nerve. The phrenic nerves contain both motor and sensory neurons, pass through the diaphragm, and divide into three branches: an anteromedial branch to the sternum, anterolateral to the costal diaphragm, and posteromedial to the crural diaphragm. This distribution should be kept in mind when an incision has to be made during an operation. Generally, an incision along the edge, with a centimeter margin to suture the diaphragm back in place, is safe and leaves the function intact [8] (Fig. 35.1).

35.7 Diaphragmatic Openings

The diaphragm has three anatomic openings: (1) the aortic hiatus, which contains the aorta, the thoracic duct, and the azygos vein; (2) the vena cava orifice, which also contains the right phrenic nerve; and (3) the esophageal hiatus. This last hiatus encloses also both vagal nerve trunks, a sensory branch of the left phrenic nerve, and branches of the left gastric vessels (Fig. 35.1). Diaphragmatic hernias occur at the esophageal opening, at the anterior sternocostal triangle, or the posterior lumbocostal triangle (the fusion lines of the diaphragm), but very rarely at the caval or aortic openings.

Small openings or "diaphragmatic pores" with a size of 2–10 mm have been described in the tendinous part of the diaphragm. These pores may be congenital, as such a defect has been described in a child operated on for a congenital defect, but most evidence suggest they are acquired. The pores become manifest in a variety of clinical conditions, such as liver cirrhosis or an ovarian tumor (Meigs' syndrome), in which the ascites is accompanied by a pleural effusion, usually on the right side. The cause of this preferential development of right hemidiaphragmatical defects is not clear. A peritoneal circulation, with an upward movement of fluid on the right side, and a pistonlike action of the liver resulting in higher local pressure have all been postulated. The existence of these diaphragmatic pores may also explain the occasional occurrence of a pneumothorax in patients who underwent laparoscopic surgery [9].

35.8 Physiology

The diaphragm is the most important muscle of inspiration, taking up to 70% of the work of breathing. Three simultaneous working mechanisms lead to inspiration: (1) Contraction of the muscle fibers produces a caudal movement of the central tendon, (2) this muscle pull creates an upward pull on the lower ribs, increasing the anterior-posterior diameter, and (3) the downward movement in turn increases abdominal pressure which pushes the lower ribs outward. The resulting negative intrathoracic pressure initiates ventilation [10].

The diaphragm, like the heart, has to work continuously. Over half of its muscle fibers are type I, highly oxidative, slow-twitch, and resistant to fatigue. These fibers are used in normal breathing. The type II fibers, fast twitch, either oxidative or glycolytic fibers, are recruited when the breathing rate increases [11]. Diseases may cause profound changes. In COPD patients, a shift from type II to type I fibers occurs, and diffuse atrophy is seen in patients on artificial ventilation [12]. This atrophy occurs much faster in the diaphragm than in other muscles [13].

The crural part of the diaphragm acts as an external sphincter of the esophagus preventing reflux. Relaxation is necessary for swallowing. This function explains why the vagal nerves innervate this part of the diaphragm. In emesis, the diaphragm is part of a complex action of abdominal muscles, gastrointestinal tract, and respiratory muscles [14]. The sensory branch of the phrenic nerve, passing through the aortic hiatus, may also play a role in this action.

35.9 Assessment of Function

Dyspnea is the most frequent symptom of respiratory muscle dysfunction, but other causes, e.g., cardiac failure, do occur. In general, if dyspnea increases in supine position, it occurs immediately in diaphragmatic paralysis and only after some time in cardiac failure. On physical examination, the lower ribs retract instead of expand (Hoover's sign) if the diaphragm moves paradoxically [15]. However, due to the anatomical location, assessment of diaphragmatic function is difficult and radiological imaging is often needed for further assessment.

Besides imaging, other investigations are available to assess function: transdiaphragmatic pressure recording, electromyography, and phrenic nerve stimulation. Transdiaphragmatic pressure recording uses balloons in the esophagus and stomach connected to pressure transducers. The change in pressure generated by contractions of the diaphragm reflects the muscle strength. The results depend on heavily on cooperation of the patient and can only be used as rough indications of diaphragmatic muscle strength. Phrenic nerve stimulation, at the cervical region, is a more objective method of investigation. The response can be recorded by pressure balloons or by EMG electrodes.

Although useful to distinguish between phrenic nerve palsy and diaphragmatic muscle disorders, these investigations are rarely used in clinical practice. They have too many artifacts, the data are difficult to obtain, and the interpretation is difficult [16].

35.10 Imaging

Due to its thinness, its dome-shaped contour, and its contiguity with the abdominal organs, visualization of the diaphragm itself is difficult. Disorders present themselves as alterations in diaphragmatic shape, position, or motion. Apart from the question of availability, the choice of the imaging technique depends much on the clinical question because each imaging technique has its advantages and disadvantages. Chest X-ray, fluoroscopy, ultrasonography, CT scanning, MR imaging are all being used. In general, dynamic investigations, such as fluoroscopy, ultrasonography, and dynamic MRI, are being used for motion disorders and multiplanar imaging CT scanning and MRI for herniation assessment. If a phrenic nerve palsy is suspected, early CT scanning is indicated to rule out tumors compressing the nerve. However, no single modality is best for all situations, and often several modalities have to be combined. Even then, it remains difficult to distinguish between herniation and eventration, between eventration and paralysis, and between herniated omental fat and paracardial lipoma [17, 18].

35.11 Diaphragmatic Dysfunction

Diaphragmatic dysfunction can be divided in two categories:

(a) The functional disorders with diminished muscle function, ranging from muscle fatigue, muscle weakness, to complete paralysis. Muscle fatigue is found in COPD patient, and muscle weakness is found in patients who have been on artificial ventilation and in muscles disease. Muscle paralysis is found in patients with phrenic nerve palsy.
(b) The anatomical causes. This second group is characterized a normal muscle function, but limited movement due to an anatomical derangement, which can vary from a herniation to diseases of neighboring organs obstructing its movement.

Research is going on to better understand the diaphragmatic muscle function, especially why the diaphragmatic muscle atrophies so quickly [19].

The increased understanding of diaphragmatic physiology has already resulted in the design of a "neurally adjusted ventilator assist" device. Using this NAVA technology, a ventilator is not triggered by a respiratory movement of the patient, generating an airflow (a late response), but by phrenic nerve impulses picked up by electrodes mounted on a nasogastric tube (Figs. 35.2 and 35.3). By using the patient's own phrenic stimuli to direct both frequency and tidal volume, some patients can be weaned off the ventilator more rapidly. This technology has also the potential to avoid diaphragm disuse atrophy in critically ill patients [20]. There is also renewed interested in the possibilities of diaphragm pacing in patients with phrenic nerve palsy [21].

There is also an increasing insight in the effects of diaphragmatic paralysis on cardiac function. Dynamic MR imaging has shown left ventricle compression in left-sided paralysis and atrial compression in right-sided paralysis. In some patients, rotation of the heart on the vascular axis due to diaphragmatic elevation even resulted in reopening of the oval foramen between the atria, leading to profound hypoxia due to right-to-left shunting between the atria [22].

Conclusion

The diaphragm is much more than just a fence separating the abdomen from the thoracic cavity. Conditions caused by defects in the anatomical integrity have always been part of the surgeons work load. Doing the same operations in a minimal invasive way is part of today's challenge. But an increasing part of our work will be formed by the increasing knowledge about the functional disorders,

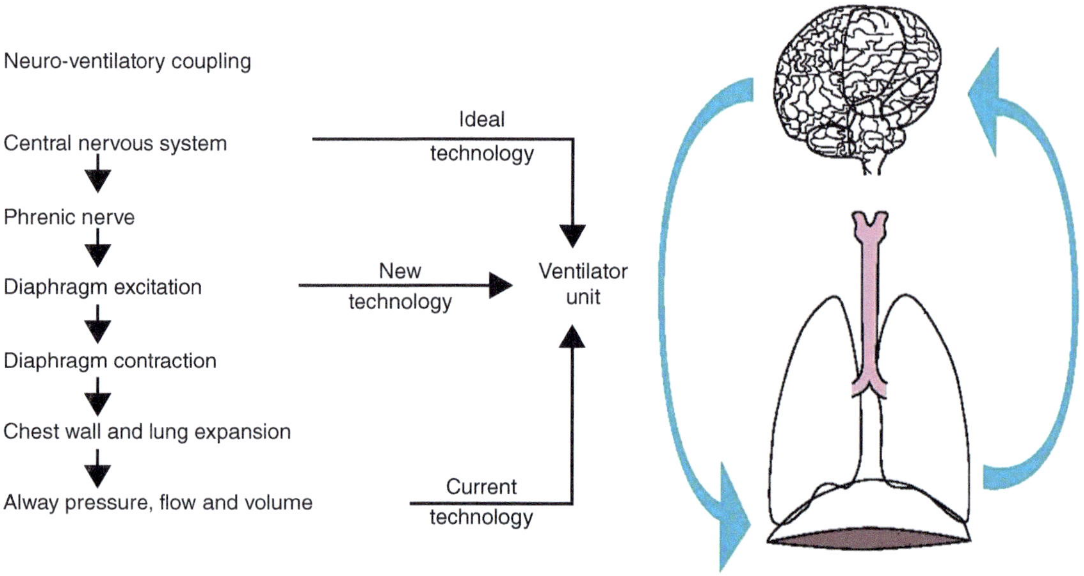

Fig. 35.2 NAVA technology triggers the ventilator by using phrenic nerve stimuli (Courtesy of Maquet Netherlands b.v.)

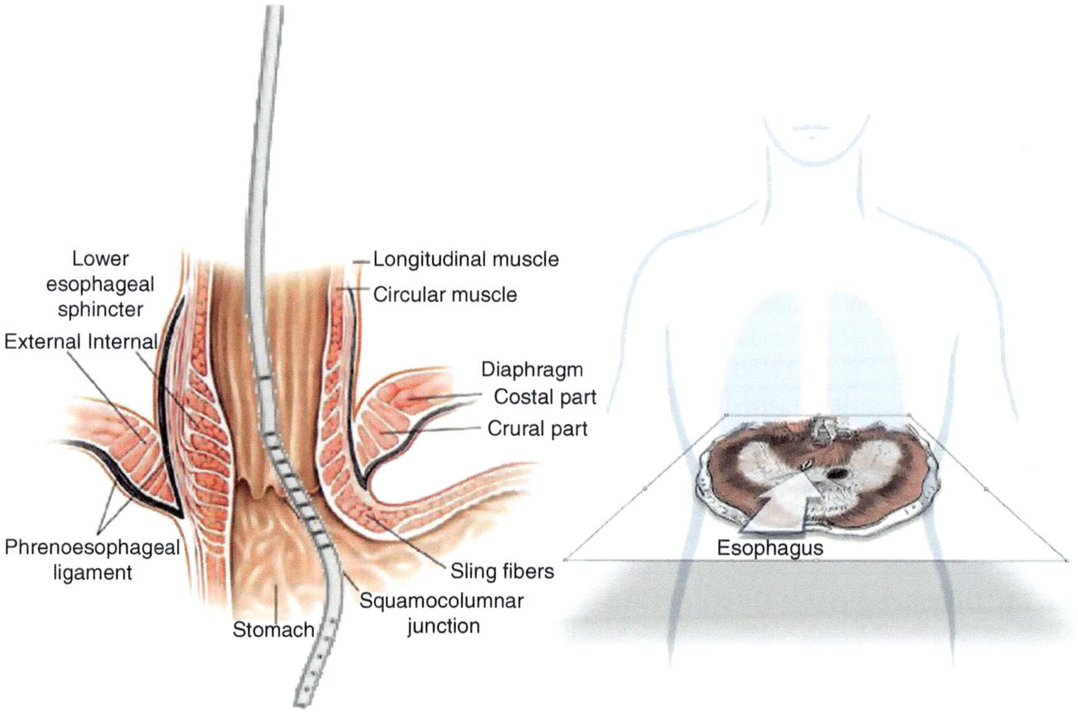

Fig. 35.3 A nasogastric tube with electrodes at the level of the diaphragm (Courtesy of Maquet Netherlands b.v.)

which ask for both new insight and for new methods to correct them. To achieve this, the expert thoracic surgeon should understand as much about the diaphragmatic functions as a chest physician and as much about its imaging as the radiologist.

References

1. Anraku M, Shargall Y (2009) Surgical conditions of the diaphragm; anatomy and physiology. Thorac Surg Clin 19:419–429
2. Epstain S (1994) An overview of respiratory muscle function. Clin Chest Med 15:619–639
3. Cruveilhier J (1834) Traite d'Anantomie descriptive. Asselin, Paris, 1827
4. McVay CB (1984) Thoracic walls: the diaphragm. In: Anson & McVay: surgical anatomy, vol I, 6th edn. WB Saunders, Philadelphia, pp 365–384
5. Loeweneck H, Feifel G (2003) Zwerchfell. In: Lanz & Wachsmuth: praktische anatomie, 2nd edn. Springer, Berlin, pp 89–103
6. Matthew LH (1958) The biology of whales. New Sci 4(107):1426–1427
7. Souilamas R, Hidden G, Riquet M (2001) Mediastinal lymphatic efferents from the diaphragm. Surg Radiol Anat 23(3):159–162
8. Merendino KA, Johnson RS, Skinner HH et al (1956) The intradiaphragmatic distribution of the phrenic nerve with particular reference to the placement of diaphragmatic incisions and controlled segmental paralysis. Surgery 39:189–198
9. Kirschner PA (1998) Porous diaphragm syndromes. Chest Surg Clin N Am 8(2):449–472
10. De Troyer A, Estenne M (1988) Functional anatomy of the respiratory muscles. Clin Chest Med 9(2):175–193
11. Geiger PC, Cody MJ, Macken RL et al (2000) Maximum specific force depends on myosin heavy chain content in rat diaphragm muscle fibers. J Appl Phys 89(2):695–703
12. Pourriat JL, Lamberto C, Hoang PH et al (1986) Diaphragmatic fatigue and breathing pattern during weaning from mechanical ventilation in COPD patients. Chest 90(5):703–707
13. Welvaart WN, Paul MA, Stienen GJ, van Hees HW, Loer SA, Bouwman R, Niessen H, de Man FS, Witt CC, Granzier H, Vonk-Noordegraaf A, Ottenheijm CA. Ann Surg. 2011 Dec;254(6):1044-9.
14. Pickering M, Jones JF (2002) The diaphragm: two physiological muscles in one. J Anat 201(4):205–212
15. Hoover CF (1913) The functions of the diaphragm and their diagnostic significance. Arch Intern Med 12:214–224
16. Pacia EB, Aldrich TK (1998) Assessment of diaphragm function. Chest Surg Clin N Am 8(2):225–236
17. Roberts HC (2009) Imaging the diaphragm. Thorac Surg Clin 19(4):431–451
18. Tarver RD, Conces DJ, Cory DA et al (1989) Imaging the diaphragm and its disorders. J Thorac Imaging 4:1–18
19. Levine S, Nguyen T, Taylor N et al (2008) Rapid disuse atrophy of diaphragm fibers in mechanically ventilated humans. N Engl J Med 358(13):1327–1335
20. Brander L, Leong-Poi H, Beck J et al (2009) Titration and implementation of neurally adjusted ventilatory assist in critically ill patients. Chest 135(3):695–703
21. Onders RP, Elmo M, Khansarinia S et al (2009) Complete worldwide operative experience in laparoscopic diaphragm pacing: results and differences in spinal cord injured patients and amyotrophic lateral sclerosis patients. Surg Endosc 23(7):1433–1440
22. Welvaart WN, Becker A, Marcus JT et al (2010) Unusual treatment of patent foramen ovale after pneumonectomy. Eur Resp J 35(4):929–931

Functional Disorders of the Diaphragm: Eventration and Acquired Paralysis

36

Willem Nicolaas Welvaart and Marinus A. Paul

Contents

W.N. Welvaart, M.D. (✉)
Department of Surgery, Rivierland Ziekenhuis Tiel, Pres. Kennedylaan 1, Tiel 4002 WP, The Netherlands
e-mail: w.welvaart@zrt.nl

M.A. Paul, M.D., Ph.D.
Department of Surgery, VU University Hospital, Boelelaan 1117, Amsterdam 1081 HV, The Netherlands
e-mail: ma.paul@vumc.nl

A paralyzed, elevated diaphragm is thought to be the result of either eventration or an acquired paralysis. Although these conditions are considered to be two separate entities, they will be discussed together because symptoms and treatment are similar. We will also give some arguments why they might even be different stages in the same process.

36.1 Etiology

Eventration (e = out, venter = belly) is defined as thinning of the diaphragm secondary to a congenital defect in the development of the muscle rim, with intact attachments to sternum, ribs, and spine [1]. It can be uni- or bilateral, total (Fig. 36.1) or localized [2]. Localized eventrations (Figs. 36.2 and 36.3) are named after the area of occurrence: anterior, posterolateral, and medial. The cause of eventration is said to be a defect in the migration of myoblasts into the pleura-parietal membranes, which normally occurs early in the development [2, 3]. The absence of muscle tissue results in a membrane-like diaphragm, in which the different parts, such as the central tendon and the affected "muscle rim," cannot be distinguished [4]. Microscopic examination shows diffuse fibroelastic changes with indeed very few muscle cells [5]. According to this hypothesis, eventration has always been present but has become symptomatic during adulthood because of additional factors, such as weight gain, or a change in lung or chest wall

R.G.C. Inderbitzi et al. (eds.), *Minimally Invasive Thoracic and Cardiac Surgery*,
DOI 10.1007/978-3-642-11861-6_36, © Springer-Verlag Berlin Heidelberg 2012

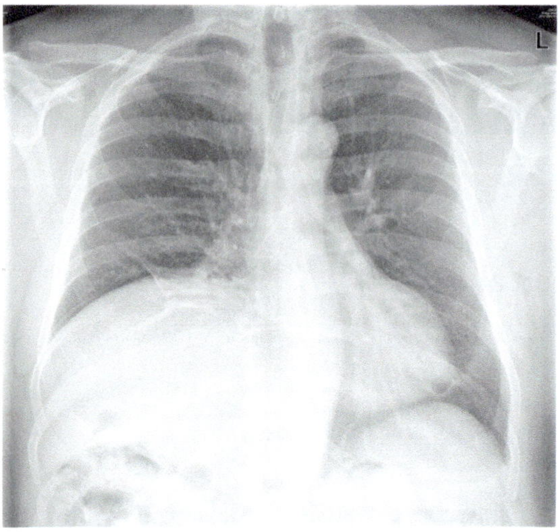

Fig. 36.1 Eventration of the right hemidiaphragm

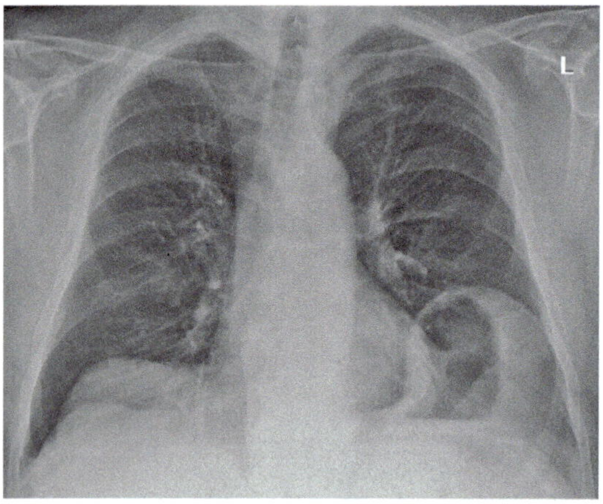

Fig. 36.2 Localized eventration of the left hemidiaphragm

compliance [4–6]. If eventration occurs, it is mostly in males and mainly on the left side [7], but the incidence is low, <0.05% [8]. For a detailed overview on the history and incidence of eventration, see Delauriers [9]. Acquired paralysis is more common. It mostly results from damage to the phrenic nerve, anywhere along its length. The differential diagnosis is broad and includes arthrosis of the cervical spine, trauma (including surgery), compression by tumor, neuropathy (diabetes mellitus), radiation therapy, and infections [10]. Despite this large list, the cause remains unknown in a large proportion of

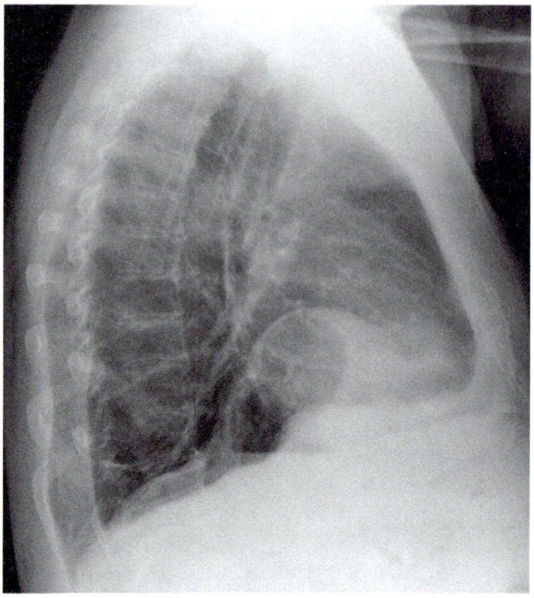

Fig. 36.3 Localized eventration of the left hemidiaphragm (lateral view)

cases. These cases are called "idiopathic." For a detailed differential diagnosis of phrenic nerve injury, see the review by Ko and Gail [11].

Myopathies, disorders affecting the diaphragmatic muscle itself, such as in thyroid disease, can also cause paresis or paralysis. If so, it often presents bilaterally.

Pseudoparalysis does also occur. Subdiaphragmatic disease may push the diaphragm upward, and pulmonary disease may pull it upward [12]. Diaphragmatic fixation due to scarring can also resemble paralysis. We have had dyspneic patients referred for plication, in whom the diaphragm was only "drawn up and fixed" to the chest wall due to scarification after a hemothorax following trauma. In these patients, there is always considerable pleural thickening. Optimal treatment consists of decortication of the lung and release of the diaphragm without plication, resulting in a functional system. Intraoperative stimulation of the phrenic nerve [13] after release of the diaphragm can be helpful to distinguish between paralysis and pseudoparalysis and prevent unnecessary and even harmful plication.

Although the literature gives arguments to distinguish between eventration and acquired paralysis [4], one might challenge this division. The following facts also need to be taken into account:

- Eventration is seen in elderly patients who never had respiratory symptoms in the past, not even on exercise. Apparently, an acquired disorder can also lead to a thin membranous diaphragm. This might be the reason that some articles start from the appearance of the diaphragm instead of etiology, calling it an eventration when it is thin and membrane-like, and then make a division between congenital and acquired eventration [14].
- The review of Revillon and Fekete showed some muscular fibers in all cases of eventration. These fibers were often replaced by scarred fibrous tissue, rich in collagen with a leukocytic infiltrate, suggesting that the thinning of the diaphragm is the end result of a wasting process [15].
- Diaphragmatic dysfunction, e.g., in ventilated patients, indeed can cause a rapid atrophy of diaphragmatic muscle [16].
- Partial eventration (anterior, posterolateral, or medial) corresponds roughly with the distribution of the phrenic nerve branches [15, 17]. The phrenic nerve is often found to be intact. The individual branches, which are deeply buried in the diaphragmatic muscle, could have been affected but were never investigated separately.

If diaphragmatic muscle may atrophy much faster than other striated muscles, then eventration can very well be the end result of an acquired paralysis. These facts together with the common symptoms and identical treatment are reason to discuss them together, as we will do.

36.2 Signs and Symptoms

The clinical presentation of diaphragm dysfunction is highly variable and depends on the degree of paralysis, whether it is unilateral or bilateral and on the presence of concomitant pulmonary disease.

In unilateral paralysis, up to half of the patients are asymptomatic, and their paralysis is often detected by chest imaging done for other reasons [18]. The symptomatic ones present with diminished exercise tolerance and dyspnea in supine position, which is called orthopnea. In newborn children with unilateral paresis, e.g., due to birth trauma, symptoms are usually much worse, due to the soft thoracic cage, weak intercostals muscles in very mobile mediastinum [9, 19]. Young children also lay supine most of the time.

Patients with bilateral diaphragm involvement are always symptomatic. Again, the most common symptom is dyspnea. Because of the gradual onset, the wide differential diagnosis of dyspnea and because the diaphragm is in a hidden position, there is often a delay of months before the diagnosis is established. Careful anamnesis will reveal that dyspnea becomes worse as soon as the patient is in supine position, whereas in cardiac disease, it takes some time before symptoms occur. On examination, Hoover's sign can be found, the lack of extension of the lower ribs on inspiration, and it can be noticed that abdominal and thoracic movements are out of synchronism.

Bilateral paralysis is difficult to detect on imaging. Both diaphragms are elevated, and paradoxical movements are absent as this phenomenon relies on the action of an intact contralateral part [12].

In all patients, the dyspnea can be explained lack of ventilation and/or by the compression of the lung, leading to atelectasis and shunting. A new factor, only recently understood, that can contribute to the diminished exercise tolerance is the compression of the heart by an elevated diaphragm, resulting in circulatory impairment [20]. A right-sided paralysis can cause compression of the atrium, reducing inflow. It can even result in rotation of the heart to the left, along the vena cava axis, with reopening of the oval foramen [21, 22]. The resulting right-to-left shunt can cause serious hypoxia. Left-sided paralysis may result in ventricular compression with diminished cardiac output. To date, although a recent series on diaphragmatic plication have reported severe dyspnea in patients who had displacement of the heart by the paralyzed diaphragm [12], this factor of diminished cardiac output is not yet mentioned [14]. There have been some case reports on car-

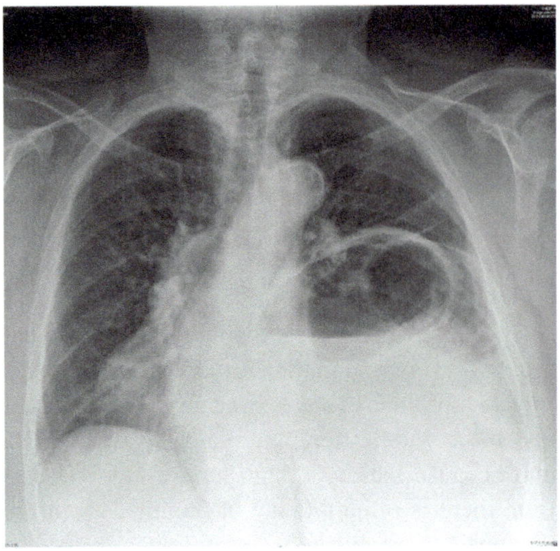

Fig. 36.4 Left-sided paralysis with gas accumulation in the fundus

diac compression, but they appeared in cardiac journals [23–25], not in reviews on diaphragm paralysis.

Besides these respiratory and circulatory symptoms, left-sided diaphragmatic dysfunction may also causes gastrointestinal complaints. The symptoms, which vary from nausea and vomiting to belching and gas bloating in adults or failure to thrive in children, can be explained by the abnormal position of the stomach. The upward position of the fundus, with the esophagogastric junction in place, results in a torsion or even a complete volvulus of the stomach [9]. The accumulation of gas in the fundus is often clearly visible on a chest X-ray (Fig. 36.4).

Pulmonary function tests are helpful but only if done in both an upright and supine position.

In supine position, a decrease of 10% of vital capacity (VC) can be noticed in healthy persons, but in unilateral paralysis, the loss is 20–30%, and in bilateral paralysis, it can be up to 50% [26, 27]. In children, the losses may be greater, up to 50% in unilateral paralysis, because in infants, the intercostal and accessory muscles of respiration do not contribute significantly to respiration. Pulmonary function tests are not very helpful to assess dyspnea because there is no good correlation between pulmonary function tests and the severity of the dyspnea. However, these tests should be done to detect concomitant pulmonary disease and to obtain an objective evaluation after surgical plication of the diaphragm [28].

Imaging is needed to establish the diagnosis. A chest X-ray will show an elevated, nonfunctioning diaphragm, especially when images are taken on inspiration and expiration. An area of atelectasis just above the diaphragm is said to be helpful to differentiate acquired paralysis from long-standing eventration. Because chest X-rays are usually taken in an upright position, the situation may be underestimated, as there is hardly any upward pressure from the abdomen. A chest X-ray in supine position should be made as well. Comparison of a chest x-ray in upright position with the scanogram of a CT scan, taken in supine position, may also reveal a striking difference.

Fluoroscopy is recommended to confirm the paradoxical movement of the diaphragm. However, false-positive and false-negative results do occur [29]. For example, in eventration, the diaphragm may not move at all, and an upward movement of the ribs by accessory respiratory muscles may give the impression that a paralyzed diaphragm is moving downward. Another method to assess diaphragmatic muscle activity is ultrasonography. During contraction, thickening of the muscle can be seen. The view, however, is limited, and the procedure is operator dependant [30]. Both investigations, fluoroscopy and ultrasonography, are difficult to interpret [31, 32].

CT scanning is used most often. Its greatest help is in revealing “pseudoparalysis” due to subpulmonic or subdiaphragmatic fluids or in showing intrathoracic causes for phrenic nerve palsy.

As mentioned before, CT scanning usually shows a higher elevation of the paralyzed diaphragm than the chest X-ray because of the abdominal pressure in supine position. Cardiac compression has been observed on CT scanning, but the incidence might be underestimated because the patient is in a resting position, without straining. Cardiac compression can, however, sometimes be observed when reviewing CT slices.

Dynamic MRI is our investigation of choice. The availability of such a scanner may be limited

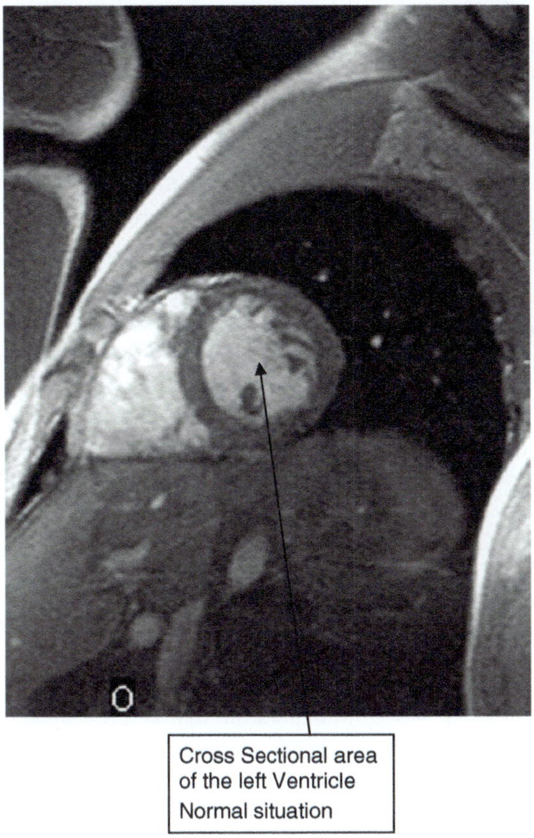

Fig. 36.5 Dynamic magnetic resonance imaging, sagittal view

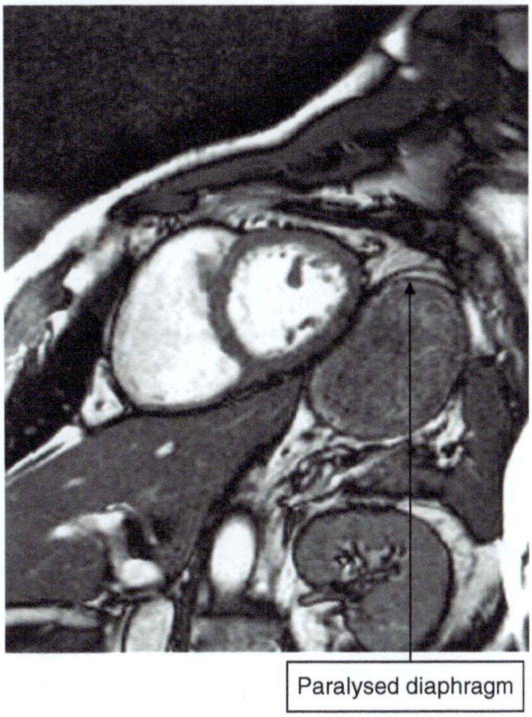

Fig. 36.6 Dynamic magnetic resonance imaging, sagittal view

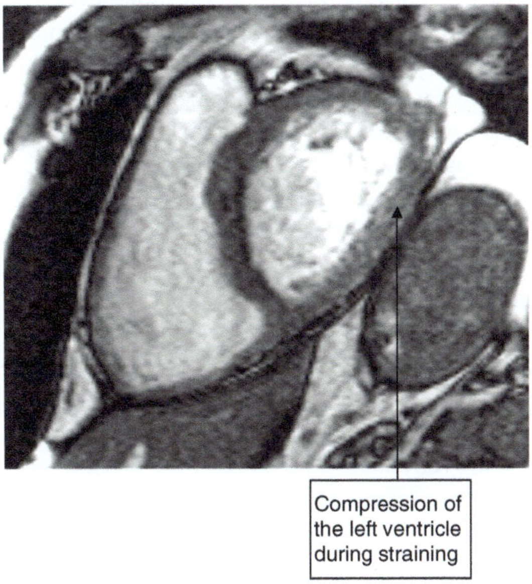

Fig. 36.7 Dynamic magnetic resonance imaging, sagittal view

in many places [12], but this investigation has revealed some new aspects in our patients, e.g., how much cardiac compression can contribute to the clinical picture. It started with a patient with a history of left pneumonectomy including phrenic nerve resection, who repeatedly fainted when digging in his garden. Pulmonary and cardiac function tests did not reveal any indication of disease nor did it explain the mechanism. Only when during a dynamic MRI investigation he was asked to lift both his legs, increasing his abdominal pressure, it was seen how the paralyzed diaphragm, being pushed upward, started to compress the left ventricle (Figs. 36.5, 36.6, and 36.7). He actually fainted during this investigation due to low cardiac output. His legs then dropped, cardiac compression stopped, and the patient woke up again. Figure 36.8 depicts his cross-sectional left ventricle surface area, which correlates with this left ventricle stroke volume over time. When the straining stopped, compression diminished, and the stroke volume returned to normal. In another,

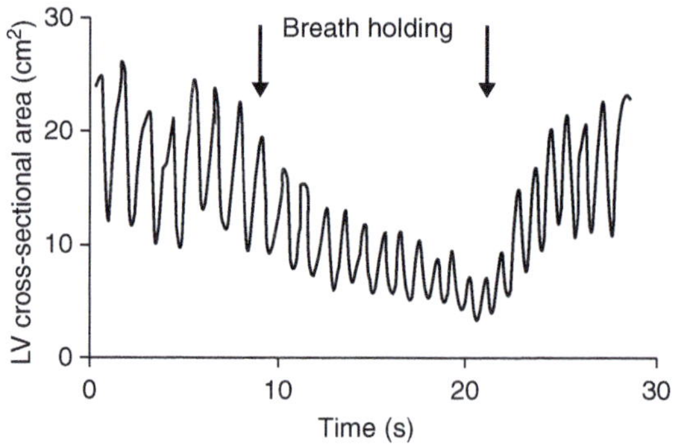

Fig. 36.8 Left ventricle cross-sectional area, reflecting cardiac output, diminishes during straining (Published in Di Giorgio et al. [33]. Reprint permission obtained (rightslink))

74-year-old, patient with right diaphragmatic paralysis after bilobectomy with pericardectomy and phrenic nerve resection, straining was seen to result in increased atrial compression, cardiac rotation, and shunting through a reopening oval foramen. Following surgical plication of the diaphragm, the heart returned to its former position, the shunting stopped, and she was no longer oxygen dependant. Initially, such cardiac compression was seen only in patients after pulmonary resection and compensatory mediastinal shift toward the paralyzed diaphragm, but we now have seen cardiac compression also in "simple eventration" patients.

The reason that many tests, and especially the pulmonary function tests, do not correlate well with the complaints and symptoms of the patient may be the fact that tests are often performed in an upright position or, if in supine position, are performed without straining. This leaves the nonfunctioning diaphragm in a "resting position." Also, the factor of cardiac compression may have been overlooked. Therefore, we now routinely perform dynamic MRI in all patients, with straining if their clinical condition permits.

36.3 Treatment

The first plication was performed in 1923 by Morrison [34], although this treatment was already suggested 7 years earlier [35]. The aim of the operation is to relieve dyspnea, so it is indicated in symptomatic patients only. A waiting time is often advised in phrenic nerve injury after cardiac surgery because nerve function may improve over time. However, many patients have already long-standing and disabling symptoms, and spontaneous recovery in this group is not to be expected. Therefore, in symptomatic patients with unilateral diaphragm paralysis, we proceed to surgical plication. The plication immobilizes the diaphragm in a lower position and reduces the paradoxical movement, making it easier for the accessory respiratory muscles to produce negative inspiratory pressure.

In bilateral diaphragmatic paralysis (BPD), the treatment is less straightforward. In many patients, symptoms can be relieved by noninvasive ventilation at night, using CPAP (continuous positive airway pressure) masks. Other methods should considered as well: Obese patients can improve with bariatric surgery [28], and some patients with motor-neuron disease are candidates for diaphragmatic pacing [36]. Complete BPD, as seen in patients with cervical spine injury, requires mechanical ventilation. Plication in BPD with good success has been described [37, 38], but all authors advise an adequate time of observation because spontaneous recovery does occur and, if so, plication impairs ventilation. In general, benefits in BPD patients are moderate and complications common [28].

At operation, a posterolateral thoracotomy through the fifth, sixth, or seventh intercostal space is the time-honored approach [4, 32, 39–43]. The access to all thoracic structures is optimal (Fig. 36.9), but the large incision itself may cause deterioration of lung function. Disabling post-thoracotomy pain syndromes are also not rare [44].

So also in diaphragm surgery, there has been a shift to less invasive procedures. Muscle-sparing anterior thoracotomy [14], minithoracotomy with thoracoscopic vision [45, 46], full thoracoscopic- [47], and laparoscopic procedures have all been described [48]. Total thoracoscopic procedures are carried out using three or four ports [49–51]. These approaches give minimal damage to the thoracic wall and rib spreading is avoided, but when large (10 mm) ports are used, there can still be

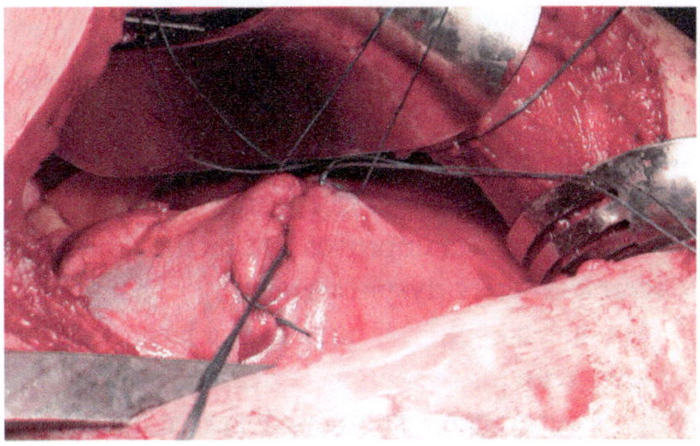

Fig. 36.9 Open plication of an eventration through a posterolateral thoracotomy

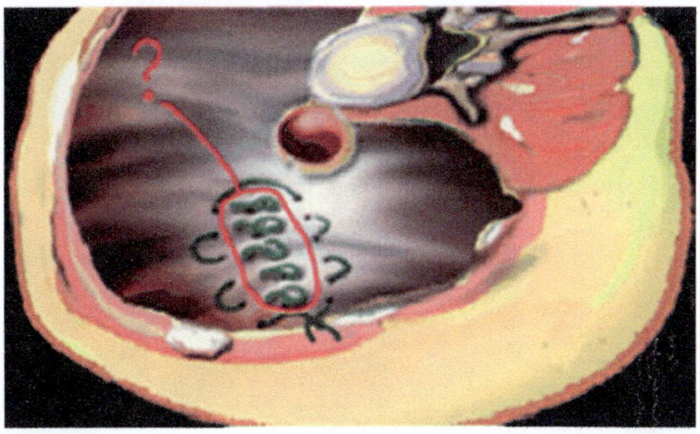

Fig. 36.10 Schematic view of a plication, using mattress sutures

long-standing disabling pain from damage of the intercostals nerves. The limited working space when the diaphragm is much elevated can make the operation a demanding procedure, although gas-insufflation may help [49, 50]. The need for selective ventilation, requiring a double-lumen tube, is another disadvantage of a thoracoscopic procedure. Many authors use a combined approach: a limited anterior thoracotomy is combined with the use of a thoracoscope for illumination and/or vision [45, 46]. They use normal surgical instruments, which can be an advantage, and if a long running suture is used, it can easily be held on tension. The most recent modification is the laparoscopic approach [48], which is the minimally invasive variant of the open abdominal approach used in children [52]. It avoids all intercostal nerve damage and seems optimal for bilateral procedures. However, for right-sided procedures, this approach can be difficult due to presence of the liver. In a recent series, however, one third of the patients underwent right-sided procedure [53].

Not only the approach, also the reefing of the diaphragm itself varied considerably. Initially, part of the excess aponeurotic part of the diaphragm is excised [2, 5], followed by a double layer closure of the muscular portion, but later the diaphragm was pulled in a radial direction and plicated, using non-resorbable mattress sutures (interrupted or continuous, with or without pledgets) [46, 51] or knife-less staplers [54, 55]. Patches are sometimes used for reinforcement [14, 56]. In general, a shift toward plication accompanies the shift toward minimal invasive procedures, and diaphragmatic resection is seldom used today (Fig. 36.10).

Due to the rarity of the disease, there are no prospective comparative trials, neither in the approach nor in the plication technique [28]. Only one institution compared plication procedures with and without a patch, but the decision to use a patch was not made beforehand but during the operation [14]. In general, most techniques seem to work well in experienced hands and much has to do with the surgeon's preference. In the literature, there is certainly a change toward minimally invasive procedures.

Our own preference used to be a small anterior thoracotomy in the 7th intercostals space. The patient is intubated with a single lumen tube and ventilated with low tidals. A nasogastric tube is in situ, which is especially important in left-sided paralysis with much air in the stomach. The table is placed in 30° downward tilt to counteract abdominal pressure upward. The assistant pushes the central part of the dome downward, creating two transverse ridges. The surgeon, who wears a headlamp for good illumination of the field and uses normal surgical instruments, sutures these ridges together with a long non-resorbable running suture, burying the surplus of the diaphragm under it. This is repeated as often as necessary to create a taut diaphragm. Since we have seen the effects of cardiac compression, special care is taken to plicate the pericardial part of the diaphragm. We have also used thoracoscopic vision through an additional port and sometimes also performed fully thoracoscopic procedures, but

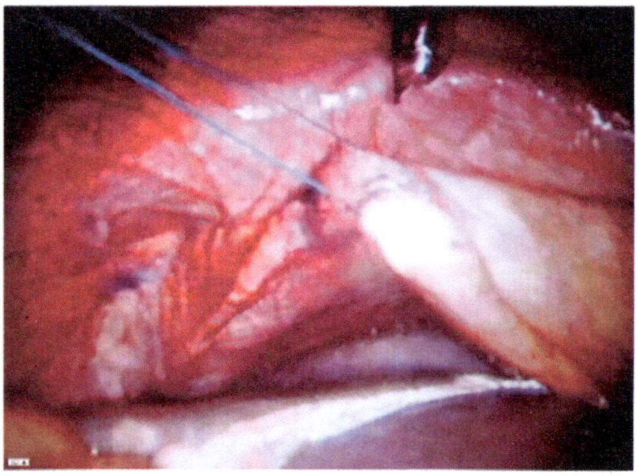

Fig. 36.11 Laparoscopic procedure. A traction suture to bring down the diaphragm greatly facilitates suturing

double-lumen intubation and selective ventilation were not always possible, and the plication sometimes really needs traction on the suture, so for convenience we returned to a low anterior thoracotomy with minimal rib spreading. The intercostal muscle is freed from the rib above it over several centimeters, and the retractor is placed between the muscle and the rib to avoid a crushing injury of the intercostal nerve. However, following the recent literature, we have successfully used the laparoscopic approach in our last patient who had a right-sided paralysis. After opening the diaphragm by cautery, the carbon dioxide enters the thoracic cavity and the diaphragm, which is no longer pushed upward, comes down and can easily be folded. Plication was performed with running sutures, using an Endo-Stitch device. The use of a traction suture can greatly facilitate the procedure (Fig. 36.11). The claim by Groth et al. [54] that the laparoscopic approach will become the most convenient is probably justified.

36.4 Results

Several authors have published their series with short- and long-term results.

In 1990, Graham et al. [39] published a series of 17 UDP patients who underwent plication by open thoracotomy. All had moderate hypoxemia that was relieved in all of them. Results remained good after 5 years. However, in six patients, there was no complete follow-up.

A series with a mean follow-up of 10 years was published by Higgs et al. [42]. Spirometric parameters improved considerably and remained so after 5 years. Most patients also reported good subjective improvement: 12 of 19 patients had more than 1-point improvement on the American Thoracic Society dyspnea scale.

Versteegh et al. [44] published a large series of patients with fluoroscopically verified paralysis in 2007. Twenty-two patients with severe dyspnea in supine position (three even needing CPAP ventilation) were treated by open plication. Three underwent a staged bilateral procedure. There was good subjective improvement: All patients could sleep supine, CPAP was no longer needed, and all improved more than five points on the transition dyspnea index scale. Pulmonary function tests also showed statistically significant improvement of FEV1 and VC (64% vs. 71% and 70% vs. 79%, respectively) at follow-up. However, there were three in-hospital deaths due to myocardial infarction, pulmonary embolism, and severe pulmonary hypertension, and four patients complained of chronic post-thoracotomy pain.

An interesting series of UDP patients was reported by Freeman et al. [56]. Interesting, because his series has control patients. Of 33 UDP patients, who all got intensive pulmonary rehabilitation, 25 patients were operated: 22 thoracoscopically, three with an open procedure (conversion needed). The seven remaining patients had declined surgery. Lung function tests improved significantly in all operated patients, while no change was seen in patients who declined surgery. The same difference was seen in the dyspnea scores. However, their follow-up is rather short, 6 months, and long-term results are awaited. Mouroux et al. [46] published the results of combined procedure in 12 patients. Approach was by a minithoracotomy without rib spreading, combined with two 5-mm thoracoscopic ports. Relieve of symptoms was seen in all patients, and lung function tests improved considerably. No relapses were seen on chest X-ray at follow-up. Recently, also data of a series of diaphragm plication by laparoscopy have become available. Groth et al. [53] published good short- and midterm results in 25 patients, nine of whom underwent a right-sided procedure. Conversion to thoracotomy was needed in only one patient. Besides these series focusing on minimal invasive procedures, one can still find series in the recent literature which use a posterolateral thoracotomy [43]. The long time period (20 years) of this study is once more an indication of the rarity of the disease.

In conclusion, diaphragmatic paralysis and eventration may be stages of the same process. Pulmonary function tests do not correlate well with the severity of the dyspnea but should be obtained to check for concomitant lung disease and to have a baseline for further testing postoperatively. Spirometry should be done both in sitting and supine position. A combination of imaging procedures is often needed to establish the correct diagnosis. Dynamic MR imaging may be the best, especially if combined with straining. Cardiac compression can be found in some patients but does not alter treatment. In symptomatic patients with unilateral disease, surgical correction may be indicated. Substantial and durable improvement can be expected. Caution is needed in recent idiopathic paralysis because spontaneous improvement might occur and in bilateral disease because improvements are limited and complications frequent.

All reported methods seem to give good results in experienced hands. There is a trend toward minimally invasive procedures, but randomized investigations are lacking due to the rarity of the disease. The laparoscopic approach seems promising.

References

1. Laxdal OE, Mc Doughall H, Mellin GW (1954) Congenital eventration of the diaphragm. N Engl J Med 250:401–408
2. Thomas TV (1968) Non-paralytic eventration of the diaphragm. J Thorac Cardiovasc Surg 55:586–593
3. Schumpelick V, Steinau G, Schluper I et al (1968) Surgical embryology and anatomy of the diaphragm with surgical applications. Surg Clin North Am 55:586–593
4. Wright CD, Williams JG, Ogilvie CM et al (1985) Results of diaphragmatic plication for unilateral diaphragmatic paralysis. J Thorac Cardiovasc Surg 90:195–198
5. Shah-Mirany J, Schmitz GL, Watson RR (1968) Eventration of the diaphragm. Physiologic and surgical significance. Arch Surg 96(5):844–850
6. Chin EF, Lynn RB (1959) Surgery of the eventration of the diaphragm. Thorax 14:311–319
7. McNamara JJ, Paulson DL, Urschel HC et al (1968) Eventration of the diaphragm. Surgery 64:1013–1021
8. Christensen P (1979) Eventration of the diaphragm. Thorax 14:311–319
9. Deslaurier J (1998) Eventration of the diaphragm. Chest Surg Clin N Am 8(2):315–330, Review
10. Fell SC (1998) Surgical anatomy of the diaphragm and the phrenic nerve. Chest Surg Clin N Am 8(2):281–294, Review
11. Ko MA, Gail ED (2009) Acquired paralysis of the diaphragm. Thorac Surg Clin 19(4):501–510
12. Gierada DS, Slone RM, Fleischman MJ (1998) Imaging evaluation of the diaphragm. Chest Surg Clin N Am 8(2):237–280
13. Michelson E (1961) Eventration of the diaphragm. Surgery 49:410–422
14. Balci AE, Özyurtkan MO (2010) Clinical and surgical specifications of adult unilateral diaphragmatic eventration according to their aetiology in 28 patients. Importance of using diaphragmatic patch and minimal thoracotomy incision. Eur J Cardiothorac Surg 37:606–612
15. Revillon Y, Fekete CN (1982) Eventration diaphragmatique chez l'enfant. Etude de trente-six cas de 1951 à 1980. Ann Chir Thorac Cardiovasc 36:71–74
16. Levine S, Nguyen T, Taylor N et al (2008) Rapid disuse atrophy of diaphragm fibers in mechanically ventilated humans. N Engl J Med 358(13):1327–1335
17. Merendino KA, Johnson RS, Skinner HH et al (1956) The intradiaphragmatic distribution of the phrenic nerve with particular reference to the placement of diaphragmatic incisions and control, ed segmental paralysis. Surgery 39:189–198
18. Piehler JM, Pairolero PC, Gracey DR (1982) et al Unexplained diaphragmatic paralysis; a harbinger of malignant disease? J Thorac Cardiovasc Surg 84:861–864
19. Ribet M, Linder JL (1992) Plication of the diaphragm for unilateral eventration or paralysis. Eur J Cardiothorac Surg 6(7):357–360
20. Hountis P, Ikonomidis P, Stamatelopoulos A, Douzinas M (2008) Compression of the right atrium due to coexistence of diaphragmatic eventration and Chilaiditi's syndrome. Thorac Cardiovasc Surg 56(6):365–367
21. Aigner C, Lang G, Taghavi S et al (2008) Haemodynamic complications after pneumonectomy: atrial inflow obstruction and reopening of the foramen ovale. Eur J Cardiothorac Surg 33(2):268–271
22. Welvaart WN, Becker A, Marcus JT et al (2010) Unusual treatment of patent foramen ovale after pneumonectomy. Eur Resp J 35:929–931
23. Kalra PR, Frymann R, Allen DR (2000) An unusual cause of cardiac compression resulting in electromechanical dissociation. Heart 83:250
24. Schoen SC, Altmann O, Strasser RH (2008) Elevation of left sided diaphragm leading to myocardial infarction by compression of the left circumflex artery. J Invasive Cardiol 20(8):E250–E252

25. Tayyareci Y, Bayazit P, Tastan CP et al (2008) Right atrial compression due to idiopathic right diaphragm paralysis detected incidentally by transthoracic echocardiography. Turk Kardiyol Dern Ars 36(6):412–414 (Engl abstr)
26. Mc Credie JM, Lovejoy FW, Kaltreider NL (1962) Pulmonary function in hemidiaphragmatic paralysis. Thorax 17:213–217
27. Clague HW, Hall DR (1979) Effect of posture on lung volume; airway closure and gas exchange in hemidiaphragmatic paralysis. Thorax 34:523–526
28. Groth SS, Andrade RS (2010) Diaphragm plication for eventration or paralysis; a review of the literature. Ann Thorac Surg 89:S2146–S2150
29. Alexander C (1966) Diaphragm movements and the diagnosis of diaphragmatic paralysis. Clin Radiol 17:79–83
30. Gottesman E, McCool FD (1997) Ultrasound evaluation of the paralysed diaphragm. Am J Respir Crit Care Med 155:1570–1574
31. Houston JG, Fleet M, Cowan MD et al (1997) Comparison of ultrasound with fluoroscopy in the assessment of suspected hemidiaphragmatic movement abnormalities. Clin Radiol 50:95–98
32. Roberts HC (2009) Imaging the diaphragm. Thorac Surg Clin 19(4):431–450, Review
33. Di Giorgio A, Cardini CL, Sammartino P et al (2006) Dual-layer sandwich mesh repair in the treatment of major diaphragmatic eventration in an adult. J Thorac Cardiovasc Surg 132:187–189
34. Morrison JM (1923) Eventration of diaphragm due to unilateral phrenic nerve paralysis. Arch Radiol Electrotherapy 28:72–75
35. Wood HG (1916) Eventration of the diaphragm. Surg Gynecol Obstet 23:244–248
36. Glenn WW, Holcomb WG, Hogan J et al (1973) Diaphragm pacing by radiofrequency transmission in the treatment of chronic ventilator insufficiency: present status. J Thorac Cardiovasc Surg 66:505–520
37. Stolk J, Versteegh MI (2000) Long-term effect of bilateral plication of the diaphragm. Chest 117(3):786–789
38. Ohta M, Ikeda N, Tanaka H et al (2007) Satisfactory results of diaphragmatic plication for bilateral phrenic nerve paralysis. Ann Thorac Surg 84(3):1029–1031
39. Graham DR, Kaplan D, Evans CC et al (1990) Diaphragmatic plication for unilateral diaphragmatic paralysis: a 10-year experience. Ann Thorac Surg 49(2):248–251
40. Kuniyoshi Y, Yamashiro S, Miyagi K et al (2004) Diaphragmatic plication in adult patients with diaphragm paralysis after cardiac surgery. Ann Thorac Cardiovasc Surg 10:160–166
41. Simansky DA, Palye M, Refaely Y et al (2002) Diaphragm plication following phrenic nerve injury; a comparison of paediatric and adult patients. Thorax 57:613–616
42. Higgs SM, Hussain A, Jackson M et al (2002) Long term results of diaphragmatic plication for unilateral diaphragm paralysis. Eur J Cardiothorac Surg 21:294–297
43. Calvinho P, Bastos C, Bernardo JE et al (2009) Diaphragmatic eventration: long-term follow-up and results of open-chest plicature. Eur J Cardiothorac Surg 36(5):883–887
44. Versteegh MI, Braun J, Voigt PG et al (2007) Diaphragm plication in adult patients with diaphragm paralysis leads to long-term improvement of pulmonary function and level of dyspnea. Eur J Cardiothorac Surg 32(3):449–456
45. Lai DT, Paterson HS (1999) Mini-thoracotomy for diaphragmatic plication with thoracoscopic assistance. Ann Thorac Surg 68:2364–2365
46. Mouroux J, Venisssac N, Leo F et al (2005) Surgical treatment of diaphragmatic eventration using video-assisted thoracic surgery: a prospective study. Ann Thorac Surg 79:308–312
47. Hüttl TP, Wichmann MW, Reichart B et al (2004) Laparoscopic diaphragmatic plication: long-term results of a novel surgical technique for postoperative phrenic nerve palsy. Surg Endosc 18(3): 547–551
48. Freeman RK, Wozniak TC, Fitzgerald EB (2006) Functional and physiologic results of video-assisted thoracoscopic diaphragm plication in adult patients with unilateral diaphragm paralysis. Ann Thorac Surg 81(5):1853–1857
49. Kim DH, Hwang JJ, Kim KD (2007) Thoracoscopic diaphragmatic plication using three 5-mm ports. Interact Cardiovasc Thorac Surg 6:280–282
50. Sato M, Hamada Y, Takada K et al (2005) Thoracoscopic diaphragmatic procedures under artificial pneumothorax. Pediatr Surg Int 21(1):34–38
51. Hwang Z, Shin JS, Cho YH et al (2003) A simple technique for the thoracoscopic plication of the diaphragm. Chest 124(1):376–378
52. Langer JC, Filler RM, Coles J et al (1988) Plication of the diaphragm for infants and young children with phrenic nerve palsy. J Pediatr Surg 23(8):749–751
53. Groth SS, Rueth NM, Kast T et al (2010) Laparoscopic diaphragm plication for diaphragmatic paralysis and eventration: an objective evaluation of short- and mid-term results. J Thorac Cardiovasc Surg 139: 1452–1456
54. Maxson T, Robertson R, Wagner CW (1993) An improved method of diaphragmatic plication. Surg Gynecol Obstet 177:620–621
55. Moon SW, Wang YP, Kim YW et al (2000) Thoracoscopic plication of diaphragmatic eventration using endostaplers. Ann Thorac Surg 70(1):299–300
56. Freeman RK, Van Woerkom J, Vyverberg A et al (2009) Long-term follow-up of the functional and physiologic results of diaphragm plication in adults with unilateral diaphragm paralysis. Ann Thorac Surg 88(4):1112–1117
57. Smulders SA, Marcus JT, Gan CT, Sutedja TG, Smeenk FW, Vonk-Noordegraaf A. Left ventricular encasement after pneumonectomy: case report. J Thorac Cardiovasc Surg. 2006 Oct;132(4):e23–4

Part VIII

Minimally Invasive Cardiac Surgery: General

37 Introduction

Roberto Pasquale Casula

Since the mid-1990s, cardiac surgery has shown a progressive and increasing interest towards the development of minimal invasive and minimal access techniques virtually worldwide.

In almost a decade, minimal access and robotic techniques have been originally described and subsequently redefined following the design of facilitating new tools and technologies and have now become established and perfectly reproducible surgical procedures.

Significantly demanding learning curves for the team and technical challenges for the operating surgeons are commonly required. Training options are available and surgical mentoring has surely become the most modern way to safely export technical knowledge and experience of new techniques to other teams in a clinical governance-based health care.

The total number of minimal access procedures (MICS) performed annually in each country represent an unfair target measure of the actual progress achieved since the 1990s in cardiac surgery given that MICS adoption remains limited to a small group of surgeons. The traditional cardiac surgical community remains concerned about the need of time-consuming and often technically demanding additional training, the increased intraoperative costs and continues practicing in a more than ever litigious society. A better picture of the present status of MICS is surely given by the presence of 'totally converted off pump' surgeon or surgeons who regularly perform their nearly entire annual case loads of isolated aortic and mitral valve procedures via a minimal access route. In the UK only, the percentage of 'off pump' coronary operation have reached a plateau of about 16% in the years 2001–2008, but in real terms, this represents not part but the entire coronary revascularisation workload for a small group of skilful cardiac surgeons.

Robotic systems represent a further adjunct in the surgical armamentarium of cardiac surgeons and probably offer important advantages when used in minimal access coronary revascularization or mitral valve repair surgery; understandably, their efficacy, precision, complication rate and reliability have all been questioned compared to conventional surgical or percutaneous alternatives. All these aspects have been evaluated favourably in various clinical trials although more evidence is required to demonstrate the superiority of patient reported and functional outcomes of robotic revascularisation procedures to justify the additional cost required. The totally endoscopic coronary revascularisation procedure with the da Vinci Si appears to be safe with low complications rate and excellent early and midterm reported graft patency rates which grant its role as a safe and efficacious alternative to a LITA to

R.P. Casula, M.D., FRCS, FETCS
Hammersmith Hospital, Imperial Healthcare College NHS Trust, London, UK

Department of Cardiothoracic Surgery, St. Mary's Hospital, Imperial College Healthcare NHS Trust, Praed Street, London, W2 1NY, UK
e-mail: roberto.casula@imperial.nhs.uk

R.G.C. Inderbitzi et al. (eds.), *Minimally Invasive Thoracic and Cardiac Surgery*,
DOI 10.1007/978-3-642-11861-6_37, © Springer-Verlag Berlin Heidelberg 2012

LAD revascularisation via a median sternotomy when performed by an experienced team.

The accessibility to robotic treatment is increasing as the technology becomes more affordable while offered in a multidisciplinary setting, and more training and mentoring opportunities are currently available for all robotic surgical techniques. However, the adoption of robotic technology in current clinical practice is not as widespread as initially anticipated due to several negative drivers and constraints. The safe adoption of all MICS and robotic techniques by cardiac surgeons requires their significant commitment to embark in further time-consuming training which is often very much dissimilar from the previously successfully acquired traditional cardiac surgical one. Robotic surgeons have to undergo a demanding learning curve to achieve clinical proficiency in these modalities. Cardiac robotic and MICS procedures should be safely performed, and reproducible clinical results should be comparable to current results reported with more conventional techniques and standard practice.

Our effort in redeveloping ourselves by approaching new technological tools and learning new techniques has to be weighted against the reality that referral practices in cardiac surgery are constantly changing and are also influenced by the presence of several different therapeutic percutaneous approaches offered by interventional cardiologists who are ultimately in competition with us for the treatment of the same patients.

Robotic surgery has been extensively applied to perform the LIMA-LAD anastomosis in the contest of a totally endoscopic or atraumatic coronary artery bypass and mitral valve repairs. Despite these clinical achievements, the actual penetration of these techniques in most of the industrialised countries remains negligible even following the 2010 publication of the European myocardial revascularisation guidelines by the European task force of the European Society of Cardiology (ESC) and the European Association for Cardiothoracic Surgery (EACTS).

Ongoing research and development will surely offer cardiac surgeons novel tools to more easily apprenticeship robotic and minimal access techniques. 'Tissue deformation tracking' is one of the exciting technologies under investigation, and it combines tracking of reference points based on stereo-thoracoscopic images and a constrained geometrical surface model that deforms with heart motion. The definition and introduction in clinical practice of similar technologies is likely to slowly return to cardiac surgeons that safety net that is lost in the large gap existing between the performances of traditional versus totally endoscopic operation at present.

This atlas presents the full range of established cardiac and thoracic minimal access and robotic enhanced procedures and offers a theoretical structured training guide for surgeons to continue their technical surgical education and learning.

Anesthesia in Minimally Invasive Cardiac Surgery

38

Fabio Guarracino and Rubia Baldassarri

Contents

Minimally invasive cardiac surgery refers to a series of surgical techniques characterized by either a limited surgical access or by a reduced operative intervention. In the last years, cardiac surgery and consequently cardiac anesthesiology have been involved with new surgical procedures and different technical approaches that have significantly changed the perioperative management of cardiac surgery patients. These procedures that shorten the length of surgery and the perioperative stress have been expanding in all surgical fields as in cardiac surgery. By limiting the surgical wounds and intraoperative stress, often avoiding cardiopulmonary bypass, the minimally invasive cardiac surgery techniques provide a more rapid patient recovery, reduce hospital length of stay, and generally improve the postoperative outcome [1–3].

Minimally invasive cardiac surgery requires an adequate anesthesiological management. During operative procedures characterized by limited surgical access and complex surgical

F. Guarracino, M.D. (✉) • R. Baldassarri, M.D.
Division of Cardiothoracic Anaesthesia and Intensive Care, Cardio-Thoracic Department, University Hospital of Pisa, Pisa, 56124, Italy
e-mail: f.guarracino@ao-pisa.toscana.it; r.baldassarri@ao-pisa.toscana.it

R.G.C. Inderbitzi et al. (eds.), *Minimally Invasive Thoracic and Cardiac Surgery*,
DOI 10.1007/978-3-642-11861-6_38,

instrumentation, intraoperative transoesophageal echocardiography (TEE) to assess cardiac function during the various phases of the operation and advanced hemodynamic monitoring with cardiovascular stability are mandatory. According to the procedural and technical characteristics of the minimally invasive cardiac procedures, the anesthesiological approach to this surgery cannot be "minimally invasive." Because the operative exposure is limited, the surgical procedure is generally complex and the eventual intraoperative complications cannot always be easily managed. In addition, in minimally invasive cardiac surgery, the myocardial protection and the perfusion techniques can be inadequate. For all these reasons, the anesthesiological approach of these patients should provide a total functional and hemodynamic monitoring to manage any possible perioperative problem [2, 4]. Anesthesiological management of the patients submitted to minimally invasive cardiac surgery is affected by the kind of surgery (coronary arteries or valve surgery), by the surgical access (sternotomy, thoracotomy, or percutaneous access), by the technical approach (port-access procedures, endovascular procedures), and obviously, by the patient's clinical conditions. An adequate anesthesiological management of patients undergoing minimally invasive cardiac surgery requires the understanding of the pathophysiological mechanisms involved in the cardiac disease and their hemodynamic implications. It should also be considered that the most of anesthetic drugs have hemodynamic effects which require to be adequately selected and titrated to limit the hemodynamic alterations [1, 2].

38.1 Pathophysiology and Anesthesia

The minimally invasive cardiac surgery techniques can be applied either to coronary artery surgery or to cardiac valve operations, either to other interventional procedures. The pathophysiological mechanisms of the various cardiac diseases, the degree of cardiac dysfunction eventually present, and the surgical technique employed require an adequate and individualized anesthesiological management to improve the perioperative outcome. Any morphological and functional change of the heart secondary to the cardiac pathology, as any increase in volume and pressure of the cardiac chambers, can determine dynamic alterations and cardiovascular instability. The cardiac anesthetist should be well aware of the patient's pathophysiological profile to choose the best perioperative monitoring and the adequate treatment.

A brief summary of the pathophysiological determinants of the most common cardiac diseases is necessary to understand the anesthesiological goals of the management of patients undergoing minimally invasive cardiac surgery [2].

38.1.1 Coronary Artery Disease

Patients affected by coronary artery disease (CAD) can be submitted to surgical myocardial revascularization to restore the coronary flow. Coronary artery bypass grafting (CABG) is a common surgical procedure for patients affected by CAD, and it is routinely performed in most of the cardiac surgical centers. In the last years, the possibility to perform CABG without using cardiopulmonary bypass (CBP) has been largely expanding [1, 5, 6]. This new technique is the so-called off-pump coronary artery bypass grafting (OPCAB).

Although the coronary blood flow (CBF) is autoregulated, it also depends on the coronary perfusion pressure [pressure differential across the coronary bed (CPP)] and on the coronary vascular resistance (CVR). In patients affected by CAD, the CVR increases and the CBF decreases due to the presence of stenosis. Off-pump coronary artery surgery is performed on a beating heart that, as it is still working, is more exposed to ischemic injuries and can be affected by any manipulation or changing position performed by the surgeon to access the coronary arteries for the revascularization. The cardiac viability and functionality depend on the adequate balance of oxygen supply and demand [2]. In critical conditions as in OPCAB, when the oxygen demand increases consequently to the surgical stress, CBF must increase to maintain an adequate oxygen supply. The main goals in patients submitted to OPCAB are the optimization of oxygen supply/demand balance providing oxygen delivery and trying to reduce myocardial oxygen consumption, and monitoring of intraoperative myocardial ischemia. Another important feature of the pathophysiological pattern of CAD is the diastolic dysfunction. Diastole is actually considered a fundamental, active phase of the cardiac cycle and of left ventricle (LV) function [3, 7]. Cardiac filling of the LV is essential to provide a normal cardiac output (CO). In cardiac surgery, the evaluation of the diastolic function is of paramount importance to provide the patient the adequate monitoring and treatment.

Diastolic impairment is characterized by the incapacity to maintain an adequate LV filling without a consequent increase in cardiac pressure secondary to the alteration of relaxation and/or compliance of the LV. Echocardiography is the best noninvasive method to asses diastolic function in clinical scenario, based on the application of spectral Doppler techniques and relatively new techniques as color M-mode and Doppler tissue imaging [3, 7, 8]. By echocardiography, it is possible to distinguish three different pathological patterns of diastolic dysfunction of increasingly severity: impaired relaxation, pseudonormal, and restrictive patterns [9].

Any type of diastolic dysfunction should be promptly recognized in cardiac surgery patients in order to provide adequate care aimed at preventing perioperative-triggering conditions from precipitating diastolic dysfunction into a diastolic failure.

Impaired relaxation is characterized by the affection of relaxation that predominates in the early phases of diastole, and it is generally well tolerated because the LV volumes and pressures are still normal as though the LV filling is prolonged. The pseudonormal pattern is considered a sort of phase of transition in the evolution of the diastolic disease when ventricular stiffness is not present yet. Generally, an increase in preload can change a pseudonormal pattern in an impaired relaxation pattern. As ventricular compliance abnormalities and chambers stiffness appear, a restrictive pattern is evaluable. Left atrial pressure (LAP) increases to maintain an adequate gradient through the mitral valve (MV) to allow LV filling. When an alteration of the LV compliance is present, the LV end-diastolic pressure (LVEDP) increases consequently to the stiffness of the ventricle and the transvalvular gradient decreases with reduction of LV filling. This pattern represents the end-stage pattern of the diastolic impairment.

The recognition of altered relaxation will prompt appropriate volume and heart rate manipulation, as well as maintenance of adequate metabolic and electrolytes profile in order to avoid tachycardia and arrhythmias to occur. These would in fact reduce filling time and coronary perfusion time, leading to reduced cardiac output and possible myocardial ischemia.

In case of altered compliance, a particular attention will be given to adequate LV filling and filling pressures: an optimal preload will require increased filling pressures, without causing pulmonary edema. Therefore, hemodynamic management will need invasive hemodynamic monitoring by pulmonary artery catheter.

38.1.2 Valvular Diseases

Cardiac valves can be affected by regurgitation and/or stenosis that can lead to a more or less significant valvular dysfunction. Abnormal valvular function imposes pressure and volume overload to the cardiac chambers resulting in morphological and functional changes of the heart. According to the underline valvular or cardiac pathology, the valvular dysfunction can onset acutely or progresses chronically. As acute valvular dysfunction generally provides a rapid impairment of the cardiac function, a chronic progression of the valvular disease lets the heart attempt to compensate the increasing pressure and volume loads imposed by the altered valve apparatus. Although each cardiac valve can be affected, the aortic valve (AV) and the mitral valve (MV) are the most frequently involved. The pathophysiological mechanisms of the AV and MV dysfunction are of paramount importance for the secondary effects induced on both systolic and diastolic function of the LV.

Aortic stenosis (AS) is the commonest cardiac valvular dysfunction. The most important pathological features of the AS are secondary to the pressure overload imposed to the LV to maintain an adequate transvalvular gradient to provide the stroke volume (SV). Although AV function is more strictly correlated with systolic phase of the cardiac cycle because in physiological conditions the LV ejects the blood into the aorta through the AV during the systole, AS affects both systolic and diastolic function of the LV. In the early stage of AS, because of the higher resistance to ejection, the LV attempts to compensate pressure overload resulting in a concentric hypertrophy: the thickness of the myocardial walls increases in absence of dilatation of the LV volume. LV increases the contractile muscle mass to maintain the SV. LV hypertrophy affects the diastolic function reducing LV filling either due to the impaired relaxation or due to the increased stiffness of the LV. Severe AS is the later stage of the disease and is characterized by elevated LV pressure and volume, by significant LV hypertrophy and by eventual LV dysfunction. The increasing in LV pressure results in left atrial enlargement and increasing LAP that can pass on the pulmonary vascular system resulting in pulmonary edema; in addition, an enlarged atrium predisposes to atrial fibrillation resulting in a further reduction of the LV filling affecting SV and CO. Patients with severe AS are generally symptomatic and recommended for surgical repair.

Aortic regurgitation (AR) provides a volume overload of the LV with consequent increase of the LVEDV. In patients with acute AR, the LV receives a sudden volume load that increases both end-diastolic and end-systolic volume of the LV chamber. The immediate attempt to compensate the volume overload and to maintain the stroke volume is the activation of the sympathetic tone resulting in tachycardia and increasing contractility. Because these compensatory mechanisms either increase myocardial oxygen demand or cannot be sufficient to provide an adequate cardiac output, the LV function can acutely deteriorate and the symptoms can require a prompt therapeutic treatment. In chronic AS, as the disease progresses and the regurgitant flow is more than 60% of the stroke volume, LVEDP increases and LV dysfunction develops. Consequently, pulmonary artery pressure increases, and patients affected by moderate AR are generally symptomatic for dyspnea and congestive heart failure. Severe aortic regurgitation is generally associated with significant LV dysfunction and pulmonary hypertension, and symptomatology is strictly correlated with poor cardiac output; myocardial ischemia can occur because of the reduction of coronary artery perfusion consequent to diastolic impairment and decrease in forward flow.

Mitral regurgitation (MR) is characterized by significant hemodynamic impairment and functional disturbance. The management of this valvular dysfunction represents really a challenge for the anesthetist because of the complexity of the pathological mechanisms involved. MR can onset acutely or develop chronically; it can be primitive or secondary to myocardial ischemia and LV remodeling. Acute MR can occur as an emergency requiring an immediate treatment. In these conditions, the sudden left atrium volume overload is followed by a rapid increase of the LAP that passes on the pulmonary vascular system. The increase in pulmonary flow determines pulmonary congestion and hypertension. As in AR, the immediate compensatory mechanism is the activation if the sympathetic tone with tachycardia and increased LV contractility resulting in increasing oxygen demand. LV

38.1.3 Hemodynamic Instability

The anesthesiological management of the patients undergoing minimally invasive cardiac surgery must consider that hemodynamic instability can occur in the perioperative period either because of the pathophysiological mechanisms of the cardiac diseases or as consequence of the surgical technique. Cardiac surgery patients are at high risk to develop cardiovascular instability because their cardiac function and dynamic reserve are often limited. Just because of its technical features and operative limitations, minimally invasive

Table 38.1 Pathophysiological conditions resulting in intraoperative hemodynamic instability

Acute coronary syndrome
RV failure
Severe sepsis or septic shock
Valvular dysfunction
Hypertension
Endocarditis
Acute myocarditis
Dysrhythmias
Pericardial effusion or tamponade
AKI
Pulmonary embolism
Aortic dissection

RV right ventricle, *AKI* acute kidney injury

cardiac surgery requires an advanced hemodynamic monitoring to promptly recognize the cause of the hemodynamic instability and to immediately provide the adequate treatment [9]. The sudden onset of hypotension, especially if it is associated with clinical signs of LV dysfunction and low cardiac output, is one of the most serious intraoperative settings. Cardiac surgery patients can develop severe hypotension because of various clinical and technical mechanisms (Table 38.1). Absolute or relative hypovolemia, massive bleeding, dysrhythmia, and myocardial ischemia are the most common causes of hemodynamic instability in patients undergoing cardiac surgery. Diastolic dysfunction is another important determinant of cardiovascular impairment especially in patients affected by CAD and valvular diseases. In patients with moderate to severe MR as in those suffering from right ventricle (RV) dysfunction, pulmonary hypertension can occur. Robotic cardiac surgery needs specific considerations according with the peculiarity of the surgical technique. This video-assisted surgery requires CO_2 inflation into the thorax to allow a better operative performance. The induced pneumomediastinum can determine hemodynamic instability by increasing the intrathoracic pressures which results in a decrease of the preload and in an increase of the afterload. This hemodynamic condition cannot always be well tolerated by the patients especially those in low cardiac output state. Despite the preoperative cardiac performance, any patient submitted to minimally invasive cardiac surgery should be monitored with intraoperative TEE to evaluate cardiac function throughout the procedure [10, 11]. Echocardiography also allows to assess the hemodynamic conditions of the patients evaluating volumes and pressures in the cardiac chambers and in the great vessels reducing significantly the use of invasive monitoring of the cardiac output. TEE can promptly recognize myocardial ischemia evaluating abnormalities of the myocardial contractility and of the regional kinetics just before ECG alterations occur [9–11]. TEE cannot provide a continuous monitoring postoperatively; however, intraoperative TEE evaluation can suggest the use of the most adequate postoperative hemodynamic monitoring, as the pulmonary artery catheter, which will be useful to optimize the hemodynamics throughout the perioperative time.

38.1.4 Monitoring

Patients submitted to minimally invasive cardiac surgery require an extensive and advanced intraoperative monitoring because they are often hemodynamically unstable and because any eventual intraoperative adverse event cannot be easily recognized and promptly treated because of the peculiarity of the minimally invasive surgical procedures. A comprehensive cardiovascular monitoring requires: (1) five-lead electrocardiogram (ECG) is necessary to monitor heart rhythm and rate and to detect intraoperative myocardial ischemia revealing any alteration of the STT tract; (2) invasive blood pressure (BP) monitoring by catheterization of the radial or femoral artery has become a standard procedure in cardiac surgery patients; continuous monitoring of the arterial pressure waves can reveal severe hypotension or hypertension throughout the surgical procedure and allows for hemodynamic evaluation in the crucial phase of surgery; (3) central venous cannulation and measure of the central venous pressure (CVP) is routinely used in cardiac surgery; nevertheless, CVP has not more considered as a significant index of loading conditions in critically ill patients, and its mean value is still measured

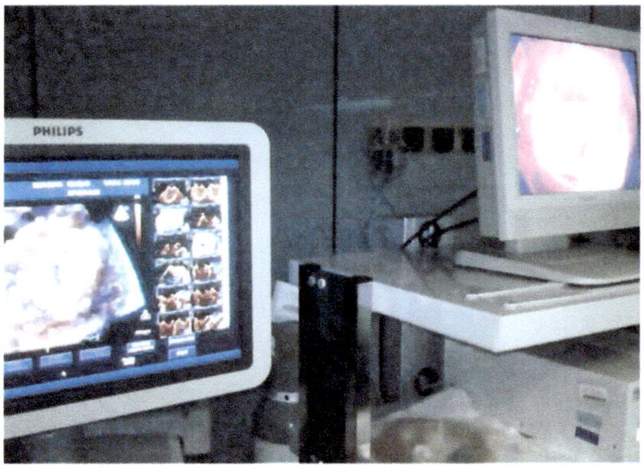

Fig. 38.1 3-D transoesophageal echocardiography during port-access mitral surgery

during cardiac surgery to evaluate the eventual variations related to changes of the loading conditions; moreover, central venous catheterization provides an adequate line for fluid administration; right jugular vein is generally preferred by the most of the anesthetist because its feasibility; in patients undergoing thoracotomy, the subclavian vein access, in the same site of surgical incision to reduce the risk of pneumothorax, should be considered; (4) peripheral veins are routinely cannulated to administer fluid and drugs; the site of catheterization depends on the patient positioning and the surgical access; (5) in selected patients, a pulmonary artery catheterization (PAC) can be required to monitor filling pressures, pulmonary pressures, and continuous cardiac output (CO); CO, or better cardiac index (CI), has been largely considered the best index of tissue perfusion. Adequate CO means adequate peripheral perfusion and flow distribution; therefore, a continuous CO monitoring is a fundamental step in patients with severe hemodynamic instability to promptly recognize any variation of cardiac output and to evaluate the adequacy of clinical treatment. Pulmonary artery catheterization by Swan-Ganz catheter has represented the only method to measure CO for many years; actually, new noninvasive or semi-invasive CO monitoring systems have been expanding in intensive care and surgical settings. PAC and the noninvasive CO monitoring systems are not generally used during surgery, because of the technical limitations of the methods especially because intraoperative TEE can adequately provide CO values throughout the procedure; (6) TEE should be performed in all patients submitted to minimally invasive cardiac surgery either as diagnostic or as hemodynamic monitoring; and (7) respiratory parameters and gas exchanges should be frequently assessed to evaluate the effectiveness of mechanical ventilation especially in patients submitted to one-lung ventilation.

38.1.5 Transoesophageal Echocardiography

Intraoperative transoesophageal echocardiography (TEE) plays a fundamental role in the diagnosis of the underline cardiac disease (Fig. 38.1), in the assessment of the effectiveness of surgery, and in the hemodynamic monitoring of unstable patients submitted to cardiac surgery [10–12]. In minimally invasive cardiac surgery, because of the small surgical accesses and the limited exposure of the heart, a semi-invasive, safe technique that provides real-time information about the heart morphology and function is of a paramount importance. Thanks to the position of the TEE probe inside the esophagus, the transducer is so close to the heart to allow an optimal visualization of the cardiac structures; for the same reason, a comprehensive TEE exam can be performed in few minutes during the surgical procedure standing by the head of the patient without disturbing the surgeon performance [13, 14]. As previously said, TEE plays an important role as hemodynamic monitoring system. Volumetric indexes are actually considered the best indicators of the preload. TEE provides the evaluation of hemodynamic parameters and of the volumes and pressures of the cardiac chambers correlated to the cardiac cycle and the loading condition. LV area and volume are good indicators of preload. Left ventricular end-diastolic area (LVEDA) seems the most appropriate parameter to evaluate LV size and changes in ventricular volume. TEE provides also a good assessment of fluid responsiveness in patients suffering from hemodynamic instability [9]; evaluating the respiratory variation of the inferior vena cava diameter, or the collapsibility of the superior vena cava, and the aortic flow VTI during inspiration under mechanical ventilation, the responsiveness to fluid administration can be adequately estimated. As previously said, echocardiography, especially the transoesophageal approach, is the only noninvasive method to study diastole (Table 38.1). In patients affected by CAD as in those suffering from valvular dysfunction, diastolic impairment can frequently occur. TEE evaluates diastolic function through the analysis of different patterns of flow velocities using two-dimensional (2D) echocardiography and specific techniques as pulsed-wave Doppler, color M-mode, and tissue Doppler. The study of the transmitral inflow velocities with the pulsed-wave echo Doppler technique identifies two waves: E wave (rapid filling) and A wave (atrial contraction) [15, 16]. On the E wave, the deceleration time (DT) can be measured. The E/A ratio (normal value ≥ 1) and DT (normal range 120–160 m) are useful parameters for the diastolic function assessment. Another method to estimate the diastolic function is Doppler evaluation of the pulmonary venous flow pattern. Recently, tissue Doppler imaging of myocardial velocities has been recognized as an important acquisition for detection of diastolic impair, as well as flow propagation velocity of the left ventricle by color M-mode analysis [17]. For all these reasons, severe hemodynamic impair occurring during minimally invasive surgery can be promptly recognized by TEE.

38.1.6 Anesthesiological Drugs

The anesthesiological management of the patients undergoing either minimally invasive or robotic cardiac surgery requires a deep knowledge of the pathophysiology of the cardiac disease involved to provide the adequate perioperative hemodynamic monitoring and the best anesthetic planning. Anesthesia should be tailored to maintain hemodynamic stability, to prevent perioperative adverse events and to allow the patient to tolerate surgery. At the same time, anesthesiological planning should provide a prompt recovery from general anesthesia at the end of the procedure or in a few hours after the operation and an adequate postoperative analgesic strategy [1, 2]. Considering that the most of the anesthesiological drugs commonly used influence hemodynamics, the pharmacological regimen should be individualized on the patient's clinical conditions, with particular regard to the homely medications, and on the surgical setting. It should be considered that the anesthesiological technique is also influenced by the anesthetist preferences. A total intravenous anesthesia (TIVA), especially when a target control anesthesia (TCI) can be performed, is actually preferred by most of the anesthetists (Fig. 38.2). The association between an anesthetic drug as propofol and an opioid as remifentanil allows to maintain anesthesia throughout the surgical procedure and to be continued in the postoperative period. The anesthetic choice can offer the advantage of pharmacological cardiac protection, as described below.

38.1.7 Postoperative Analgesia

According to the fast-track principles of minimally invasive cardiac surgery, adequate anesthesiological technique and postoperative analgesia strategy are required to allow a rapid emergence from general anesthesia and a prompt weaning from mechanical ventilation [1]. Despite the small surgical accesses and the reduced intraoperative stress, postoperative pain score seems to be quite similar in patients sub-

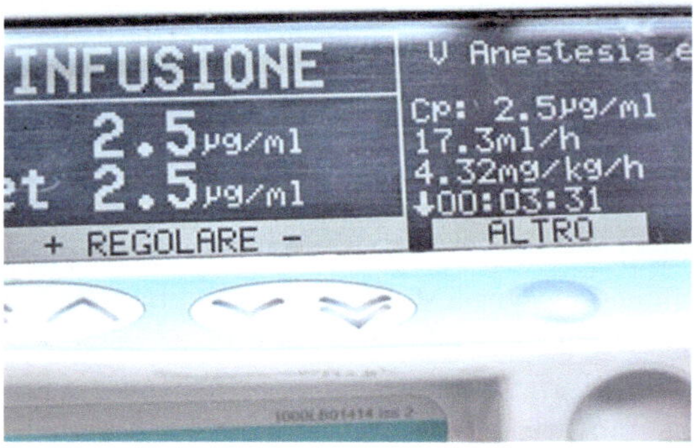

Fig. 38.2 Plasmatic concentration of anesthetic drugs on TCI system

mitted to minimally invasive cardiac surgery and in those undergoing conventional surgery. This is especially true for patients submitted to minithoracotomy. Intravenous continuous infusion of a short-acting opioid as remifentanil, especially if associated with nonsteroidal anti-inflammatory agents, is generally sufficient to maintain an adequate analgesic level in the immediate postoperative period. Low doses of remifentanil do not affect significantly either consciousness or the respiratory rate and are well tolerated by elder patients. High-thoracic epidural catheterization has also been proposed. The positioning of a high-thoracic epidural catheter allows to provide peripheral anesthesia and perioperative analgesia by the administration of continuous infusion of local anesthetics and sedative drugs. High-thoracic anesthesia-analgesia has been especially used in patients submitted to minithoracotomy access to provide a satisfactory postoperative analgesia [18]. The administration of local anesthetic drugs through the epidural catheter allows to stop the perioperative stress response induced by neuroendocrine activation. The abolition of the stress-induced effects as tachycardia and hypertension are fundamental to reduce the oxygen consumption of a beating heart, so providing cardioprotection. Moreover, such a protective effect is provided by an epidural block at T1–T3 level, which provides cardiac sympathetic block with reduced heart rate.

The appropriate analgesia management, through any technique, plays a major role in preventing myocardial ischemia by avoiding the deleterious effects of perioperative tachycardia, which is one of the most important determinants of myocardial ischemia in the surgical patient.

38.2 Anesthesiological Management for Minimally Invasive Valve Surgery

Minimally invasive valve surgery requires the use of endoscopic instrumentations through small ports and limited sternotomy or thoracotomy. The so-called port-access procedures allow the surgeon to perform valve repair or replacement as in conventional cardiac surgery with peripheral CPB [1]. The minimally invasive valve surgery requires general anesthesia, endotracheal intubation, and mechanical ventilation with the exception of the aortic valve percutaneous procedures that can be performed under local anesthesia or mild sedation.

38.2.1 Minimally Invasive Mitral Valve Surgery

Patients affected by MV disease can be submitted to port-access valve surgery and to robotic cardiac surgery to repair or to replace the diseased MV. The port-access procedures have been developed by a group of physicians of the Stanford University and later by Heartport, in attempt to reduce the surgical stress correlated with sternotomy [1, 2]. MV minimally invasive surgery (MVMIS) requires general anesthesia and one-lung ventilation.

The pathophysiological mechanism of the valvular dysfunction, the severity of the valvular regurgitation or stenosis, and the preoperative cardiac function as the hemodynamic effects induced by the valvular disease should be well known by the anesthetist [19]. The anesthesiological management of these patients should be the same of those submitted to conventional mitral valve surgery, but some specific considerations should be done:

1. The supine position is generally used in patient submitted to minithoracotomy incision, but a semilateral position can be requested, and it may be necessary to elevate one arm above the head or to place a support under the patient's side or back for a better surgical exposition. The peripheral and central venous cannulation and the arterial catheterization can be influenced by the patient's position on the operatory bed.
2. The port-access surgery requires selective endotracheal intubation when minithoracotomy incision is performed; in these cases the correct position of the selective endotracheal tube should be assessed before the incision to allow a safe intrathoracic access and to avoid dangerous and challenging repositioning of the tube during the surgical procedure. One-lung ventilation requires a continuous monitoring of the gas exchanges to provide the patient with the adequate respiratory support.
3. The patients undergoing port-access valve surgery need a temporary cardiac pacing (generally placed through a central venous catheter before surgery) to perform heart stimulation if a significant bradycardia or cardiac block occurs; considering that a direct cardioversion of the heart is not possible in these patients in presence of atrial or ventricular fibrillation, skin patches should be placed on the thorax before the induction of the anesthesia [2]. The main goals of the anesthesiological planning for MVMIS are the hemodynamic stability, the preservation of the sinus rhythm or of an adequate heart rate, the optimization of the contractile function of the LV, and the intraoperative assessment either of the valve dysfunction and cardiac functionality either of the effectiveness of the valve repair. An advanced hemodynamic monitoring is required, and the use of intraoperative TEE (Class I, a) is recommended by the European and American guidelines. The port-access procedures require CPB as in conventional MV surgery, but the bypass cannulae are usually positioned through the femoral vessels, so performing a peripheral CPB. The aortic cross-clamping was performed through an endoaortic clamp since a few years ago. Recently, a direct aortic clamping is preferred through the minithoracotomy.

Because of the lack of a direct visualization of the heart, TEE is fundamental to evaluate the correct position of the venous and arterial cannulae and of the endoaortic clamp [20–22].

An extensive hemodynamic monitoring requires (1) electrocardiogram and (2) invasive blood pressure monitoring, central venous catheterization, peripheral oxygen saturation, and serial gas exchanges evaluation. Patients hemodynamically unstable or affected by severe MV dysfunction with pulmonary hypertension and right ventricle dysfunction may require a pulmonary artery catheterization (PAC) to evaluate the filling pressure and to monitor cardiac output.

General anesthesia is generally induced and maintained by the association between a hypnotic agent and an analgesic-sedative drug that provides a safe and deep anesthesia without significant hemodynamic effects. A total intravenous anesthesia (TIVA) with propofol and remifentanil administration can be safely used to induce and to maintain the surgical anesthesia. Because of their pharmacokinetics profile, the infusion of propofol and remifentanil can be continued in intensive care unit (ICU). A rapid weaning from general anesthesia occurs just after stopping propofol infusion, and low-dose infusion of remifentanil provides a good postoperative analgesia even in patients with thoracotomy. The use of an inhalatory anesthesia can be considered in patients with coexisting CAD. Hemodynamic management of the patients submitted to MVMIS requires an adequate assessment of the volemic status to optimize the preload and to modulate the afterload. Increasing preload in patients with MV dysfunction can be helpful to maintain the forward flow, but considering the atrial dilation and the high LA and LV pressures, an excess of fluid administration can deteriorate cardiac output.

38.2.2 Minimally Invasive Aortic Valve Surgery

Aortic valve surgery can be safely performed by minimally invasive surgical procedures with benefits for the patient correlated to the limited surgical incision. A limited superior median sternotomy allows good exposure of the aortic valve providing all the advantages of the open heart surgery, reducing the intraoperative stress and postoperative pain. Minimally invasive surgery has been reported effective for aortic valve replacement as in conventional aortic valve surgery [23, 24]. Limited surgical incision provides a more rapid weaning from mechanical ventilation because of the preserved respiratory function, less postoperative pain, and reduced CBP time. For these reasons, patients submitted to minimally invasive aortic valve replacement emerge earlier from general anesthesia and the hospital length of stay is reduced. The anesthesiological management of patients undergoing minimally invasive aortic valve replacement does not differ from that used in conventional valve surgery. Anesthesia should be tailored to achieve hemodynamic stability and a prompt recovery from general anesthesia. A careful optimization of the load conditions and of the heart rhythm and rate is mandatory in patients that are significantly affected by chronic pressure overload and in whom sinus rhythm is fundamental to maintain an adequate LV filling [2, 3]. Intraoperative TEE is surely useful to assess cardiac function and hemodynamic profile in order to provide the adequate therapeutic support as inotropic agents or fluid administration and to check the effectiveness of valve replacement [9, 20, 21]. The fast-track goals of minimally invasive cardiac surgery should be observed providing a safe anesthetic technique and an adequate hemodynamic management.

38.2.3 Transcatheter Aortic Valve Implantation

Transcatheter aortic valve implantation (TAVI) has been recognized as a safe and effective alternative to surgical aortic valve replacement in high-risk patients affected by aortic valve stenosis. Actually, aortic valve replacement is considered the only adequate therapy for patients affected by severe aortic valve stenosis [24]. Patients with moderate to severe and severe aortic valve stenosis, recommended for valve replacement but considered at high risk for surgery, can be scheduled for transapical or percutaneous (transfemoral and subclavian) procedures of valve implantation. TAVI provides an adequate treatment of aortic stenosis avoiding the risks correlated to sternotomy, CPB, and cardiac arrest. It represents an advantage for critically ill patients that cannot tolerate a significant surgical stress because of the associated comorbidities and the severity of the clinical conditions. TAVI is generally performed in the cath-lab or in the hybrid operatory room with a cardiac surgeon actively present during the procedure or ready to operate if necessary [25]. TAVI can be performed either under general anesthesia or local anesthesia plus mild sedation according to the procedural technique and the patient conditions [26–28].

In patients with severe respiratory comorbidity leading to orthopnea, a new approach with noninvasive ventilation (NIV) has been reported. NIV helps in maintaining a supine position throughout the procedure and in preventing respiratory depression associated with sedation [29].

Hemodynamic monitoring consists of basic ECG, invasive BP, central venous pressure, and pulse oximetry. Urine output and body temperature are generally investigated throughout the procedure [30]. All patients receive echocardiographic evaluation by transthoracic or transoesophageal approach in order to investigate cardiac function and to evaluate the various steps of the procedure and the effectiveness of the valve implantation. In all cases, it is worth monitoring the patient in ICU for at least 6 h. A cautious approach suggests longer ICU stay in patients with severe LV dysfunction, who often require pharmacological support with cardioactive drugs.

38.2.4 Transcatheter Mitral Valve Repair

In the recent years, the MitraClip® system (Evalve Inc., Menlo Park, California) has been expanding as an emergent alternative to surgery in the MR repair in patients at too high risk for surgery. The MitraClip® consists in a percutaneous edge-to-edge repair of the mitral valve, mimicking the surgical procedure. A double-arm clip mounted on a catheter is advanced into the left atrium through a transeptal puncture and then in the LV beyond the tip of the leaflets. The clip is positioned between the anterior and posterior leaflet to reduce the valve regurgitation.

The MitraClip procedure requires TEE examination as long as the procedure lasts. For this reason, general anesthesia is required. The anesthetic management of these patients is the same as in patients submitted to open heart MV surgery. Patients are monitored in ICU postoperatively. Once the patients' postoperative clinical conditions have been well balanced and a good hemostasis at femoral site is achieved, the sedation is stopped and the patients undergo ventilatory weaning and tracheal extubation.

During such procedures, TEE examination is needed from the beginning to the end of the MitraClip procedure. After the TEE probe had been placed into the esophagus, a comprehensive baseline TEE examination is performed in order to confirm the presence and the severity of MR, to evaluate cardiac function and ventricular performance, and to acquire the adequate TEE views and cardiac chambers measurements to guide the procedure. TEE monitoring allows to guide the procedure and to detect any eventual impairment of the system throughout the steps of the percutaneous valve repair.

38.3 Robotically Assisted Cardiac Surgery

Robotically assisted cardiac surgery has been continuously expanding since the first experiences in the 1990s. Actually, the robotic procedures are most commonly employed for MV repair and CABG [31, 32]. The anesthesiological management of the patients undergoing robotically assisted cardiac surgery is strongly conditioned by the presence and by the specific technical characteristic of the machine [2, 18]. Firstly, when the robotic system is fully positioned on the patient and is docked, no further changes in patient positioning are possible during the surgical procedure. Secondly, once the machine is on site, the direct access to the patient is limited that any anesthesiological intervention can be not easy to perform. For all these reasons, a complete interaction between the anesthetist and the robotic system is absolutely necessary to allow the patient to tolerate surgery and to improve the outcome [18, 33, 34]. Before the robotic machine is physically placed on the patient, the anesthetist should contribute to assess that the patient positioning is adequate for the surgical procedure and safe for the patient itself (Fig. 38.3); that any peripheral and central infusion line, any monitoring system and the skin patches are correctly positioned and available throughout the operatory time. Specific care about the possibility that the robotic arms can accidentally contact the patient with consequent pressure or crush injuries is mandatory. A constant and careful vigilance during the procedure is generally sufficient to avoid traumatic lesions as injuries caused by the patient positioning. The robotically assisted cardiac surgery is necessarily affected by cardiovascular and respiratory perturbances that can result in hemodynamic impairment. The anesthetist should well know the complexity of the robotic system and the physiological alterations that can occur during the robotic procedure to provide the adequate anesthetic planning and to maintain the hemodynamic stability throughout the procedure. The physiological effects induced by robotically assisted cardiac surgery are the same as described in patients undergoing thoracoscopy. A combination of patient positioning, one-lung ventilation, surgical manipulation, and occult blood loss can significantly alter ventilation and perfusion with consequent respiratory and hemodynamic instability. It should also be considered that the most of the surgical procedures require the continuous insufflation of carbon dioxide (CO_2) into the chest to facilitate surgery providing a better exposure or the operatory field. The impact of the CO_2 pneumothorax on the cardiovascular and respiratory systems strongly affects the hemodynamic stability. The CO_2 increases airway pressure in the ventilated lung and intrathoracic pressures.

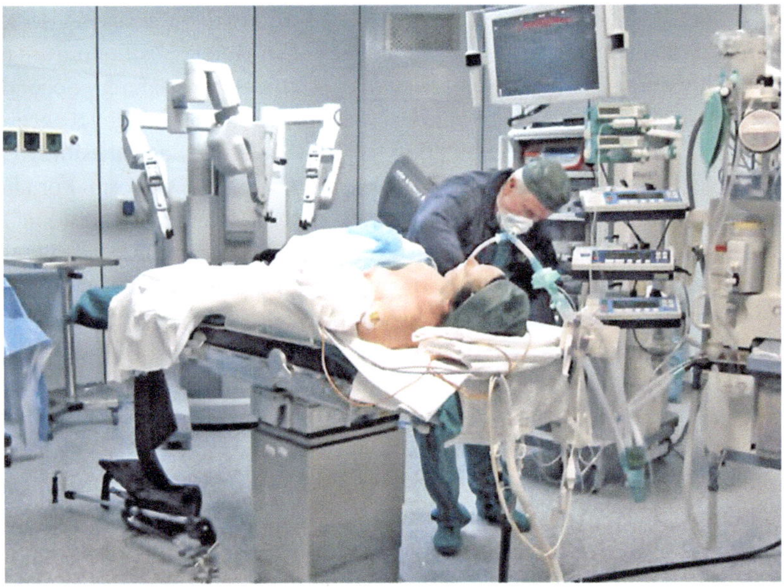

Fig. 38.3 A patient during anesthetic preparation for robotic cardiac surgery

As intrathoracic pressures increase, venous return to the heart and ventricle compliance decrease resulting in low cardiac output and hemodynamic instability. At the same time, mechanical ventilation can become more difficult by the increasing airway pressure and by the continuous absorption of the intrathoracic CO_2. The accidental injury of the contralateral pleura can lead to a pneumothorax in the dependent lung with consequent impairment of ventilation and alteration of the gas exchanges. This event must be promptly diagnosed and treated, stopping the CO_2 insufflation because of the significant hemodynamic and respiratory dysfunction.

38.3.1 Robotically Assisted MV Repair

The surgical access requires small incisions to introduce the endoscopic instrumentation that are connected to the robotic arms [35–37]. The patient is generally positioned supine. Double-lumen endotracheal tube is placed, and one-lung ventilation is performed. Hemodynamic monitoring with ECG, invasive BP, CVP, and SaO_2 is commonly employed. In selected patients, a PAC can be inserted to provide more information. Each patient receives a transoesophageal probe and is submitted to a comprehensive intraoperative TEE examination [22, 35]. Peripheral and central infusion lines are positioned, and end-tidal CO_2 is continuously monitored. The anesthetic technique is decided on the basis of the anesthetist personal experience and on the clinical condition of the patient with particular regard to cardiac function and respiratory performance. TEE is of a paramount importance to guide the surgical procedure and to assess the effectiveness of the MV repair at the end of surgery. TEE provides also much information about cardiac function and hemodynamic profile. Although there are not randomized controlled trials comparing robotically assisted MV surgery with other video-assisted procedures or conventional surgery, several investigations have demonstrated that robotically enhanced MV repair is associated with a low incidence of perioperative bleeding and with a better postoperative outcome [31].

38.3.2 Robotically Assisted Coronary Artery Surgery

Robotically assisted coronary artery surgery has been formerly employed to harvest left internal mammary artery (IMA) [6, 31]. Once the IMA has been harvested, a small (3–4 cm) anterior thoracotomy allows the coronary anastomosis to be performed. The use of robotic-enhanced surgery to perform all the bypasses grafting has been recently proposed [38].

38.4 Anesthesia for Off-Pump Coronary Artery Bypass Grafting

Generally, the coronary artery surgery requires sternotomy and cardiopulmonary bypass (CBP). Sternotomy is associated with postoperative morbidity (infection, disruption of the sternum) as well as pain; CPB can cause postoperative complications due to manipulation, cannulation, and cross-clamping of the aorta (embolism, dissection) and to the CPB-induced inflammatory stress response with consequent coagulation disorders and possible multiple organ dysfunction. In the last years, many efforts have been done to reduce perioperative morbidity and mortality in CABG [1]. Alternative surgical incisions have been suggested. Among them, the left-anterior thoracotomy, the right thoracotomy, and various parasternal and partial sternotomy incisions can be recognized. The left-anterior thoracotomy provides the direct access to the left-anterior descending coronary artery (LAD) and to the diagonal vessels. This surgical approach is the so-called minimally invasive direct coronary artery bypass (MIDCAB) and has been of the most popular in these few last years [5]. Although the surgical approach can be considered a major concern, the avoidance of CPB has been one of the main goals to improve postoperative outcome. This surgical procedure requires a careful preoperative selection of the patients.

38.4.1 Anesthesiological Management

Off-pump coronary artery surgery requires a continuous monitoring of cardiac function and hemodynamic parameters to promptly recognize any adverse event correlated with surgery. Depending on the preexisting cardiac function and coronary anatomy, the heart can poorly tolerate prolonged ischemia of the target vessels or significant modification of the heart normal position, with eventual myocardial injury, cardiac dysfunction, and hemodynamic instability [2, 18]. For these reasons, the anesthesiological management of patients undergoing OPCAB is focused either on efficient technical monitoring or on adequate strategies to prevent myocardial damages. Avoiding CBP during coronary artery surgery can significantly reduce the incidence of systemic complications, CBP-correlated, but a beating heart is surely exposed to ischemic damages because it is still working during surgical manipulations with possible unbalance of the adequate oxygen demand-supply ratio. For these reasons, during OPCAB, it is extremely necessary to apply any strategy to protect the heart from myocardial ischemia either increasing oxygen supply or reducing oxygen consumption or using pharmacological approach to cardioprotection.

38.4.2 Cardioprotection

Performing OPCAB means to significantly reduce the perioperative ischemic-/reperfusion-induced myocardial damage occurring during CPB [39]. As the risk of perioperative myocardial ischemia is surely lower than in on-pump surgery, during beating heart surgical procedure, myocardial protection is however necessary to provide the adequate balance between oxygen supply and demand throughout the procedure [1, 2]. During OPCAB, the heart is continuously perfused because an adequate perfusion pressure can be quite easily achieved.

The critical phases of the surgical procedure are essentially two: (1) the bypass grafting because the coronary is generally closed and the forward blood flow is stopped with consequent transitory ischemia of the tributary myocardial territory and (2) the displacing of the heart to perform the distal anastomosis, due to the mechanical effects on either venous return or ejection flow with possible reduction of the coronary flow. In these crucial steps of OPCAB, the risk of myocardial hypoperfusion can be significantly reduced by an accurate manipulation of the heart by the surgeon and the use of intracoronary shunts that allow for preservation of the coronary flow during the bypass performance, with the exception of a brief period that is generally well tolerated by critical patients too [39, 40]. Providing an adequate oxygen supply by maintaining coronary flow throughout surgery and high levels of blood hemoglobin and providing adequate oxygenation by mechanical ventilation is a fundamental goal of intraoperative myocardial protection of a beating heart. Providing oxygen supply/demand balance also means decrease myocardial oxygen consumption by avoiding *dysrhythmias*, tachycardia, and bradycardia and maintaining a mild intraoperative hypothermia. Tachycardia is actually considered the most important predisposing factor for intraoperative myocardial ischemia because an accelerated heart rate from one site increases myocardial oxygen demand and from the other reduces diastolic time impairing LV filling and SV. Patients undergoing coronary surgery are generally preoperatively treated with beta-blockers to achieve safe values of heart rate and blood pressure. A target of 70 beats for minutes and a systolic pressure ≥100 mmHg is generally considered adequate to decrease the cardiac risk and to provide good cardiac performance.

38.4.3 Myocardial Preconditioning

Perioperative ischemia can occur in patients undergoing cardiac surgery, and it is not infrequently in those submitted to OPCAB. As well known, the direct access to coronary artery as well as the heart displacing to perform the grafts, as well as the lateral aortic cross-clamping on a beating heart, can result in myocardial ischemia. For this reason, many efforts have been done to find a cardioprotective approach for the management of these patients. In the last years, the role of some anesthetics drugs, especially volatile agents, have been recognized in protecting the myocardium from ischemia/reperfusion damage [41–43]. Myocardial lesions are time correlated. Myocytes suffer from ischemia, reducing their contractility till stopping contracting in a few minutes after a reduction of oxygen supply. If ischemia lasts more than 15 min, the myocardial cells go into necrosis. A persisting ischemia causes a loss of the myocardial contractility following the extension of tissue damage. The heart function gradually decreases under ischemia, and even when reperfusion occurs, cardiac dysfunction is still present. As well demonstrated in several investigations, a transient ischemia would be protective for ischemic damage caused by subsequent longer ischemic events. The exposition to a relatively short period of reduction in oxygen supply would protect myocytes from anatomical and functional alterations [44, 45]. This phenomenon, the so-called preconditioning effect, has been largely studied in animal models, and the main pathophysiological mechanisms of cardioprotection have been recognized in several experimental investigations. Some anesthetic drugs, firstly volatile agents, have been recognized to have a cardioprotective action when administered for the induction and the maintenance of general anesthesia. An adequate plasmatic concentration of these drugs would be able to reduce ischemic/reperfusion damage of the myocardium and to limit the extension of the ischemic/infarction areas.

38.4.4 Technical and Pharmacological Approaches

The so-called anti-ischemic drugs as nitroglycerin or calcium channels blockers have been largely used in the past years. Actually, their effectiveness to reduce ischemic risk during cardiac surgery is object of discussion. The prophylactic use of vasodilating and negative inotrope drugs can induce hemodynamic instability in patients whose cardiovascular response is not usually predictable [2].

Some surgical techniques have been proposed to reduce ischemic myocardial injury during OPCAB. Among them, the use of intracoronary shunts and the performance of the proximal grafts before the distal one to assure an immediate flow through the coronary artery are the most common. In patients with poor cardiac functionality or bad anatomy of the coronary flow, a perfusion assistance can be performed. This technique provides an extracorporeal circulation while the heart is beating. It requires arterial-venous cannulation and complete heparinization. This procedure provides a high blood flow during the graft performance and allows the surgeon to safely manipulate the heart and the great vessels. The writer's opinion is that the perfusion assistance combines the disadvantages of both on-pump and off-pump techniques. From one side, it presents the CPB collateral effects, and from the other side, it does not provide a complete cardioprotection.

38.4.5 Hemodynamic Assessment

Patients submitted to OPCAB can suffer from hemodynamic instability throughout the surgical procedure but especially when the bypasses are performed. A severe hypotension that is not immediately responsive to fluid administration or to the head-down maneuver must be promptly investigated to be adequately treated as soon as possible. When there is not an immediately evident cause of hypotension, as massive fluid loss, acute dysrhythmia, or extended displacing of the heart, TEE can provide specific information about cardiac function and hemodynamic profile of the patient, evaluating the causes of the hemodynamic instability and suggesting the appropriate therapy. In the coronary patients, the fluid administration must be adjusted on the cardiac function and on the hemodynamic profile of the patient. When severe cardiac dysfunction, enlargement of the cardiac chambers, and significant myocardial hypertrophy are present, the fluid administration must be regulated on the pressure-volume loop to not exceed the volume expansion providing the adequate volemia. Off-pump surgery is generally characterized by limited blood loss, but sometimes the OPCAB patients receive blood transfusion to optimize the oxygen delivery, providing adequate hemoglobin blood levels.

38.5 Minimal Access Atrial Fibrillation Surgery

Atrial fibrillation (AF) is one of the most common rhythm disturbances with an incidence of 1–2% of the general population. Therapy management of AF includes strategies to reduce the embolic risk and pharmacological therapies to regulate rhythm and heart rate. The surgical treatment of AF provides the atrioventricular nodal ablation [31, 32]. The Cox-Maze procedure has been largely considered the only effective surgical treatment for AF nevertheless its complexity, length, and the incidence of correlated adverse events. The Cox-Maze approach is generally performed in patients undergoing mitral valve repair with significant increase of CPB and surgery length. Actually, some experiences of AF surgical ablation in beating heart have been performed; robotically assisted procedures for AF treatment are in a very initial phase, but they are full of promises. AF ablation procedures require general anesthesia and advanced hemodynamic monitoring; the anesthesiological and hemodynamic management is strongly conditioned by the surgical approach and by the presence of CPB. Robotically assisted procedure is in the very initial phase of the learning curve; therefore the patients submitted to this surgical technique require a careful anesthesiological management and hemodynamic monitoring.

38.6 Biventricular Resynchronization

In patients affected by symptomatic severe cardiac failure and delayed intraventricular conduction despite an optimal medical therapy, cardiac function can be improved by ventricular resynchronization. LV lead placement reduces significantly morbidity and mortality and affects positively the outcome of these patients [46]. The procedure is generally performed by percutaneous access from the coronary sinus, but because of anatomic and technical characteristics cannot be applied in all patients and is associated with a high percentage of failure. Surgical implantation of epicardial LV lead has becoming a new therapeutic chance performed either by minithoracotomy or video-assisted thoracoscopy. Recently, robotically assisted surgery has been successfully proposed to place LV lead in patients in whom percutaneous access was not available [31, 32]. The anesthesiological management of patients submitted to LV lead placement is tailored to provide general anesthesia and hemodynamic stability as in any other minimally invasive or robotically assisted procedure.

38.7 Aortic Arch Surgery

Aortic arch surgery is extremely complex and associated with high perioperative morbidity and mortality. A minimally invasive approach to this surgery is an emergent technical chance to reduce the risk of adverse events and complications. Patients undergoing ascending aorta and aortic arch surgery require an advanced intraoperative hemodynamic and neurological monitoring to assess either cardiovascular instability or cerebral hypoperfusion. Aortic arch surgery is frequently affected by significant hemodynamic impairment and by the risk of neurological complications because the supra-aortic branches are usually involved. Cerebral injuries may develop either from cerebral hypoperfusion or from embolic mechanisms and consequent focal ischemia. Neurological symptoms can be divided in four groups: (1) toxic and metabolic neurological injury characterized by delayed awakening, (2) ischemic injuries as TIA and stroke, (3) early and late neurocognitive symptoms, and (4) peripheral nerve injuries [47, 48].

Despite the intraoperative advanced neurological monitoring and the routine use of techniques providing cerebral protection in the crucial phase of the deep hypothermic circulatory arrest (DHCA), the incidence of postoperative neurological disturbs is still high. Actually, new hybrid open and endovascular surgical procedures have been proposed as a valid alternative to conventional aortic arch surgery. They result in supra-aortic branches revascularization associated with endovascular repair of aortic arch disease [49, 50]. These less invasive techniques could significantly reduce the perioperative complications, limiting the surgical trauma and the extension of the resection [51]. Aortic arch surgery requires a continuous neurological monitoring throughout the procedure to promptly recognize any impairment of cerebral perfusion.

Actually, no advanced neurological monitoring system can be considered absolutely adequate because of either technical limitations or complexity of the technique. Among the various monitoring system, the use of intraoperative near-infrared spectroscopy (NIRS) has been largely expanding in the last years with promising results. NIRS evaluates cerebral flow by transcutaneous electrodes applied on the head of the patient in frontal region. It seems to be an effective and safe method to assess any variation in cerebral perfusion compared to the basal value in awake condition. Other neurological monitoring systems (EEG, transcranial Doppler) have been proposed, but their effective usefulness is still debated. Transcranial Doppler may be used to detect cerebral flow abnormalities.

At the moment, the best neuromonitoring strategy would be a multimodal approach, combining different techniques providing information on both brain perfusion and function.

References

1. Fedorow C, Grocott HP (2010) Cerebral monitoring to optimize outcomes after cardiac surgery. Curr Opin Anaesthesiol 23(1):89–94
2. Hensley FA, Martin DE, Gravlee GP (2003) A practical approach to cardiac anesthesia, 3rd edn. Lippincott Williams and Wilkins, Philadelphia
3. Fuchs KH (2002) Minimally invasive surgery. Endoscopy 34:154–159

4. Rosenhek R, Binder T, Maurer G (2002) Intraoperative transesophageal echocardiography in valve replacement surgery. Echocardiography 19(8):701–707
5. Schaff HV (1997) New surgical techniques: implications for the cardiac anesthesiologist: mini-thoracotomy for coronary revascularization without cardiopulmonary bypass. J Cardiothorac Vasc Anesth 11(2 Suppl 1):6–9
6. Atluri P, Kozin ED, Hiesinger W, Woo YJ (2009) Off-pump, minimally invasive and robotic coronary revascularization yield improved outcomes over traditional on-pump CABG. Int J Med Robot 5:1–12
7. Guarracino F (2008) Ecocardiografia transesofagea in area critica. Elsevier, Milano
8. Achong N, Wahi S, Marwick TH (2009) Evolution and outcome of diastolic dysfunction. Heart 95:813–818
9. Appleton CP, Hatle LK, Popp RL (1998) Relation of transmitral flow velocity patterns to left ventricle diastolic function: new insights from a combined hemodynamic and Doppler echocardiographic study. J Am Coll Cardiol 12:426
10. Shanewise JS, Kodali SK, Billings FT (2009) Transcatheter aortic valve implantation: anesthetic considerations. Anesth Analg 108:1453–1462
11. Cheitlin MD, Armstrong WF, Aurigemma GP, Beller GA, Bierman FZ, Davis JL, Douglas PS, Faxon DP, Gillam LD, Kimball TR, Kussmaul WG, Pearlman AS, Philbrick JT, Rakowski H, Thys DM, American College of Cardiology (2003) ACC/AHA/ASE 2003 guideline update for the clinical application of echocardiography: a report of the American College of Cardiology/American Heart Association Task Force on Practice Guidelines (ACC/AHA/ASE Committee to update the 1997 guidelines for the clinical application of echocardiography). Circulation 108(9):1146–1162
12. Mattew JP, Ayoub CM (2005) Clinical manual and review of transesophageal echocardiography. McGraw-Hill, USA
13. Click RL, Abel M, Schaff HV (2000) Intraoperative transesophageal echocardiography: 5-year prospective review of impact on surgical management. Mayo Clin Proc 75:241–247
14. Fanshawe M, Ellis C, Habib S, Konstandt SN, Reich DL (2002) A retrospective analysis of the costs and benefits related to alterations in cardiac surgery from routine intraoperative transesophageal echocardiography. Anesth Analg 95(4):824–827
15. Guarracino F (2001) The role of transesophageal echocardiography in intraoperative hemodynamic monitoring. Minerva Anestesiol 67(4):320–324
16. Garcia MJ, Thomas JD, Klein AL (1998) New Doppler echocardiographic applications for the study of diastolic function. J Am Coll Cardiol 32(4):865–875
17. Arques S, Roux E, Luccioni R (2007) Current clinical application of spectral tissue Doppler echocardiography (E/E ratio) as a noninvasive surrogate for left ventricular diastolic pressures in the diagnosis of heart failure with preserved left ventricular systolic function. Cardiovasc Ultrasound 26(5):16
18. Sullivan MJ, Frost EAM, Lew MW (2008) Anesthetic care of the patient for robotic surgery. Middle East J Anesthesiol 19(5):967–982
19. Ambler G, Omar RZ, Royston P, Kinsman R, Keogh BE, Taylor KM (2005) Generic, simple risk stratification model for heart valve surgery. Circulation 112:224–231
20. Vahanian A, Baumgartner H, Bax J, Butchart E, Dion R, Filippatos G, Flachskampf F, Hall R, Iung B, Kasprzak J, Nataf P, Tornos P, Torracca L, Wenink A (2007) Task force on the management of valvular heart disease of the European Society of Cardiology; ESC Committee for practice guidelines. Guidelines on the management of valvular heart disease: the Task Force on the Management of Valvular Heart Disease of the European Society of Cardiology. Eur Heart J 28:230–268
21. Bonow RO, Carabello B, Kanu C et al (2006) ACC/AHA 2006 guidelines for the management of patients with valvular heart disease: a report of the American College of Cardiology/American Heart Association Task Force on Practice Guidelines (writing committee to revise the 1998 guidelines for the management of patients with valvular heart disease): developed in collaboration with the Society of Cardiovascular Anesthesiologists: endorsed by the Society for Cardiovascular Angiography and Interventions and the Society of Thoracic Surgeons. Circulation 114(5):e84–e231
22. Grossi EA, Galloway AC, LaPietra A et al (2002) Minimally invasive mitral valve surgery: a 6-year experience with 714 patients. Ann Thorac Surg 74:660–664
23. Koch CG, Milas BL, Savino JS (2003) What does transesophageal echocardiography add to valvular heart surgery? Anesthesiol Clin North America 21(3):587–611
24. Liu J, Sidiropoulos A, Konertz W (1999) Minimally invasive aortic valve replacement (AVR) compared to standard AVR. Eur J Cardiothorac Surg 16:80–83
25. Guarracino F, Baldassarri R (2009) Transesophageal echocardiography in the OR and ICU. Minerva Anestesiol 75(9):518–529
26. Covello RD, Ruggieri L, Landoni G, Guarracino F, Bignami E, Gonfalini M, Virzo I, Michev I, Colombo A, Zangrillo A (2010) Transcatheter implantation of an aortic valve: anesthesiological management. Minerva Anestesiol 76:100–108
27. Shanewise JS, Cheung AT, Aronson S, Stewart WJ, Weiss RL, Mark JB, Savage RM, Sears-Rogan P, Mathew JP, Quinones MA, Cahalan MK, Savino JS (1999) ASE/SCA guidelines for performing a comprehensive intraoperative multiplane transesophageal Intraoperative Echocardiography and the Society of Cardiovascular Anesthesiologists Task Force for Certification in Perioperative Transesophageal Echocardiography. Anesth Analg 89(4):870–884
28. Sellevold OF, Guarracino F (2010) Transcutaneous aortic valve implantation: recent advances and future. Curr Opin Anaesthesiol 23(1):67–73

29. Guarracino F, Cabrini L, Baldassarri R, Petronio S, De Carlo M, Covello RD, Landoni G, Gabbrielli L, Ambrosino N (2011) Noninvasive ventilation for awake percutaneous aortic valve implantation in high-risk respiratory patients: a case series. J Cardiothorac Vasc Anesth 25(6):1109–1112
30. Billings FT, Kodali SK, Shanewise JS (2009) Transcatheter aortic valve implantation: anesthetic considerations. Anesth Analg 108:1453–1462
31. Modi P, Rodriguez E, Chitwood WR Jr (2009) State-of-the-art – cardiac general robot-assisted cardiac surgery. Interact Cardiovasc Thorac Surg 9:500–505
32. Woo YJ (2006) Robotic cardiac surgery. Int J Med Robot 2:225–232, Review Article
33. Czibik G, D'Ancona G, Donias HW, Karamanoukian HL (2002) Robotic cardiac surgery: present and future applications. J Cardiothorac Vasc Anesth 16:495–501
34. Lanfranco AR, Castellanos AE, Desai JP, Meyers W (2004) Robotic surgery: a current perspective. Ann Surg 239(1):14–21
35. Tatooles AJ, Pappas PS, Gordon PJ, Slaughter MS (2004) Minimally invasive mitral valve repair using the da Vinci robotic system. Ann Thorac Surg 77(6):1978–1982
36. Chitwood WR Jr, Nifong LW, Elbeery JE et al (2000) Robotic mitral valve repair: trapezoidal resection and prosthetic annuloplasty with the Da Vinci surgical system. J Thorac Cardiovasc Surg 120:1171–1172
37. Grossi EA, LaPietra A, Ribakove GH et al (2001) Minimally invasive versus sternotomy approaches for mitral reconstruction: comparison of intermediate-term results. J Thorac Cardiovasc Surg 121:708–713
38. Subramanian VA, Patel NU, Patel NC, Loulmet DF (2005) Robotic assisted multivessel minimally invasive direct coronary artery bypass with port-access stabilization and cardiac positioning: paving the way for outpatient coronary surgery? Ann Thorac Surg 79(5):1590–1596
39. Chitwood WR Jr, Wixon CL, Elbeery JR, Francalancia NA, Lust RM (1999) Minimally invasive cardiac operation: adapting cardioprotective strategies. Ann Thorac Surg 68(5):1974–1977
40. Campos JC (2010) An update on robotic thoracic surgery and anesthesia. Curr Opin Anaesthesiol 23:1–6
41. De Hert SG, Turani F, Mathur S, Stowe DF (2005) Cardioprotection with volatile anesthetics: mechanisms and clinical implications. Anesth Analg 100:1584–1593
42. Stowe DF, Kevin LG (2004) Cardiac preconditioning by volatile anesthetic agents: a defining role for altered mitochondrial bioenergetics. Antioxid Redox Signal 6:439–448
43. De Hert SG, Van der Linden PJ, Cromheecke S et al (2004) Choice of primary anesthetic regimen can influence intensive care unit length of stay after coronary surgery with cardiopulmonary bypass. Anesthesiology 101:9–20
44. Kloner R, Jennings R (2001) Consequences of brief ischemia: stunning, preconditioning, and their clinical implications Part 1. Circulation 104:2981–2989
45. Kloner R, Jennings R (2001) Consequences of brief ischemia: stunning, preconditioning, and their clinical implications Part 2. Circulation 104:3158–3167
46. Derose JJ Jr, Belsley S, Swistel DG, Shaw R, Ashton RC (2004) Robotically assisted left ventricular epicardial lead implantation for biventricular pacing: the posterior approach. Ann Thorac Surg 77:1472–1474
47. Clements F, Shanewise J (2001) Minimally invasive cardiac and vascular surgical techniques. Society of cardiovascular anesthesiologists monograph. Lippincott Williams and Wilkins, Philadelphia
48. Murkin JM (2009) NIRS: a standard of care for CPB vs. an evolving standard for selective cerebral perfusion? J Extra Corpor Technol 41(1):P11–P14
49. Schoder M, Lammer J, Czerny M (2009) Endovascular aortic arch repair: hopes and certainties. Eur J Vasc Endovasc Surg 38(3):255–261
50. Chan YC, Cheng SV, Ting AC, Ho P (2008) Supra-aortic hybrid endovascular procedures for complex thoracic aortic disease: single center early to midterm results. J Vasc Surg 48(3):571–579
51. Antoniou GA, El Sakka K, Hamady M, Wolfe JHN (2010) Hybrid treatment of complex aortic arch disease with supra-aortic debranching and endovascular stent graft repair. Eur J Vasc Endovasc Surg 39:683–690

Part IX

Minimally Invasive Cardiac Surgery: The Heart

Minimal Access Mitral Valve Surgery 39

Thierry A. Folliguet

Contents

T.A. Folliguet, M.D., FACS
Chirurgie Cardiaque Vasculaire & Transplantation,
Institut Lorrain du Coeur et des
Vaisseaux Louis Mathieu,
CHU Brabois-Nancy, France
e-mail: t.folliguet@chu-nancy.fr

39.1 Clinical Background

Alternative incisions to expose the mitral valve have included upper partial sternotomy, parasternal incisions and minithoracotomies. The annulus of the mitral valve is nearly the sagittal plane of the body making a posterior mini right thoracotomy the optimal approach to the valve. This approach provides direct access to the mitral valve through a left atriotomy. The addition of video assistance into the right chest allows better visualization and minimal incision size. Initial reports of successful mitral valve repair using video assistance and a right minithoracotomy were published in 1996 [1, 2]. This technique of "port-access" mitral valve surgery has been extensively performed across the world. Similar results can be obtained in experienced teams as compared with median sternotomy [3–9]. Most of the complex repair can be repaired through these incisions with excellent result [8–10]. Clearly, the results are operator dependent, and both a solid experience of mitral valve repair and of video surgery are needed to obtain good results [7].

Robotic surgery has been introduced in 2002 and provides the surgeon with optimal 3D imaging, magnification, miniaturized instruments, and mobility through seven degrees of freedom mimicking the human wrists. The instruments are placed directly through 10-mm trocars which are positioned in a triangular fashion with the 3-D camera, apart from the minithoracotomy. When comparing both techniques, the robotic platform allows "novice" endoscopic surgeons to perform

R.G.C. Inderbitzi et al. (eds.), *Minimally Invasive Thoracic and Cardiac Surgery*,
DOI 10.1007/978-3-642-11861-6_39, © Springer-Verlag Berlin Heidelberg 2012

complex task more rapidly and more efficiently. The surgeon's vision and method of operating is more "intuitive" as the surgeon is seating and controls the instruments through three fingers in each hand. However, the cost of the platform and of each instrument represents and increased cost as compared to port access [11], and the surgeon depends more of the overall team including nurses and assistant in order to perform the surgery [12]. Feasibility of robotic mitral valve repair has been demonstrated in both simple and complex repairs [13–17]. Despite a longer aortic and cross clamp time than through a sternotomy, excellent immediate and long-term repair can be achieved in experienced teams [17–22]. More rapid return to work, diminished blood loss, and reduced length of hospitalization have been measured following robotic mitral valve surgery [23].

39.2 Patient Selection and Assessment

Patient selection depends of the team experience. At the beginning "easy repair" should be performed, and as experience is gained more complex repair can be attempted. All patients should have a surgical and an anesthesiologist consult. Exclusion criteria should include: emergency, pulmonary disease, atherosclerotic and enlarged ascending aorta, aortic insufficiency, peripheral vessel disease including femoral and iliac disease, prior right chest surgery, or major trauma. Poor ejection fraction, multiple valve repair or replacement, and associated coronary revascularization should be excluded as it exposes the patient to prolonged operating and CPB time, and it adds to the complexity of the procedure.

Therefore, a complete preoperative checklist should be done including chest X-ray, EKG, echocardiogram, coronary angiogram, complete pulmonary function tests, and peripheral arterial and venous Doppler. Also of interest, a CT scan of the chest will evaluate the degree of aortic calcification, the presence of emphysema, and the anatomy of the patient (left atrial enlargement, right and left ventricular dimension). Finally, a signed consent from each patient should be obtained, explaining that other techniques are possible (median sternotomy, port access).

39.3 Technique (Patient Positioning, CPB, Anesthetic)

As with elective cardiac procedures, standard hemodynamic monitoring lines, including central venous lines and arterial lines, should be placed. A double lumen endotracheal tube is necessary to allow for left single lung ventilation during the preparation phase. A trans-esophageal echocardiogram is also necessary to check the placement of the cannulas and also to assess the mitral valve repair and the ventricular function after declamping. External defibrillator cardioversion pads are placed on the patient behind the right scapula and on the left anterolateral chest wall.

The patient is placed supine with a small pillow placed under the right scapula in order to elevate the right hemithorax, and then the right arm is positioned along the side of the patient with the elbow slightly flexed in order to have access to the right axillary area. Small inflatable pillow are also placed under the ankles and the knees to avoid compression point on the table. The patient should be prepped from the neck to the knees, and access to the chest, to both groins, and to the right neck should be available.

Cannulation of the femoral vessels can be individualized as experienced is gained. Usually, a right cutdown is made in the inguinal area, and the femoral or iliac vessels are exposed and cannulated percutaneously. A 17- or 18-mm wire-wrapped cannula is inserted in the artery, and a 27- or 29-mm wire-wrapped double-staged cannula is inserted in the vein and placed in the right atrium under echo guidance. Most of the time, this will allow adequate drainage; however, sometimes it can be necessary to place percutaneously in the right jugular vein either a 17- or an 18-mm wire-wrapped cannula. This will provide optimal venous drainage. An active aspiration on the reservoir should be added with a biocentrifugal pump, and direct control of the cavas is not necessary unless the right chest is entered [24].

Cardioplegia is performed antegrade with a long cannula placed either through the minithoracotomy or separately in the 2nd or 3rd intercostal space. Aortic occlusion can be done either with a transaortic clamp placed in the 2nd intercostal space mid posterior axillary line or with an endoartic clamp. Both techniques have advantages and disadvantages [25, 26]. The direct transthoracic clamp is an easy technique to perform which does not require specific training; however, it can be traumatic to the left atrial appendage. Therefore, clamping should be performed with optimal visualization. The endoaortic balloon requires an additional arterial line in the right radial artery in order to recognize balloon migration. Also, it requires another groin access, but it provides both occlusion and cardioplegia and does not require aortic manipulation and has been associated with decreased cerebral microemboli compared with the transaortic clamp [27]. Finally, cases of aortic dissection have been reported with this endoclamp balloon. We usually decrease body temperature to 32°C and repeat blood cardioplegia every 10–15 min without removing the atrial retractor.

The robot is positioned on the left side of the table and should be positioned securely after groin preparation has been made.

Prior to incision in the right chest, the right lung is deflated, a 4-cm submammary posterolateral incision is performed, and the chest is entered in the 4th interspace. CO_2 is insufflated either directly with the camera port or through a separate stab wound placed posteriorly in the 7th intercostal space. The diaphragm is retracted inferiorly with a stitch brought in the 7th intercostal space as to create a working space. The robotic camera is placed in the more medial part of the incision or through a separate port median to the thoracotomy. Robotic trocars are positioned in triangular fashion one or two interspaces above and below the thoracotomy, slightly more inferior to the incision.

The pericardium is entered and opened in a longitudinal fashion from the diaphragm to the aorta. Traction sutures are placed usually at the level of the pulmonary veins and brought inferior to the cannulas and the incision, in order to "bring the heart" toward the chest wall. The inferior vena cava is dissected from the pericardium and the interatrial groove clearly dissected exposing the left atrium. This allows opening the left atrium more toward the mitral valve and will facilitate greatly the exposure.

The robotic fourth arm dynamic left atrial retractor is placed either through the incision or through a separate port in the 3rd intercostal space medial to the incision but away from the camera in order to avoid any conflict. If a fourth arm is not available, an endoscopic retractor is placed through the left atriotomy and brought parasternal in the 4th intercostal space. It should be secure to the chest either with a clamp or with a flexible retractor. The second solution allows some flexibility and mobility of the endoscopic retractor. If the camera was well positioned, minimal traction with the retractor is needed to allow optimal mitral valve visualization. We then place three annular stitches at the commissures and at the level of P2, which are brought through the incision. This provides traction on the annulus and "brings" the valve toward the incision, which facilitates repair. A left ventricular vent is positioned in the atrium toward the pulmonary veins to provide a dry field.

Standard techniques of valve repair can then be employed.

After repair, the left atrium is closed with two 4-0 monofilament sutures starting at each extremity. We recommend Goretex sutures as these can be pulled with the robot and tied more efficiently then Prolene because they offer greater resistance. Before purging, left ventricular wires should be placed on the right inferior part of the ventricle. Air is purged through the aortic hole and under TEE guidance. Aorta is then declamped and the cardioplegia suture should be secure before ECC is completed.

Two chest tubes are inserted through the thoracotomies and placed over the diaphragm and at the apex of the right chest. A transthoracic intercostal catheter is placed posteriorly in the incision prior to closure.

Then, the patient should be reintubated with a regular endotracheal tube before brought to the intensive care unit.

39.4 Summary

Robotic mitral valve repair can be performed in experience teams. The results are clearly center and operator dependent. Before embarking on a robotic program, training of the entire staff has to be performed. Modification of the anesthesiology and of the extracorporeal circulation is essential in order to obtain good results. Also regular practice is needed in order to keep the team efficient, and therefore this technique should be applied only in high volume centers. Compared with median sternotomy, most studies have shown decreased blood loss, more rapid recovery, and shorter hospitalization with the robotic approach. However, increased operative time including cardiopulmonary and aortic cross clamp times, as well as an increase in cost, is associated with robotic surgery. Short-term results are acceptable and compared with median sternotomy in terms of mortality and morbidity; however, long-term results show a slight increase in reoperation with the robotic approach. Again, this may be related to the learning curve since experience is extremely important in order to obtain good results.

References

1. Vanermen H, Wellens F, De Geest R, Degrieck I, Van Praet F (1999) Video-assisted port-access mitral valve surgery: from debut to routine surgery. Will Trocar-Port-Access cardiac surgery ultimately lead to robotic cardiac surgery? Semin Thorac Cardiovasc Surg 11:223–234
2. Mohr FW, Falk V, Diegeler A, Walther T, van Son JA, Autschbach R (1998) Minimally invasive port-access mitral valve surgery. J Thorac Cardiovasc Surg 115:567–574; discussion 574–566
3. Raanani E, Spiegelstein D, Sternik L, Preisman S, Moshkovitz Y, Smolinsky AK, Shinfeld A (2010) Quality of mitral valve repair: median sternotomy versus port-access approach. J Thorac Cardiovasc Surg 140:86–90
4. Aybek T, Dogan S, Risteski PS, Zierer A, Wittlinger T, Wimmer-Greinecker G, Moritz A (2006) Two hundred forty minimally invasive mitral operations through right minithoracotomy. Ann Thorac Surg 81:1618–1624
5. Casselman FP, La Meir M, Jeanmart H, Mazzarro E, Coddens J, Van Praet F, Wellens F, Vermeulen Y, Vanermen H (2007) Endoscopic mitral and tricuspid valve surgery after previous cardiac surgery. Circulation 116:I270–I275
6. Casselman FP, Van Slycke S, Dom H, Lambrechts DL, Vermeulen Y, Vanermen H (2003) Endoscopic mitral valve repair: feasible, reproducible, and durable. J Thorac Cardiovasc Surg 125:273–282
7. Galloway AC, Schwartz CF, Ribakove GH, Crooke GA, Gogoladze G, Ursomanno P, Mirabella M, Culliford AT, Grossi EA (2009) A decade of minimally invasive mitral repair: long-term outcomes. Ann Thorac Surg 88:1180–1184
8. Modi P, Rodriguez E, Hargrove WC 3rd, Hassan A, Szeto WY, Chitwood WR Jr (2009) Minimally invasive video-assisted mitral valve surgery: a 12-year, 2-center experience in 1178 patients. J Thorac Cardiovasc Surg 137:1481–1487
9. Seeburger J, Borger MA, Falk V, Kuntze T, Czesla M, Walther T, Doll N, Mohr FW (2008) Minimal invasive mitral valve repair for mitral regurgitation: results of 1339 consecutive patients. Eur J Cardiothorac Surg 34:760–765
10. Lapenna E, Torracca L, De Bonis M, La Canna G, Crescenzi G, Alfieri O (2005) Minimally invasive mitral valve repair in the context of Barlow's disease. Ann Thorac Surg 79:1496–1499
11. Morgan JA, Thornton BA, Peacock JC, Hollingsworth KW, Smith CR, Oz MC, Argenziano M (2005) Does robotic technology make minimally invasive cardiac surgery too expensive? A hospital cost analysis of robotic and conventional techniques. J Card Surg 20:246–251
12. Folliguet T, Vanhuyse F, Constantino X, Realli M, Laborde F (2006) Mitral valve repair robotic versus sternotomy. Eur J Cardiothorac Surg 29:362–366
13. Jones BA, Krueger S, Howell D, Meinecke B, Dunn S (2005) Robotic mitral valve repair: a community hospital experience. Tex Heart Inst J 32:143–146
14. Chitwood WR Jr, Kypson AP, Nifong LW (2003) Robotic mitral valve surgery: a technologic and economic revolution for heart centers. Am Heart Hosp J 1:30–39
15. Chitwood WR Jr, Nifong LW, Elbeery JE, Chapman WH, Albrecht R, Kim V, Young JA (2000) Robotic mitral valve repair: trapezoidal resection and prosthetic annuloplasty with the da vinci surgical system. J Thorac Cardiovasc Surg 120:1171–1172
16. Rodriguez E, Nifong LW, Chu MW, Wood W, Vos PW, Chitwood WR (2008) Robotic mitral valve repair for anterior leaflet and bileaflet prolapse. Ann Thorac Surg 85:438–444; discussion 444
17. Murphy DA, Miller JS, Langford DA (2007) Endoscopic robotic mitral valve surgery. J Thorac Cardiovasc Surg 133:1119–1120; author reply 1120
18. Akpinar B, Guden M, Sagbas E, Sanisoglu I, Caynak B, Bayramoglu Z (2006) Robotic-enhanced totally endoscopic mitral valve repair and ablative therapy. Ann Thorac Surg 81:1095–1098
19. Smith JM, Stein H, Engel AM, McDonough S, Lonneman L (2007) Totally endoscopic mitral valve repair using a robotic-controlled atrial retractor. Ann Thorac Surg 84:633–637

20. Reade CC, Johnson JO, Bolotin G, Freund WL Jr, Jenkins NL, Bower CE, Masroor S, Kypson AP, Nifong LW, Chitwood WR Jr (2005) Combining robotic mitral valve repair and microwave atrial fibrillation ablation: techniques and initial results. Ann Thorac Surg 79:480–484
21. Chitwood WR Jr, Rodriguez E, Chu MW, Hassan A, Ferguson TB, Vos PW, Nifong LW (2008) Robotic mitral valve repairs in 300 patients: a single-center experience. J Thorac Cardiovasc Surg 136:436–441
22. Nifong LW, Chitwood WR, Pappas PS, Smith CR, Argenziano M, Starnes VA, Shah PM (2005) Robotic mitral valve surgery: a United States multicenter trial. J Thorac Cardiovasc Surg 129:1395–1404
23. Woo YJ, Nacke EA (2006) Robotic minimally invasive mitral valve reconstruction yields less blood product transfusion and shorter length of stay. Surgery 140:263–267
24. Sobieski MA 2nd, Slaughter MS, Hart DE, Pappas PS, Tatooles AJ (2003) Peripheral cardiopulmonary bypass with modified assisted venous drainage and transthoracic aortic crossclamp: optimal management for robotic mitral valve repair. Perfusion 18:307–311
25. Dogan S, Aybek T, Risteski PS, Detho F, Rapp A, Wimmer-Greinecker G, Moritz A (2005) Minimally invasive port access versus conventional mitral valve surgery: prospective randomized study. Ann Thorac Surg 79:492–498
26. Reichenspurner H, Detter C, Deuse T, Boehm DH, Treede H, Reichart B (2005) Video and robotic-assisted minimally invasive mitral valve surgery: a comparison of the Port-Access and transthoracic clamp techniques. Ann Thorac Surg 79:485–490; discussion 490–481
27. Maselli D, Pizio R, Borelli G, Musumeci F (2006) Endovascular balloon versus transthoracic aortic clamping for minimally invasive mitral valve surgery: impact on cerebral microemboli. Interact Cardiovasc Thorac Surg 5:183–186

Minimally Invasive Mitral Valve Surgery via Right Minithoracotomy

40

Jamshid H. Karimov and Mattia Glauber

Contents

J.H. Karimov, M.D., Ph.D. (✉) • M. Glauber, M.D.
Department of Cardiothoracic Surgery,
Heart Hospital, "G. Monasterio" Tuscany Foundation for Research and Health, Via Aurelia Sud, 54100 Massa, Italy
e-mail: asr_uz_2003@yahoo.com;
mattia.glauber@ftgm.it

40.1 Introduction

Mitral valve (MV) disease is known to be the most common valve lesion [1, 2] resulting from degenerative valve disease, ischemia, infective endocarditis, and other causes [3, 4]. Heart valve diseases are highly prevalent and are independent determinants of subsequent mortality in a patient population [1, 2, 5]. Surgical valve repair or replacement continues to be the only treatment for MV disease with defined clinical success [4, 6]. Currently, the full median sternotomy with an incision of the left atrium remains a standard approach for surgery on the MV and the valve apparatus as the incision is easily opened and closed, and access to the entire heart is possible [7]. Despite the fact that conventional MV surgery has been well established as safe and effective, the procedure is still invasive and carries a risk of significant complications due to the surgical trauma, especially in patients with serious comorbidities [4, 8].

Years of research and development [9–11] led to the introduction of minimally invasive MV surgery concepts into clinical practice in the mid-1990s [12–14] and have grown in popularity since then [15]. The first complex mitral repair under videoscopy was performed by Carpentier through a minithoracotomy (5×4 cm) in a 30-year-old female [12]. The concept of minimally invasive surgery has been driven by a desire to translate the benefits observed in minimal invasive general surgery access to the cardiac

R.G.C. Inderbitzi et al. (eds.), *Minimally Invasive Thoracic and Cardiac Surgery*,
DOI 10.1007/978-3-642-11861-6_40, © Springer-Verlag Berlin Heidelberg 2012

surgical arena [16] using different strategies with variable results [17]. The port-access system concepts were developed and introduced in collaboration with industry (HeartPort, Inc., Redwood City, CA, now Edwards Lifesciences, Irvine, CA, USA) [18]. A separate set of instruments was designed to provide intracardiac retraction and to allow surgeon to work through small incisions or so called "ports" [13, 14, 17, 18]. The system initially consisted of cardioplegia delivery either through the proximal port of a balloon catheter or through a percutaneously placed coronary sinus catheter. The port-access approach was developed in order to offer an integrated solution for a cardiac surgical procedure [19] and initially consisted of small thoracotomy, endoscopy-enhanced field visualization [12, 13], and dedicated perfusion systems, allowing various direct and peripheral cannulation as well as aortic cross-clamping options [16, 20]. The port-access surgery has undergone many changes [21–24] and continues to be optimized by surgeons according to their needs and preferences. With this system, a surgeon can establish standard myocardial protection and perform precise cardiac operations without a sternotomy [17, 18, 25, 26]. As an alternative to the standard, median sternotomy access, the clinical benefits of the port-access technique include a reduction of surgical trauma, increased patient comfort, and shorter hospital stay which is based on the assumption that smaller incisions should lead to less postoperative pain and rapid return to full activity [27]. The development of a system for cardiopulmonary bypass (CPB) and cardioplegic arrest that did not require a median sternotomy incision [16] was a major breakthrough that helped to widen the application of minimally invasive mitral valve surgery [18].

When first introduced, minimally invasive surgery critics questioned the compromise of potentially longer operations with greater risk and more complications for the advantage of better cosmetic result [28]. They stated concern that the learning curve associated with this technique may be challenging even for the experienced surgeons, because of femoral cannulation, use of guidewires and endoaortic occlusion balloons [29], small incisions [30], and decreased surgical maneuverability compared with the conventional approach [31]. However, this method has been proven to require no longer than a conventional procedure, and the patients have a lower transfusion rate, better respiratory function, shorter length of hospital stay, less postoperative pain, and the same rate of recurrent mitral regurgitation after repair [28]. Additionally, the most common pain reported by median sternotomy patients is back pain, largely due to traction of the ribs and thoracic ligaments [7]. This and other postoperative discomforts are greatly reduced in minimally invasive operations performed through small incisions [27, 32]. The smaller incision(s) also reduces the risks for wound infection and blood loss. Patients recover more rapidly [33] and are discharged from the hospital sooner, thus reducing the hospital costs [34].

Because minimally invasive cardiac surgery is a relatively new method however and does have limitations and certain inherent complications discussed below, a gradual transition of conventional skills to this new approach and establishment of experienced extended team support are imperative to avoid unnecessary problems related to the surgery itself and technical complications associated with the technology [30].

The realization of the significant advantages to the minimally invasive approach has driven innovation and considerable progress in developing new operating techniques [16, 20, 35, 36] and dedicated instruments and devices [37] for minimally invasive valve repair options. These include an array of valvular, subvalvular, and annular procedures aimed at restoration of leaflet coaptation [4]. With these advances, minimally invasive MV surgery was widely introduced into clinical practice [12–14] and is now considered one of the most innovative methods adopted in the spectrum of minimally invasive surgical techniques [38, 39].

Minimally invasive MV surgery has evolved into a safe and effective surgical option for thousands of patients and represents a significant recent paradigm shift in modern cardiac surgery [40].

This approach has been introduced in experienced centers worldwide as an alternative therapeutic option for isolated MV disease and concomitant procedures [14, 17, 18, 26, 41–46] and has proven to be a safe, reproducible technique [47] with low preoperative morbidity and mortality and with late outcomes that are equivalent to conventional MV surgeries [17, 41, 48]. Recent further advances in technology and surgical methods have also expanded its application to the repair of complex valves [31, 40] and the performance of concomitant procedures [49, 50].

As patients, in turn, become aware of the potential advantages of less invasive approaches to treating valve diseases, they are increasingly requesting less invasive MV procedures [28], and this is becoming their treatment of choice. Due to the previously stated advantages of minimally invasive techniques over the standard approach and to the increasing comorbidities in a continuously aging patient population [1, 6] in need of MV repair or replacement, the minimally invasive approach for isolated valve surgery has been shown to be a safe option with excellent results [8] and with less potential for serious complications in patients with high and prohibitive operative risk and is also recommended as an approach for patients who have had previous cardiac procedures [47, 51–53]. The minimally invasive approach also appears to yield equivalent safety and efficacy outcomes to that reported for conventional surgical repair of atrial septal defects and atrial tumors [38].

In this chapter, we present our approach to MV repair or replacement performed through a single-access right minithoracotomy in the third or fourth intercostal space. This is the most commonly employed minimally invasive incision for mitral valve surgery [39] and can be performed under direct vision by utilizing alternate arterial and venous perfusion techniques. In our institution, we have extended use of this approach from isolated mitral valve procedures to more complex cases requiring concomitant procedures such as aortic and/or tricuspid valve operations [50, 54], as well as atrial fibrillation ablations in selected cases [55].

40.2 Patient Selection and Assessment

Patients should be carefully screened, and candidates for an isolated MV surgery must meet the selection criteria for each procedure to be performed. All patients undergo a routine chest X-ray and transthoracic echocardiography. Assessing the position of the right atrium and ascending aorta over the projection of the intercostal spaces on the chest X-ray is critical [35] to imagine the incision site and potential exposure. Patients must also undergo extensive preoperative evaluation for the presence of significant vascular disease [56]. Previous right chest trauma and right-sided mastectomy with chest wall radiation [57] may be considered contraindications for this approach in selected patients. Anatomic abnormalities (pectus excavatum), ascending aortic aneurysm, aortic arch aneurysm, highly calcified aortic valve or MV annulus, severe peripheral arterial vessel disease [58], indications for aortic root reconstruction, and significant multivessel coronary disease are considered as contraindications for this approach. Treatments of atrial fibrillation [59] and concomitant aortic and/or tricuspid surgery are not contraindications [49, 50]; however, they are recommended only after a high level of expertise is achieved with isolated and uncomplicated MV surgeries.

Good exposure of the MV is one of the most important factors for performing repair or replacement [7]. A very deep chest (deep anteroposterior diameter) and those with unusual cardiac orientation (extremely vertical or horizontal, leftward shift) [35] can be considered as a contraindication because a central aortic cannulation and MV exposure is particularly difficult. These patients can be excluded, at least during initial experiences with this method, but can be managed more easily when experience grows. Central aortic cannulation should be avoided by use of peripheral aortic cannulation in patients with a short ascending aorta which limits space for direct aortic cross-clamping. Obtaining the adequate exposure can also be difficult in markedly obese patients. While advanced age per se is not considered as exclusion criteria for port-access MV surgery, minimally invasive MV surgery can be indicated in high risk elderly patients [60], when a median sternotomy together with other concomitant diseases may result in increased operative risk, postoperative wound infection, and pulmonary complications.

40.3 Anesthesia and Patient Preparation

The procedure is performed in a standard operating room with each team member positioned according to existing protocols for conventional MV surgery. The basic operative setting we use to place the equipment and position the surgical team members is illustrated in Fig. 40.1. Special attention should be taken to organize the operating room architecture and establish correct patient positioning as the surgeons' position and working comfort can ultimately influence the quality and extent of this type of operation.

General intravenous anesthesia using the standard techniques [61] is provided according to the standard protocol used for conventional MV repair or replacement. Peripheral arterial and venous accesses are established for patient hemodynamic monitoring and IV infusion. Two percutaneous sheath introducers are placed in the jugular vein. A standard 4-lumen (7.0 or 8.5 Fr) venous introducer is used for drug administration and central venous pressure monitoring. Another percutaneous sheath (8.5 Fr) introducer is placed in the same right jugular vein for eventual insertion of endocavitary pacemaker leads, when necessary. In cases where endoaortic balloon occlusion is expected to be employed, both right and left radial artery monitoring lines are placed for immediate warning of balloon migration

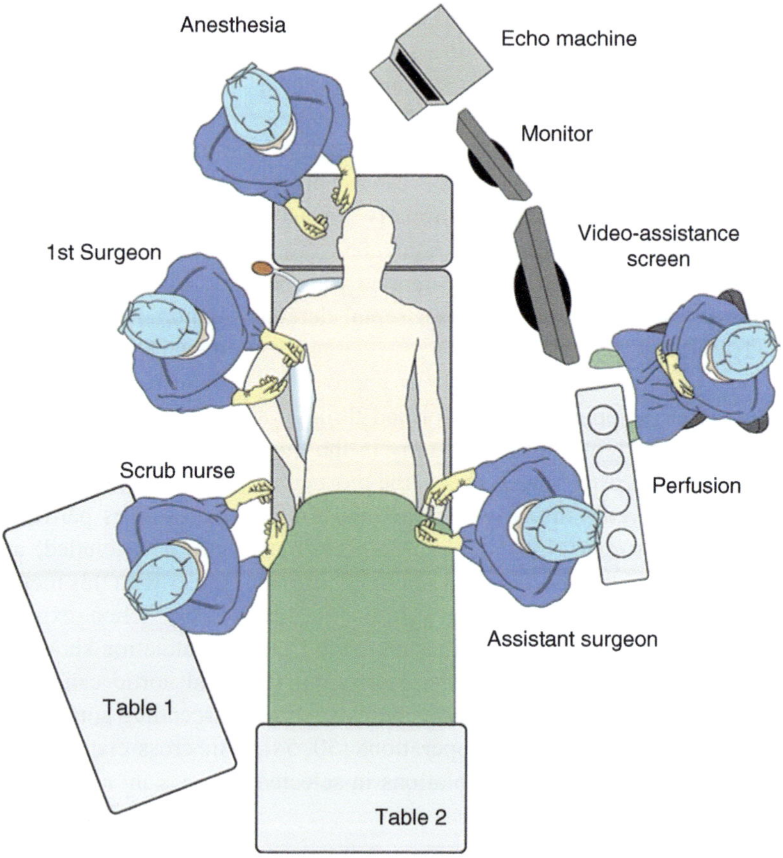

Fig. 40.1 Positioning of the surgical team in the operating room

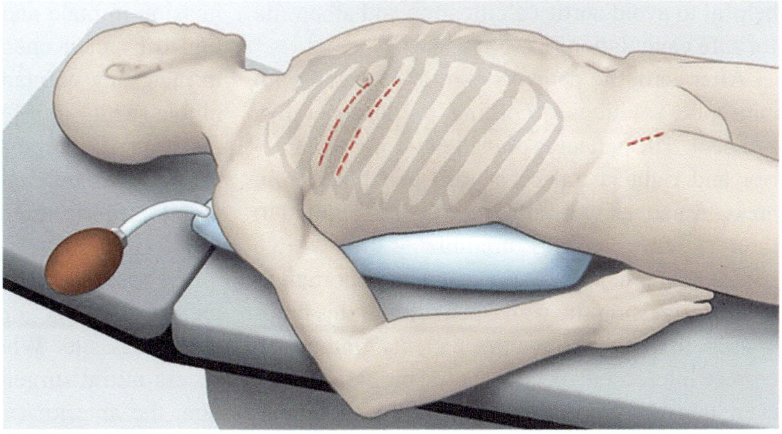

Fig. 40.2 Patient positioning for a right-sided single-access mitral valve procedure. Right hand is moderately displaced, laterally from patients' body. An inflatable air sack is positioned under right subscapular area, and the patients' right chest is elevated accordingly

resulting in the innominate artery obstruction [39]. If the endoaortic balloon is not used, one radial artery line and two jugular venous sheaths are sufficient. The responsibility of anesthesiologist may also include superior vena cava cannulation and insertion of a coronary sinus catheter for cardioplegia delivery through the right jugular vein under the TEE guidance [62]. The advantage of not having any additional catheter in the operating field [63] by use of a cardioplegia catheter must be weighed against the risk of sinus perforation (especially in elderly patients) and is not considered an absolutely necessary procedure [64]. We have abandoned coronary sinus catheter placement because of unpredictable coronary sinus anatomy, potential risk of sinus injury [30], a significant learning curve, and other difficulties encountered during placement which may significantly prolong the intraoperative preparation time.

The patient is intubated and anesthetized after arterial and venous lines are placed. Both single- and double-lumen endotracheal tubes can be used [65]. The use of a left double-lumen endotracheal tube is not mandatory [30], but can facilitate the procedure [66] if a challenging surgical preparation (difficult cannulation, pleural adhesions) is expected when the minithoracotomy is made. We prefer a single-lumen tube for routine intubation, but in patients with a deep chest or those undergoing reoperative surgery, the role of double-lumen tube may be particularly important. When a double-lumen endotracheal tube is used or if a difficult intubation is expected, a McGRATH® video laryngoscope (Aircraft Medical Ltd., Edinburgh, UK) or a regular bronchoscope can be used to facilitate the procedure and confirm the correct position of the endotracheal tube.

Two defibrillator pads are placed across the chest wall with the right pad placed under the patients' right shoulder and left pad over the anterior left chest wall [39, 66]. Attention is paid to these pads after skin preparation when occasionally the pads may be detached from the skin in case of very abundant application of antiseptic solutions. The patient is placed in a supine position, and an inflatable balloon is placed under the right scapula to elevate the patient's right chest slightly [61] for better working field exposure as shown on Fig. 40.2. This can be useful particularly in patients with a deep chest. The balloon can be inflated or deflated to adjust (raise and lower) the right chest position as needed. This balloon should be secured in order to prevent any dislodgement during operation. The patient's right hand should be slightly displaced laterally from the body; this allows space for working port placement and also allows the surgeon to take a more comfortable position during his approach to the patient.

Transesophageal echocardiography (TEE) is used for assessment of MV and cardiac function, ventricular filling, intracardiac air, and peripheral venous cannula insertion. The TEE may also be helpful to avoid aortic calcification and atheroma for safe cannulation [67, 68].

Afterward, the patient's skin is prepared with antiseptic solutions according to intraoperative protocol. The patient is draped exposing the anterior and right lateral chest wall and both groin areas. An adhesive aseptic strip is then applied to the exposed areas, thus, minimizing the possible risk of contamination. It may also be important to mark the incision site with a pen prior to this preparation. In a majority of male patients, finding the correct intercostal space is not a problem; however, this can be difficult at times in a female patient, so marking the submammary crease can be particularly important to following the right surgical plane. Also, in women, it is recommended to lift the right mammary with the assistants' free hand prior to aseptic strip application. The large mammary may become difficult to mobilize which can influence the operating visual field and render a procedure more difficult.

In case of the need for concomitant atrial fibrillation radiofrequency ablation, additional pads are placed along the patient's right scapular area and left side of the thorax. If a bipolar irrigated ablation device is to be applied, the external pads are not necessary.

40.4 Surgical Techniques

40.4.1 Incision and Exposure

The MV visualization is obtained through a limited access, single-access right minithoracotomy. Generally, two types of incisions (anterior and anterolateral) can be employed to access the valve and subvalvular structures. Incision options are shown in Fig. 40.3. Both incisions can be performed in the third or fourth intercostal spaces. The choice is primarily based on expected type of cannulation and patients' chest conformation. An incision in the third intercostal space is preferred if direct ascending aorta cannulation is planned. Also, MV visualization is more direct, and a video-assistance may be of secondary importance in cases when the minithoracotomy incision is constructed more laterally. The difference of incision in male and female patients is predetermined by their chest conformation: the incision in men may be made either above or below the nipple, while in a female patient, the incision is made in the submammary crease [39]. When femoro-femoral cannulation for CPB is planned, then the fourth intercostal space may be used as an alternative.

Preoperative chest X-ray helps to evaluate the incision construction and the potential quality of the access site. When minimally invasive port-access mitral surgery was started in our institution, the anterior (more medial) incision was a preferred option in a majority of cases. Then, the anterolateral incision has become more popular however due to more direct MV exposure and much more comfortable working conditions. The standard 5 Fr venous introducer sheath is placed percutaneously in a right femoral vein prior to incision. This is done before systemic heparinization and helps to avoid undesirable bleeding from possible femoral artery punctures made before heparin administration. A prepared right femoral vein introducer sheath allows direct venous cannula insertion without any delay, when the patient's systemic anticoagulation is confirmed.

The procedure is carried out through a 5–7-cm incision in the third or fourth intercostal space, centered on the midclavicular line or more laterally. The intercostal muscles are dissected from the upper and lower ribs or in any preferred manner, but preferably closer to the margin of the lower rib, in order to avoid intercostal arterial and venous branches and to obtain a secure hemostasis. A partial rib resection may be performed [19] to facilitate the exposure, but this is not common and may require the isolation and subsequent ligation of the right internal mammary artery. Attention should be paid to meticulous hemostasis at this point as it appears to be much easier to identify and cauterize any oozing vessels at this point in the procedure than prior to thoracotomy closure when many of these vessels may become "silent" and are not always easily recognizable during hemostasis of the incision site before closure.

The medium width of available multiuse retractor blades is approximately 4–5 cm, and the

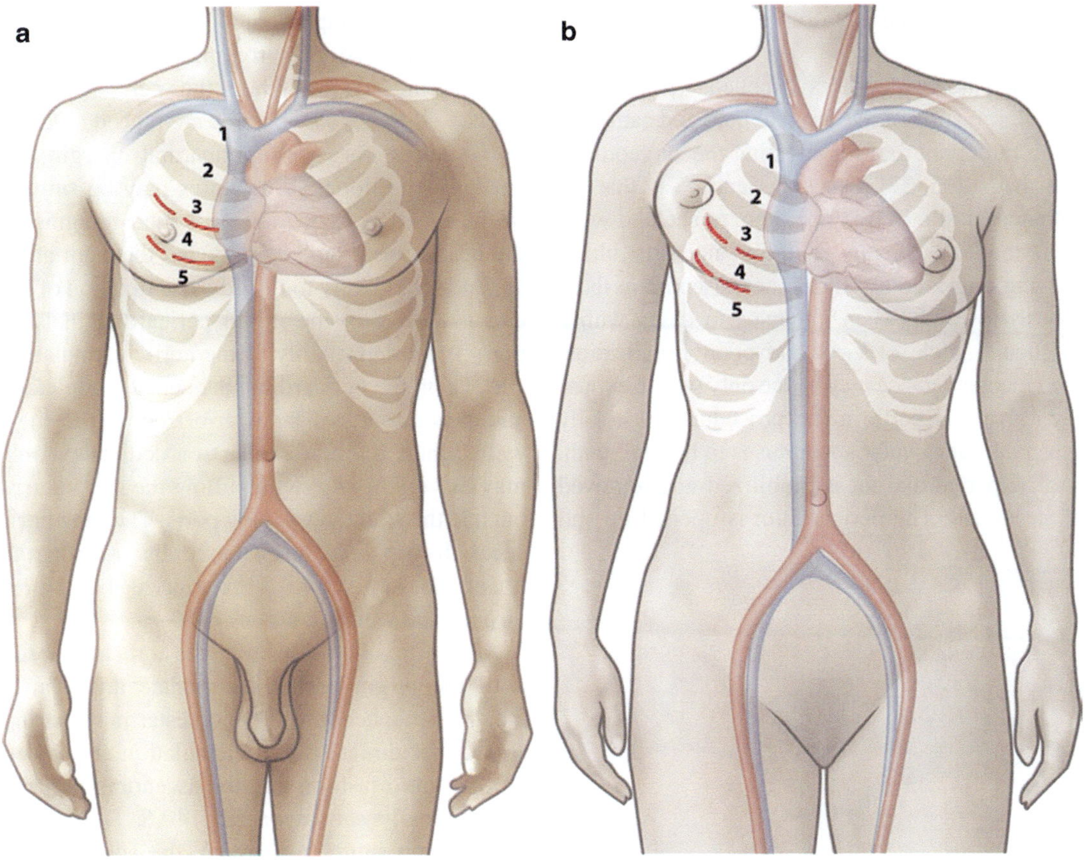

Fig. 40.3 Incision options in a male (**a**) and female (**b**) patient made in the third or fourth intercostal space. An incision in the submammary crease in female patient can be facilitated by pulling the right mammary upward and placing adhesive aseptic strip in the operative room

incision length is usually around 5–7 cm of length. The length of the incision is not critical during the initial procedures and can be made smaller with additional experience. The incision length itself is qualitatively based first on the minimum necessary surgical access to implement a procedure with a good visualization and working comfort. The right minithoracotomy is made such that the medial angle (end) of incision is positioned approximately at 4–6 cm from the sternal edge. We started our experience with a more anterior incision and then gradually switched to the more lateral, submammary crease incision in almost all patients, which gives better visualization of the field and perfect valve exposure.

In our department, we practice a single-access minithoracotomy approach; all the routines of CPB, perfusion, and manipulations are implemented through the minithoracotomy incision. Once the minithoracotomy is made, two auxiliary working ports are placed through the right chest wall. Each working port is provided with trocar that facilitates a port insertion through a stab skin incision, as demonstrated in Fig. 40.4.

One 5.5-mm working port is used for video-assistance and stay sutures. The port is placed in the same intercostal space with the minithoracotomy incision but at a lower level by the anterior axillary line. Another 10.5-mm port is placed in the fifth to seventh intercostal space at the midaxillary line. These ports are used for the cardiotomy vent, CO_2 insufflation, and exteriorization of pericardial stay sutures. The soft tissue retractor and metallic multiuse retractors allow optimal exposure through the small incision [57].

An example of the metallic retractor is shown in Fig. 40.5.

Video-assistance gives excellent visualization and illumination of the surgical field and can serve as an important tool for assisting the surgeon and anesthetist [35, 37]. Our experiences say that the port-access allows first operators to see and work with the MV directly, without any difficulties, making the video-assistance not essential in these cases. However, when it comes to cases with a "difficult" angle of view and poor visualization, the video-assistance may be the only way to expose the valve and perform the procedure, especially when the subvalvular apparatus is to be dealt with.

The pericardial fat is mobilized and removed as necessary. The pericardium is opened up and down from the diaphragm to the ascending aorta, keeping the incision approximately 3–4 cm above the phrenic nerve. When the pericardium is opened, 2–0 silk stay sutures are placed (usually two sutures for each pericardial margin) as needed. Additional stay sutures may be sutured to the inner thoracic wall or wound margins. If the heart appears to be bulky and the right atrial appendage is likely to impede visualization of the cannulation site, the initial pericardial incision may be limited mainly to the aortic cannulation site. Then, the pericardium is opened completely, and the stay sutures are exteriorized via the chest wall. Small hooks (crochet) or dedicated tools may be very helpful with pulling the stay sutures outside through the working ports. The long port-access forceps may be also used, by grabbing the tip of the stay suture to exteriorize the sutures through the working ports.

Under direct visualization, the aorta is exposed until the origin of the innominate artery after which two concentric 2–0 polyester purse-string sutures for direct arterial cannulation are placed in a standard fashion into the ascending aorta as schematically shown on Fig. 40.6. During the purse-string suture placement, the aorta can be kept steady using locking forceps to reduce the physiological motion.

The cannulation site is generally chosen according to the following consideration: operator should identify the transverse sinus as the orientation where the aortic cross-clamp will be

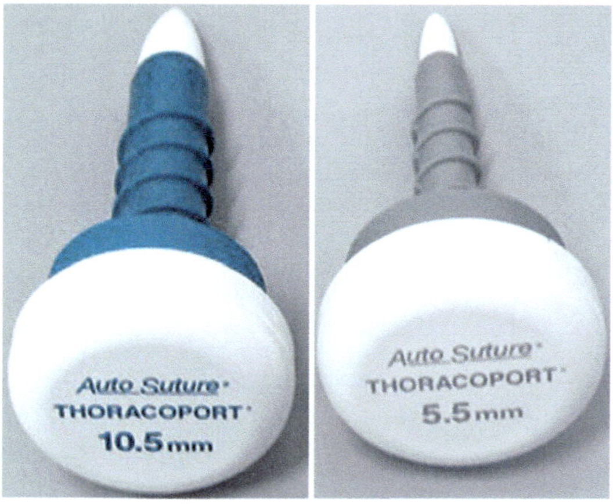

Fig. 40.4 A 10.5-and a 5.5-mm single-use thoracic working port with trocars

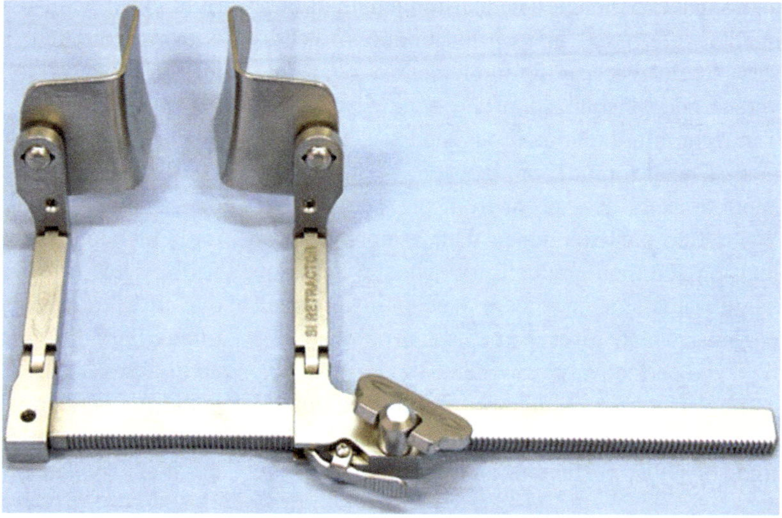

Fig. 40.5 Metallic multiuse retractor for minithoracotomy incision (Estech, San Ramon, CA, USA)

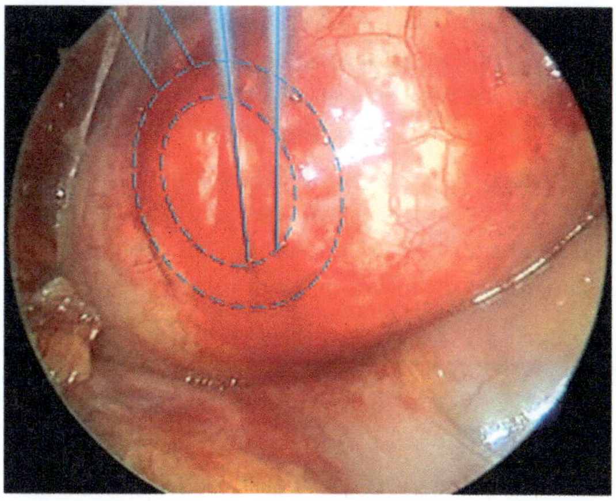

Fig. 40.6 Videoscopic view of two purse-string sutures laterally placed on ascending aorta in a standard concentric fashion

placed. It is sufficient if the cannulation site stays at some distance above the cross-clamp level. The purse-strings may be reinforced with pledgets if needed. Some surgeons prefer using pledgets (usually one is enough) placed on the outer suture only. Purse-string sutures are left long enough to be managed easily and exteriorized outside the chest wall via minithoracotomy incision. We do not recommend exteriorizing the purse-string sutures through small working ports; it may be difficult to pull or tie the sutures immediately when needed, if the tourniquets are to be released from the ports.

The operative field may be exposed poorly in patients with a high diaphragmatic dome: in these cases, a thick silk stay suture can be placed on the central tendon of the diaphragm and pulled out of the thorax through the lower working port. This stitch should not be released, but be tied tightly at the end of the operation, in order to close any oozing diaphragmatic vessels injured by a needle tip during the stitch placement.

40.4.2 Venous Cannulation

Once the purse-strings on the ascending aorta are ready, preparation of the groin is started. Most venous cannula sets presently available on the market include a low-profile cannula, guidewire, and a range of introducers (venous dilators). Generally, the femoral vein should be punctured 6–8 cm below the inguinal ligament line using the Seldinger technique: this permits a straighter introduction of the venous cannula into the right femoral vein and prevents guidewire kinking during the cannula insertion. The guidewire is placed through the venous introducer sheath and is advanced to the right atrium under visualization with the TEE probe adjusted to a bicaval view (~90–120°). In this particular view, the superior vena cava is on the right and inferior vena cava on your left as you view them; at the top of the screen near the probe is the left atrium. With the guidewire held in place, the introducer sheath is removed. The puncture site is then enlarged with a #11 blade on the skin, and successively larger dilators are inserted over the guidewire to enlarge the percutaneous tunnel and facilitate easy advancement of the venous cannula. The venous return cannula is then advanced into the femoral vein and positioned so that the tip of a double-stage cannula is above the cavoatrial junction in the superior vena cava. The guidewire is slowly withdrawn while holding the cannula in place. The venous cannula is then de-aired by partially unclamping and expelling blood and any residual air from the lumen before connecting to the venous line of the CPB circuit. One silk stay suture is placed on the skin as a tourniquet over the cannula body to fix it in place and prevent dislodgement. This tourniquet may be easily released and refixed if we need to adjust (push or pull) the cannula during the procedure.

The venous cannula can also be inserted using an open technique as shown in Fig. 40.7. The femoral vein and artery are isolated according to standard technique. One 5–0 polypropylene purse-string suture is placed on the femoral vein. The vein is punctured with an introducer needle through the purse-string, and a guidewire is advanced into the right atrium after the introducer is removed. The venous cannula is directly introduced over the guidewire, similarly to the percutaneous technique as described above in the text.

The choice of the venous cannula is based on the patient's weight and the surgeon's personal preferences; in our institution, we employ a range of 22–25 Fr for the venous cannulae in almost all patients, with a 21 Fr cannula used in the smallest adult patients. Different manufacturers present various product features; all of them have their advantages and disadvantages regarding the device characteristics (low-profile body, available size range, included supplemental material, and pricing). Some typical venous cannulae that can be used are: 22 and 25 Fr QuickDraw® venous cannulae (Edwards Lifesciences, Irvine, CA, USA); 19, 21, and 25 Fr Bio-Medicus® multistage venous cannulae (Medtronic, Minneapolis, MN, USA); RAP (remote access perfusion) double-stage 22–22 Fr and 23–25 Fr venous cannulae (Estech, San Ramon, CA, USA). Venous cannulation options may include an additional right jugular vein cannulation kit which is placed by the anesthesiologist before the operation if it is considered necessary. In our early experience, this was mostly necessary when concomitant tricuspid valve surgery was scheduled. Modern double-stage low-profile venous cannulae can maintain the venous return without any compromise and are more than sufficient in size for appropriate CPB [39]; therefore, jugular vein cannulation was completely abandoned in our department, even in double mitral-tricuspid operations.

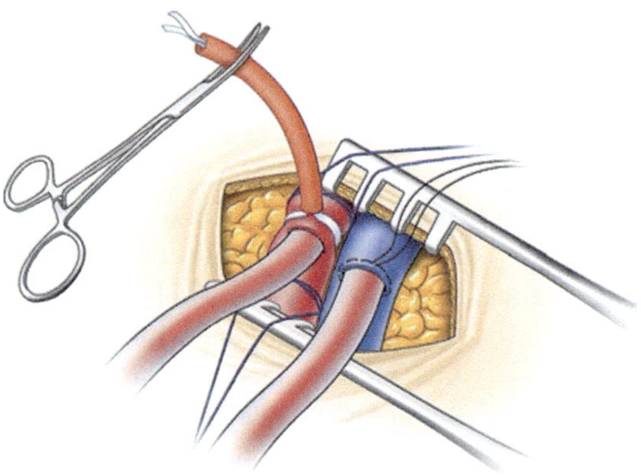

Fig. 40.7 An open femoro-femoral cannulation. After isolation of both artery and vein, the cannulae are inserted. The arterial cannula position is secured by snaring a tourniquet

40.4.3 Aortic Cannulation

The direct cannulation of the ascending aorta is accomplished under direct vision using one of the available aortic cannulae. The Direct Arterial Cannula (Edwards Lifesciences, Irvine, CA, USA) is a port-access cannula with the AutoIncisor Introducer, which aids aortic cannula insertion as shown in Fig. 40.8. Central aortic cannulation can provide superior myocardial protection [69] and eliminates the potential issues of obstructive peripheral disease, small femoral vessel size (especially in women), groin-related complications, limb ischemia, and femoral artery injury [20].

The Direct Arterial Cannula handle contains a plunger that advances the blade and provides

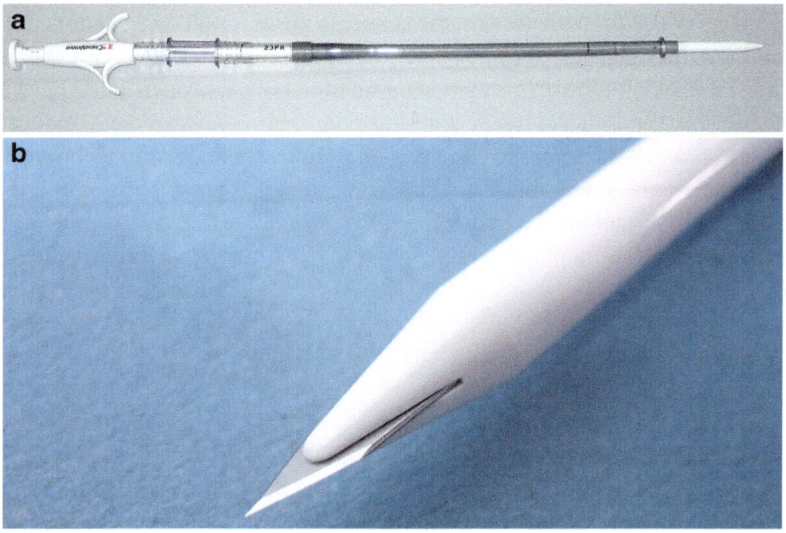

Fig. 40.8 The Direct Arterial Cannula (Edwards Lifesciences, Irvine, CA, USA) is shown (**a**). A spring-loaded tip-mounted blade (**b**) is used to make an incision in the aorta, and the tapered tip allows for easy and nearly bloodless introduction of the aortic cannula into the vessel lumen

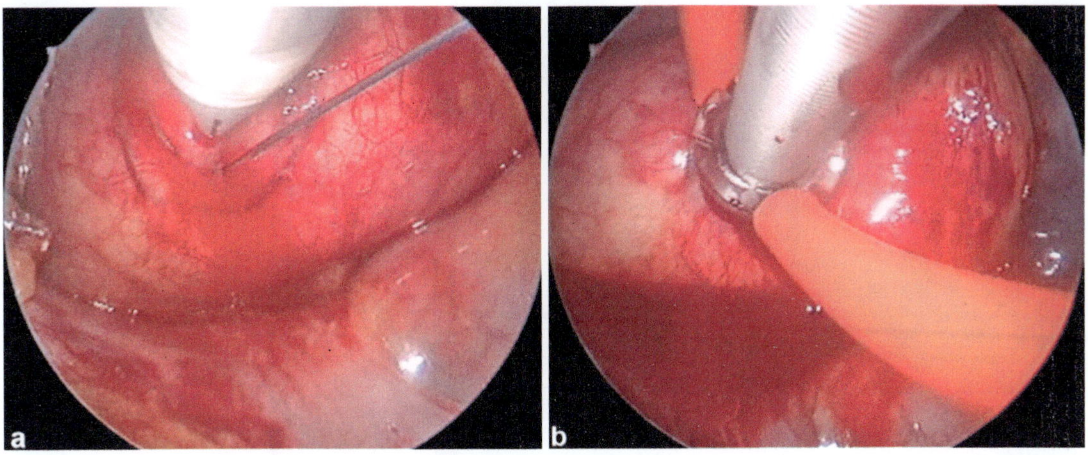

Fig. 40.9 Direct ascending aorta cannulation. The cannula tip is placed in the center of a concentric purse-string (**a**). The plunger is pressed, and the cannula tip is advanced into the aortic wall and secured with two tourniquets in a conventional manner (**b**)

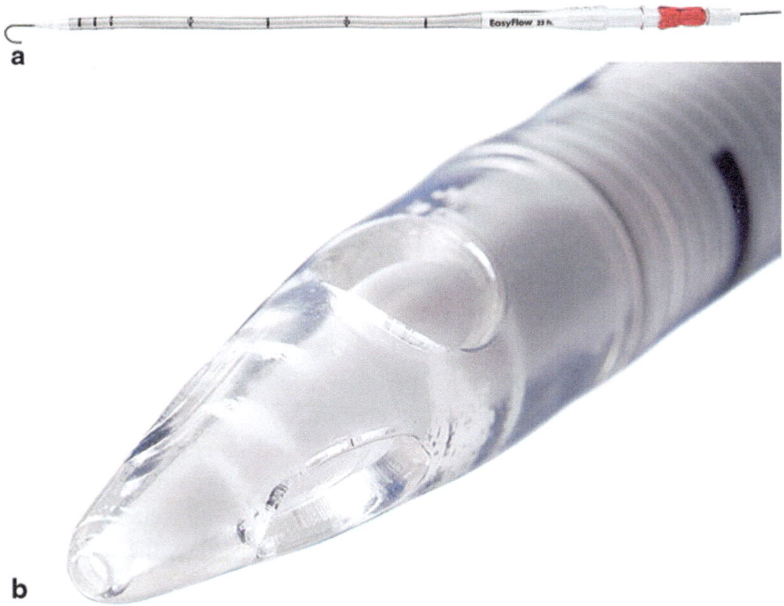

Fig. 40.10 The EasyFlow® Aortic cannula (Estech, San Ramon, CA, USA) is shown (**a**). The cannula is provided with an obturator (**b**) designed to facilitate insertion of the tip

feedback (a "click") indicating the automatic retraction of the blade after plunger advancement. This feedback and automatic retraction are important in that if the cannula plunger is advanced further into the aorta after puncture, puncturing of the posterior aortic wall may occur, leading to the aortic dissection and its associated complications. The videoscopic view of aortic cannula insertion is demonstrated in Fig. 40.9. In our opinion, in patients with a small ascending aorta, the Direct Arterial Cannula application should be avoided.

Another type of aortic cannula that can be used is the EasyFlow® (Estech, San Ramon, CA, USA). The principal difference between this cannula and the one described above is the absence of the AutoIncisor mechanism. This cannula has an advanced tip and obturator designed to allow easier aortic insertion with superior flexibility within the thorax as presented in Fig. 40.10. The EasyFlow® cannula tip has to be secured with a cannula ring (which is not prefixed by the manufacturer) as shown in Fig. 40.11. We always place

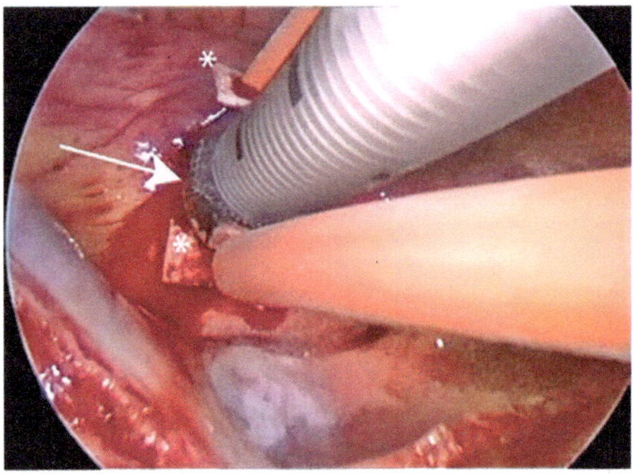

Fig. 40.11 Aortic cannulation. *White arrow* shows where the black silk suture is placed to fix the cannula ring at the desired level. Two Teflon pledgets are shown by *asterisks*

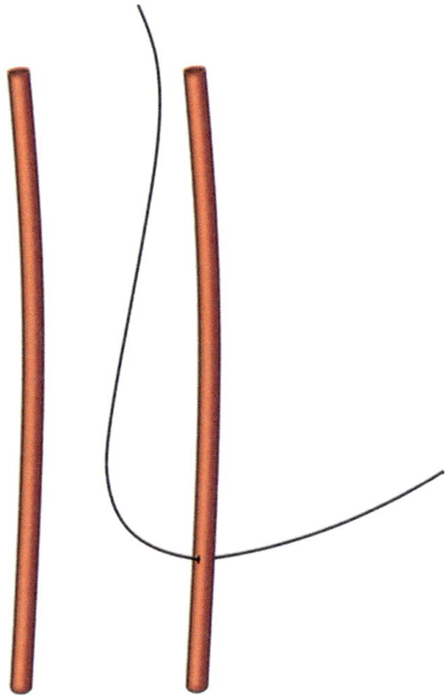

Fig. 40.12 A silk suture is pre-placed through a standard rubber tourniquet before its insertion into the chest to facilitate fastening the aortic cannula inside the chest

silk suture reinforcement in order to prevent ring dislocation after the cannula tip enters the aortic wall. This can be important to remember, because it is not always possible to control how far the cannula tip enters the aortic wall, and the only orientation available is defined by the cannula ring. After experiencing aortic dissection in one patient due to posterior wall puncture with the cannula tip, we always use silk suture reinforcement of the cannula ring and have not experienced this complication since.

The lungs must be deflated prior to aortic cannulation, and the right lung must be off if a left-sided double-lumen endotracheal intubation was performed. When the aortic cannula is advanced into the aorta, excessive tension on the purse-string sutures must be avoided during insertion. After deployment and while the assistant surgeon holds the cannula, the first operator must secure the cannula with two tourniquets using a silk suture. This can be difficult in cases of a deep chest and distant cannulation sites. In these cases, a silk suture pre-placed previously through one of the tourniquets can facilitate knotting inside the chest. The schematic rendering of these standard tourniquets is displayed in Fig. 40.12. Tourniquets themselves are secured with a stitch on the skin margin in order to avoid any possible dislocation and to gain maximum working space. The cannula is de-aired and connected to the CPB arterial line.

Arterial cannulation via an open technique consists of femoral artery preparation through a small transverse or oblique incision in the groin as previously shown in Fig. 40.7. When both femoral arterial and venous cannulation are used, a transverse 3–4-cm incision along the inguinal fold over the pulsating femoral artery projection is made to expose the vessels [57]. Both artery and vein are encircled with two Silastic sutures distally and proximally, and generally the right femoral artery and vein are cannulated in an open technique. Also, the artery is surrounded with an umbilical tape proximally. The umbilical tape is enclosed into a tourniquet. When heparin is administered, the arteriotomy is made, and the femoral artery cannula is inserted into the vessel. The cannula is then secured over the vessel with a tourniquet and connected to the CPB arterial line.

The aortic cannula size usually depends on the patients' weight, and the type is the surgeon's choice. For patients with a weight below 80 kg, we prefer a 21 Fr-size cannula, and 23 Fr for those of ≥90 kg, respectively. The EasyFlow® (Estech, San Ramon, CA, USA) and the Direct Arterial Cannula (Edwards Lifesciences, Irvine, CA, USA) are available in 23 Fr size.

40.4.4 Procedure

After initiation of the CPB, venous drainage is achieved with vacuum assistance of approximately −40 mmHg. We usually can regulate the venous flow by using negative pressures up to −70 to −80 mmHg to maintain desired flows. Also, after the CPB is established, a combined Y-shape cardioplegia/aortic vent catheter is placed into the ascending aorta, and cardioplegia lines are connected in the usual manner. The surgery proceeds from this point following the typical stages of a conventional valvular procedure. The aorta is directly clamped with a flexible cross-clamp as demonstrated in Fig. 40.13. Currently, several options are available for aortic cross-clamping. An external Cosgrove flexible or a Chitwood clamp can be used [34]. In our institution, we apply two kinds of external clamps. One is a flexible Cygnet® clamp (Novare Surgical Systems Inc, Cupertino, CA, USA) as shown in Fig. 40.14.

The suction tip is relatively safe and could be very helpful for manipulating the aorta during the cross-clamp application, as demonstrated in Fig. 40.15. The surgeon can slightly elevate the aorta by pushing it with suction tip in a contralateral direction, to provide better visualization of the clamping area. The rigid shaft of this clamp enables tunneling and accurate placement of the clamping jaws. Once properly placed on the aorta, the rigid shaft retracts leaving a flexible neck on the cross-clamp as presented in Fig. 40.16. Another clamping instrument recently

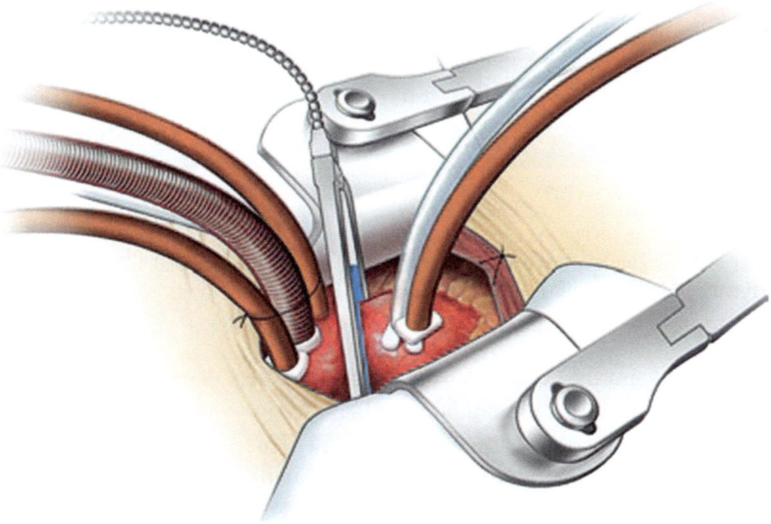

Fig. 40.13 Aortic cross-clamping; for a better control, the straight limb of the device is placed under the ascending aorta in the transverse pericardial sinus

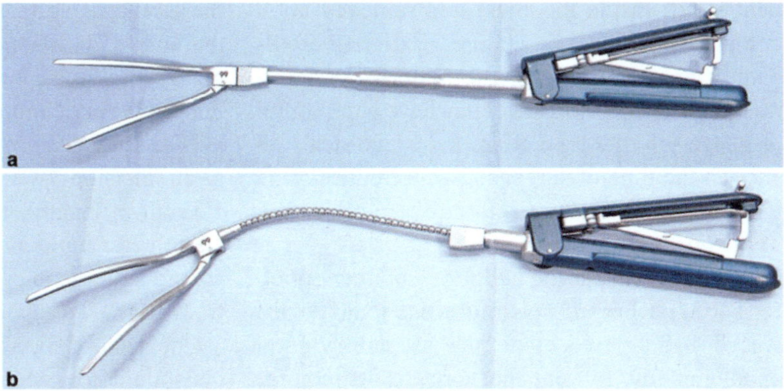

Fig. 40.14 The Cygnet® clamp (Novare Surgical Systems Inc, Cupertino, CA, USA). Options for a straight (rigid) shaft (**a**) and a flexible shaft (**b**) are shown

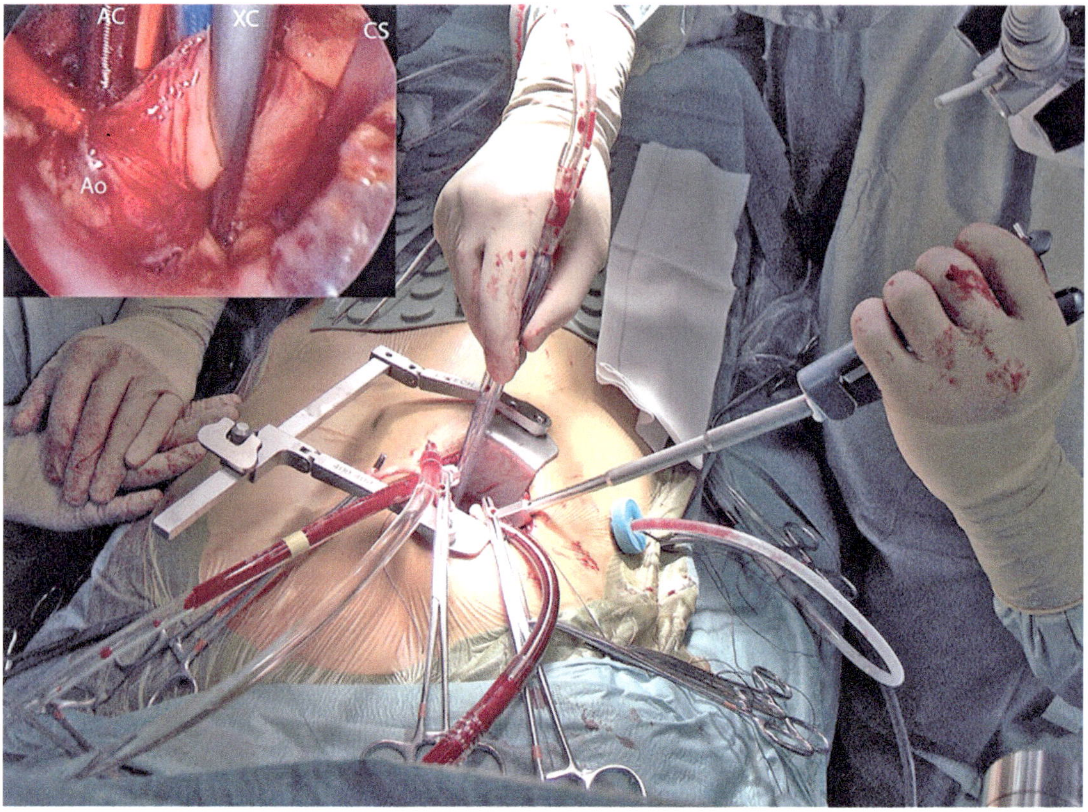

Fig. 40.15 Aortic cross-clamping: placing the cardiotomy suction tip (*CS*) at the level of the transverse pericardial sinus can be very useful for lifting the aorta (*Ao*) slightly, thus facilitating the visualization of the area available for aortic cross-clamping (*XC*) (straight limb of the cross-clamping device is partially visualized); *AC* aortic cannula

introduced is the CardioVision® MIC-Aortic Clamp [70], (Cardiomedical GmbH, Langenhagen, Germany) as is seen in Fig. 40.17. This cross-clamping instrument is provided with completely detachable clamping jaws. This clamp is mounted on a delivery shaft and applied to the aorta with the jaws; the clamping component is left inside the chest and removed upon completion of the procedure. External cross-clamps are applicable in the majority of minimally invasive operations. They have a minimum presence on the operative field and tend to shorten the time of surgery [24], to reduce costs and perioperative complications by simplification of the operative procedure [34].

Use of an endoaortic balloon is another option for aortic occlusion. This multifunctional device was designed to occlude the ascending aorta endoluminally, to vent the aortic root, monitor aortic root pressure and deliver cardioplegia solution to the coronary ostia. A schematic illustration of the EndoClamp Aortic Catheter (Edwards Lifesciences, Irvine, CA, USA) is presented in Fig. 40.18. Contraindications for the use of the EndoClamp may consist of more than mild aortic regurgitation, patent coronary grafts attached to the ascending aorta, and extensive calcification of the aorta [71]. A small femoral artery size (less than 21 Fr) may be a contraindication [20] for femoral artery cannulation as well.

The EndoClamp used for insertion through a groin incision is a 10.5 Fr wirebond (65 and 100 cm in length), three-lumen catheter with an elastomeric balloon on its tip for occluding the ascending aorta in order to separate the aortic root from arterial circulation. This balloon can occlude a wide range of aorta diameters, usually 30–35 mm, but should not exceed 40-mm limit. This balloon

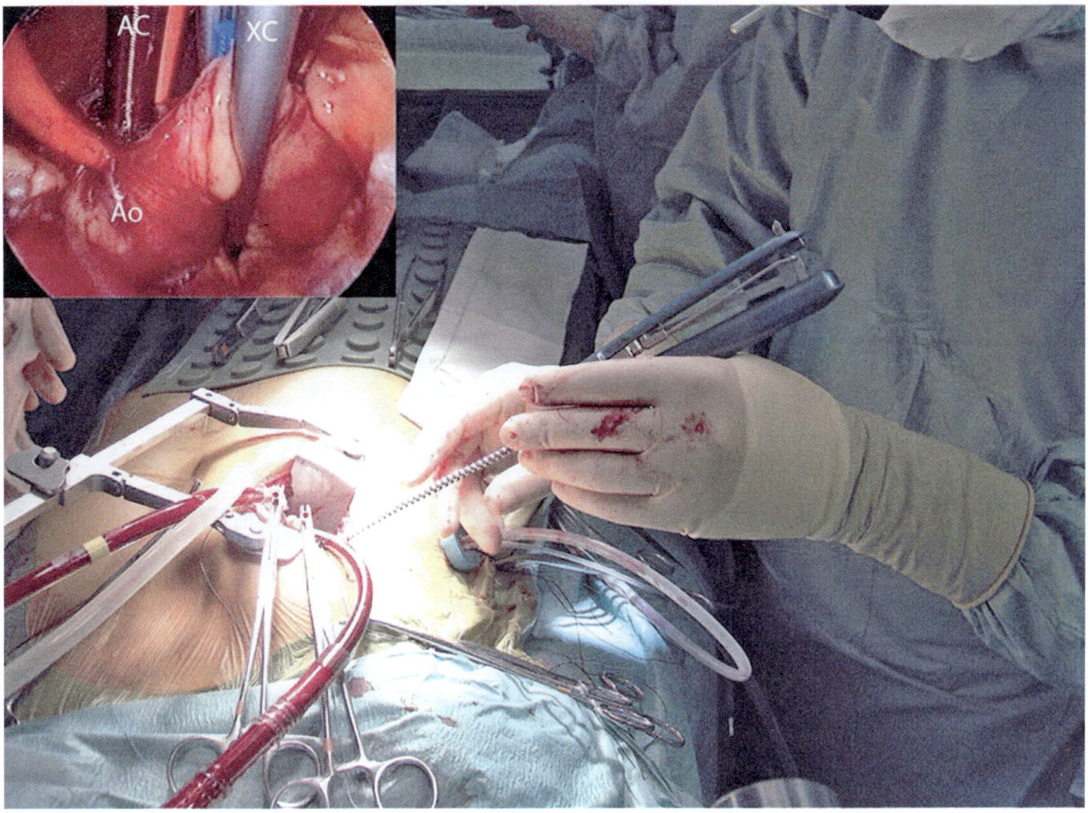

Fig. 40.16 Aortic cross-clamping: when clamp shaft is open and becomes flexible, it can be exteriorized from thoracotomy remote from the surgeon's working field; *AC* aortic cannula, *XC* cross-clamp, *Ao* aorta

is inserted from the open femoral artery access site through the EndoReturn Arterial Cannula (21 or 23 Fr) (Edwards Lifesciences, Irvine, CA, USA) and advanced into the ascending aorta under echo guidance, ensuring that the balloon is correctly placed in the aorta under the origin of the brachiocephalic artery. Under TEE control, the balloon is rapidly inflated to create an occlusive seal (as a rough guide, 1 ml of sterile saline per 1 mm of aortic size is required for inflation; total inflation volume is 20–35 ml). The gradient created between the aortic root and mean arterial pressure is an indicator of a complete aortic occlusion. The stability of EndoClamp catheter is ensured by tightening the rotating hemostatic valve of the EndoReturn cannula. When balloon inflation is complete with total occlusion accomplished, the cardioplegia solution is gradually infused. Currently, we use the EndoClamp Catheter mostly in redo operations, when direct aortic cross-clamping may be more cumbersome to accomplish.

Mitral procedures and/or concomitant tricuspid repair can also be performed [72] without aortic cross-clamping under cold fibrillatory arrest [41, 73–75]. The key principle for myocardial protection is to keep the heart completely decompressed by opening the left atrium immediately upon fibrillation to prevent the left ventricle from distending [73]. Since coronary perfusion is dependent on oxygenated blood flow against intact aortic valve, the method is contraindicated with incompetent aortic valve.

The cardioplegia in all types of cross-clamping is initially delivered as a single bolus (20 ml/kg) of cold crystalloid solution (Custodiol), (Dr.Franz Köhler Chemie GmbH, Alsbach-Hähnlein, Germany) antegrade into the aortic root which provides the optimal myocardial protection throughout the procedure [76, 77]. Cardioplegia administration is controlled under TEE. The patient is cooled, and the temperature is maintained in mild hypothermia at 34 °C. If a multidose

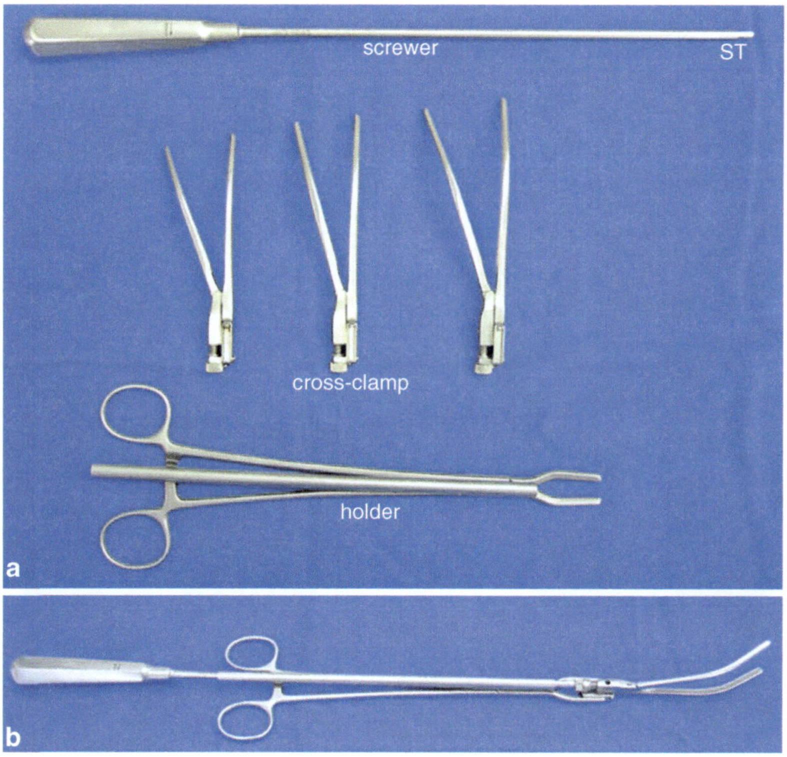

Fig. 40.17 The CardioVision® MIC-Aortic Clamp (Cardiomedical GmbH, Langenhagen, Germany) consists of a holder, screwer, and a variety of detachable clamping limbs (**a**). The completely assembled aortic clamping device (**b**)

cardioplegia administration is chosen, it should be considered that with the minimally invasive approach, the ventricles stay in contact with surrounding structures and may have a tendency to rewarm faster after cooling [13] which may require more frequent cardioplegia administration.

Carbon dioxide (CO_2) flow used to fill the pleural cavity and reduce the volume of retained intracardiac gas usually is run at 0.5–1 l/min and, however, can be maintained at higher levels [78, 79]. As mentioned earlier, the 10.5-mm port placed in the fifth to seventh intercostal space at the midaxillary line is used for CO_2 gas insufflation and afterward also for cardiotomy suction. Because of its high solubility in blood, any residual carbon dioxide gas in the left side of the heart is easily absorbed, thereby minimizing the risk of air embolism [10, 39].

During the procedure, the surgeon has a choice between direct and indirect video-assisted visualization. Total endoscopic repair is also feasible [80] and performed through a smaller (4-cm) incision with the rest of technique similar to the direct or video-assisted approach [23]. In all approaches, proper pericardial retraction gives a perfect view of the operative field and must not be underestimated.

When myocardial standstill is established, dissection of the Sondergaard's plane is made near the interatrial groove. A special atrial retractor and obtainable MV exposure are illustrated in Fig. 40.19. The surgeon should size the atrial retractor blade to properly elevate the intra-atrial septum anteriorly and slightly to the patients left in order to expose the anterior mitral annulus [36]. A stab incision is made over the right sternal margin, and the retractor handle is bluntly passed though skin, between the sternal edge and the right internal mammary artery, and then screwed to the blade which is manually introduced into the chest. The blade is elevated by pulling the handle from outside of the chest and

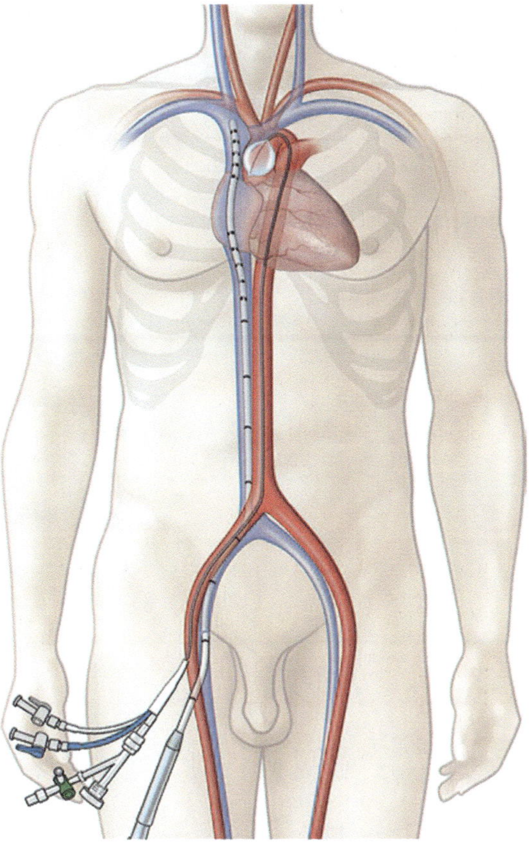

Fig. 40.18 Place of insertion and positioning of the EndoClamp endoaortic Catheter. The balloon tip is recognizable inside the ascending aorta

locked at the desired level. Other types of the atrial retractors may be used as an alternative in selected cases [81]. Special instruments developed for a minimally invasive surgery are employed throughout the operation as presented in Figs. 40.20 and 40.21.

When the MV is exposed, the type of repair is decided based on direct visualization of the valve. For the valve replacement, the procedure is accomplished in a standard manner. If annuloplasty is indicated, the surgeon can place initial sutures (2–0 polyester braided sutures) on the mitral valve annulus. The valve is then inspected again with hooks and a water probe as needed. The mitral annulus size is determined using dedicated ring sizer, and sutures are passed through the mitral ring, knotted with a knot pusher and excised [36]. A water probe is applied again to confirm valve competence with lowered open mitral ring. A video-assisted view of an annuloplasty using the C-G Future Band Mitral Annuloplasty Ring (Medtronic, Minneapolis, MN, USA) is shown in Fig. 40.22.

During MV repair, air may be entrained into the left atrium, ventricle, and aorta; after the completion of the procedure, the left ventricular vent is positioned across the MV, and the left atrial incision is closed. The remaining residual air is aspirated by aortic root and ventricular vents and by inflation of the lungs to clear the pulmonary veins of air [36, 61]. The heart is then filled with blood by reducing venous drainage. The patient may be also placed in the Trendelenburg position during this maneuver. Once the intracardiac air removal is confirmed by TEE, ventricular and aortic vents are removed and the left atriotomy closure is finalized. Finally, the cross-clamp is fully released, and the patient is cardioverted if needed. After rewarming and appropriate reperfusion, the patient is weaned from CPB, and the venous cannula is removed after reversal of heparinization with protamine. After the percutaneous venous cannula is withdrawn, the femoral vein access site is temporarily (10–15 min) placed under compression to secure hemostasis [20]; and the cannula insertion site (stab incision) is closed with a single mattress stitch.

If the open femoro-femoral cannulation was performed through a groin incision, the venous cannula is removed, the purse-string is tightened, and hemostasis is secured. Aortic cannula is subsequently removed, and the arterial wall is reconstructed in a standard fashion.

If direct aortic cannulation was used, the two tourniquets can be removed simultaneously and tied after the cannula is removed. If the purse-strings are extremely distant from the minithoracotomy incision making access to the sutures challenging, the inner purse-string tourniquet can be removed first by a first operator and made ready for a first knot. The second tourniquet is released by the assistant surgeon, making it ready to be closed immediately after the cannula removal.

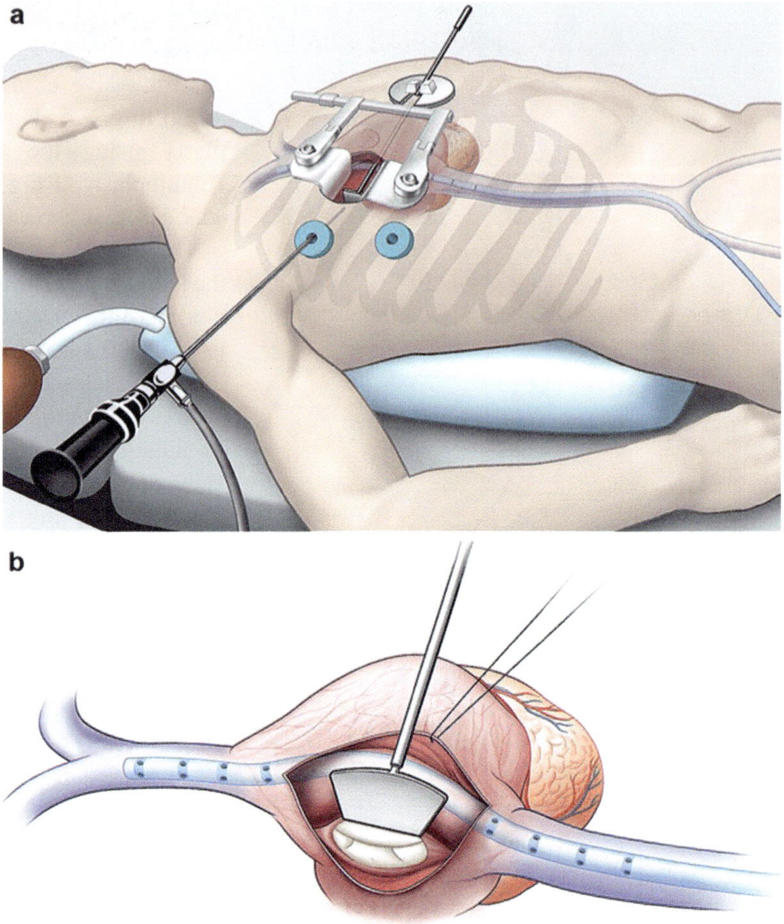

Fig. 40.19 The site of atrial retractor placement. (**a**) The tip of the videoscope is directed toward the area of interest (mitral valve), and the MV is exposed; (**b**) the flexibility of a double-stage venous cannula enables its adaptation to the anatomy and shape of the surrounding structures with no alteration to the venous return during the atrial retraction

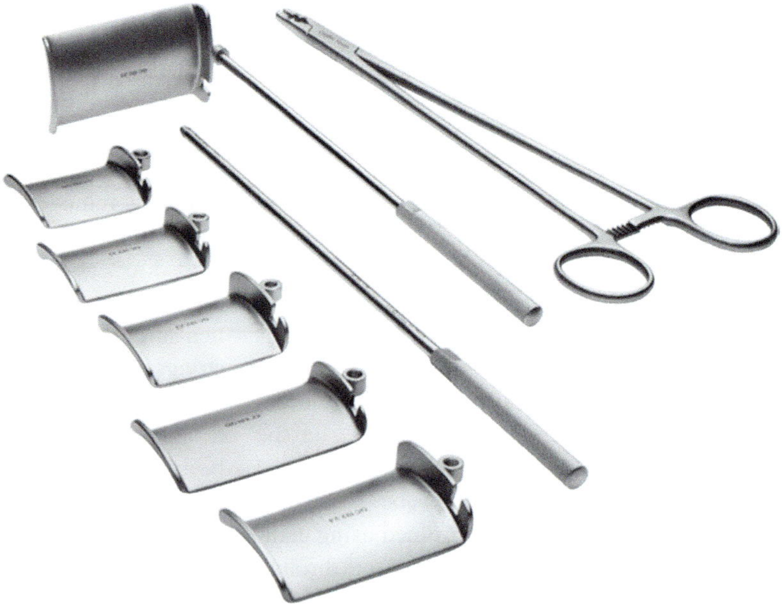

Fig. 40.20 Typical minimally invasive surgery kit with atrial retractors (Cardiomedical GmbH, Langenhagen, Germany)

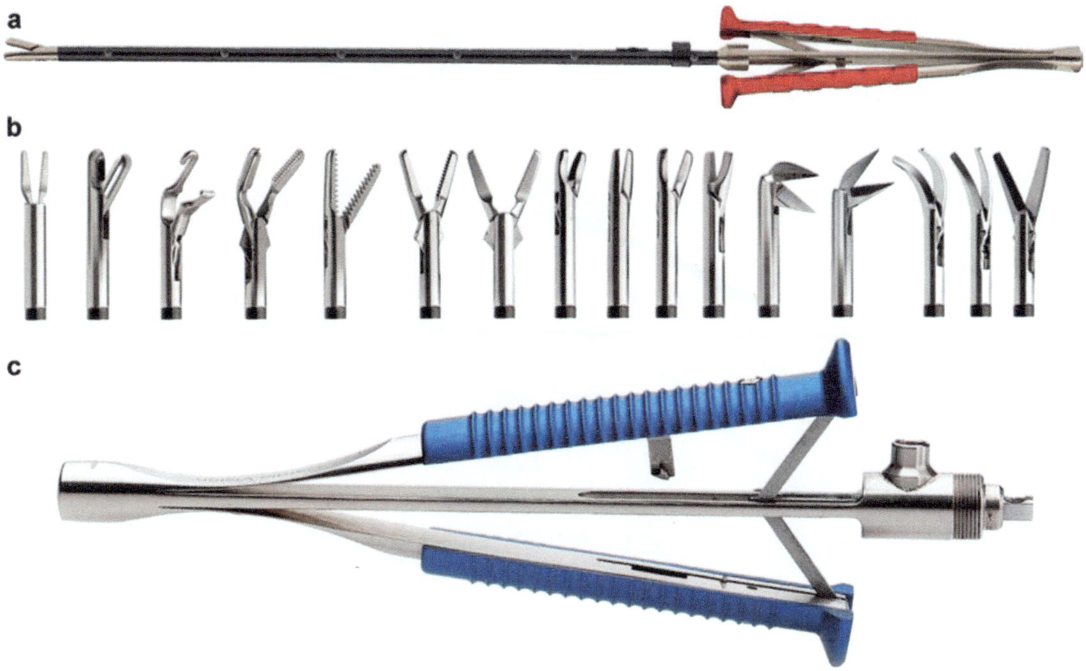

Fig. 40.21 Typical instrumentation used for the minimally invasive procedures, a complete needle holder (**a**), range of end-effectors (**b**), and a bi-leaf instrument handle assembly (**c**)

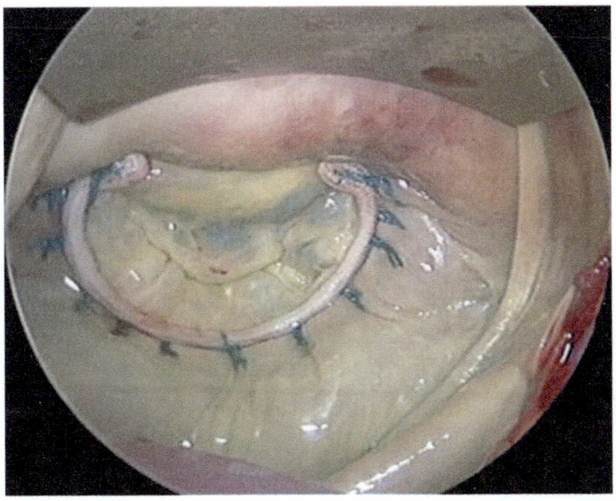

Fig. 40.22 A mitral valve exposure as seen on video-assistance monitor. The annuloplasty ring is sutured, and the valve is checked for the quality of the repair in a standard manner

When the cannula is then removed from the aorta by the first operator, he ties the first purse-string and then switches to the second purse-string. The second tourniquet is then removed, and the purse-string suture is tightened in the same manner. Any possible sutures interference should be avoided at this stage. A hand tightening of the sutures is preferred to a knot-pusher suture lowering technique when it comes to aortic sutures. The cannula insertion site is meticulously controlled for bleeding and secured with sutures reinforced with pledgets if necessary.

In the majority of cases postoperatively, the bleeding comes from the chest wall, thus careful hemostasis is crucial and must be checked before chest closure; videoscope and a dental mirror may be useful tools for this purpose [58]. When the hemostasis is secured, two 28 Fr chest Blake® silicone drains (Ethicon, Sommerville, NJ, USA) are placed through the 5.5-mm and 10.5-mm ports into the pericardium and right pleural space as rendered in Fig. 40.23. The pericardium is closed with 2–3 single sutures. Temporary atrial pacing wires are usually not placed unless the patient is especially vulnerable to rhythm disturbances. The ribs can be approximated by placing 1 or 2 nonabsorbable braided (0 or 1 Ethibond)

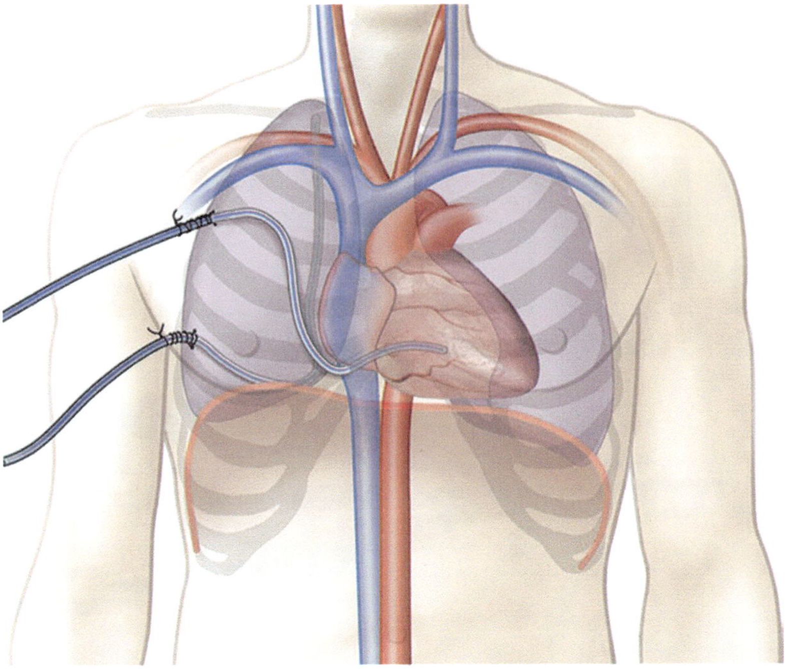

Fig. 40.23 Two Blake® pericardial silicone drains (Ethicon, Somerville, NJ, USA) are placed into the right pleural cavity (through a lower working port) and into the pericardium (upper working port)

sutures, (Ethicon, Somerville, NJ, USA) and pulled together to restore their position prior to minithoracotomy retraction. The minithoracotomy incision is then closed in anatomical layers. Skin is approximated in a traditional manner with intradermic absorbable sutures according to the operative protocol.

Standard postoperative care is provided, and most patients are usually extubated in intensive care unit and transferred to the ward on a postoperative day 1. Patients usually have less discomfort and fewer postoperative complications [32, 64] than with conventional MV surgeries and thus get back to a normal activity soon. Postoperative follow-up is managed according to the hospital protocol, with the goal of speeding up hospital discharge [35].

40.5 Reoperative Surgery

Reoperative sternal splitting is primarily a blind procedure and carries high risk for damage to the underlying structures [82]. With increasing number of patients being referred for reoperative surgery, minimally invasive approaches are increasingly being considered for this patient population as well [83]. The approach has been explored by several different groups [51, 52, 75, 84, 85] as an alternative to a conventional median sternotomy reoperation [86, 87] to minimize dissection of tissue adhesions and reduce bleeding [53, 82, 88].

The reoperative surgical technique is generally similar to that used in the primary minimally invasive operations described above. In redo cases, double-lumen intubation is extremely helpful for effective tissues dissection [85], and preference is given to peripheral (femoro-femoral) cannulation, though direct aortic cannulation is possible in selected cases [89]. The aortic cross-clamping can be safely accomplished using either the endoaortic balloon [86] or via direct (external) clamping [90, 91]. The central aortic cannulation and cross-clamping usually require extra dissection around the aorta [52]. The choices for the type of cardioplegia and the need for vacuum-assisted venous drainage for CPB are not altered in reoperative MV surgery [90]. Fibrillatory arrest is used when there is a patent mammary artery [52, 53]. In reoperative surgery, effective de-airing should be accomplished with care as adhesions may tilt the left ventricular apex above the outflow tract in the supine position, thus favoring air entrapment [82].

Visualization is performed using direct or video-assisted methods [84], and the surgical exposure of the MV does not compromise access for all cases [82, 91] allowing the performance of all types of complex procedure without additional risk [83, 85, 88].

The outcomes of reoperative surgery via minithoracotomy are comparable with those over the conventional approach in terms of less bleeding, lower need for transfusion, low rate of wound infection, short intensive care unit and hospital stays, and reduced use of hospital resources [82, 89, 91, 92].

40.6 Summary

Minimally invasive cardiac surgery represents a significant change in the way cardiac surgeons treat their patients today. The described surgical techniques via right minithoracotomy in the third and fourth intercostal space and application of custom-designed armamentarium of surgical tools and aides provide excellent MV exposure and working field and can be performed with low perioperative complication rates and good durability [31]. This approach permits treatment of patients with less invasiveness; yields better cosmetic results, improved comfort, and less postoperative pain; and provides a faster overall rehabilitation and shorter hospital stay [16, 18, 39, 48]. All known types of surgical correction for MV disease and concomitant procedures (valve repair, replacement, neochordae placement, valve leaflet resection, reductive annuloplasty, patch repair, myectomy, etc.) are feasible through a single-access minithoracotomy approach. The kind of repair technique and replacement options depends on assessment of the valve dysfunction, the surgeons' personal preferences, and the patient's choice, as during any conventional valvular operation.

The MV repair or replacement via right minithoracotomy has already become a routine procedure in many experienced centers [14, 17, 18, 26, 41–46]. Since port-access surgery was adopted as a treatment of choice, various technical details of this approach underwent multiple improvements [93] in order to further reduce the complication rate and simplify the procedure. These include (1) preferred use of the direct aortic cannulation with percutaneous venous return cannula insertion over the femoro-femoral cannulation via open access in the groin [56] in order to reduce the risk of vascular complications and stroke [94], (2) replacing the endoaortic clamp with direct cross-clamping techniques which makes the procedure less complicated [30] and reduces the procedure costs [24], and (3) the placement of a coronary sinus catheter for retrograde cardioplegia in experienced centers [63], with the alternative (less complex) cardioplegia administration methods retained in others due to the significant learning curve, unpredictable coronary anatomy, and potential sinus injury [30] which is the most feared complication of endovascular insertion of these catheter [63].

The minimally invasive approach brings new challenges to the surgeon as well as the anesthesiologist. Proper anesthesia preparation is crucial to obtaining better exposure enabling the performance of complex procedures [95]. Double-lumen intubation controlled by bronchoscope, selective one-lung ventilation, and placement of endovascular CPB devices and specialized catheters [63] under TEE guidance [67, 96] are a few of the many skills required from the anesthesiologist for the minimally invasive surgery team [95]. The TEE is essential in minimally invasive valve surgery, to detect problems that require immediate remedy [67]. Probe placement allows real-time assessment of MV and cardiac function, ventricular filling, and intracardiac air. TEE guidance is necessary for percutaneous venous cannulation, placement of an endoaortic occlusion balloon, as well as confirmation of valvular pathology and the efficacy of the repair or replacement MV surgical procedure [96].

While the right minithoracotomy approach has become somewhat standardized and reproducible and is preferred by more surgeons, surgeons today have an armamentarium of possibility devices and instruments to select from to make individual modifications to the surgical techniques upon their own preferences.

Minimally invasive MV surgery approaches has been further developed into a reliable technique for reoperative cases as well as for concomitant involving other valves and/or the treatment of atrial fibrillation [59]. The use of minimally invasive techniques has also been extended for the elderly population [97], even those with moderately elevated perioperative risk [60]. The approach appears to be feasible and easily reproducible with outcomes comparable to standard approaches in terms of morbidity and mortality and has a potential for significant reductions in resource usage [8, 16, 89].

The purpose of minimally invasive surgery is to provide the morbidity and mortality rates of open cardiac surgical procedures with the advantages of decreased pain, morbidity, and recovery time [11]; however, these advantages are realized after a significant learning curve [98] for the whole surgical team [39].

In our institution, we are currently performing all isolated MV procedures in a right minithoracotomy approach and applying the same minithoracotomy approach for concomitant tricuspid valve disease and surgical treatment of atrial fibrillation. The MV repair and replacement via right minithoracotomy is a feasible method that can be performed safely and effectively. The method allows use of the vast range of the valve repair techniques and the use of new innovative devices which can be employed with similar success. With the growing commitment of the overall surgical community to the adoption and routine application of this approach, it may have even more impact on the patient population offering better value to patients with technological improvements. Carefully designed prospective studies will continue to better define the limits of the procedure in respect to establishing the right patient population.

With both isolated mitral or concomitant valve and/or ablation operations, as well as for primary and reoperative surgeries, there can exist increased risks in performing suboptimal reconstruction using a right minithoracotomy compared with the conventional approach [75]. No compromise should be accepted [34] in this regard, and the surgeon should not hesitate to enlarge the incision if the approach compromises the quality of the operation [13].

40.6.1 Surgical Perspectives

Recently, several minimally invasive approaches have been proposed for isolated heart valve surgery. These methods have been introduced in order to provide acceptable exposure of the heart valves with less invasive surgical trauma. Minimally invasive valve surgery has become a routine procedure for isolated MV operations, and the operative possibilities are being rapidly expanded; the right minithoracotomy is being evaluated for concomitant atrial fibrillation treatment in cardiac double and triple valve disease surgeries. Minimally invasive MV surgery is technically more complex compared to that in a full median sternotomy; however, the current technological innovations allow operative conditions and surgeon comforts similar to those in a standard approach. These include a bloodless operative field, good valve exposure, either direct or video-enhanced visualization (excellent luminosity, image magnification options, and high-definition camera), instruments adjustable in length, smart solutions such as a flexible and completely detachable aortic cross-clamps, vacuum-assisted venous drainage, low-profile venous cannulae, and long and flexible aortic cannulae, along with many other technical solutions.

The minimally invasive approach to MV disease has moved treatment of MV disease toward improved surgical outcomes. It is important however to keep in mind that it is mainly the smaller incision, i.e., less surgical trauma, that has decreased the intensive care unit and hospital length of stay and allowed for earlier patient mobilization and not the other components of the surgical procedure that are essentially unchanged from the conventional approach. These, as always, will depend entirely on the technical performance of surgical team.

It is our belief that the number of complex surgical procedures utilizing a less invasive approach will increase with expanding indications and selection criteria. In experienced centers, minimally invasive MV surgery will gradually become the conventional approach with fewer contraindications due to the complexity of the valve repair. As experience grows, the specific indications for the minimally invasive MV therapies will be better defined, and the operative technical possibilities performed through a minithoracotomy will be extended.

As the general tendency in cardiac valve therapies moves toward less invasive procedures, it appears likely that percutaneous transcatheter valve devices will play a significant role in the future treatment of valvular heart disease. The new transcatheter technologies may enhance MV repair and replacement through right minithoracotomy, by significantly minimizing the CPB and operative times. It also is inevitable that these innovative valve therapies will be extended to lower risk populations where all currently known technical and clinical issues associated with minimally invasive approaches would be put under more intense examination than they have in the high-risk, elderly population with short life expectancy and poorer predicted outcomes.

It is inevitable that therapeutic tendencies will increasingly shift toward less invasive implementation of all known cardiac surgical routines due to an aging population and increasing demand for them by patients as a procedure of choice. It must be noted however that with the successful introduction of any less invasive and/or transcatheter valve delivery techniques, it will always be important to ensure and enhance the safety and effectiveness of complex minimally invasive surgical procedures and techniques, involving multiple valve repair, great vessels, and other cardiac and interventional procedures. Appropriate patient selection, preoperative screening and careful conduct of the procedure and postoperative management should remain a priority.

References

1. Nkomo VT, Gardin JM, Skelton TN, Gottdieneri JS, Scott CG, Enriquez-Sarano M (2006) Burden of valvular heart diseases: a population-based study. Lancet 368(9540):1005–1011
2. Iung B, Baron G, Butchart EG, Delahaye F, Gohlke-Bärwolf C, Levang OW, Tornos P, Vanoverschelde JL, Vermeer F, Boersma E, Ravaud P, Vahanian A (2003) A prospective survey of patients with valvular heart disease in Europe: the euro heart survey on valvular heart disease. Eur Heart J 24(13):1231–1243
3. Chandrashekhar Y, Westaby S, Narula J (2009) Mitral stenosis. Lancet 374(9697):1271–1283
4. Enriquez-Sarano M, Akins CW, Vahanian A (2009) Mitral regurgitation. Lancet 373(9672):1382–1394
5. Rankin JS, Hammill BG, Ferguson TB Jr, Glower DD, O'Brien SM, DeLong ER, Peterson ED, Edwards FH (2006) Determinants of operative mortality in valvular heart surgery. J Thorac Cardiovasc Surg 131(3):547–557
6. Roger VL, Go AS, Lloyd-Jones DM, Benjamin EJ, Berry JD, Borden WB, Bravata DM, Dai S, Ford ES, Fox CS, Fullerton HJ, Gillespie C, Hailpern SM, Heit JA, Howard VJ, Kissela BM, Kittner SJ, Lackland DT, Lichtman JH, Lisabeth LD, Makuc DM, Marcus GM, Marelli A, Matchar DB, Moy CS, Mozaffarian D, Mussolino ME, Nichol G, Paynter NP, Soliman EZ, Sorlie PD, Sotoodehnia N, Turan TN, Virani SS, Wong ND, Woo D, Turner MB, American Heart Association Statistics Committee and Stroke Statistics Subcommittee (2012) Heart disease and stroke statistics – 2012 update: a report from the American Heart Association. Circulation 125(1):e2–e220
7. Navia JL, Cosgrove DM 3rd (1996) Minimally invasive mitral valve operations. Ann Thorac Surg 62(5):1542–1544
8. Grossi EA, Galloway AC, Ribakove GH, Buttenheim PM, Esposito R, Baumann FG, Colvin SB (1999) Minimally invasive port access surgery reduces operative morbidity for valve replacement in the elderly. Heart Surg Forum 2(3):212–215
9. Pompili MF, Stevens JH, Burdon TA, Siegel LC, Peters WS, Ribakove GH, Reitz BA (1996) Port-access mitral valve replacement in dogs. J Thorac Cardiovasc Surg 112(5):1268–1274
10. Peters WS, Smith JA, Preovolos A, Rabinov M, Buckland MR, Rosenfeldt FL (1997) Mitral valve replacement via a right mini-thoracotomy in the dog: use of carbon dioxide to reduce intracardiac air. Eur J Cardiothorac Surg 11(6):1067–1073
11. Schwartz DS, Ribakove GH, Grossi EA, Buttenheim PM, Schwartz JD, Applebaum RM, Kronzon I, Baumann FG, Colvin SB, Galloway AC (1997) Minimally invasive mitral valve replacement: port-access technique, feasibility, and myocardial functional preservation. J Thorac Cardiovasc Surg 113(6):1022–1030; discussion 1030–1031
12. Carpentier A, Loulmet D, Carpentier A, Le Bret E, Haugades B, Dassier P, Guibourt P (1996) Open heart operation under videosurgery and minithoracotomy. First case (mitral valvuloplasty) operated with success. C R Acad Sci III 319(3):219–223
13. Loulmet DF, Carpentier A, Cho PW, Berrebi A, d'Attellis N, Austin CB, Couëtil JP, Lajos P (1998)

Less invasive techniques for mitral valve surgery. J Thorac Cardiovasc Surg 115(4):772–779
14. Greco E, Zaballos JM, Alvarez L, Urso S, Pulitani I, Sàdaba R, Juaristi A, Goiti JJ (2008) Video-assisted mitral surgery through a micro-access: a safe and reliable reality in the current era. J Heart Valve Dis 17(1):48–53
15. Iribarne A, Russo MJ, Easterwood R, Hong KN, Yang J, Cheema FH, Smith CR, Argenziano M (2010) Minimally invasive versus sternotomy approach for mitral valve surgery: a propensity analysis. Ann Thorac Surg 90(5):1471–1477; discussion 1477–1478
16. Iribarne A, Easterwood R, Chan EY, Yang J, Soni L, Russo MJ, Smith CR, Argenziano M (2011) The golden age of minimally invasive cardiothoracic surgery: current and future perspectives. Future Cardiol 7(3):333–346
17. Schroeyers P, Wellens F, De Geest R, Degrieck I, Van Praet F, Vermeulen Y, Vanermen H (2001) Minimally invasive video-assisted mitral valve surgery: our lessons after a 4-year experience. Ann Thorac Surg 72(3):S1050–S1054
18. Galloway AC, Shemin RJ, Glower DD, Boyer JH Jr, Groh MA, Kuntz RE, Burdon TA, Ribakove GH, Reitz BA, Colvin SB (1999) First report of the port access international registry. Ann Thorac Surg 67(1):51–56; discussion 57–58
19. Mohr FW, Falk V, Diegeler A, Walther T, van Son JA, Autschbach R (1998) Minimally invasive port-access mitral valve surgery. J Thorac Cardiovasc Surg 115(3):567–574; discussion 574–576
20. Glower DD, Clements FM, Debruijn NP, Stafford-Smith M, Davis RD, Landolfo KP, Smith PK (1999) Comparison of direct aortic and femoral cannulation for port-access cardiac operations. Ann Thorac Surg 68(4):1529–1531
21. Chitwood WR Jr, Elbeery JR, Moran JF (1997) Minimally invasive mitral valve repair using transthoracic aortic occlusion. Ann Thorac Surg 63(5): 1477–1479
22. Aybek T, Dogan S, Wimmer-Greinecker G, Westphal K, Mortiz A (2000) The micro-mitral operation comparing the port-access technique and the transthoracic clamp technique. J Card Surg 15(1):76–81
23. Casselman FP, Van Slycke S, Wellens F, De Geest R, Degrieck I, Van Praet F, Vermeulen Y, Vanermen H (2003) Mitral valve surgery can now routinely be performed endoscopically. Circulation 108(Suppl 1): II48–II54
24. Reichenspurner H, Detter C, Deuse T, Boehm DH, Treede H, Reichart B (2005) Video and robotic-assisted minimally invasive mitral valve surgery: a comparison of the port-access and transthoracic clamp techniques. Ann Thorac Surg 79(2):485–490; discussion 490–491
25. Gulielmos V, Wagner FM, Waetzig B, Solowjowa N, Tugtekin SM, Schroeder C, Schueler S (1999) Clinical experience with minimally invasive coronary artery and mitral valve surgery with the advantage of cardiopulmonary bypass and cardioplegic arrest using the port access technique. World J Surg 23(5):480–485
26. Gulielmos V, Tugtekin SM, Kappert U, Cichon R, Matschke K, Karbalai P, Schueler S (2000) Three-year follow-up after port-access mitral valve surgery. J Card Surg 15(1):43–50
27. Grossi EA, Zakow PK, Ribakove G, Kallenbach K, Ursomanno P, Gradek CE, Baumann FG, Colvin SB, Galloway AC (1999) Comparison of post-operative pain, stress response, and quality of life in port access vs. standard sternotomy coronary bypass patients. Eur J Cardiothorac Surg 16(Suppl 2):S39–S42
28. Svensson LG, Atik FA, Cosgrove DM, Blackstone EH, Rajeswaran J, Krishnaswamy G, Jin U, Gillinov AM, Griffin B, Navia JL, Mihaljevic T, Lytle BW (2010) Minimally invasive versus conventional mitral valve surgery: a propensity-matched comparison. J Thorac Cardiovasc Surg 139(4):926-32.e1–926-32.e2
29. Dogan S, Aybek T, Risteski PS, Detho F, Rapp A, Wimmer-Greinecker G, Moritz A (2005) Minimally invasive port access versus conventional mitral valve surgery: prospective randomized study. Ann Thorac Surg 79(2):492–498
30. Wimmer-Greinecker G, Matheis G, Dogan S, Aybek T, Kessler P, Westphal K, Moritz A (1999) Complications of port-access cardiac surgery. J Card Surg 14(4):240–245
31. Seeburger J, Borger MA, Falk V, Kuntze T, Czesla M, Walther T, Doll N, Mohr FW (2008) Minimal invasive mitral valve repair for mitral regurgitation: results of 1339 consecutive patients. Eur J Cardiothorac Surg 34(4):760–765
32. Walther T, Falk V, Metz S, Diegeler A, Battellini R, Autschbach R, Mohr FW (1999) Pain and quality of life after minimally invasive versus conventional cardiac surgery. Ann Thorac Surg 67(6):1643–1647
33. Glower DD, Landolfo KP, Clements F, Debruijn NP, Stafford-Smith M, Smith PK, Duhaylongsod F (1998) Mitral valve operation via port access versus median sternotomy. Eur J Cardiothorac Surg 14(Suppl 1): S143–S147
34. Chitwood WR Jr, Wixon CL, Elbeery JR, Francalancia NA, Lust RM (1999) Minimally invasive cardiac operation: adapting cardioprotective strategies. Ann Thorac Surg 68(5):1974–1977
35. Aklog L, Adams DH, Couper GS, Gobezie R, Sears S, Cohn LH (1998) Techniques and results of direct-access minimally invasive mitral valve surgery: a paradigm for the future. J Thorac Cardiovasc Surg 116(5):705–715
36. Grossi EA, Ribakove G, Schwartz DS, Galloway AC, Colvin SB (1998). Port-access approach for minimally invasive mitral valve surgery. Operative Techniques in Cardiac and Thoracic Surgery 2;3(1):32–46.
37. Yozu R, Okamoto K, Kudo M, Nonaka H, Adams DH (2012) New innovative instruments facilitate both direct-vision and endoscopic-assisted mini-mitral valve surgery. J Thorac Cardiovasc Surg 143(4 Suppl):S82–S85
38. Greco E, Barriuso C, Castro MA, Fita G, Pomar JL (2002) Port-access cardiac surgery: from a learning

process to the standard. Heart Surg Forum 5(2):145–149
39. Woo YJ, Rodriguez E, Atluri P, Chitwood WR Jr (2006) Minimally invasive, robotic, and off-pump mitral valve surgery. Semin Thorac Cardiovasc Surg 18(2):139–147
40. Schmitto JD, Mokashi SA, Cohn LH (2011) Past, present, and future of minimally invasive mitral valve surgery. J Heart Valve Dis 20(5):493–498
41. Grossi EA, Galloway AC, LaPietra A, Ribakove GH, Ursomanno P, Delianides J, Culliford AT, Bizekis C, Esposito RA, Baumann FG, Kanchuger MS, Colvin SB (2002) Minimally invasive mitral valve surgery: a 6-year experience with 714 patients. Ann Thorac Surg 74(3):660–663; discussion 663–664
42. Aybek T, Dogan S, Risteski PS, Zierer A, Wittlinger T, Wimmer-Greinecker G, Moritz A (2006) Two hundred forty minimally invasive mitral operations through right minithoracotomy. Ann Thorac Surg 81(5):1618–1624
43. Chu JJ, Chang CH, Lin PJ, Liu HP, Tsai FC, Wu D, Chiang CW, Lin FC, Su WJ, Tan PP (1998) Video-assisted cardiac surgery: preliminary results in Chang Gung Memorial Hospital. Chin Med J (Engl) 111(5):422–427
44. Poffo R, Pope RB, Selbach RA, Mokross CA, Fukuti F, Id SJ, Agapito A, Cidral I (2009) Video-assisted cardiac surgery: results from a pioneer project in Brazil. Rev Bras Cir Cardiovasc 24(3):318–326
45. Raanani E, Spiegelstein D, Sternik L, Preisman S, Moshkovitz Y, Smolinsky AK, Shinfeld A (2010) Quality of mitral valve repair: median sternotomy versus port-access approach. J Thorac Cardiovasc Surg 140(1):86–90
46. Glauber M, Karimov JH, Farneti PA, Cerillo AG, Santarelli F, Ferrarini M, Del Sarto P, Murzi M, Solinas M (2008) Minimally invasive mitral valve surgery via right minithoracotomy. Multimedia Man Cardiothorac Surg. doi:10.1510/mmcts.2008.003350
47. Mishra YK, Khanna SN, Wasir H, Sharma KK, Mehta Y, Trehan N (2005) Port-access approach for cardiac surgical procedures: our experience in 776 patients. Indian Heart J 57(6):688–693
48. Schroeyers P, Wellens F, De Geest R, Degrieck I, Van Praet F, Vermeulen Y, Vanermen H (2001) Minimally invasive video-assisted mitral valve repair: short and mid-term results. J Heart Valve Dis 10(5):579–583
49. Kypson AP, Glower DD (2002) Port-access approach for combined aortic and mitral valve surgery. Ann Thorac Surg 73(5):1657–1658
50. Karimov JH, Solinas M, Latsuzbaia K, Murzi M, Cerillo AG, Glauber M (2009) Surgical treatment of double and triple heart valve disease through a limited single-access right minithoracotomy. Multimedia Man Cardiothoracic Surg. doi:10.1510/mmcts.2009.004036
51. Trehan N, Mishra YK, Mathew SG, Sharma KK, Shrivastava S, Mehta Y (2002) Redo mitral valve surgery using the port-access system. Asian Cardiovasc Thorac Ann 10(3):215–218
52. Meyer SR, Szeto WY, Augoustides JG, Morris RJ, Vernick WJ, Paschal D, Fox J, Hargrove WC 3rd (2009) Reoperative mitral valve surgery by the port access minithoracotomy approach is safe and effective. Ann Thorac Surg 87(5):1426–1430
53. Murzi M, Kallushi E, Tiwari KK, Cerillo AG, Bevilacqua S, Karimov JH, Solinas M, Glauber M (2009) Minimally invasive mitral valve surgery through right thoracotomy in patients with patent coronary artery bypass grafts. Interact Cardiovasc Thorac Surg 9(1):29–32
54. Karimov JH, Bevilacqua S, Solinas M, Glauber M (2009) Triple heart valve surgery through a right antero-lateral minithoracotomy. Interact Cardiovasc Thorac Surg 9(2):360–362
55. Solinas M, Bevilacqua S, Karimov JH, Glauber M (2010) A left atrial ablation with bipolar irrigated radio-frequency for atrial fibrillation during minimally invasive mitral valve surgery. Eur J Cardiothorac Surg 37(4):965–966
56. Jeanmart H, Casselman FP, De Grieck Y, Bakir I, Coddens J, Foubert L, Van Vaerenbergh G, Vermeulen Y, Vanermen H (2007) Avoiding vascular complications during minimally invasive, totally endoscopic intracardiac surgery. J Thorac Cardiovasc Surg 133(4):1066–1070
57. Saunders PC, Grossi EA, Sharony R, Schwartz CF, Ribakove GH, Culliford AT, Delianides J, Baumann FG, Galloway AC, Colvin SB (2004) Minimally invasive technology for mitral valve surgery via left thoracotomy: experience with forty cases. J Thorac Cardiovasc Surg 127(4):1026–1031; discussion 1031–1032
58. Modi P, Rodriguez E, Hargrove WC 3rd, Hassan A, Szeto WY, Chitwood WR Jr (2009) Minimally invasive video-assisted mitral valve surgery: a 12-year, 2-center experience in 1178 patients. J Thorac Cardiovasc Surg 137(6):1481–1487
59. Onnasch JF, Schneider F, Falk V, Mierzwa M, Bucerius J, Mohr FW (2002) Five years of less invasive mitral valve surgery: from experimental to routine approach. Heart Surg Forum 5(2):132–135
60. Holzhey DM, Shi W, Borger MA, Seeburger J, Garbade J, Pfannmüller B, Mohr FW (2011) Minimally invasive versus sternotomy approach for mitral valve surgery in patients greater than 70 years old: a propensity-matched comparison. Ann Thorac Surg 91(2):401–405
61. Mishra YK, Malhotra R, Mehta Y, Sharma KK, Kasliwal RR, Trehan N (1999) Minimally invasive mitral valve surgery through right anterolateral minithoracotomy. Ann Thorac Surg 68(4):1520–1524
62. Grossi EA, Ribakove G, Galloway AC, Colvin SB (2000) Minimally invasive mitral valve surgery with endovascular balloon technique. Operative Techniques in Thoracic and Cardiovascular Surgery 8;5(3): 176–89.
63. Lebon JS, Couture P, Rochon AG, Laliberté E, Harvey J, Aubé N, Cossette M, Bouchard D, Jeanmart H, Pellerin M (2010) The endovascular coronary sinus

catheter in minimally invasive mitral and tricuspid valve surgery: a case series. J Cardiothorac Vasc Anesth 24(5):746–751
64. Colvin SB, Grossi EA, Ribakove G, Galloway AC (2000) Minimally invasive aortic and mitral valve operation. Oper Tech Card Thorac Surg 5:212–220
65. Chaney MA, Nikolov MP, Tuchek M, Bakhos M (1998) An institution's initial experience with port-access minimally invasive cardiac surgery. J Cardiothorac Vasc Anesth 12(6):617–619
66. Saroul C, Keller G, Benaissa M, Lehot JJ (2011) Anesthesia for minimally invasive cardiac procedure. Ann Fr Anesth Reanim 30(Suppl 1): S38–S43
67. Secknus MA, Asher CR, Scalia GM, Cosgrove DM 3rd, Stewart WJ (1999) Intraoperative transesophageal echocardiography in minimally invasive cardiac valve surgery. J Am Soc Echocardiogr 12(4): 231–236
68. Lecharny J-B, Paquin S, de Vaumas C, Philip I (1998) Monitoring by transoesophageal echocardiography in minimally invasive cardiac surgery. Baillière's Clin Anaesthesiol 12:637–646
69. Schmitz C, Ashraf O, Bimmel D, Welz A (2002) Direct aortic cannulation in minimally invasive mitral-valve operations. Heart Surg Forum 5(4):370–372
70. Glauber M, Karimov JH (2010) A completely detachable aortic clamping instrument for minimally invasive cardiac surgery. Innovations 5(4):309–310
71. Glower DD, Desai B (2010) Transaortic endoclamp for mitral valve operation through right minithoracotomy in 369 patients. Ann Surg 5(6):394–399
72. Lee TC, Desai BS, Milano C, Jaggers J, Glower DD (2010) Comparison of minithoracotomy versus sternotomy in 304 consecutive tricuspid valve operations. Innovations (Phila) 5(1):3–6
73. Umakanthan R, Leacche M, Petracek MR, Kumar S, Solenkova NV, Kaiser CA, Greelish JP, Balaguer JM, Ahmad RM, Ball SK, Hoff SJ, Absi TS, Kim BS, Byrne JG (2008) Safety of minimally invasive mitral valve surgery without aortic cross-clamp. Ann Thorac Surg 85(5):1544–1549; discussion 1549–1550
74. Kumar S, Petracek MR, Greelish JP, Ahmad RM, Balaguer JM, Byrne JG (2007) Ultra minimally invasive mitral valve surgery without aortic cross-clamp. Heart Lung Circ 16(Suppl 1):S16
75. Svensson LG, Gillinov AM, Blackstone EH, Houghtaling PL, Kim KH, Pettersson GB, Smedira NG, Banbury MK, Lytle BW (2007) Does right thoracotomy increase the risk of mitral valve reoperation? J Thorac Cardiovasc Surg 134(3):677–682
76. Braathen B, Jeppsson A, Scherstén H, Hagen OM, Vengen Ø, Rexius H, Lepore V, Tønnessen T (2011) One single dose of histidine-tryptophan-ketoglutarate solution gives equally good myocardial protection in elective mitral valve surgery as repetitive cold blood cardioplegia: a prospective randomized study. J Thorac Cardiovasc Surg 141(4):995–1001
77. Viana FF, Shi WY, Hayward PA, Larobina ME, Liskaser F, Matalanis G (2012) Custodiol versus blood cardioplegia in complex cardiac operations: an Australian experience. Eur J Cardiothorac Surg [Epub ahead of print] PubMed PMID: 22665382
78. Chaudhuri K, Guddati R, Nawata K, Bhuyan R, Sawada T, Crouch G, Worthington M, Stuklis R, Edwards J (2011) Technical aspects of CO_2 gas insufflation in minimally invasive mitral valve surgery. Heart Lung Circ 20:794
79. Chaudhuri K, Storey E, Lee GA, Bailey M, Chan J, Rosenfeldt FL, Pick A, Negri J, Gooi J, Zimmet A, Esmore D, Merry C, Rowland M, Lin E, Marasco SF (2012) Carbon dioxide insufflation in open-chamber cardiac surgery: a double-blind, randomized clinical trial of neurocognitive effects. J Thorac Cardiovasc Surg [Epub ahead of print] PubMed PMID: 22578685
80. Casselman FP, Van Slycke S, Dom H, Lambrechts DL, Vermeulen Y, Vanermen H (2003) Endoscopic mitral valve repair: feasible, reproducible, and durable. J Thorac Cardiovasc Surg 125(2):273–282
81. Murzi M, Solinas M, Bevilacqua S, Gasbarri T, Glauber M, Cerillo AG (2009) A new left atrial retractor for minimally invasive mitral valve surgery. J Card Surg 24(2):175–177
82. Ricci D, Pellegrini C, Aiello M, Alloni A, Cattadori B, D'Armini AM, Rinaldi M, Viganò M (2010) Port-access surgery as elective approach for mitral valve operation in re-do procedures. Eur J Cardiothorac Surg 37(4):920–925
83. Mihaljevic T, Cohn LH, Unic D, Aranki SF, Couper GS, Byrne JG (2004) One thousand minimally invasive valve operations: early and late results. Ann Surg 240(3):529–534; discussion 534
84. Seeburger J, Borger MA, Falk V, Passage J, Walther T, Doll N, Mohr FW (2009) Minimally invasive mitral valve surgery after previous sternotomy: experience in 181 patients. Ann Thorac Surg 87(3): 709–714
85. Bolotin G, Kypson AP, Reade CC, Chu VF, Freund WL Jr, Nifong LW, Chitwood WR Jr (2004) Should a video-assisted mini-thoracotomy be the approach of choice for reoperative mitral valve surgery? J Heart Valve Dis 13(2):155–158; discussion 158
86. Sharony R, Grossi EA, Saunders PC, Schwartz CF, Ursomanno P, Ribakove GH, Galloway AC, Colvin SB (2006) Minimally invasive reoperative isolated valve surgery: early and mid-term results. J Card Surg 21(3):240–244
87. Karimov JH, Piagneri V, Murzi M, Latsuzbaia K, Tiwari K, Cerillo AG, Solinas M, Glauber M (2010) Multiple recurrent periprosthetic leak after a mitral valve replacement in a 30-year-old man. J Cardiovasc Med (Hagerstown) 11(4):288–290
88. Onnasch JF, Schneider F, Falk V, Walther T, Gummert J, Mohr FW (2002) Minimally invasive approach for redo mitral valve surgery: a true benefit for the patient. J Card Surg 17(1):14–19

89. Iribarne A, Easterwood R, Russo MJ, Chan EY, Smith CR, Argenziano M (2012) Comparative effectiveness of minimally invasive versus traditional sternotomy mitral valve surgery in elderly patients. J Thorac Cardiovasc Surg 143(4 Suppl):S86–S90
90. Burfeind WR, Glower DD, Davis RD, Landolfo KP, Lowe JE, Wolfe WG (2002) Mitral surgery after prior cardiac operation: port-access versus sternotomy or thoracotomy. Ann Thorac Surg 74(4): S1323–S1325
91. Arcidi JM Jr, Rodriguez E, Elbeery JR, Nifong LW, Efird JT, Chitwood WR Jr (2012) Fifteen-year experience with minimally invasive approach for reoperations involving the mitral valve. J Thorac Cardiovasc Surg 143(5):1062–1068
92. Murzi M, Solinas M, Glauber M (2009) Is a minimally invasive approach for re-operative mitral valve surgery superior to standard resternotomy? Interact Cardiovasc Thorac Surg 9(2):327–332
93. Mohr FW, Onnasch JF, Falk V, Walther T, Diegeler A, Krakor R, Schneider F, Autschbach R (1999) The evolution of minimally invasive valve surgery – 2 year experience. Eur J Cardiothorac Surg 15(3):233–238; discussion 238–239
94. Grossi EA, Loulmet DF, Schwartz CF, Ursomanno P, Zias EA, Dellis SL, Galloway AC (2012) Evolution of operative techniques and perfusion strategies for minimally invasive mitral valve repair. J Thorac Cardiovasc Surg 143(4 Suppl):S68–S70
95. Noiseux N, Ruel M, Hemmerling TM (2008) Minimally invasive cardiac surgery: new challenges for the surgeon and the anesthesiologist. Tech Reg Anesth Pain Manag 12:72–79
96. Aybek T, Doss M, Abdel-Rahman U, Simon A, Miskovic A, Risteski PS, Dogan S, Moritz A (2005) Echocardiographic assessment in minimally invasive mitral valve surgery. Med Sci Monit 11(4): MT27–MT32
97. Passage J, Seeburger J, Doll N, Czesla M, Walther T, Falk V, Mohr FW (2010) Minimally invasive mitral valve surgery in octogenarians. Heart Lung Circ 19:503
98. Gillinov AM, Banbury MK, Cosgrove DM (2000) Hemisternotomy approach for aortic and mitral valve surgery. J Card Surg 15(1):15–20

Robotic Mitral Valve Surgery

41

Thierry A. Folliguet and François Laborde

Contents

T.A. Folliguet, M.D., FACS (✉)
Chirurgie Cardiaque Vasculaire & Transplantation, Pole Territorial Lorrain, Chirurgie Cardiaque Vasculaire et Transplantations, ILCV, CHU Brabois Nancy, France
e-mail: t.folliguet@chu-nancy.fr

F. Laborde, M.D.
Institut Mutualiste Montsouris, 42 Boulevard Jourdan, 75014 Paris, France
e-mail: francois.laborde@imm.fr

41.1 Clinical Background

Alternative incisions to expose the mitral valve have included upper partial sternotomy, parasternal incisions, and minithoracotomies. The annulus of the mitral valve is nearly the sagittal plane of the body, making a right posterior minithoracotomy the optimal approach to the valve. This approach provides direct access to the mitral valve through a left atriotomy. The addition of video assistance into the right chest allows better visualization and minimal incision size. Initial reports of successful mitral valve repair using video assistance and a right minithoracotomy were published in 1996 [1, 2]. This technique of "port-access" mitral valve surgery has been extensively performed across the world.

Similar results can be obtained in experienced teams as compared with median sternotomy [3–9]. Most of the complex repair can be repaired through these incisions with excellent result [8–10]. Clearly the results are operator dependent and a solid experience both of mitral valve repair and of video surgery is needed to obtain good results [7].

Robotic surgery has been introduced in 2002 and provides the surgeon with optimal 3D imaging, magnification, miniaturized instruments, and mobility through seven degrees of freedom mimicking the human wrists. The instruments are placed directly through 10-mm trocars which are positioned in a triangular fashion with the 3D camera, apart from the minithoracotomy. When comparing both techniques, the robotic platform allows "novice" endoscopic surgeons to perform

R.G.C. Inderbitzi et al. (eds.), *Minimally Invasive Thoracic and Cardiac Surgery*,
DOI 10.1007/978-3-642-11861-6_41, © Springer-Verlag Berlin Heidelberg 2012

complex task more rapidly and more efficiently. The surgeon's vision and method of operating is more "intuitive" as the surgeon is seating and controls the instruments through three fingers in each hand (Fig. 41.1).

However, the cost of the platform and of each instrument represents an increased cost as compared to port access [11], and the surgeon depends more on the overall team including nurses and assistant in order to perform the surgery [12]. Feasibility of robotic mitral valve repair has been demonstrated in both simple and complex repairs [13–17]. Despite a longer aortic and cross clamp time than through a sternotomy, excellent immediate and long-term repair can be achieved in experienced teams [17–22]. More rapid return to work, diminished blood loss, and reduced length of hospitalization have been measured following robotic mitral valve surgery [23] (Fig. 41.2).

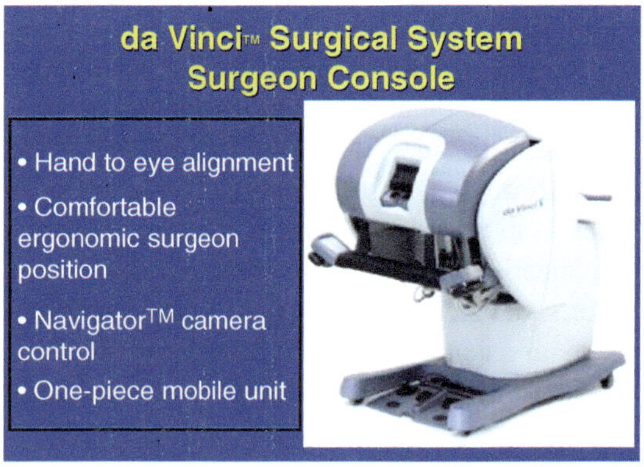

Fig. 41.1 da Vinci console

41.2 Patient Selection and Assessment

Patient selection depends on the team experience. At the beginning, "easy repair" should be performed, and as experience is gained, more complex repair can be attempted. All patients should have a surgical and an anesthesiologist consult. Exclusion criteria should include emergency, pulmonary disease, atherosclerotic and enlarged ascending aorta, aortic insufficiency, peripheral vessel disease including femoral and iliac disease, prior right chest surgery, or major trauma. Poor ejection fraction, multiple valve repair or replacement, and associated coronary revascularization should be excluded as it exposes the patient to prolonged operating and CPB time and it adds to the complexity of the procedure.

Therefore a complete preoperative checklist should be done including a chest X ray, EKG, echocardiogram, coronary angiogram, complete pulmonary function tests, and peripheral arterial and venous Doppler. Also of interest is a CT scan of the chest that will evaluate the degree of aortic calcification, the presence of emphysema, and the anatomy of the patient (left atrial enlargement, right and left ventricular dimension). Finally a signed consent from each patient should

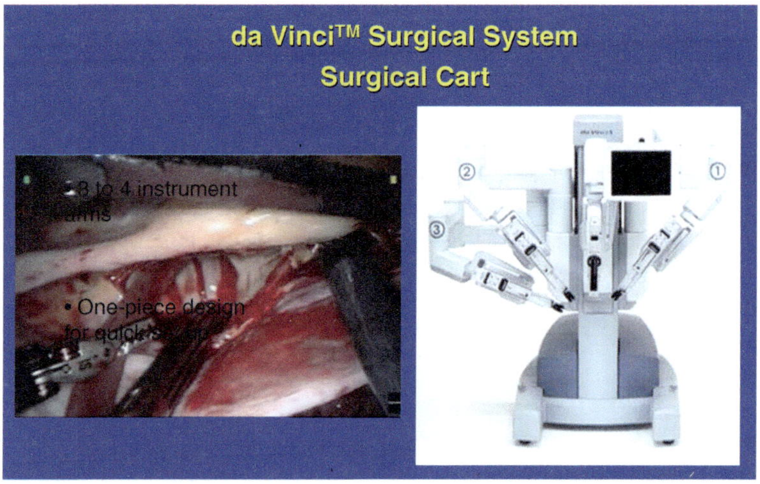

Fig. 41.2 da Vinci surgical system. One camera, three surgical arms

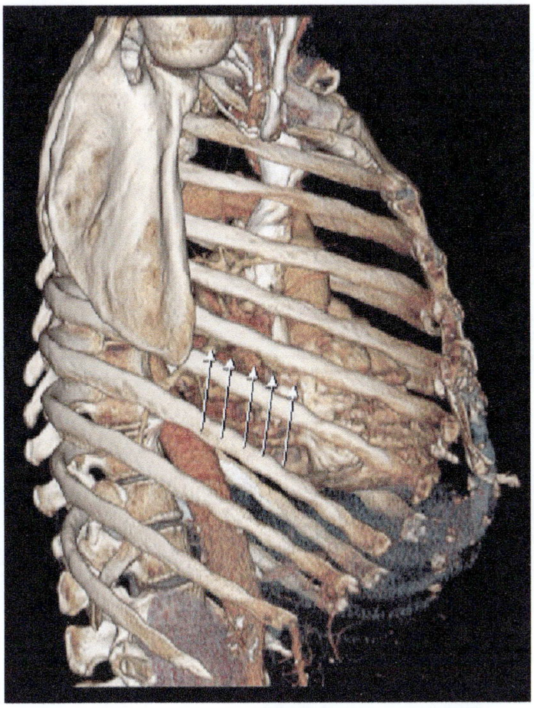

Fig. 41.3 CT scan of the chest allows projecting the heart on the costochondral cartilage

be obtained, explaining that other techniques are possible (median sternotomy, port access). Also a CT scan of the chest can help in assessing the morphology of the patient and help in choosing the right intercostal space incisions (Fig. 41.3).

41.3 Technique (Patient Positioning, CPB, Anesthetic)

As with elective cardiac procedures, standard hemodynamic monitoring lines, including central venous lines and arterial lines, should be placed. A double lumen endotracheal tube is necessary to allow for left single lung ventilation during the preparation phase (Fig. 41.4).

A transesophageal echocardiogram is also necessary to check the placement of the cannulas and also to assess the mitral valve repair and the ventricular function after declamping. External defibrillator cardioversion pads are placed on the patient behind the right scapula and on the left anterolateral chest wall. The patient is placed supine with a small pillow placed under the right scapula in order to elevate the right hemithorax, and then the right arm is positioned along the side of the patient with the elbow slightly flexed in order to have access to the right axillary area. Small inflatable pillow are also placed under the ankles and the knees to avoid compression point on the table (Fig. 41.5).

The patient should be prepped from the neck to the knees and access to the chest, to both groins, and to the right neck should be available. Cannulation of the femoral vessels can be individualized as experience is gained. Usually a right cut down is made in the inguinal area, and the femoral or iliac vessels are exposed and cannulated percutaneously. A 17- or 18-mm wire-wrapped cannula is inserted in the artery, and a 27- or 29-mm wire-wrapped double-staged cannula is inserted in the vein and placed in the right atrium under echo guidance. Most of the time this will allow adequate drainage; however sometimes it can be necessary to place percutaneously in the right jugular vein either a 17- or an 18-mm wire-wrapped cannula. This will provide optimal venous drainage. An active aspiration on the reservoir should be added with a biocentrifugal pump, and direct control of the cavas is not necessary unless the right chest is entered [24].

Cardioplegia is performed antegrade with a long cannula placed either through the minithoracotomy or separately in the 2nd or 3rd intercostal space. Aortic occlusion can be done either with a transaortic clamp placed in the 2nd intercostal space midposterior axillary line or with an endoaortic clamp. Both techniques have advantages and disadvantages [25, 26]. The direct transthoracic clamp is an easy technique to perform which does not require specific training; however it can be traumatic to the left atrial appendage. Therefore clamping should be performed with optimal visualization. The endoaortic balloon requires an additional arterial line in the right radial artery in order to recognize balloon migration. Also it requires another groin access, but it provides both occlusion and cardioplegia and does not require aortic manipulation and has been associated with decreased cerebral microemboli compared with the transaortic clamp [27]. Finally cases of aortic

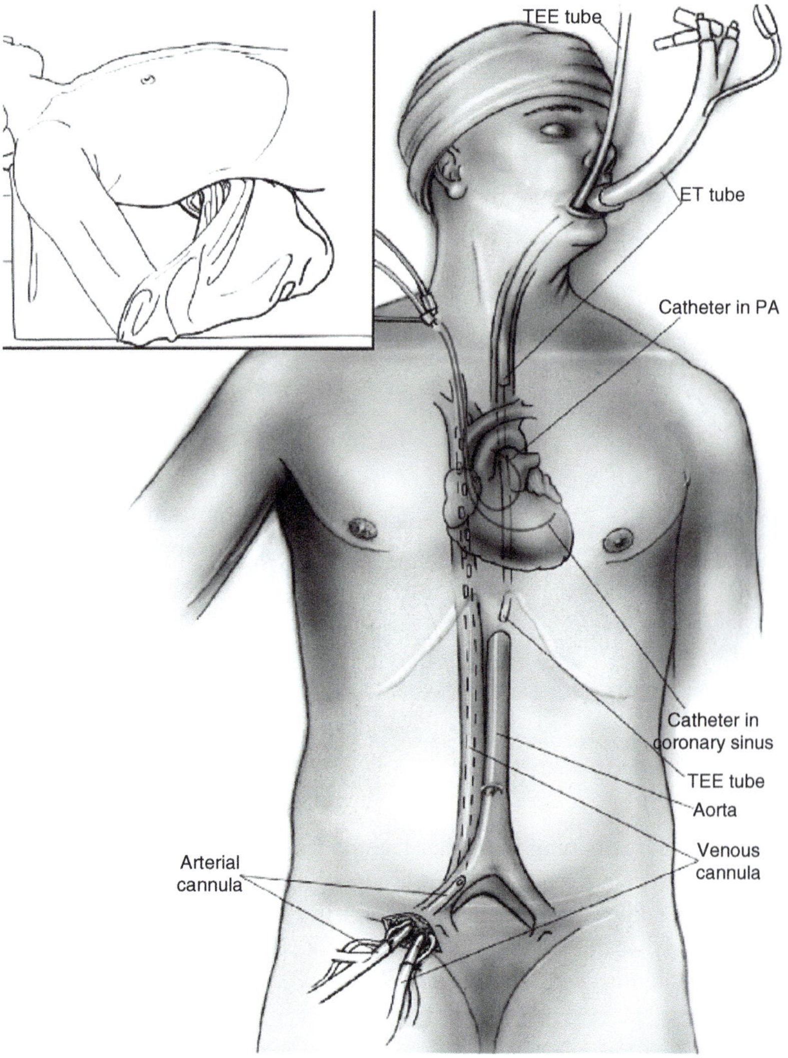

Fig. 41.4 Anesthesia with double lumen tube and peripheral femoral vessels cannulation. Patient is positioned at the right edge of the table with the right arm placed in a sling slightly lower than the edge of the table. A roll is placed behind the shoulders

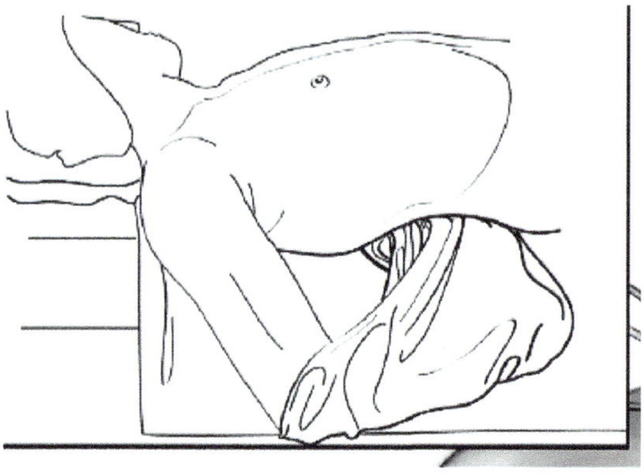

Fig. 41.5 Positioning on the table with a subscapular roll and arm protection

dissection have been reported with this endoclamp balloon. We usually decrease body temperature to 32°C and repeat blood cardioplegia every 10–15 min without removing the atrial retractor. The robot is positioned on the left side of the table and should be positioned securely after groin preparation has been made (Fig. 41.6).

Prior to incision in the right chest, the right lung is deflated, a 4-cm submammary posterolateral incision is performed, and the chest is entered in the 4th interspace. The incision should be posterolateral rather then anterolateral. This provides direct access to the mitral valve and facilitates repair (Fig. 41.7).

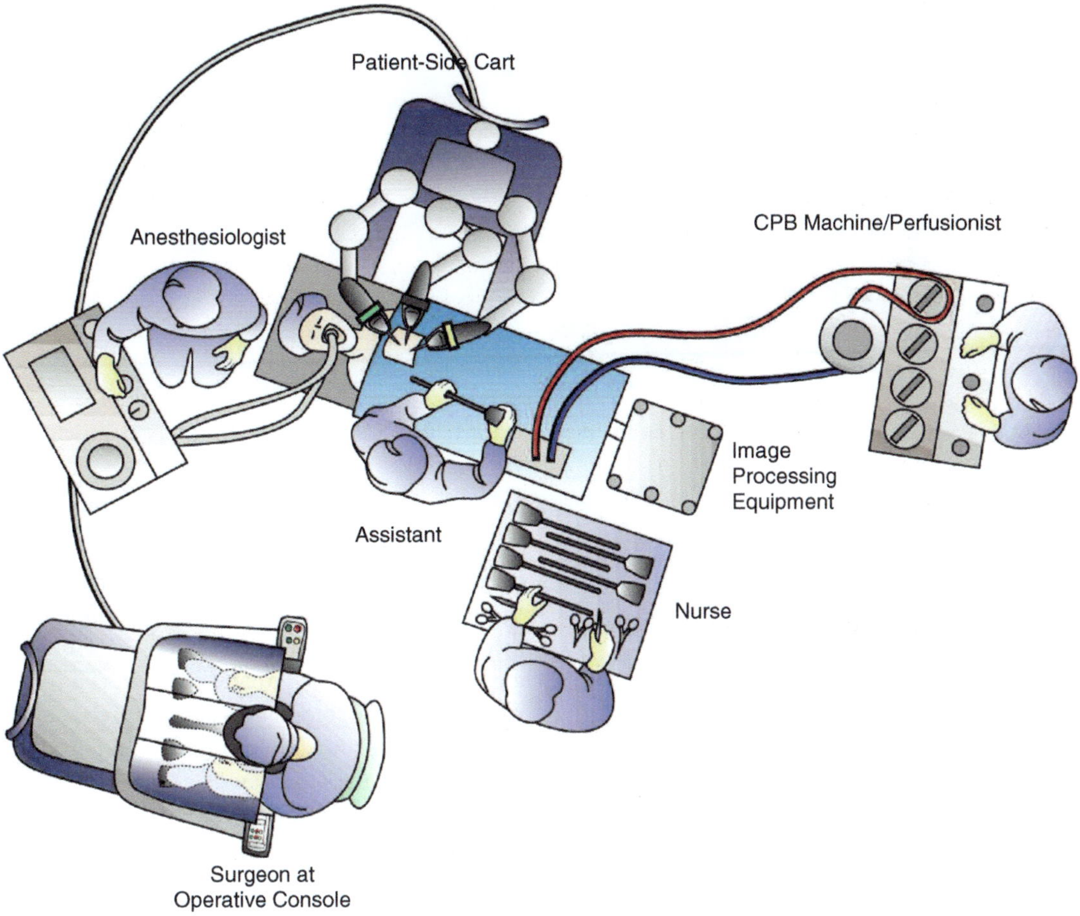

Fig. 41.6 Robot positioning

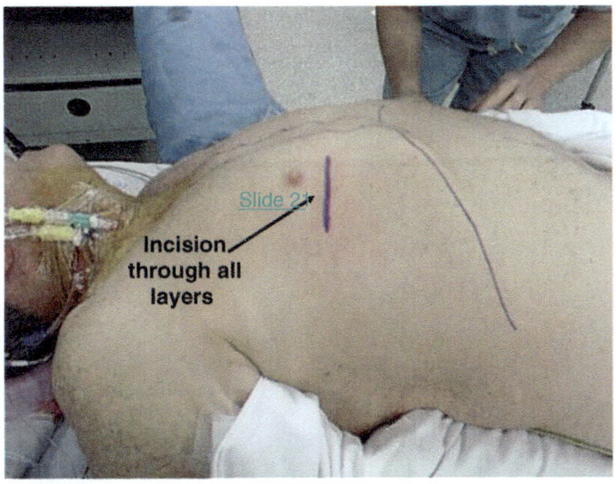

Fig. 41.7 Minithoracotomy incision in 5th or 4th intercostal space

Co_2 is insufflated either directly with the camera port or through a separate stab wound placed posteriorly in the 7th intercostal space between 8 and 10 l/min.

The diaphragm is retracted inferiorly with a stitch brought in the 7th intercostal space as to create a working space. The robotic camera is placed in the more medial part of the incision or through a separate port median to the thoracotomy (Fig. 41.8).

Robotic trocars are positioned in triangular fashion one or two interspaces above and below the thoracotomy, slightly more inferior to the incision, usually in the third and seven or six intercostal space. Robotic trocars are 8 mm and

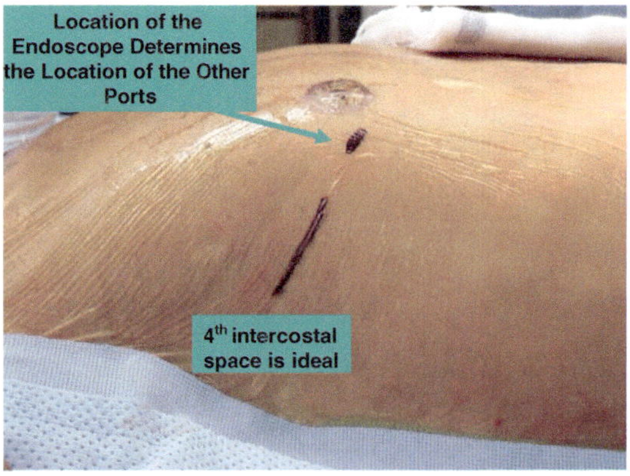

Fig. 41.8 Positioning of the camera more medial than the incision

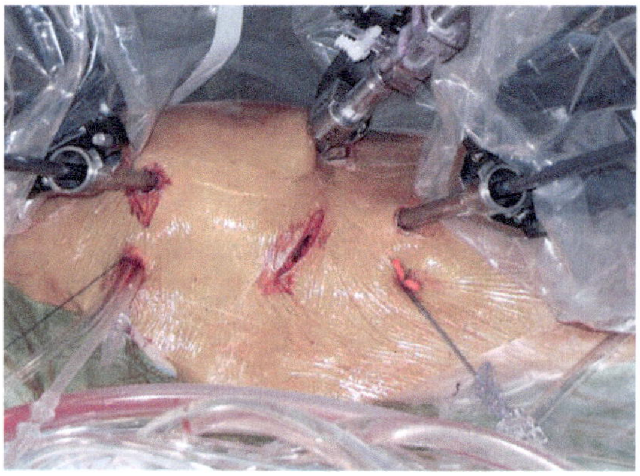

Fig. 41.10 Positioning of the camera, trocars left vent, and CO_2 line

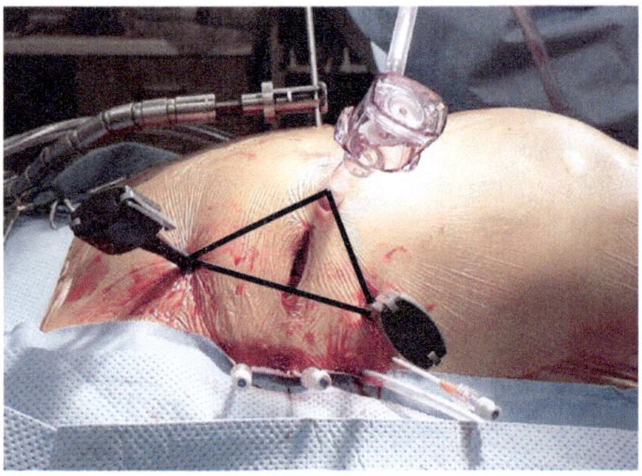

Fig. 41.9 Positioning of the robotic trocars in a triangular fashion. Also note CO_2 injection and vent line positioned lateral

allow 5-mm instruments (Figs. 41.9, 41.10, and 41.11).

The pericardium is entered and opened in a longitudinal fashion from the diaphragm to the aorta (Fig. 41.12).

Traction sutures are placed usually at the level of the pulmonary veins and brought inferior to the cannulas and the incision in order to "bring the heart" toward the chest wall (Fig. 41.13).

The inferior vena cava is dissected from the pericardium and the interatrial groove clearly dissected exposing the left atrium (Fig. 41.14).

This allows opening the left atrium more toward the mitral valve and will facilitate greatly the exposure (Fig. 41.15).

The robotic fourth arm dynamic left atrial retractor is placed either through the incision or through a separate port in the 3rd intercostal space medial to the incision but away from the camera in order to avoid any conflict. If a fourth arm is not available, an endoscopic retractor is placed trough the left atriotomy and brought parasternal in the 4th intercostal space. It should be secure to the chest either with a clamp or with a flexible retractor. The second solution allows some flexibility and mobility of the endoscopic retractor. If the camera was well positioned, minimal traction with the retractor is needed to allow optimal mitral valve visualization (Fig. 41.16).

We then place three annular stitches at the commissures and at the level of P2, which are brought through the incision. This provides traction on the annulus and "brings" the valve toward the incision, which facilitates repair. A left ventricular vent is positioned in the atrium toward the pulmonary veins to provide a dry field.

Standard techniques of valve repair can then be employed (Fig. 41.17).

All annular sutures are brought through the incision and positioned properly (Figs. 41.18 and 41.19).

Special robotic instruments are used, usually one or two needle holders and a hook retractor (Fig. 41.20).

After repair, the left atrium is closed with two 4–0 monofilament sutures starting at each extrem-

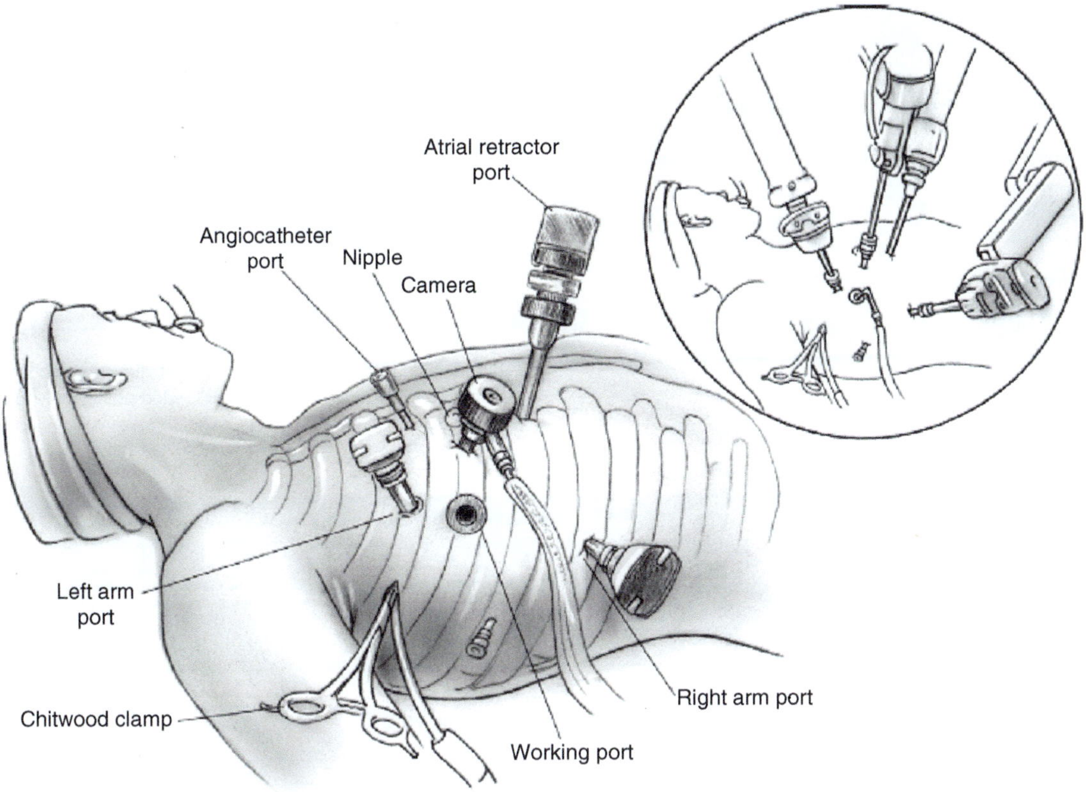

Fig. 41.11 Port placement. The camera is usually positioned below the right nipple and in the fifth intercostal space. The working port is made in the same intercostal space more posterolaterally. Two robotic trocars are positioned in a triangular fashion from the camera, one or two intercostal spaces above and below the incision. The left port is placed one interspace above and the right port two intercostal space below. A transthoracic clamp is inserted through a stab wound made below the axilla in the 2nd intercostal space and a left vent is also brought out from the same incision.

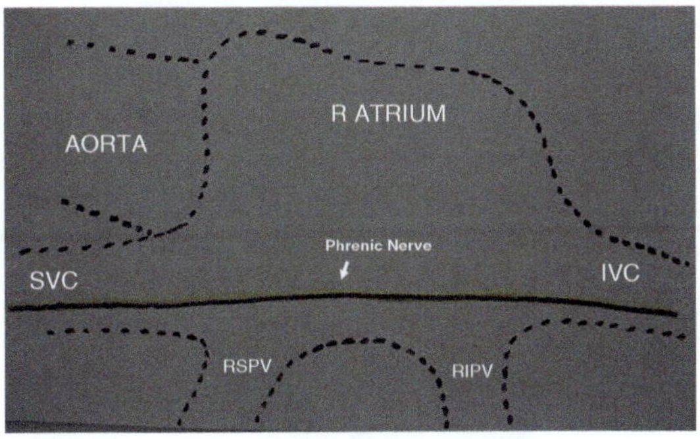

Fig. 41.12 Opening of the pericardium along the phrenic nerve

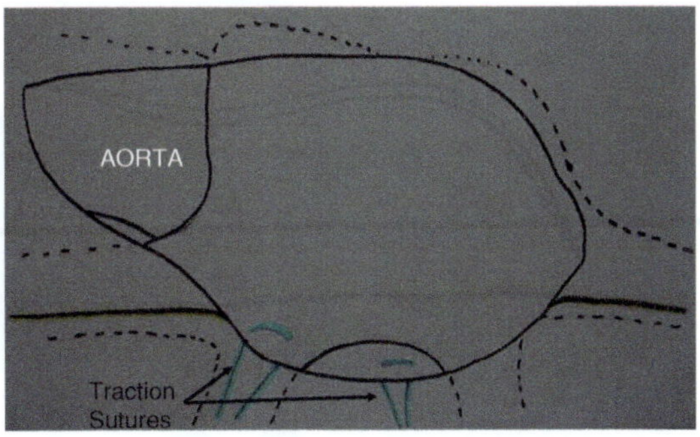

Fig. 41.13 Traction sutures are placed on the pericardium and brought through the medial part of the incision

ity. We recommend Gore-Tex sutures as these can be pulled with the robot and tied more efficiently then Prolene because they offer greater resistance. Before purging, left ventricular wires should be placed on the right inferior part of the ventricle. Air is purged through the aortic car-

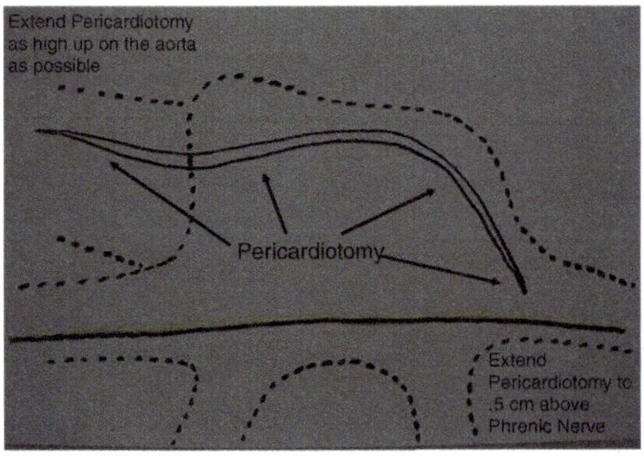

Fig. 41.14 Pericardiotomy extends as high as possible on the aorta and 5 cm above phrenic nerve

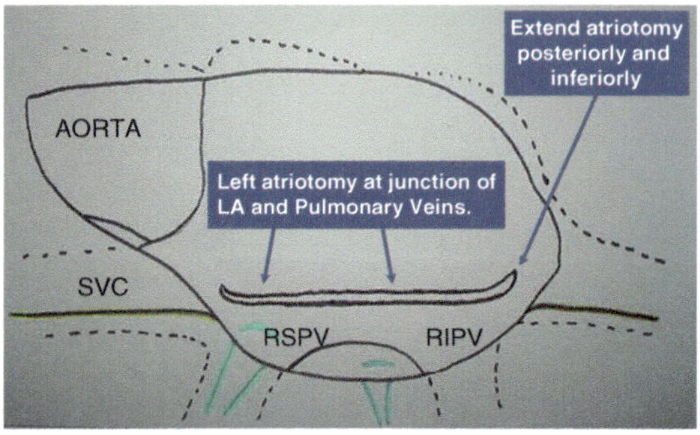

Fig. 41.15 Left atriotomy opened at junction of left atrium and pulmonary veins and extended posteriorly and inferiorly

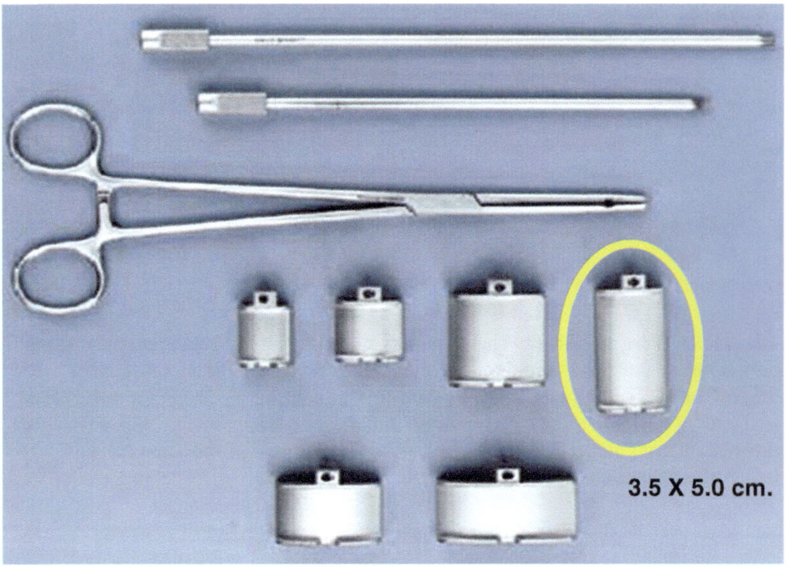

Fig. 41.16 Atrial retractors, different sizes according to size and length of the left atrium

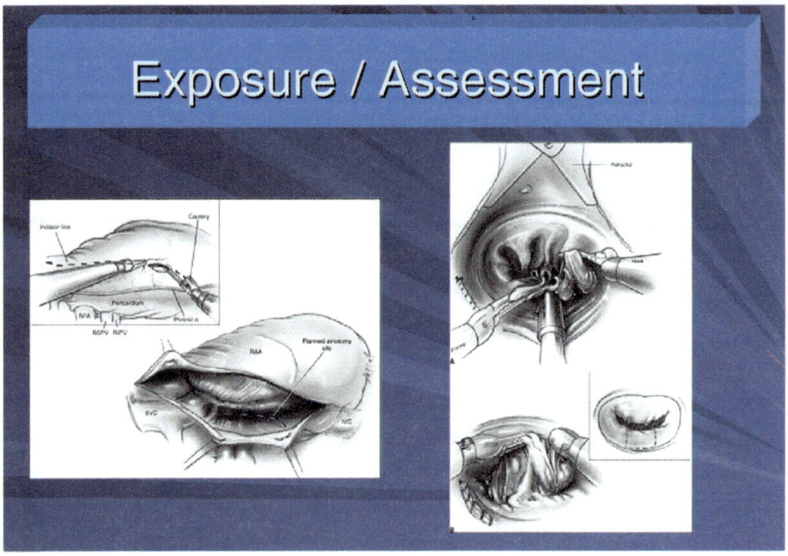

Fig. 41.17 Opening of the pericardium (1.2 *left*), flail posterior leaflet, and quadrangular resection (*superior* and *inferior right*)

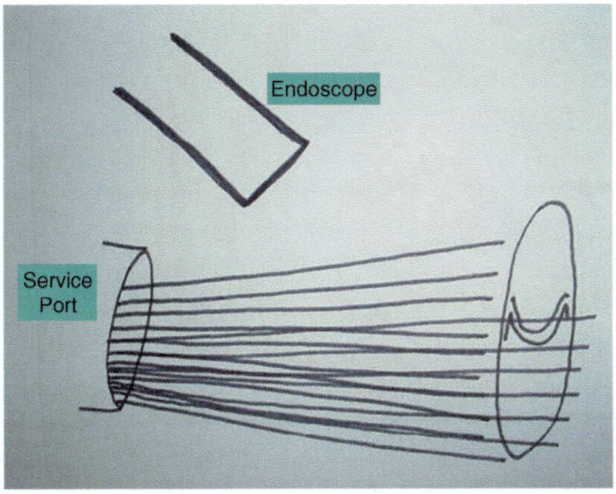

Fig. 41.18 Sutures brought through the working port or incision after being placed in the annulus

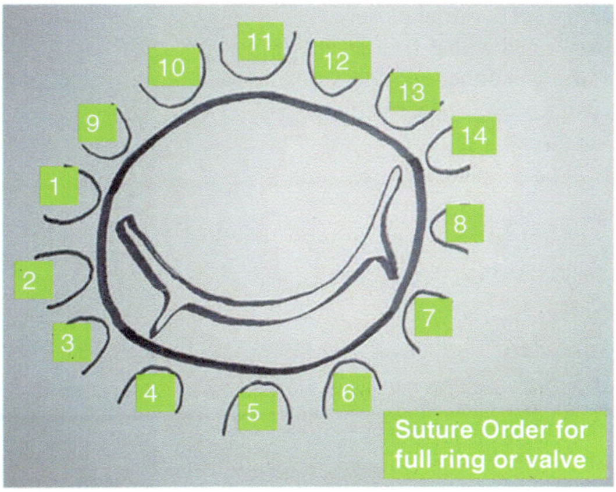

Fig. 41.19 Suture order for full ring or valve

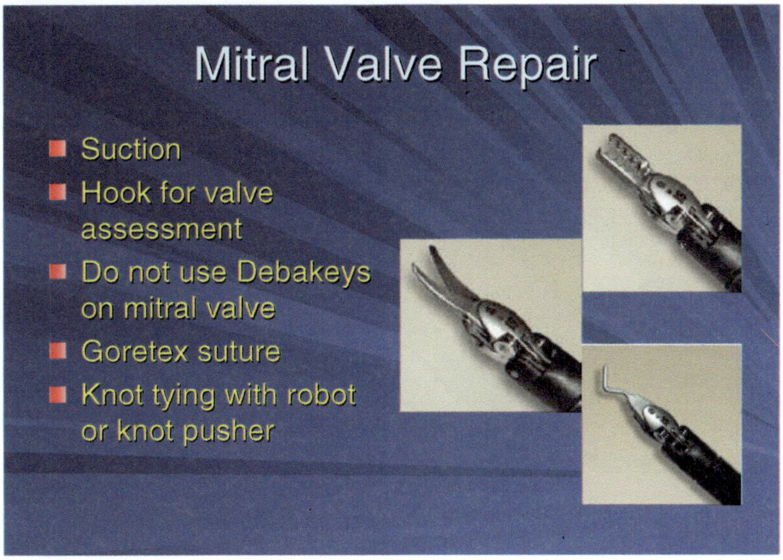

Fig. 41.20 Robotic instruments

dioplegia hole and under TEE guidance as the ventricle is filled with blood and both lungs are being ventilated. The table is titled in Trendelenburg with the head of the patient down. Aorta is then declamped and the cardioplegia suture should be secure before ECC is completed (Figs. 41.21 and 41.22).

Two chest tubes are inserted through the thoracotomies and placed over the diaphragm and at the apex of the right chest. A transthoracic intercostal catheter is placed posteriorly in the incision prior to closure and continuous Marcaine is given for the first 48 h.

Then the patient should be reintubated with a regular endotracheal tube before being brought to the intensive care unit (Fig. 41.23).

41.4 Summary

Robotic mitral valve repair can be performed by experienced teams. The results are clearly center and operator dependent. Before starting a robotic program, training of the entire staff has to be performed. Modification of the anesthesiology and of the extracorporeal circulation is essential in

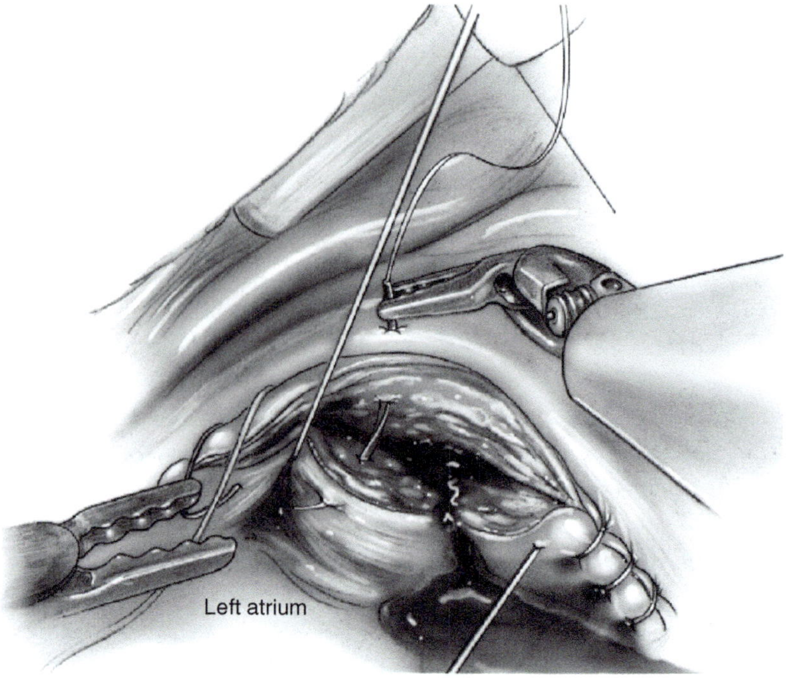

Fig. 41.21 Atrial closure performed with 4-0 Gore-Tex starting at either end and running toward the middle of the atrium

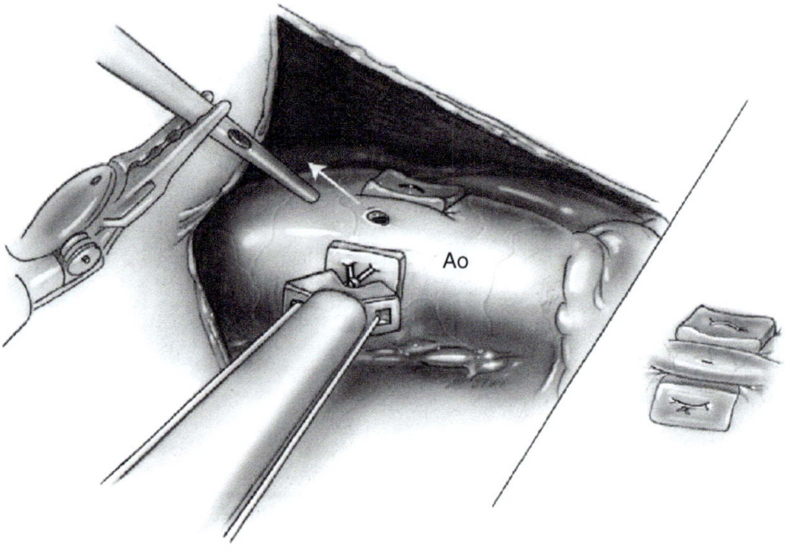

Fig. 41.22 The cardioplegia is removed, air is purged before tying with pledgeted sutures of 4-0

order to obtain good results. Also regular practice is needed in order to keep the team efficient, and therefore this technique should be applied only in high-volume centers. Compared with median sternotomy, most studies have shown decreased blood loss, more rapid recovery, and shorter hospitalization with the robotic approach. However increased operative time including cardiopulmonary and aortic cross clamp times, as well as an increase in cost, is associated with robotic surgery. Short-term results are acceptable and compared with median sternotomy in terms of mortality and morbidity; however long term-results show a slight increase in reoperation with the robotic approach. Again this may be related to the learning curve since experience is extremely important in order to obtain good results (Tables 41.1, 41.2, 41.3, and 41.4).

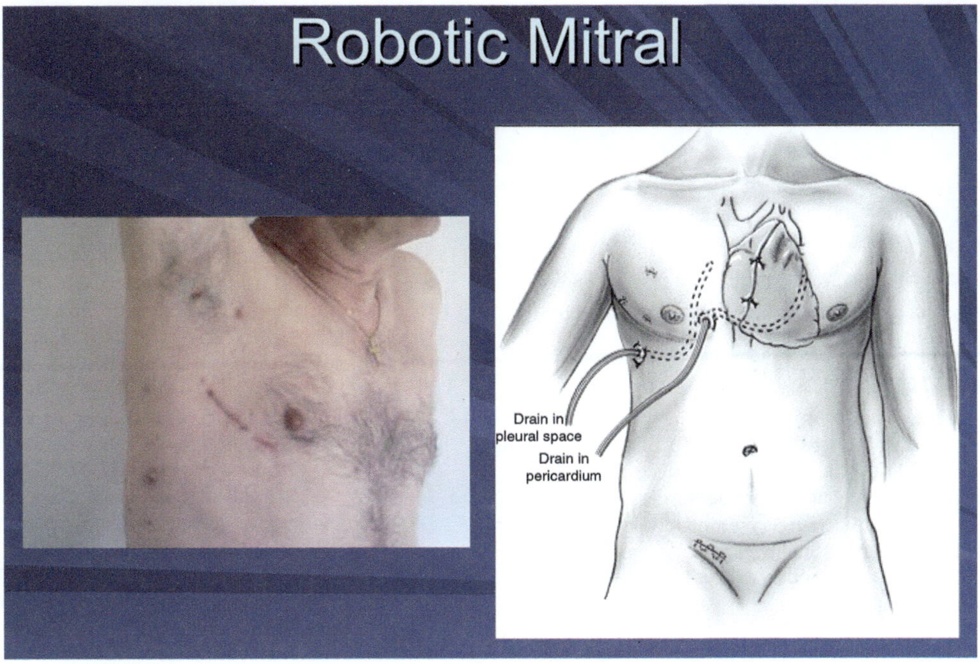

Fig. 41.23 Incisions and drains placement after closure

Table 41.1 Demographic data

Age 47 (17–81)	
H 14 F 16	
Euroscore 3	
FEVG 55	
Mitrale 30	
26 Prolapsus P2	
1 Prolapsus P1	
1 Cleft grande valve mitrale	
1 Mitrale ischémique (redux)	
1 CAV partiel	
Characteristic	Robotic ($n = 30$)
Age (years) mean	47.3 ± 11.2
Sex	
Female	14 (36%)
Male	16 (64%)
EF mean	0.55
MR grade	
3+	16 (44%)
4+	14 (56%)
NYHA	
Class I	17 (68%)
Class II	11 (24%)
Class III	2 (8%)
Euroscore	3.18 ± 10.3
Rhythm	
Sinus	29 (96%)
Arrhythmias	1 (4%)

Table 41.2 Operative data

Variable mean ± SD	Robotic ($n = 30$)
Procedure time (min)	241 ± 53.3
CPB (min)	123.1 ± 25.7
Cross clamp (min)	98.1 ± 24.3
Ring annuloplasty (min)	49.3 ± 3.8
Leaflet repair (min)	36.1 ± 6.8

Table 41.3 Postoperative data

Variable	Sternotomy ($n = 25$)	Robotic ($n = 25$)	p
Intubation time (min)	12.8 ± 6.1	11.4 ± 6.5	0.8
ICU (h)	48.5 ± 4.3	35.7 ± 4.8	0.3
Bleeding (ml)	566.2 ± 201.8	477.2 ± 212.5	0.2
PRBC transfusion	4 (16%)	2 (8%)	0.8
Length of stay (d)	9	7	0.05

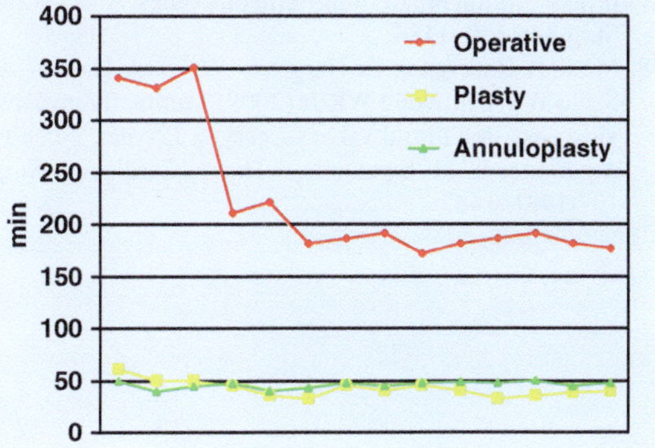

Table 41.4 Postoperative complications

Variable	Robotic (n=30)
Conversion thoracotomy	1 (4%)
Reoperations for bleeding	2 (8%)
TIA	1 (4%)
Groin lymphocele	3 (12%)
Pleural effusion	3 (12%)
Reoperations for MR	1 (4%)
Peripheral embolus	1 (4%)

TIA transient ischemic attack, *MR* mitral regurgitation

References

1. Vanermen H, Wellens F, De Geest R, Degrieck I, Van Praet F (1999) Video-assisted port-access mitral valve surgery: from debut to routine surgery. Will trocar-port-access cardiac surgery ultimately lead to robotic cardiac surgery? Semin Thorac Cardiovasc Surg 11:223–234
2. Mohr FW, Falk V, Diegeler A, Walther T, van Son JA, Autschbach R (1998) Minimally invasive port-access mitral valve surgery. J Thorac Cardiovasc Surg 115:567–574; discussion 574–566
3. Raanani E, Spiegelstein D, Sternik L, Preisman S, Moshkovitz Y, Smolinsky AK, Shinfeld A (2010) Quality of mitral valve repair: median sternotomy versus port-access approach. J Thorac Cardiovasc Surg 140:86–90
4. Aybek T, Dogan S, Risteski PS, Zierer A, Wittlinger T, Wimmer-Greinecker G, Moritz A (2006) Two hundred forty minimally invasive mitral operations through right minithoracotomy. Ann Thorac Surg 81:1618–1624
5. Casselman FP, La Meir M, Jeanmart H, Mazzarro E, Coddens J, Van Praet F, Wellens F, Vermeulen Y, Vanermen H (2007) Endoscopic mitral and tricuspid valve surgery after previous cardiac surgery. Circulation 116:I270–I275
6. Casselman FP, Van Slycke S, Dom H, Lambrechts DL, Vermeulen Y, Vanermen H (2003) Endoscopic mitral valve repair: feasible, reproducible, and durable. J Thorac Cardiovasc Surg 125:273–282
7. Galloway AC, Schwartz CF, Ribakove GH, Crooke GA, Gogoladze G, Ursomanno P, Mirabella M, Culliford AT, Grossi EA (2009) A decade of minimally invasive mitral repair: long-term outcomes. Ann Thorac Surg 88:1180–1184
8. Modi P, Rodriguez E, Hargrove WC 3rd, Hassan A, Szeto WY, Chitwood WR Jr (2009) Minimally invasive video-assisted mitral valve surgery: a 12-year, 2-center experience in 1178 patients. J Thorac Cardiovasc Surg 137:1481–1487
9. Seeburger J, Borger MA, Falk V, Kuntze T, Czesla M, Walther T, Doll N, Mohr FW (2008) Minimal invasive mitral valve repair for mitral regurgitation: results of 1339 consecutive patients. Eur J Cardiothorac Surg 34:760–765
10. Lapenna E, Torracca L, De Bonis M, La Canna G, Crescenzi G, Alfieri O (2005) Minimally invasive mitral valve repair in the context of Barlow's disease. Ann Thorac Surg 79:1496–1499
11. Morgan JA, Thornton BA, Peacock JC, Hollingsworth KW, Smith CR, Oz MC, Argenziano M (2005) Does robotic technology make minimally invasive cardiac surgery too expensive? A hospital cost analysis of robotic and conventional techniques. J Card Surg 20:246–251
12. Folliguet T, Vanhuyse F, Constantino X, Realli M, Laborde F (2006) Mitral valve repair robotic versus sternotomy. Eur J Cardiothorac Surg 29:362–366
13. Jones BA, Krueger S, Howell D, Meinecke B, Dunn S (2005) Robotic mitral valve repair: a community hospital experience. Tex Heart Inst J 32:143–146
14. Chitwood WR Jr, Kypson AP, Nifong LW (2003) Robotic mitral valve surgery: a technologic and economic revolution for heart centers. Am Heart Hosp J 1:30–39
15. Chitwood WR Jr, Nifong LW, Elbeery JE, Chapman WH, Albrecht R, Kim V, Young JA (2000) Robotic mitral valve repair: trapezoidal resection and prosthetic annuloplasty with the da Vinci surgical system. J Thorac Cardiovasc Surg 120:1171–1172
16. Rodriguez E, Nifong LW, Chu MW, Wood W, Vos PW, Chitwood WR (2008) Robotic mitral valve repair for anterior leaflet and bileaflet prolapse. Ann Thorac Surg 85:438–444; discussion 444
17. Murphy DA, Miller JS, Langford DA (2007) Endoscopic robotic mitral valve surgery. J Thorac Cardiovasc Surg 133:1119–1120; author reply 1120
18. Akpinar B, Guden M, Sagbas E, Sanisoglu I, Caynak B, Bayramoglu Z (2006) Robotic enhanced totally endoscopic mitral valve repair and ablative therapy. Ann Thorac Surg 81:1095–1098
19. Smith JM, Stein H, Engel AM, McDonough S, Lonneman L (2007) Totally endoscopic mitral valve repair using a robotic-controlled atrial retractor. Ann Thorac Surg 84:633–637
20. Reade CC, Johnson JO, Bolotin G, Freund WL Jr, Jenkins NL, Bower CE, Masroor S, Kypson AP, Nifong LW, Chitwood WR Jr (2005) Combining robotic mitral valve repair and microwave atrial fibrillation ablation: techniques and initial results. Ann Thorac Surg 79:480–484
21. Chitwood WR Jr, Rodriguez E, Chu MW, Hassan A, Ferguson TB, Vos PW, Nifong LW (2008) Robotic mitral valve repairs in 300 patients: a single-center experience. J Thorac Cardiovasc Surg 136:436–441

22. Nifong LW, Chitwood WR, Pappas PS, Smith CR, Argenziano M, Starnes VA, Shah PM (2005) Robotic mitral valve surgery: a United States multicenter trial. J Thorac Cardiovasc Surg 129:1395–1404
23. Woo YJ, Nacke EA (2006) Robotic minimally invasive mitral valve reconstruction yields less blood product transfusion and shorter length of stay. Surgery 140:263–267
24. Sobieski MA 2nd, Slaughter MS, Hart DE, Pappas PS, Tatooles AJ (2003) Peripheral cardiopulmonary bypass with modified assisted venous drainage and transthoracic aortic crossclamp: optimal management for robotic mitral valve repair. Perfusion 18:307–311
25. Dogan S, Aybek T, Risteski PS, Detho F, Rapp A, Wimmer-Greinecker G, Moritz A (2005) Minimally invasive port access versus conventional mitral valve surgery: prospective randomized study. Ann Thorac Surg 79:492–498
26. Reichenspurner H, Detter C, Deuse T, Boehm DH, Treede H, Reichart B (2005) Video and robotic-assisted minimally invasive mitral valve surgery: a comparison of the Port-Access and transthoracic clamp techniques. Ann Thorac Surg 79:485–490; discussion 490–481
27. Maselli D, Pizio R, Borelli G, Musumeci F (2006) Endovascular balloon versus transthoracic aortic clamping for minimally invasive mitral valve surgery: impact on cerebral microemboli. Interact Cardiovasc Thorac Surg 5:183–186

Minimal Access Aortic Valve Surgery

42

Roberto Pasquale Casula

Contents

R.P. Casula, M.D., FRCS, FETCS
Department of Cardiothoracic Surgery, St. Mary's Hospital, Imperial College Healthcare NHS Trust, Praed Street, London, W2 1NY, UK

Hammersmith Hospital, Imperial Healthcare College NHS Trust, London, UK
e-mail: roberto.casula@imperial.nhs.uk

42.1 Clincal Background

Aortic valve replacements (AVRs) amount to the second most common cardiac surgical procedures performed worldwide, their indication been mainly represented by symptomatic severe aortic valve stenosis (AS). The most common cause of AS is the calcific degeneration of the anatomically normal tri-cusp aortic valve which becomes increasingly common after the seventh decade of life.

The UK sixth National Adult Cardiac Surgical 2008 report shows a mortality rate 1.8% in nearly 5,000 patients aged 60–70 years old operated in 2004–2008, while it increases to 5.5% for 420 patients over the age of 85 who had isolated aortic valve surgery in the same time frame. Despite these excellent surgical results, it was observed once more that 'older' age remains strongly associated with an increased morbidity and mortality following first time AVR surgery. Very limited surgical data is available to assess any potential benefits of minimal access procedures compared to conventional surgery in these older patients population despite the understandable working hypothesis that older and fragile patients would potentially benefits also in terms of mortality from less invasive procedures.

Most commonly aortic valve surgery is performed via a median sternotomy and on cardiopulmonary bypass, and this type of conventional aortic valve replacement following excision of the native aortic valve can be performed solely on cardiopulmonary bypass. The median sternotomy

R.G.C. Inderbitzi et al. (eds.), *Minimally Invasive Thoracic and Cardiac Surgery*,
DOI 10.1007/978-3-642-11861-6_42, © Springer-Verlag Berlin Heidelberg 2012

incision provides surgeons with the best exposure to all heart structures and great vessels but is associated with a significant post-operative morbidity and is also responsible for the slow patients' recovery post-cardiac surgery commonly seen in the elderly.

In most recent times, trans-aortic valve implantation (TAVI) has allowed both cardiologists and surgeons' teams to deploy sutureless aortic prosthesis following AV balloon valvuloplasty leaving the native calcific valve in situ and without cardiopulmonary bypass.

From the early 1990s, many surgical disciplines have been shaken by advent of potentially less invasive procedures performed via a minimal access approach of which the laparoscopic cholecystectomy probably represents a milestone. Also, cardiac surgery has seen several attempts to perform well-established procedures via less invasive surgical approaches in the 1990s.

Cardiac surgery has been the last to adopt minimal access surgical approaches to perform established cardiac surgical procedures compared to most of the other surgical specialties probably due to the technical complexity of most of these cardiac procedures. Minimal access operations performed via a 'non-distensible' chest are more likely to require not just a modification of the surgical equipment used but also a thorough process of adaptation from surgeons towards the new techniques via a 'learning curve' which will require a considerable number of procedures to be acquired.

Minimal access AVR potentially offers several advantages to the patients but none to the surgeon who requires some specific time consuming retraining to perform a significantly large number of procedures in order to become as familiar with these procedures as when he or she is operating via the widely used 'sternotomy approach'.

Since 1996, many minimal access approaches have been explored and many terms have been coined such as 'ministernotomy', 'hemisternotomy', 'upper sternotomy' and 'partial or limited sternotomy'. We will mainly refer to the longitudinal division of the sternal manubrium and part of the body of the sternum which is completed laterally by dividing the sternum at the level of the 3rd or 4th IC space as a 'limited upper sternotomy' (LUS). At present, this technique is the most widely used for minimal access aortic surgery worldwide.

In 1996, Cosgrove and Sabik described a minimal access approach to perform aortic valve surgery consisting of a right para-sternal incision; since then, another three different minimal access surgical approaches to the aortic valve have been described, and several clinical series have been reported for each one of them:

- The right para-sternal approach
- The transverse sternotomy
- The minimal right thoracotomy
- The limited upper sternotomy

The first two of them do only retain historic value while the limited upper sternotomy (LUS) approach has certainly become the gold standard technique for many surgeons around the world including the authors, and it will be part of a more extensive description and discussion in this chapter.

42.2 Patient Selection and Assessment

Every patient undergoing isolated aortic valve surgery is clinically assessed, and his or her suitability for a minimal access approach should be considered according to the competence level of the operating surgeon. Patients' morphological features such as chest size and chest wall abnormalities are carefully assessed and matched to both lateral and postero-anterior chest x-ray findings.

Absolute contraindications are uniquely represented by the presence of important chest wall (i.e. pectus type) or vertebral spine deformities and by the case of severe obesity. Large patients with an uncommonly large antero-posterior chest dimension also represent a technical challenge. In those cases, an unpredictable variation from the normal internal anatomy can be responsible for an excessive distance and tackling angle between the surgical incision and the location of the aortic valve plane resulting with an inadequate surgical exposure.

Re-operations to the aortic valve via a limited upper sternotomy have been reported and should only be performed when a large experience with the 'first time' procedures has been safely acquired. In case of previous coronary surgery, the presence of a patent left internal mammary artery to the left anterior descending coronary artery does not represent a contraindication since the operation can be performed with at least moderate hypothermia and by delivering regular doses of cardioplegia without need for LIMA mobilisation and clamping just as many surgeons would do also in the case of a redo full median sternotomy.

The need for coronary artery bypass grafting remains a limitation for a minimal access approach since no target coronary artery can be appropriately visualised or exposed. As an alternative in these cases, a hybrid approach could be considered which combines a single or double vessel percutaneous coronary intervention with coronary stents usually performed prior to the minimal access AVR. Feasibility and safety of the hybrid approach have been extensively reported; individual cases should be assessed also according to the skills and experience of each individual cardiac team.

In the case of a limited upper sternotomy (LUS), the patient is prepared on the operating table in a supine position just as in a case of a median sternotomy, and similarly the chest skin is prepped and draped including the routine preparation of one or both the groin areas.

External defibrillating equipment use is mandatory, and defibrillating pads are carefully positioned over the left anterior and posterior thorax. Accurate placements and waterproof isolation are advisable for their perfect function since neither adult standard nor paediatric defibrillation hand-held pads can be fitted in a suitable location if a correct minimal access approach had been performed (Table 42.1).

Anaesthesia is induced and the patient is intubated with a single-lumen tube as in conventional sternotomy surgery.

Intra-operative trans-oesophageal echocardiography (TOE) is mandatory in all cases of aortic valve surgery, and all parameters assessed in a conventional aortic valve operation performed via a median sternotomy should be equally assessed in a minimal access procedure. TOE retains paramount importance in the cases of minimal access AVR particularly for the following reasons:

- In the event in which femoral vein cannulation is required, TOE guidance will assist the surgeon in accurately positioning a double stage femoral venous cannula to reach up to the origin of the superior vena cava for perfect venous drainage.
- It allows monitoring of any left ventricular distension during the delivery of antegrade cardioplegia.
- It is mandatory to assist the surgeon with a thorough de-airing process after releasing the aortic cross-clamp.
- In order to assist both the surgeon and the anaesthesiologist during the weaning of the patient from cardiopulmonary bypass. In the case of truly minimal access, no visual or conventional manual assessment of right ventricular preload and overall ventricular contractility can be made.

Table 42.1 Ten technical steps/guides to LUS AVR approach

1. Avoid extreme obese or very tall patients at the beginning of your experience
2. Start by performing the reverse 'J' into the 4th IC space and move up to 3rd once more experienced
3. Use a flat Medtronic bi-caval venous cannula centrally when possible
4. If point 3 is not possible, then percutaneous cannulation (Estech Femoral venous cannula; REF 200–100; 200–150)
5. Use 'head light' routinely
6. Position accurately defibrillation pads since no alternative internal pads can be fitted via a truly LUS incision
7. Open widely the right pleura and drain both pleural space and pericardium
8. Position ventricular temporary pacing leads before releasing the aortic cross-clamp
9. Do not use upper pulmonary vein vent and allow bleeding via aortotomy when suturing aorta back
10. Allow antegrade extensive de-airing via ascending aorta under TOE guidance

In the patients' consent discussion, a less than 3% risk of conversion to median sternotomy and for the uncommon need of peripheral femoral arterial and/or venous cannulation should be mentioned.

Despite in experienced hands, the conversion rate to a full sternotomy is very low at less than 3%; it is advisable to safely convert to a full sternotomy in the case of poor exposure in the early stage of each surgeon experience.

42.3 Surgical Techniques

42.3.1 The Limited Upper Sternotomy Approach (LUS)

Several clinical series reported have shown that the reversed 'J' approach for minimal access aortic valve surgery is as safe and effective as the conventional sternotomy approach, and at present it represents the gold standard minimal access approach for aortic valve surgery.

The limited upper sternotomy (LUS) (Fig. 42.1a) was initially described by Gundry et al. in 1998. In an adult patient, the skin incision can be often limited to 6–8 cm circa in length starting at the Luis sternal angle and continuing longitudinally over the middle of the sternum.

In its original description, the sternum is divided in a reverse 'T' fashion; this can be achieved with a redo oscillating saw and ideally with a narrow blade. The sternal incision is completed to the left and right transversally into the intercostal space chosen. The decision to which intercostal space to enter should be facilitated by a careful chest x-ray assessment. It is advisable to enter the 4th space in order to allow a more generous exposure in patients with severe emphysema or when the chest x-ray shows that the heart lies transversally onto the diaphragm.

Gundry et al. suggested to locate the distance of the annulus of the aortic valve with TOE probe from the upper manubrium of the sternum in order to chose if entering the 3rd or 4th IC space which can surely be of advisable during the initial phase of a surgeon learning curve.

The upper sternum is divided longitudinally from the top of the manubrium, and the sternal incision is completed as a 'T' laterally to the right and left at the level of the 3rd or 4th IC space with the use of an oscillating saw.

This approach has been modified by Svensson's and Tam's separate groups in the way that a sternal 'reversed J' incision is performed as an alternative to the original description of a complete transverse sternotomy. In this case, the redo oscillating saw is used to start the longitudinal sternal

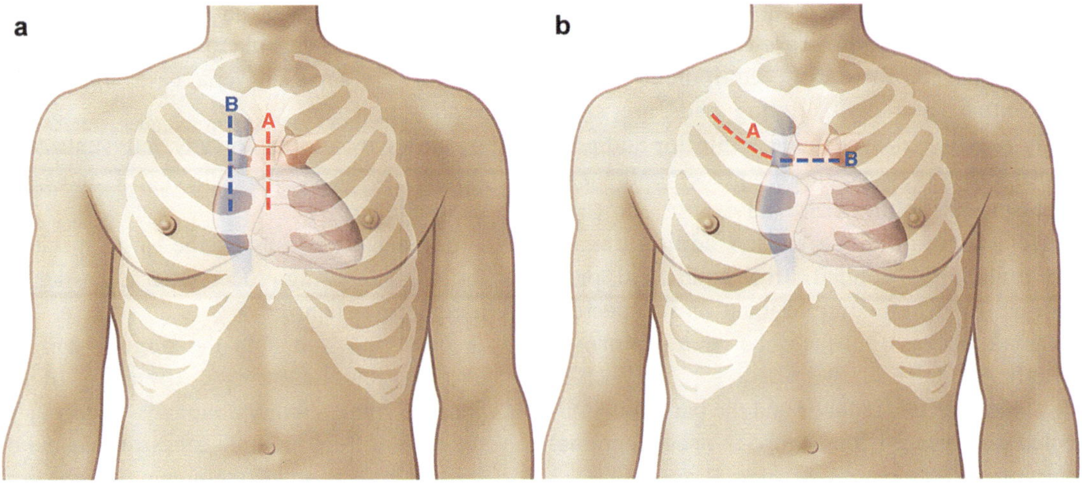

Fig. 42.1 (**a**) LUS and para-sternal approaches skin incisions and (**b**) transverse sternotomy and right mini-thoracotomy skin incisions

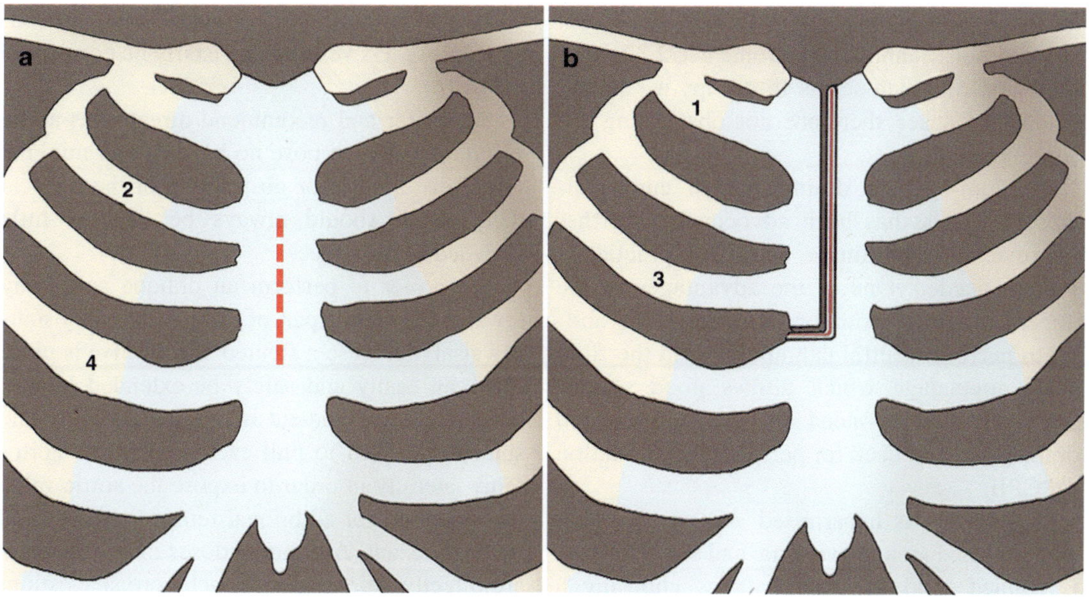

Fig. 42.2 Skin incision (**a**) and sternal incision (**b**) in the case of limited upper sternotomy

incision which is then completed solely to the right into the 3rd or 4th intercostal space.

Alternatively, a traditional sternal saw is engaged in the upper manubrium, directed caudally and eventually turned aside to the right into the 3rd or 4th intercostal space (Fig. 42.2).

The limited upper sternotomy approach allows a good surgical exposure of the ascending aorta down to the aortic root and of the right atrial appendage allowing central cannulation for cardiopulmonary bypass in the vast majority of cases. Several groups have described more complex aortic procedures including aortic root surgery and homografts or stentless valve replacements via the limited upper sternotomy.

We use an Estech (San Ramon, CA) minimal invasive retractor which is positioned to spread the two upper halves of the sternum apart, and the maximum spread length achievable is about 6 cm wide. The thymic fat is dissected off the pericardium and resected up to the brachio-chephalic vein. The pericardium is opened similarly to the sternum in a longitudinal fashion from the brachio-chephalic vein down, just to expose the right appendage, and it is left to great extent intact and surrounding left and right ventricles. The pericardial hedges are carefully pulled by retraction sutures in order to gently pull the aortic valve and root plane closer to the surgical incision (Fig. 42.3).

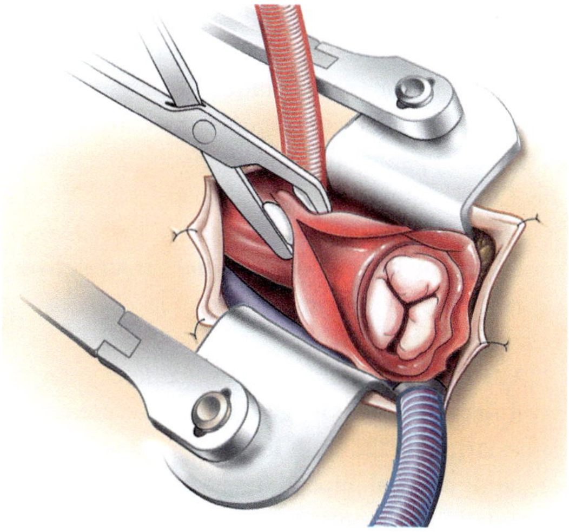

Fig. 42.3 LUS drawing from operative site showing both arterial and 2-stage venous cannulae in place. The aortic valve is seen via the aortotomy

3/0 or 4/0 Prolene cannulation sutures are placed in the distal ascending aorta for securing in place the arterial cannula and to position an aortic cardioplegia cannula with a lateral arm for the vent site. Our preference is to cannulate the aorta with a Medtronic Iopa 774 and to cannulate the right atrial appendage with a bi-caval oval shape venous cannula (Medtronic MC2 32/40 or MC2 36/46) which seems to occupy a minimal amount of space therefore not obstructing the aortic valve view.

Vacuum-assisted drainage with cardiopulmonary bypass has been advocated to further improve venous drainage but in our practice is seldom needed. One of the advantages of the upper limited sternotomy approach is the ability to perform central cannulation via the right atrial appendage which allows good venous drainage with no need for vacuum-assisted drainage and no need for peripheral cannulation for CPB.

The patient is heparinised and an umbilical tape is placed around the aorta, and some traction is applied caudally which allows choosing a higher position for aortic cannulation. After aortic cross-clamping which can be carried out with a conventional right-angled aortic cross-clamp without disturbing the working field, cardioplegia is delivered into the aortic root in case of aortic stenosis or regurgitation no more than moderate. Trans-oesophageal echocardiography (TOE) is of paramount importance in assessing if any LV dilatation occurs while cardioplegic solution has been delivered. In case LV distension is observed, the aorta is opened and direct delivery of cardioplegia is administered via each of the coronary ostia.

A retrograde cardioplegia catheter can be positioned under TOE guidance after creating a purse string on the right lateral aspect at the base of the right atrial appendage just below the atrial cannulation site only in the case the chest had been entered via the 4th IC space. A few published reports highlighted the risk of atrial perforation, therefore it is advisable to avoid this technique altogether and to limit cardioplegia solution delivery directly into the coronary ostia. Gundry et al. reported that in 8% of cases, a retrograde catheter could not be successfully positioned.

After commencing cardiopulmonary bypass, LV venting can be achieved either via the right upper pulmonary vein which is safely reachable only once the heart is decompressed on CPB or uncommonly via the left atrial appendage (LAA). PA venting can easily be performed as well.

We prefer and recommend direct trans-aortic LV venting which pose no hazards and minimal visual disturbance or obstruction of the surgical field which should always be kept as little crowded as possible.

We prefer to perform an oblique aortotomy towards the middle part of the non-coronary sinus of valsalva in case a stented aortic valve is used. This can easily and safely be extended in case aortic root enlargement is required. 4/0 Prolene sutures are used to pull each side of the aortotomy laterally in order to expose the aortic valve without need for additional retractors to be held by an assistant. Additional doses of cardioplegia are directly delivered into each coronary ostium at regular 30-min intervals.

We start by positioning 2/0 Ethibond stay stitches to each commeasure in order to gently pull the aortic valve plane closer to the incision and further improve valve exposure.

The risk of air embolism due to poor ability to de-air has been advocated as a potential limitation in the case of any type of minimal invasive approach. CO_2 continuous insufflation directly onto the surgical field has been claimed to reduce intracardiac air trapping.

Cardiac de-airing starts with removal of the trans-aortic LV vent while closing the aortotomy and positioning the patient in anti-Trendelenburgh position to allow filling of the LV apex with blood. Ascending aorta venting is started at completion of the aortotomy, and air evacuation is facilitated by manual lungs ventilation and gentle heart filling under TOE guidance. In the authors' experience, a prolonged antegrade suctioning at the ascending aorta level has been a safe a reliable technique even in the in absence of CO_2 surgical field insufflation.

The aortotomy is closed with running 4/0 Prolene in one or two layers, and in our practice we stopped using CO_2 irrigation of the surgical field in 2003 with no clinical consequences in our patients neurological outcome.

Positioning of ventricular pacing wires is difficult and hazardous if accomplished after removal of the aortic cross-clamp with a non-decompressed heart. It is recommended to gently expose the right ventricular free wall and position epicardial temporary pacing wires while the heart is still cardioplegic and obviously decompressed. It is our preference to open the right pleura at the end of the procedure and the pacing wires being passed outside the chest via the 4th right IC space laterally to the RIMA.

The pericardial retraction sutures should be released before coming off cardiopulmonary bypass.

A 28-F curved chest drain is left in situ to drain the right pleural space which we routinely open at the end of the procedure to reduce the risk of cardiac tamponade since the pericardium surrounding the left and right ventricles is always left intact. A second curved 28-F chest drain is inserted into the chest medially to the previous one and positioned over the ascending aorta and pulmonary artery and with its tip reaching the pericardium rapping the apex of the heart.

The chest drains are exteriorised in a cosmetically appropriate position underneath and laterally to the right nipple in men while in the sub-mammary fold in women. The upper sternum is re-approximated with sternal steel wires or Ethibond sternal sutures transversally which allows optimal stability of the sternum of which its lower end remains intact (Fig. 42.4).

Advantages of this approach are that the internal mammary arteries are not sacrificed and conversion to a full sternotomy can be easily and rapidly performed if required. Furthermore, the full stability of the sternum is maintained also in the uncommon case for a conversion to a full sternotomy. An advantage compared to the other minimal access techniques described is the ability to perform central aortic and right atrium cannulation in the vast majority of cases. In the authors experience in a very minority of cases, femoral either arterial or venous cannulation or both is required in order to maximise the working space through the limited incision.

A sternal saw should be kept in the sterile surgical field until the end of the procedure, and a battery-operated saw should be kept readily available in the cardiac recovery area in case of cardiac arrest requiring internal cardiac massage should present.

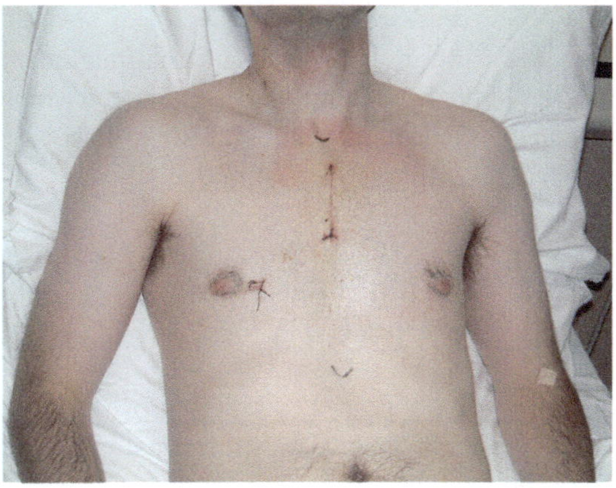

Fig. 42.4 Cosmetic result after a limited upper sternotomy (LUS) aortic valve replacement

42.3.2 The Transverse Sternotomy

This minimal access approach (Fig. 42.1b) to the aortic valve was originally used in the late 1990s but currently no longer utilised. It requires a 10–12-cm skin incision most commonly performed transversally above the sternum which is usually transversally sewn at the level of the 2nd IC or 3rd IC spaces. The pericardium above the aorta can be opened longitudinally, and its edges are pulled up to improved the aortic root exposure. Central venous cannulation by use of a two-stage right atrial cannula is most commonly achievable while femoral aortic cannulation may be required. Exposure of the aortic valve, part of the ascending aorta, and right atrium can usually be achieved, and the sternum is re-approximated by a figure of ‘eight’ or two separate sternal wires at the end of the procedure.

If a conversion to a full longitudinal sternotomy is required, this would result in four sternal fragments which even after careful closure could be responsible for an increased sternal instability at the end of the procedure.

Further drawbacks of this approach are also the need for transecting both internal mammary arteries at the level of the entered IC space which would preclude their future utilisation in case surgical revascularisation will be required.

42.3.3 The Right Para-Sternal Approach

It was originally described by Cosgrove in 1996 and at present maintains only historical value and is no longer in use (Fig. 42.1a).

An 8–10-cm skin incision circa is required which extends from over the second costal cartilage to the fifth. The muscle plane is divided and both the third and fourth IC cartilages are excised. The right internal mammary artery is most commonly transected while sometimes can be carefully retracted laterally. Both the pericardium and right pleural spaces are entered, and usually exposure of the aortic valve, most of the ascending aorta, and right atrium can be achieved. The pericardial edges are pulled in order to better expose the aortic root. Central venous and arterial cannulation is not easily achievable, and in most of the cases both arterial and venous femoral cannulation is required.

A limitation of this approach has been the consequent anterior chest wall instability which can result from the excision of costal cartilages. The sacrifice of the right internal mammary artery and the need for femoral arterial and venous cannulation make this approach a less attractive surgical option. Degenerative aortic valve disease is independently associated to aortic atherosclerosis which makes femoral arterial cannulation and retrograde perfusion less than ideal compared to direct ascending aorta cannulation and antitrade arterial perfusion by increasing the risks of embolism and peripheral vascular complications.

Furthermore, in the case of poor exposure or the need for an emergency conversion, the performance of a sternotomy is not practical and more likely to leave the patient with chest wall potential instability. Increased rate of wound complication has been reported.

42.3.4 The Right Anterior Mini-thoracotomy

It was initially described by Benetti et al. in 1997 and then popularised by the New York University Medical Centre surgeons since the late 1990s (Fig. 42.1b). This surgical approach is uncommonly used at present.

The patient is most commonly positioned supine on the operating table, and the entire chest and groins are prepared and draped as for a conventional approach. The right chest can be somewhat elevated by inflating a pressure bag underneath the right scapula.

The skin incision can be limited to 6–8 cm (Fig. 42.1) and is performed laterally to the sternum over the 3rd IC space. The subcutaneous tissue and muscle planes are divided, and the chest is entered most commonly via the 2nd or 3rd IC space which is opened, and gentle rib spreading is achieved via a small thoracotomy spreader. Removal of costal cartilages is not required, and the limited length of skin incision prevents excessive rib spreading.

Femoral cannulation is most commonly required while direct aortic cross-clamping and antegrade cardioplegia delivery are feasible in the vast majority of patients. Limitations of this approach are potential limited exposure since rib fractures have to be avoided if the benefits of a minimal invasive approach have to be maintained. Furthermore, conversion to a median sternotomy would be less than practical and lead to a larger degree of surgical trauma than predicted.

In 2001, Kort et al. highlighted the need for femoral cannulation in half of their cases.

In 2003, Colvin group reported that in a case-match analysis conducted on a comparative retrospective study of 169 patients, central direct aortic cannulation was feasible in 89.4% and femoral arterial in the remaining while femoral vein cannulation in 69%. Colvin and his group showed that their minimal access AVR patients were comparable to the sternotomy ones in terms of post-operative mortality and morbidity at 36 months follow-up. The minimal access patients appeared to have a significantly shorter hospital stay, and a higher proportion of them were sent directly home rather than to a rehabilitation facility or nursing home (52.6% vs. 38.6%; $p=0.03$).

42.4 Discussion

We would expect that cardiac surgeons do perform their continuous surgical training in order also to tailor their surgical incisions to the procedure to be carried out regardless their own comfort zone. The aim of a minimal access approach should be to minimise the amount of surgical trauma and try to preserve the integrity of the rib cage as much as feasible by limiting the amount of skin, soft tissue, muscle and bone structures trauma and moreover reducing the level of sternal spread required during surgery.

Several clinical series reported in the late 1990s have mostly described surgical initial experiences and retrospective limited clinical series comprising a small number of operations. Cardiac surgeons who have performed many hundred operations via a full sternotomy are used to see every part of the heart and great vessels even if they do not have to operate on all of them as in the case of isolated valve surgery. Understandably, surgeons have developed a natural sense of confidence since almost any unexpected complication can be rapidly and easily controlled while operating passing through a fully open sternum. Moving away from this safe platform into a much smaller incision obviously requires further training, a certain degree of psycho-physical adaptation and an increased level of surgical dexterity. In the case of minimal access valve surgery, the completion of its learning curve could require a few hundred cases to be performed. Most of the series reported do not seem to take into consideration any issue relative to the learning curve involved, and consequently numerical variables such as operative, cardiopulmonary and aortic cross-clamp times have often resulted to be longer compared to the ones recorded with conventional procedures performed using a sternotomy.

Minimal access AV surgery requires small changes in the routinely used instrumentation with no added cost of disposables but mostly a period of technical training.

In aortic redo surgery performed via a ‘redo’ median sternotomy, it is common practice for many experienced surgeons to leave the left ventricle and part of the RV un-dissected from surrounded structures such as the pericardium or left lung. Exposure of mainly the cannulation sites and ascending aorta is commonly achieved while the rest of the heart such as the left and right ventricles are not dissected off their surrounding structures while operating on a redo AVR. Similarly, we could argue that there is no need to see all cardiac structures apart from the right atrium, ascending aorta and aortic root when performing a first time aortic valve replacement.

The Brigham and Women Hospital group’s experience does confirm that the upper limited sternotomy approach is safe and effective and can be offered to the vast majority of patients with few exclusion criteria which will reduce dramatically the need for conversion to sternotomy due to poor surgical exposure.

In 2006, the same Brigham group reported of 861 minimal access aortic valve replacements performed via a limited upper sternotomy approach of which 117 were re-operations. Their experience clearly confirms that all valve substitutes could be used including homografts and stentless prosthesis.

Despite some limited series published in the late 1990s have shown a marginally longer aortic cross-clamp and/or cardiopulmonary bypass (CPB) times, once the full learning curve of such a minimal access procedure is acquired, both aortic cross-clamp, cardiopulmonary bypass and also overall procedure duration times will not be significantly increased compared to the ones of similar operations performed with a conventional sternotomy approach. This is evidently shown by the Brigham group who showed an improvement over the time; their aortic cross-clamp and CPB times were 91 and 124 min, respectively, in the first 365 patients operated upon while in the entire series of 861 cases, they were 79 and 109, respectively.

Brown et al. in a systematic review and meta-analysis published in 2009 and comprising 2,054

Table 42.2 Time to extubation (in hours)

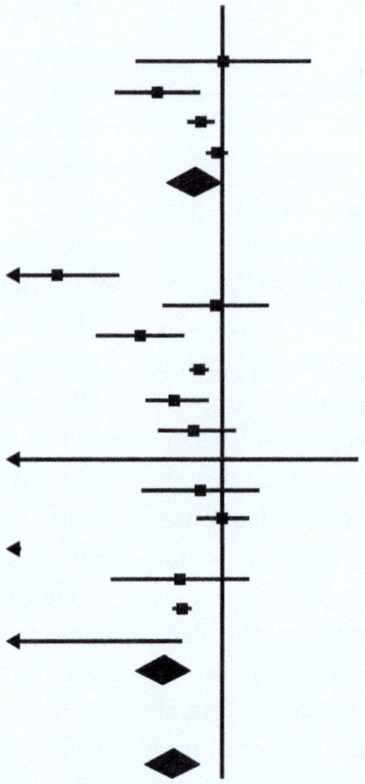

Study	WMD (random) 95%	Weight %	WMD (random) 95% CI
Randomized			
Aris		2.98	0.00 [−4.02, 4.02]
Machler		6.62	−3.00 [−4.91, −1.09]
Bonacchi		9.66	−0.90 [−1.52, −0.28]
Dogan		9.18	−0.20 [−1.07, 0.67]
Subtotal (95% CI)		28.44	−0.96 [−1.93, 0.01]
Observational			
Chang		4.52	−7.60 [−10.50, −4.70]
Christiansen		5.40	−0.30 [−2.74, 2.14]
Liu		6.50	−3.83 [−5.78, −1.88]
Szwerc		10.0	−1.10 [−1.49, −0.71]
Ehrlich		7.98	−2.20 [−3.57, −0.83]
Detter		6.99	−1.20 [−2.96, 0.56]
Doll		0.14	−16.00 [−38.16, 6.16]
Lee		4.73	−1.00 [−3.78, 1.78]
Masiello		8.31	0.00 [−1.24, 1.24]
Corbi		1.93	−21.38 [−26.72, −16.04]
Farhat		4.09	−2.00 [−5.16, 1.16]
Suenega		9.96	−1.85 [−2.28, −1.42]
Bakir		1.02	−9.60 [−17.35, −1.85]
Subtotal (95% CI)		71.56	−2.71 [−3.80, −1.62]
Total (95% CI)		100.00	−2.13 [−2.95, −1.30]
Test for heterogeneity: Chi^2 = 109.99, df = 16 ($P < 0.00001$), $I^2 = 85.5\%$			
Test for overall effect: $Z = 5.06$ ($P = 0.00001$)			

Taken from Brown et al. (2009)
Systematic review of 17 studies shows decreased time to extubation in minimal access group vs. conventional sternotomy. Time to extubation in hours after operation
This table demonstrates pooled estimates for time to extubation. Estimates less than 1 indicate decreased time to extubation with ministernotomy approach (*MINI*). This is divided into randomized and observational studies
WMD weighted mean difference, *CI* confidence interval, *df* degrees of freedom, *FULL* full sternotomy

limited upper sternotomy cases showed that the aortic cross-clamp and total cardiopulmonary bypass duration were an average of 7.9 and 11.5 min longer compared to the same parameters in the conventional sternotomy. This difference is likely to carry no clinical significances (Tables 42.2 and 42.3).

Limited access is not a synonym of poor access. An adequate volume of cases will allow an experienced surgeon to increase his or her skills and surgical dexterity in order to operate through a limited access with good exposure.

42.4.1 Pain Perception and Use of Analgesics

One of the aims of minimal access aortic valve surgery is to reduce post-operative pain and consequently reduce the need for analgesics.

Less wound discomfort facilitates a deeper, more efficient breathing and more effective coughing which allows early mobilisation which has been proven to prevent lung atelectatic changes and reduce the risk of lung infections.

Table 42.3 Blood loss after operation (in milliliters per 24 h)

Study	WMD (random) 95%	Weight %	WMD (random) 95% CI
Randomized	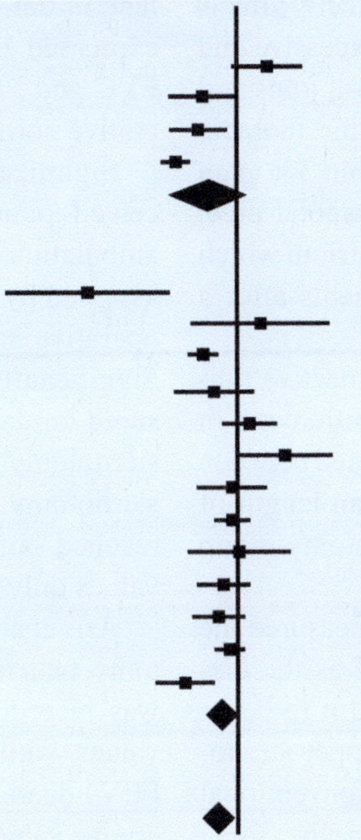		
Aris		5.71	124.00 [−14.84, 262.84]
Machler		5.83	−150.00 [−284.40, −15.60]
Bonacchi		6.55	−164.90 [−274.96, −54.84]
Dogan		7.47	−255.00 [−333.38, −176.62]
Subtotal (95% CI)		25.56	−117.90 [−268.82, 33.03]
Nonrandomized			
Byrne		2.28	−613.00 [−934.33, −291.67]
Christiansen		2.80	85.00 [−192.73, 362.73]
Liu		7.88	−140.00 [−202.62, −77.38]
Szwerc		5.17	−102.50 [−261.04, 56.04]
Ehrlich		6.68	45.00 [−60.63, 150.63]
Doll		4.49	191.00 [5.36, 376.64]
Lee		5.84	−29.00 [−163.04, 105.04]
Masiello		7.68	−31.00 [−101.60, 39.60]
Corbi		3.99	1.00 [−207.10, 209.10]
Farhat		6.64	−71.00 [179.02, 36.02]
De Smet		6.64	−85.00 [−192.05, 22.05]
Suenega		8.08	−11.00 [94.69, 12.69]
Bakir		6.29	−220.00 [−338.97, −101.03]
Subtotal (95% CI)		74.44	−63.90 [−120.38, −7.42]
Total (95% CI)		100.00	−79.37 [−135.78, −22.96]
Test for heterogeneity: $Chi^2 = 69.99$, $df = 16$ ($P < 0.00001$), $I^2 = 77.1\%$			
Test for overall effect: $Z = 2.76$ ($P = 0.006$)			

Taken from Brown et al. (2009)

Systematic review of 17 studies shows decreased time to extubation in minimal access group vs. conventional sternotomy. Blood losses after operation

This table demonstrates pooled estimates for blood loss after operation. Estimates less than 1 indicate lower volume of blood loss with ministernotomy (*MINI*) approach. This is divided into randomized and observational studies

WMD weighted mean difference, *CI* confidence interval, *df* degrees of freedom, *FULL* full sternotomy

Unfortunately, not many studies have been conducted to address these issues in an appropriately powered prospective randomised fashion to show if any significant difference exists in terms of post-operative pain between patients undergoing aortic valve replacements performed with a conventional sternotomy or by means of a limited upper sternotomy.

Perception of pain post-cardiac surgery is likely to be multi-factorial, and many factors can be intuitively alleged as been responsible for pain such as:

- The extent of the skin, soft tissue and muscles surgical incisions
- The extent of sternal bone and periostium severed both intentionally or unintentionally during surgery
- The fracture of ribs and the dislocation of costo-condral junctions
- The degree of sternal spreading

While most of the factors listed above are likely to be responsible for pain perceived at the level of and mainly in direct proximity of the surgical incision, other factors could be responsible for pain and discomfort in sites located far from the surgical incision.

The degree of sternal spreading directly affects the rib cage integrity and causes an excessive and pathologic strain on the costo-vertebral joins and stretching of the brachial plexus at the thoracic inlet joins. The latest are responsible for pain referred to areas such as the inter-scapular area, the back, the shoulders and the epigastrium which are very commonly suffered by patients after a full median sternotomy.

In 2002, Bonacchi et al. in a prospective randomised study found a significant difference in the length of the skin incision as expected between the minimal access AVR group (mean length of 8.2 cm) compared to their full sternotomy group (mean length of 23.7 cm).

In the same year, Candaele et al. measured the degree of sternal spreading reported as the distance of the sternal halves and found it to be an average of 68 mm in their limited upper sternotomy patients and 114 mm in the conventional sternotomy patients ($p<0.0001$). In the same prospective study also elegantly showed that limited upper sternotomy patients suffered a significantly less intense degree of pain at rest compared to the sternotomy patients which continued up to 1 month post-surgery. More importantly, a significant lower proportion of minimal access patients suffered from 'moderate' or 'severe' pain assessed by means of a V.A.S. score (Visual Analogue Scale) at rest, after coughing or after performing a standard spirometry. In addition, the pain distribution significantly differed between the two groups studied since 79% of the patients post-sternotomy complained also of pain referred to other site other than the sternum while only 33% of the limited upper sternotomy ones reported pain in other site other than the sternum.

42.4.2 Pulmonary Function

It is recognised that a full median sternotomy does compromise the chest wall integrity with a consequent initial impairment of respiratory function. Few studies have appropriately addressed this important aspect, and all confirmed that patients post-sternotomy do show an important initial deterioration of their lung function expressed by a decrease of up to 40% in their FVC and FEV1 values compared to their preoperative normal levels.

Significant differences in the level of perceived pain are likely to equally affect early ambulation and respiratory function which was assessed by several studies both in the early post-operative stage and at 1 month post-discharge. Significantly higher FEV1 and FVC were measured on day 4 post-surgery in the limited upper sternotomy patients compared to the conventional sternotomy patients. In the latest, their FVC reached both absolute and relative preoperative values only at 1 month post-surgery.

Aris et al. found that their limited upper sternotomy patients showed a decreased FEV1 which was recorded at 62% compared to preoperative values while their sternotomy ones suffered a FEV1 decrease to 52.6% compared to their preoperative values. This results did not quite reach statistical significance ($p=0.08$) in their 20 patient prospectively randomised. Furthermore, their same study showed a trend towards less post-operative pain in the upper sternotomy patients which once more did not reach statistical significance. A larger group of patients studied could have indeed shown a significant difference.

A recent systematic review and meta-analysis of 26 studies which allowed to retrospectively compare 2,054 limited upper sternotomy AVRs to 2,532 sternotomy AVRs have shown that both ventilation time post-surgery, total post-operative blood losses, intensive care unit length of stay and hospital length of stay were all shorter in the upper sternotomy group vs. the sternotomy one. Furthermore, major limitations highlighted were the small number of patients enrolled in each published study and the inclusion of each of the surgeon's initial experience and learning curve. The same systematic review confirmed that the upper sternotomy patients had a marginally longer aortic cross-clamp time averaging less than 8 min duration longer than the conventional group.

Future studies should assess the speed of our patients' recovery including their time of return to work or normal preoperative daily physical activities. Doll et al. have shown that limited upper sternotomy AVR patients were less likely to have a delayed (8%) or severely delayed (1%) time to ambulation when compared to those undergoing a conventional sternotomy AVR (25% and 5% respectively, $p=0.002$).

Randomised clinical trials have shown no difference between limited upper sternotomy and conventional sternotomy patients in terms of mortality and major post-operative complications. This confirms that a minimal access upper sternotomy can be safely performed by experienced surgeons who were adequately trained in this specific procedure.

In the future, both better designed and statistically powered studies could show if the positive trends shown in the minimal access group of patients are actually significant or may become significant if an older and/or higher risk patient population is chosen for randomisation.

In the specific case of sternal infection or sternal mal-union, the minimal access upper sternotomy is likely to produce a contained sternal infection and would not result in a full sternal instability by definition.

Cardiac surgeons have historically been unwilling to move from their safe platform so hardly conquered over many years of work operating with the comfort of a sternotomy. This surgical access offers wide exposure to the whole of the heart and great vessels with ability to handle the heart during common traditional de-airing manoeuvres and visual assessment of left and right ventricular distension and preload subjective assessment via pulmonary artery manual palpation. Stepping off this stable platform obviously represents an important 'jump' into a less known surgical world in which the use of the trans-oesophageal echocardiography is the only guidance to an exclusively but effective antegrade de-airing process and where no direct heart manipulation is possible. Previously acquired surgical skills have to be refined while using marginally modified instruments passed via less accessible surgical incisions. Direct surgical vision is often good but unusually limited to our targets aortic valve and root instead of the entire heart.

Suggested Reading

Aris A, Camara ML, Montiel J, Delgado LJ, Galan J, Litvan H (1999) Ministernotomy versus median sternotomy for aortic valve replacement; a prospective randomized study. Ann Thorac Surg 67:1583–1588

Benetti FJ, Mariani MA, Rizzardi JL, Benetti I (1997) Minimally invasive aortic valve replacement [published erratum appears in J Thorac Cardiovasc Surg 1997;114:947]. J Thorac Cardiovasc Surg 113: 806–807

Black D, Pearson M (2002) Average length of stay, delayed discharge, and hospital congestion. BMJ 325:610–611

Bloomstein LZ, Gielchinsky I, Bernstein AD et al (2001) Aortic valve replacement in geriatric patients: determinants of in-hospital mortality. Ann Thorac Surg 71:597–600

Bonacchi M, Prifti E, Giunti G et al (2002) Does ministernotomy improve postoperative outcome in aortic valve operation? A prospective randomized study. Ann Thorac Surg 73:460–465; discussion 465–466

Brown M, McKellar SH, Sundt TM, Schaff H (2009) Ministernotomy versus conventional sternotomy for aortic valve replacement: a systematic review and meta-analysis. J Thorac Cardiovasc Surg 137: 670–679

Byrne JG, Hsin MK, Adams DH et al (2000a) Minimally invasive direct access heart valve surgery. J Card Surg 15:21–34

Byrne JG, Karavas AN, Cohn LH et al (2000b) Minimal access aortic root, valve, and complex ascending aortic surgery. Curr Cardiol Rep 2:549–557

Byrne JG, Leacche M, Unic D et al (2005) Staged initial percutaneous coronary intervention followed by valve surgery ('hybrid approach') for patients with complex coronary and valve disease. J Am Coll Cardiol 46(9):1782–1783

Candaele S, Herijgers P, Demeyere R et al (2003) Chest pain after partial upper versus complete sternotomy for aortic valve surgery. Acta Cardiol 58:17–21

Chang YS, Lin PJ, Chang CH et al (1999) "I" ministernotomy for aortic valve replacement. Ann Thorac Surg 68:40–45

Cohn LH (2001) Minimally invasive valve surgery. J Card Surg 16:260–265

Cohn LH, Adams DH, Couper GS, Bichell DP, Rosborough DM, Sears SP et al (1997) Minimally invasive cardiac valve surgery improves patient satisfaction while reducing costs of cardiac valve replacement and repair. Ann Surg 226:421–428

Colvin SB, Galloway AC, Ribakove G et al (1998) Port-Access mitral valve surgery: summary of results. J Card Surg 13:286–289

Cosgrove DM 3rd, Sabik JF (1996) Minimally invasive approach for aortic valve operations. Ann Thorac Surg 62:596–597

Cosgrove DM 3rd, Sabik JF, Navia JL (1998) Minimally invasive valve operations. Ann Thorac Surg 65:1535–1538; discussion 1538–1539

Dogan S, Dzemali O (2003) Minimal invasive versus conventional aortic valve replacement: a prospective randomized trial. J Heart Valve Dis 12:76–80
Doty DB, DiRusso GB, Doty JR (1998) Full-spectrum cardiac surgery through a minimal incision: mini-sternotomy (lower half) technique. Ann Thorac Surg 65:573–577
Gillinov AM, Banbury MK, Cosgrove DM (2000) Hemisternotomy approach for aortic and mitral valve surgery. J Card Surg 15:15–20
Greelish JP, Ailiwadi M, Balaguer JM et al (2006) Combined percutaneous coronary intervention and valve surgery. Curr Opin Cardiol 21:113–117
Grossi EA, Zakow PK, Ribakove G et al (1999) Comparison of post-operative pain, stress response, and quality of life in port access vs. standard sternotomy coronary bypass patients. Eur J Cardiothorac Surg 16(suppl 2):S39–S42
Gundry SR, Shattuck OH, Razzouk AJ et al (1998) Facile minimally invasive cardiac surgery via ministernotomy. Ann Thorac Surg 65:1100–1104
Jones JM, O'Kane H, Gladstone DJ et al (2001) Repeat heart valve surgery: risk factors for operative mortality. J Thorac Cardiovasc Surg 122:913–918
Kasegawa H, Shimokawa T, Matsushita Y, Kamata S, Ida T, Kawase M (1998) Right-sided partial sternotomy for minimally invasive valve operation: "open door method". Ann Thorac Surg 65:569–570
Lazzara RR, Kidwell FE (1998) Right parasternal incision: a uniform minimally invasive approach for valve operations. Ann Thorac Surg 65:271–272
Liu J, Sidiropoulos A, Konertz W (1999) Minimally invasive aortic valve replacement (AVR) compared to standard AVR. Eur J Cardiothorac Surg 16(suppl 2):S80–S83
Lund O, Flo C, Jensen FT et al (1997) Left ventricular systolic and diastolic function in aortic stenosis. Prognostic value after valve replacement and underlying mechanisms [see comments]. Eur Heart J 18:1977–1987
Machler HE, Bergmann P, Anelli-Monti M et al (1999) Minimally invasive versus conventional aortic valve operations: a prospective study in 120 patients. Ann Thorac Surg 67:1001–1005
Masiello P, Coscioni E, Panza A et al (2002) Surgical results of aortic valve replacement via partial upper sternotomy: comparison with median sternotomy. Cardiovasc Surg 10:333
Mihaljevic T, Cohn LH, Unic D et al (2004) One thousand minimally invasive valve operations: early and late results. Ann Surg 240:529–534; discussion 534
Minale C, Reifschneider HJ, Schmitz E, Uckmann FP (1997) Single access for minimally invasive aortic valve replacement. Ann Thorac Surg 64:120–123
Mistiaen WP, Van Cauwelaert P, Muylaert P et al (2001) Determinants of survival after aortic valve replacement as treatment for symptomatic aortic valve disease in the elderly. J Heart Valve Dis 10:354–360
Moreno-Cabral RJ (1997) Mini-T sternotomy for cardiac operations. J Thorac Cardiovasc Surg 113:810–811
Rodriguez JE, Cortina J, Perez de la Sota E, Maroto L, Ginestal F, Rufilanchas JJ (1998) A new approach to cardiac valve replacement through a small midline incision and inverted L shape partial sternotomy. Eur J Cardiothorac Surg 14(suppl 1):S115–S116
Sundt TM, Bailey MS, Moon MR et al (2000) Quality of life after aortic valve replacement at the age of 80 years. Circulation 102:III70–III74
Svensson LG (1997) Minimal-access "J" or "j" sternotomy for valvular, aortic, and coronary operations or reoperations. Ann Thorac Surg 64:1501–1503
Svensson LG, Nadolny EM, Kimmel WA (2001) Minimal access aortic surgery including re-operations. Eur J Cardiothorac Surg 19:30–33
Szwerc MF, Benckart DH, Wiechmann RJ et al (1999) Partial versus full sternotomy for aortic valve replacement. Ann Thorac Surg 68:2209–2213; discussion 2213–2214
Tam RK, Almeida AA (1998) Minimally invasive aortic valve replacement via partial sternotomy. Ann Thorac Surg 65:275–276

Transcatheter Aortic Valve Implantation

43

Volkmar Falk and Thomas Walther

Contents

V. Falk, M.D. (✉)
Division of Cardiovascular Surgery, University of Zürich, Rämistrasse 100, Zürich CH-8091, Switzerland
e-mail: volkmar.falk@usz.ch

T. Walther, M.D., Ph.D.
Department of Cardiac Surgery, Kerckhoff Heartcenter, Benekestrasse 2-8, Bad Nauheim 61231, Germany
e-mail: t.walther@kerckhoff-klinik.de

43.1 Introduction

Transcatheter aortic valve implantation was first described by Cribier in 2002 [1] and since then has evolved as a routine procedure for high-risk patients with aortic stenosis [2, 3]. As by June 2010, 10,000 transfemoral (TF) implants of the CoreValve™ prosthesis (Medtronic Inc., Minneapolis, MN, USA) and approximately a similar number of TF and transapical (TA) implants of the Edwards Sapien™ prosthesis (Edwards Lifesciences Inc., Irvine, CA, USA) have been reported. While most centers report encouraging procedural results, mid- and long-term data are sparse. No randomized trials have been conducted to prove similar or better outcomes with transfemoral (TF) or transapical (TA) aortic valve implantation (AVI) compared to conventional aortic valve replacement (AVR). Appropriate indications, patient selection and risk assessment, the ideal setting to perform TF/TA-AVI, the involved imaging techniques, and periprocedural treatment are currently under investigation. A high incidence of paravalvular leaks and AV-block, challenges in device positioning, and procedure-related and previously unknown complications have stimulated new design concepts for transcatheter valves that are currently undergoing clinical trials.

R.G.C. Inderbitzi et al. (eds.), *Minimally Invasive Thoracic and Cardiac Surgery*,
DOI 10.1007/978-3-642-11861-6_43, © Springer-Verlag Berlin Heidelberg 2012

43.2 Indication and Patient Selection for Transcatheter Valve Implantation

Without doubt, patient screening and selection is crucial for success. The best source for appropriate patient selection is a joint statement published on behalf of the European Society of Cardiology (ESC), the European Association of Cardiothoracic Surgery, and the European Association of Percutaneous Cardiovascular Interventions (EAPCI) [4].

Accordingly, TAVI is indicated in patients with calcified pure or predominant AS. Patients therefore need to have confirmed severe and symptomatic aortic stenosis with an established indication for aortic valve surgery according to current guidelines [5]. Aortic stenosis needs to be verified by measurements of valve area and flow-dependent indices. For the growing number of patients with low ejection fraction, low-dose dobutamine echocardiography should be used to differentiate between severe and the rare "pseudo severe" AS in patients with low LV ejection fraction.

Since TF and TA-AVI are still at an early clinical phase, analysis of the risk of conventional aortic valve surgery needs to be assessed. There is general consensus that in order to justify transcatheter valve implantation, the risk of conventional surgery should exceed a perioperative mortality of 10% as predicted by the logistic Euroscore or the STS score. It is well recognized that these widely applied surgical scoring systems were not primarily designed to predict the risk of catheter-based interventions. Since high-risk patients were underrepresented in the populations the scores were derived from, they cannot adequately predict outcome in very high-risk patients either. In addition, not all comorbidities such as severe aortic calcification or liver cirrhosis are captured with conventional scoring systems, and therefore an individual assessment of surgical risk is mandatory. More recently, frailty scores have been used in an effort to address the risk of elderly patients. There is agreement that patients should be at least 70 years of age or older and have a life expectancy of more than 1 year to qualify for transcatheter valve implantation. Patient desire is as yet not acceptable as an indication for this relatively new technique.

Specific indications for a TF or a TA approach relate to anatomical considerations. In general, severe atherosclerosis of peripheral vessels is a contraindication for a TF approach, as there is an excess risk of vascular complications. A minimal luminal diameter of 6 mm is required for transfemoral access with the CoreValve™ while 6–8 mm are required for TF implantation of the Edwards Sapien™ valve, and others may need larger vessel diameters. Aortic aneurysms or severe atherosclerosis of the aortic arch are considered additional risk factors for a retrograde approach, as retrograde passage of a stiff guidewire may dislodge debris with the potential for cerebral embolism.

Aneurysm of the left ventricular apex or left ventricular thrombus and severe pericardial calcification preclude a transapical approach. Pulmonary insufficiency defined as a forced expiratory volume in 1 s (FEV1) <1 l may result in prolonged postoperative ventilatory support with any approach and thus is an important risk factor.

General contraindications for TAVI include aortic valve annular diameters of less than 18 mm. For different valves, the maximum of aortic annular diameter varies but should not exceed 27 mm [4]. A 29-mm version of the Edwards SAPIEN will soon be available expanding the indication for bigger annuli.

Transcatheter treatment of bicuspid valves is still not recommended (although occasionally performed) because of the risk of incomplete deployment. Presence of asymmetric heavy valvular calcification may lead to complications during TAVI. Eccentric local plaque burden can lead to paravalvular leak due to incomplete expansion of the implant. The atrioventricular (AV) node and its left bundle branch pass adjacent to the noncoronary cusp of the aortic valve within the central fibrous body. Especially in settings with heavy calcification of the noncoronary cusp, local compression of the AV-node by an expanding stent can lead to permanent third-degree AV-block necessitating pacemaker implantation in up to one-third of the patients. Excessive calcification can also lead to partial or complete coronary occlusion. Therefore, it is important to assess the distance from the aortic annulus to the coronary ostia. As a rule of thumb, the distance from the coronary ostium to the annulus should not be less than 10 mm. Aortic root dimension should not exceed 45 mm at the aorto-tubular junction for self-expandable prostheses as the implant can otherwise not be positioned in a stable position. Very narrow tubular aortic roots with small or absent sinuses increase the risk of coronary occlusion as there is little room for the relocation of calcified cusps. Patients with severe left ventricular hypertrophy and small left ventricular cavities might be at an increased risk for cardiac perforation by the extra-stiff guidewire used to stabilize the prosthesis during implantation.

A multidisciplinary decision-making process is required for transcatheter valve implantation. Ideally, a valve team includes an interventional cardiologist, a cardiac surgeon, and an anesthesiologist. Primary care physicians and geriatricians should play an important role in determining the indication for transcatheter valve implantation in high-risk elderly patients.

43.3 Imaging

Preoperative and intraoperative imaging is of utmost importance for procedural planning and execution. Preoperatively information on (1) vascular access sites; (2) quality and tortuosity of the femoral, iliac vessels, and the whole aorta; (3) relation of the apex to the chest wall; (4) angulation of the left ventricle and left ventricular outflow tract in relation to the aortic root; (5) aortic valve leaflets and leaflet calcification; (6) aortic valve annular dimension, geometry, and calcification; (7) distance of coronary ostia from aortic annulus; (8) the extent of concomitant coronary artery disease; (9) concomitant valvular pathology; and (10) left ventricular function need to be determined.

Intraoperatively, fluoroscopy and transesophageal echocardiography (TEE) are used to (1) guidewire placement, (2) perform root angiography, (3) guide positioning of the balloon for balloon valvuloplasty, and (4) position the implant and for (5) quality control. There is consensus that for intraoperative guidance, both high-resolution fluoroscopy and TEE are required.

43.3.1 Coronary Angiography

A preoperative coronary angiogram should be obtained in all patients to rule out significant coronary artery disease. In patients with contraindication for conventional open surgery, feasibility of PCI should be addressed. Visualization of femoral and iliac arteries allows assessment of possible vascular access.

43.3.2 Echocardiography

Echocardiography is used to confirm the diagnosis of aortic stenosis and to determine aortic annular and root dimensions. Confirmation of tricuspid configuration and local calcium burden of the native aortic valve cusps are best seen in short axis views. Transesophageal echocardiography (TEE) is used to measure the diameter of the aortic root (long axis view) and to evaluate the extent and pattern of calcification (short axis). The diameter of the aortic annulus is measured, including all cusp calcifications, at mid-systole from the insertion of the right coronary cusp at the junction between interventricular septum, aortic annulus, and aortic root and the insertion of the left coronary cusp just opposite at the junction between the anterior mitral leaflet, aortic annulus, and aortic root [6]. In cases with severe annular calcification, echocardiographic measurement of annular dimension can, however, be misleading. The diameters of the aortic root are taken during systole at the level of the LVOT, aortic annulus, sinus, sinutubular junction, and proximal ascending aorta. Both self-expanding and balloon expandable devices are on purpose oversized (by 10%) relative to the aortic valve annulus as they rely in part on sufficient radial force for anchoring the valve within the aortic root. In addition, some oversizing may lead to better apposition at the annular level in order to prevent higher degrees of paravalvular leakage. Oversizing needs to be considered when assessing aortic root dimensions during preoperative screening. While undersizing, the prosthesis relative to the aortic valve annulus may increase the likelihood of paravalvular aortic regurgitation or prosthetic valve embolization with the need to implant a second valve excessive oversizing the balloon for aortic valvuloplasty, and prosthesis by underestimation of the diameter of the aortic valve annulus can increase the risk of aortic root rupture.

TEE is used intraoperatively to monitor cardiac function (especially after balloon dilatation when acute aortic insufficiency can dramatically impact ventricular function). Positioning and placement of the implant can be guided by TEE, but most centers rely on fluoroscopy as the artifacts caused by the stent as well as excessive calcifications can impair the image quality and thus the precision of TEE visualization. TEE is also important to watch for the position of guidewires and to watch for pericardial effusion and cardiac tamponade which can result from perforation of both the right (temporary pacemaker) and left ventricle (stiff guidewire). Functional assessment of the implant and diagnosis of the presence and extent of paravalvular leakage can guide the decision for post-dilatation after initial implantation. Hemodynamics and valve function can be immediately assessed after valve implantation.

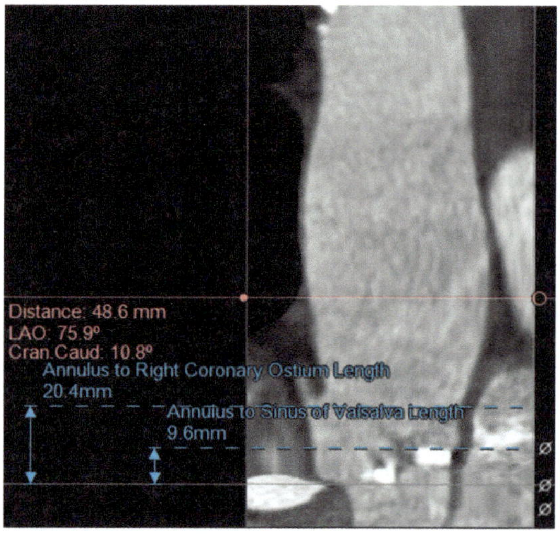

Fig. 43.1 Multislice detector CT scan of the aortic root indicating distance from aortic annulus to the right coronary ostium

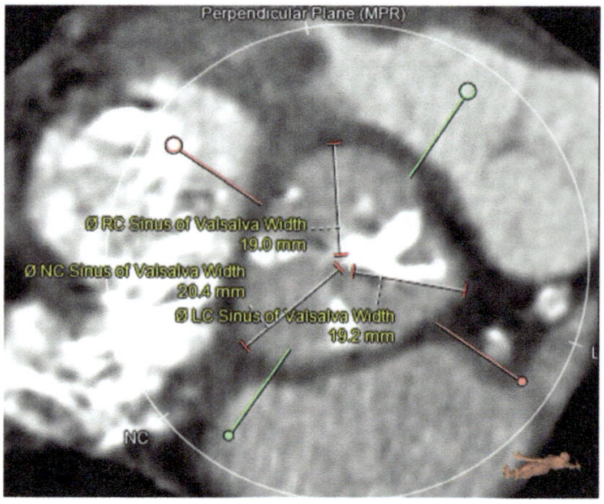

Fig. 43.2 MSCT showing aortic annulus dimensions and asymmetric calcification pattern

43.3.3 Computed Tomography

Multislice computer tomography (MSCT) is useful for procedural planning. The pattern of aortic valve calcification can be clearly visualized. The geometry of the aortic valve and aortic root and all critical dimensions are readily available. Angulation of the left ventricle and left ventricular outflow tract in relation to the aortic root is easily visualized, and the distance of the coronary ostia from the aortic annulus can be adequately measured. The right coronary orifice is usually located more distally (Fig. 43.1), thus the distance from the annulus to left coronary orifice becomes the critical measure and should be at least 10 mm. If heavy eccentric calcification is present in the left coronary cusp and if in addition the aortic root is narrow, the safety margin becomes limited. Three-dimensional reconstruction of the root may be useful for enhanced planning algorithms (Fig. 43.2). Based on MSCT images, the accuracy of implant size selection for the CoreValve™ prosthesis can be increased when considering the elliptic shape of the aortic root and left ventricular outflow tract. It has been suggested that the mean area at the level of the aortic annulus rather than one diameter is more appropriate to optimize valve selection and may be used to minimize the risk of paravalvular leakage or AV-block [7].

In the absence of angina, clinical evidence, or a positive history for coronary artery disease, cardiac MSCT may also be used to rule out coronary artery disease. In case of high calcium load or significant stenosis visible on CT, a coronary angiogram should nevertheless be performed.

Access planning for transfemoral access is best performed by using an angio-CT (Fig. 43.3). Advanced software intuitively encodes diameters and tortuosity for easy assessment of the feasibility of a femoral approach. Especially in redo situations, thoracic CT will allow to determine the best intercostal space for transapical access.

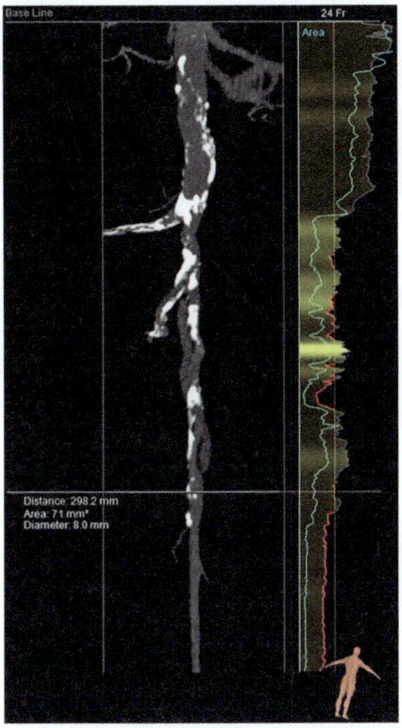

Fig. 43.3 Multislice angio-CT of the femoral and iliac vessels. Note severe calcification. Tortuosity (*yellow bands*) and critical diameters as set by the operator (*red line*) are automatically displayed

43.3.3.1 Intraoperative Fluoroscopy

Intraoperative fluoroscopy is applied to guide catheter placement, balloon dilation, valve positioning, and implantation. Different projections are used to visualize the aortic root. It is essential to understand the impact of different projections on the fluoroscopic view. The ventriculo-aortic angle can only be appreciated in the RAO view, but not in the LAO view, since the latter looks at this angulation en face (Fig. 43.4). The annular plane is sometimes visible depending on the amount of annular calcification. Indirect clues are provided by the position of the pigtail catheter, which should be placed at the bottom of the right coronary sinus.

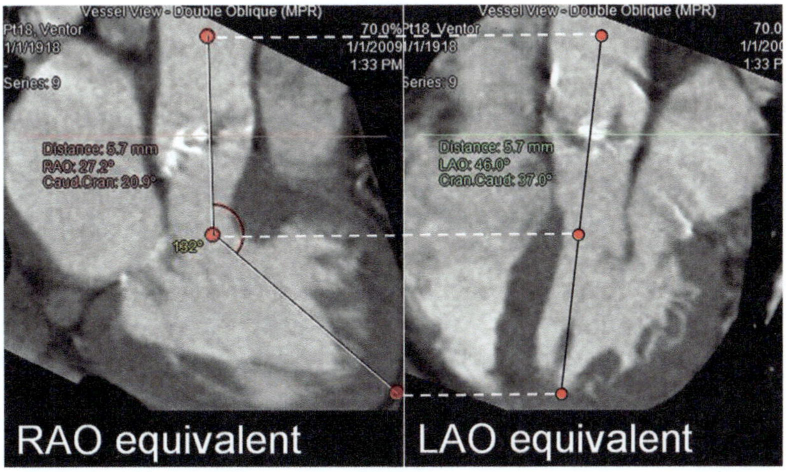

Fig. 43.4 CT example showing that the ventriculo-aortic angle will be apparent in the RAO but not the LAO equivalent of the corresponding angiographic projections

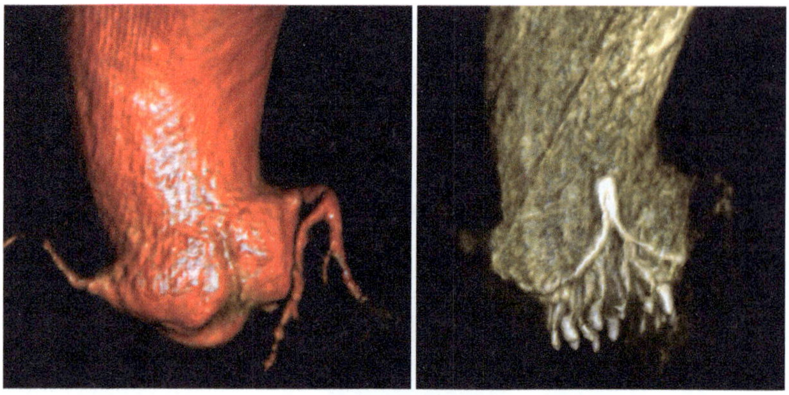

Fig. 43.5 Intraoperative rotational angiography before and after implantation of a Ventor Embracer-valve

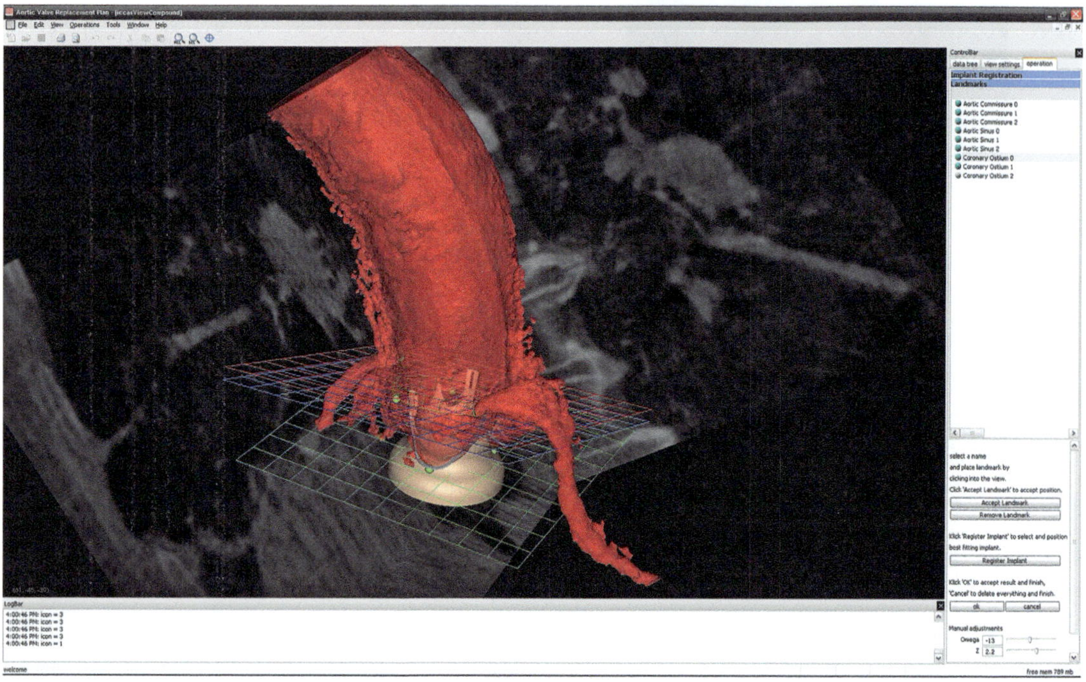

Fig. 43.6 Augmented reality using a virtual valve template that is projected on *top* of the reconstructed aortic root (intraoperative reconstruction)

43.3.3.2 Image-Based Planning

Based on CT images, two possible methods of image guidance can be applied to overlay a three-dimensional reconstruction of the aortic root with two-dimensional angiographic images: (1) A three dimensional reconstruction of the aortic root is segmented from a preoperative CT-data set. This reconstrcution is then registered with the intraoperative fluoroscopy. (2) Intraoperatively, a rotational angiography also known as dynamic CT is performed. After injecting dye into the aortic root under rapid pacing (prevents rapid dilution), sequential frames are collected while the detector rotates around the patient. From these images, a 3D reconstruction can be performed (Fig. 43.5) [8]. Registering is in this case not necessary as the patient has not moved between exams. For enhanced planning, templates of implants can be virtually placed into the reconstructed root (Fig. 43.6). Information from a planning CT or dynamic intraoperative CT can be used to guide the procedure and help to calculate

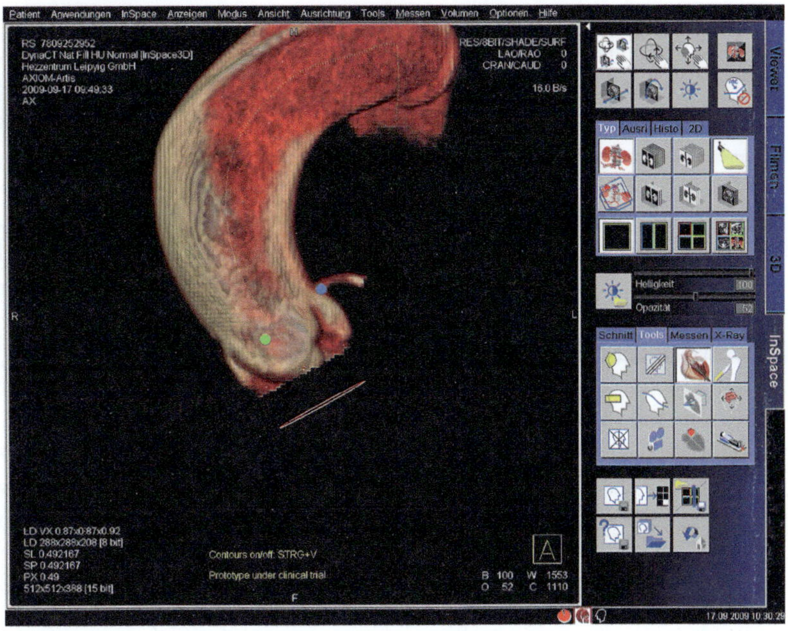

Fig. 43.7 Root reconstruction with automated coronary ostia detection and indicator of subannular plane as a guiding tool for valve implantation

the best possible fluoroscopic view for the implantation (usually orthogonal) and automatically adjust the angulation of the C-arm (Fig. 43.7).

One principle problem when using image guidance results from inaccuracies due to motion artifacts. When the heart is beating, root reconstructions are currently not synchronized and prone for geometric error. One potential solution is to track the aortic root by native markers such as leaflet calcifications. These algorithms are currently under investigation. If augmented reality and live mode overlay will impact the complication rate remains to be seen [9].

43.4 Institutional Requirements

Consensus exists that TF- and TA-AVI are best performed in a hybrid suite equipped for both catheter intervention including percutaneous coronary intervention as well as for open heart surgery. Laminar airflow is recommended to secure a sterile environment during the implant procedure. Besides, a high-resolution angiography unit and availability of transesophageal echocardiography and immediate access to cardiopulmonary bypass are required. Although presence of an ECMO may be regarded sufficient for immediate circulatory support, a full CPB set may be preferable as massive bleeding in the rare event of ventricular or annular rupture can be best managed with additional suction lines and autotransfusion. The number and arrangement of monitors is still under debate, but operators should have immediate and unobstructed view of fluoroscopic, echocardiographic, and hemodynamic data simultaneously from a comfortable working position. Inappropriate imaging and lack of a safety net will lead to inferior results and are therefore not acceptable.

43.5 Operator Skills

Ideally, transcatheter valve interventions are performed by a team of interventional cardiologists and cardiac surgeons. The complexity of the procedure and the severity of potential complications demand for an interdisciplinary approach and appropriate training. The team should also include a dedicated anesthesiologist, perfusionist, and nurses trained for catheter interventions and open surgery. With rapidly expanding indications and more widespread use also in younger patients, it is not acceptable to deny patients the safety net of a skilled team and to perform these interventions without on-site surgical backup.

43.6 Implantation Procedures

43.6.1 Transapical Implantation

For most valves, the technique of transapical access is similar until the valve is finally deployed, and hence this is a generic description of the approach following the recommendations by Walther [6]. Variations may apply for the different implants and are discussed in more detail below. Technical details are taken mostly from the available literature which is quoted in the respective paragraphs.

All procedures should be performed with the patient prepped and draped as required for full sternotomy and cardiopulmonary bypass in standby. External defibrillator pads should be placed. For transapical access, the patient is placed in a supine position with the left chest slightly elevated. A 6-F femoral arterial sheath is inserted into the right femoral artery, and a pigtail catheter is placed into the aortic root for contrast aortography. A 6-F introducer sheath is inserted into the right femoral vein and a guidewire placed in the right atrium to establish access for fast percutaneous cannulation in case conversion to extracorporeal circulation becomes necessary (safety precaution). Low-dose heparin is given with a target-activated clotting time of 150 s (for some valves, an ACT of >300 is recommended). An incision (5–7 cm) is performed in the 5th or 6th intercostal space for transapical access. An epicardial temporary pacemaker wire is sutured to the left ventricle and tested. The pericardium is incised and fixed with stay sutures. Two apical felt pledgeted purse-string sutures are placed slightly lateral and above the true apex with an inner diameter of approximately 2–3 cm. Rotational angiography for 3D reconstruction of the aortic root was performed in some cases as previously described [8]. This technique facilitates orthogonal orientation of the C-arm and improves the ease of anatomically orientating the implant if necessary. The left ventricular apex is punctured with an 18-G Seldinger-type needle. A 14-F soft sheath is introduced and positioned across the aortic valve. A 6-F right Judkins catheter is placed in the descending aorta, and through this, a 035″ super-stiff guidewire is positioned across the aortic arch. A balloon valvuloplasty catheter of appropriate size is positioned under fluoroscopic and echocardiographic guidance, and balloon valvuloplasty is performed under a brief period of rapid ventricular pacing at a rate of 180 bpm. Effective pacing is verified by a low output state but should be limited in time because hemodynamic function can easily deteriorate especially with acute AI resulting from balloon valvuloplasty.

Details of actual valve implantation are described below for the different valves.

After implantation and confirmation of appropriate positioning and functioning of the implant by fluoroscopy and echocardiography, all sheaths and guidewires are pulled and the apex secured by tightening the purse-string sutures. Intercostal blockade is applied using a local anesthetic. The pericardium is partially closed over the apex, and a left lateral chest tube is inserted. The intercostal incision is closed in a standard fashion. Finally, the femoral sheaths and catheters are removed [6].

43.6.2 Transfemoral Access

All transfemoral procedures should also be performed with the patient prepped and draped as required for full sternotomy and cardiopulmonary bypass in standby. External defibrillator pads should be placed. For transfemoral access, the patient is placed in a supine position. A 6-F femoral arterial sheath is inserted each into the right and left femoral artery, and a pigtail catheter is placed from the contralateral site into the aortic root for contrast aortography. During the intervention, the patient is heparinized to achieve an activated clotting time of 300–350 s (CoreValve). A pacemaker lead is placed in the right ventricular apex through either the femoral or the internal jugular vein. This will serve two purposes: (a) for rapid (~180 bpm) ventricular pacing during aortic valve balloon valvuloplasty (and valve implantation for some

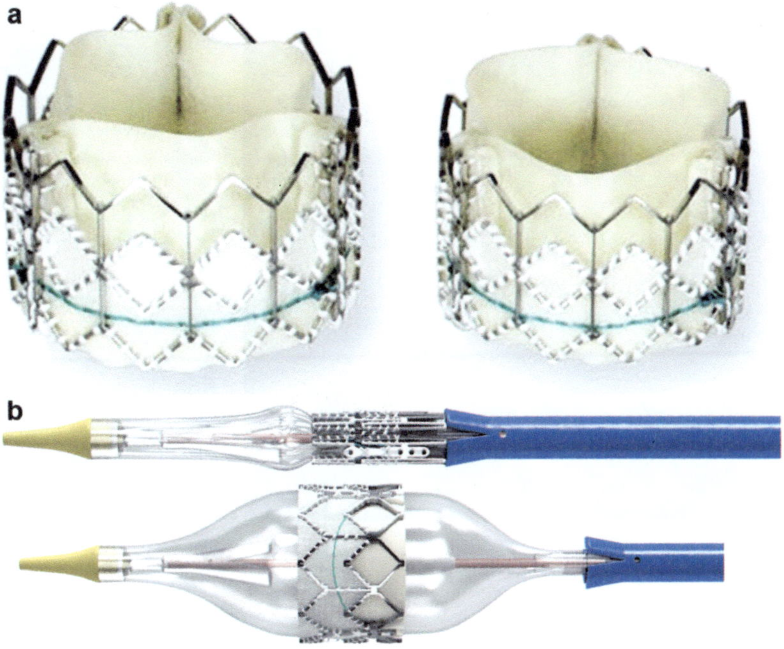

Fig. 43.8 Sapien XT Valve (Edwards Life Science) (**a**) and ballon expandable delivery system (**b**)

implants) and (b) as a temporary pacemaker until permanent pacemaker implantation (should it become necessary). The left ventricle is wired, usually with the help of an AL1 or AL2 diagnostic catheter using a hydrophilic guidewire. A 0.035-in. super-stiff guidewire is advanced into the left ventricular apex over a pigtail catheter [10].

43.6.3 Trans-Subclavian Access

In patients with severe peripheral artery disease, severe calcification, tortuosity, or small diameter <6 mm of the femoral and iliac arteries, femoral vascular access may not be feasible even for the 18-F delivery system. This also applies to patients with previous aortofemoral bypass, severe atherosclerosis of the arch, coarctation, or abdominal aortic aneurysms with mural thrombus.

An alternative access for retrograde aortic valve implantation is the left subclavian artery. The vessel should have a diameter >6–7 mm, and absence of ostial calcification at its origin from the aortic arch should be documented. Presence of a patent left internal mammary artery (LIMA) graft is considered a relative contraindication.

The procedure taken is performed under general anesthesia. Standard surgical cutdown of the left axillary/subclavian artery is performed, and an end-to-side 8-mm Dacron graft is placed. Through this graft, an initial 9-Fr and, after exchange for a stiff wire, an 18-Fr sheath are inserted. Alternatively, direct sheath insertion may be performed in larger vessels. After positioning of the stiff guidewire, aortic valvuloplasty is performed. Advancement of the prosthesis through the 18-Fr sheath, the aortic arch, and finally through the valve is accomplished using the push-and-pull technique over the super-stiff guidewire under fluoroscopic guidance. The artery is surgically repaired, and angiography of the subclavian artery is performed to rule out dissection or other complications [11].

43.6.4 Sapien™ Valve

The Edwards Sapien Valve (lately Sapien XT) is a balloon expandable bovine pericardial valve mounted on a stainless steel (cobalt chromium – SAPIEN XT) frame (Fig. 43.8a Sapien Valve). CE mark approval for TA-AVI of the Sapien valve

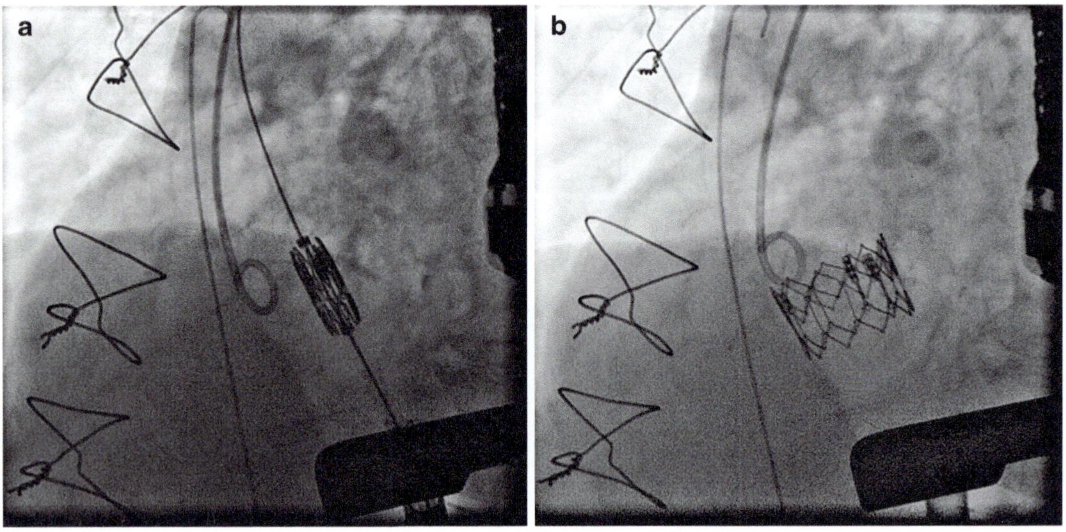

Fig. 43.9 Positioning of the Sapien XT Valve in the aortic annulus, fluoroscopic view (**a**); implanted valve (**b**)

(Edwards Lifesciences, Irvine, CA) was granted in January 2008. The valve can be implanted both transfemorally as well as transapically.

For TA implantation, the delivery sheath is inserted, in a blunt fashion following balloon angioplasty. Optimal sheath position is reached 4–5 cm below the aortic annulus. The valve is introduced into the annulus and the pusher retrieved back into the delivery sheath. This is necessary as balloon expansion cannot be performed properly with the pusher in place. The valve is ideally implanted with one-third of the stent above and two-thirds of the stent below the level of the aortic annulus. Axial motion of the implant during positioning and deployment can be monitored and counterbalanced under fluoroscopic guidance. Since a non-axial position of the valve can lead to misplacement, the valve should be oriented in line with the long axis of the aortic root and perpendicular to the aortic annulus (Fig. 43.9a). Coaxial positioning can be achieved by slowly manipulating the sheath and straightening or loosening the stiff guidewire. Under rapid ventricular pacing, valve implantation is performed by gradually inflating the balloon (Fig. 43.9b). Depending on the local calcium burden, dilatation of the balloon can be incomplete or asymmetric potentially leading to valve misplacement.

After full dilatation the balloon is deflated and retrieved. The guidewire is usually left in place until the need for repeat balloon dilatation is ruled out. Repeat dilatation with an extra balloon filling of 1–2 ml can be considered in the presence of moderate (2+) paravalvular leak and if there is an angiographic evidence of incomplete expansion.

For transfemoral access, a steerable delivery system is used (NovaFlex) that can be introduced through an 18-Fr sheath (8b).

43.6.5 Symetis™ Valve

The Symetis Accurate Valve is a porcine trileaflet valve mounted on a self-expanding nitinol stent (Fig. 43.10). The stent comprises the body of the stent at the inflow portion and an upper anchoring crown and stabilization arches that self-align the valve in the ascending aorta. The delivery sequence releases first the stabilization arms, then the superior crown, and lastly the body of the stent (Fig. 43.11). Clinical results are limited to 35 patients, the feasibility trial will be finished soon, and a multicenter pivotal study is being planned.

43.6.6 Direct Flow™ Valve

The Direct Flow Valve is a trileaflet bovine pericardial tissue valve that is attached to a balloon inflatable stent with a slightly tapered, conformable polyester fabric cuff (Fig. 43.12). The upper and lower margins of the cuff consist of two independently inflatable rings connected by a tubular system. The upper aortic ring is connected to three evenly distributed detachable positioning/fill lumens (PFLs) which are used to inflate and deflate the valve, as well as to accurately position it inside the native annulus. The folded valve is loaded into a 22-F sheath at the end of a 15-F delivery catheter with an olive-shaped tip designed to seal the distal end of the delivery sheath and to facilitate an atraumatic passage through the aorta. The loaded delivery system is advanced over a guidewire placed transvalvular in the left ventricle. A basketlike nitinol recovery system can be introduced into the delivery sheath to retrieve the valve if required (Fig. 43.13).

After balloon inflation of the native aortic valve, a stiff wire is placed in the left ventricle. The loaded delivery catheter is advanced over the wire through the aorta. After the device crosses the native valve, the delivery catheter is pulled back, and the deflated valve is unfolded in the left ventricle. After inflation of the ventricular ring with 50:50 saline/contrast, the pericardial leaflets are immediately competent. By adjusting the positioning/fill lumens, the ventricular ring is positioned and aligned in the native aortic annulus and the left ventricular outflow tract. Then, the upper (aortic) ring and the transverse tubes are inflated. This pushes the calcified native valve against the aortic wall thereby covering the native annulus. The prosthetic valve is then tested for correct sub-coronary position, proper function, and paravalvular leakage by TEE, fluoroscopy, and aortography. If necessary, repositioning can be performed after partial deflation, or if needed the valve can be completely removed and exchanged for a valve of a different size. When correct position and function was achieved, the saline contrast mix is replaced by a fluid polymer under constant pressure of 8–10 atm. The curing process of the polymer takes up to 24 h, but a firm gel is present already after 90 min. The positioning/fill lumens are then detached from the upper ring and the delivery system removed.

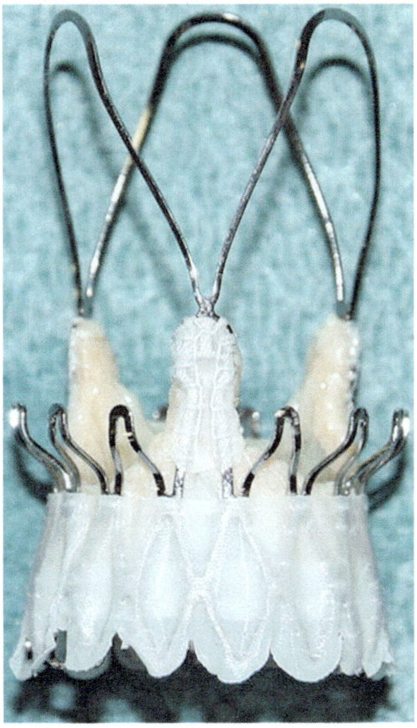

Fig. 43.10 Symetis Accurate Valve

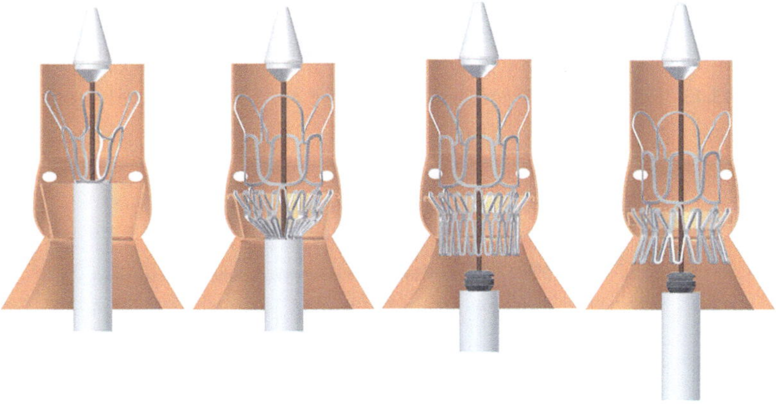

Fig. 43.11 Stepwise implantation of the self-expanding Symetis Accurate Valve

Limited clinical data are available. For the first-in-man trial, 31 patients were included. The device could be correctly positioned in 22 patients. Fourty-two percent of the patients had paravalvular leakage I, AV-block occurred in 3/22, coronary occlusion occurred in 1 patient (treated with PCI), and over-all MACCE rate was 12.9%. Eighteen patients were discharged with a permanent implant. Three and 6 month survival were 87.1% and 80.6%, respectively [12]. Long-term follow-up data are not available.

43.6.7 CoreValve™

The CoreValve (Medtronic, Inc., Minneapolis, Minnesota) aortic valve prosthesis is a trileaflet bioprosthetic porcine pericardial tissue valve that is mounted in a self-expanding nitinol stent (Fig. 43.14). The stent has an overall length of 50 mm. The distal portion of the multilevel support frame provides a low radial force area that orients the valve in the ascending aorta. The constrained area is designed to minimize the risk of coronary occlusion. High radial force at the proximal portion of the stent provides secure anchoring. While the first-generation 24-F device often required surgical cutdown of the common iliac artery for vascular access, the second-generation (21-F) and third-generation (18-F) devices are now routinely used percutaneously. As an alternative to femoral artery access, the subclavian artery can be used for retrograde valve placement. The CoreValve design allows a deployment error margin and device retrieval until partial implantation of the first two-thirds of the prosthesis. After balloon valvuloplasty with a 20- to 23-mm balloon under rapid pacing, the device is deployed retrogradely under fluoroscopic guidance. An incremental deployment technique allows for safe positioning. After deployment of the distal two-thirds of the prosthesis, the valve is already functioning, while device position can still be adjusted. Up to this point, the valve can still be retrieved if positioning is not optimal. The valve is available in two sizes: 26 mm (for aortic annulus diameters from 20 to 23 mm) and 29 mm (for aortic annulus diameters from 23 to 27 mm). Acetylsalicylic acid (100 mg/day) is administered before the procedure and continued indefinitely. In the early series, all patients received clopidogrel (300-mg loading dose), followed by 75 mg daily for at least 6–12 months.

Procedural success substantially increased over the last couple years. In the first series reported on the 2nd- and 3rd-generation devices, procedural success was only 88% and secondary

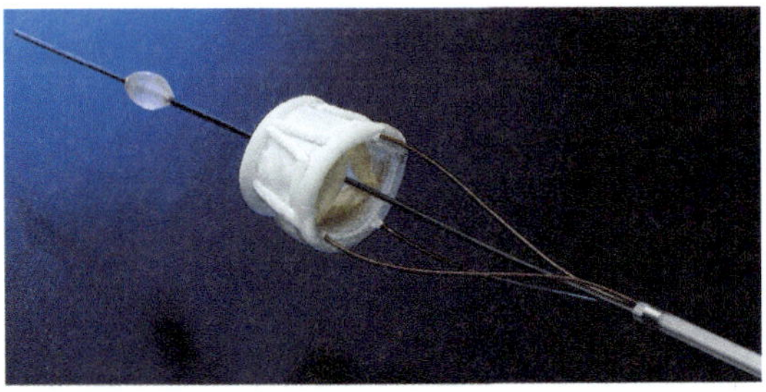

Fig. 43.12 Direct Flow Valve

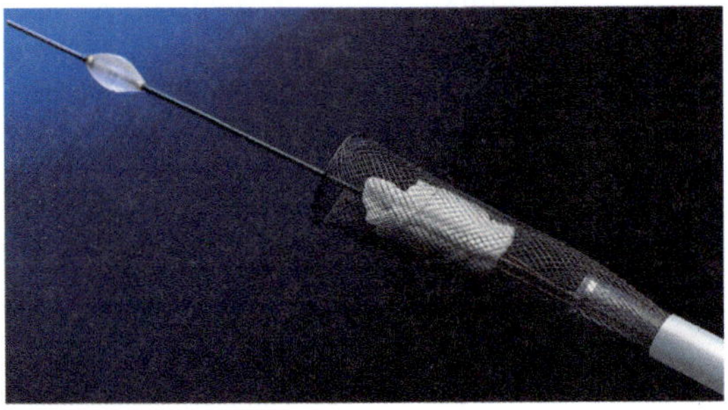

Fig. 43.13 Retrieval system for Direct Flow Valve

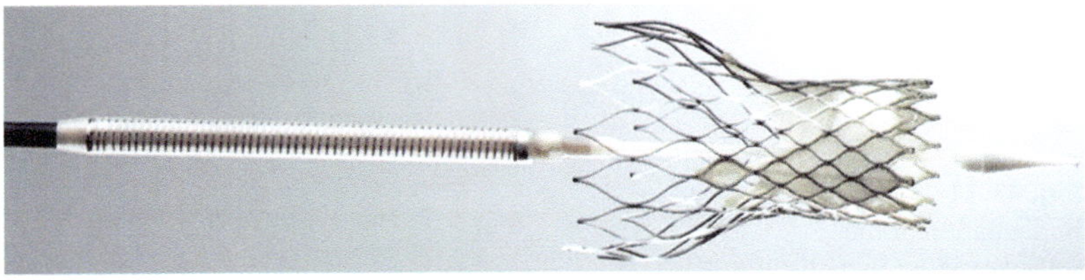

Fig. 43.14 Medtronic CoreValve

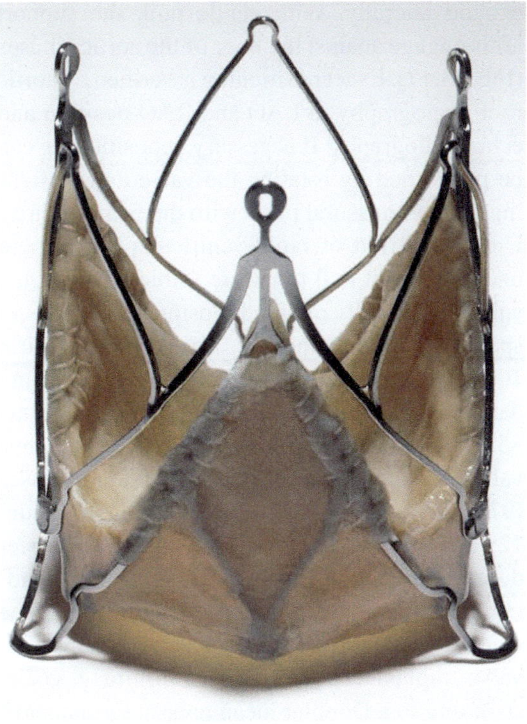

Fig. 43.15 Jena Valve

interventions (second valve or surgery) were frequently required. With the current 18-F delivery system, procedural success is reported in up to 98% [10].

43.6.8 Jena™ Valve

The Jena Valve (Jena Valve, Munich, Germany) is a tricuspid pericardial tissue valve mounted on a self-expanding nitinol stent (Fig. 43.15). The valve can be inserted transapically or transfemorally. The JenaClip stent is unique in that it comprises a double layer system of three clips aligned in two rows: one used to affix the valve tissue onto the stent (via sutures) and the other for precise positioning and anchoring into the native diseased aortic valve annulus and leaflets. This clipping mechanism enabled shortening of the stent length to about 30 mm. The stent also features a maximum diameter of 32 mm upon expansion and a minimum diameter of 6 mm when compressed. Upon advancement of the device above the aortic valve annulus, the catheter sheath is pulled back (transfemoral) or pushed forward (transapical) to release three "positioning feelers" that are then maneuvered by the operator in the sinus region and behind the native cusps of the diseased aortic valve. The feelers provide a tactile feedback to the physician to facilitate accurate positioning of the valve prosthesis. When the feelers are properly seated, the catheter sheath is further advanced to release the annular anchoring mechanism followed by full release of the prosthesis. Once released, the JenaClip stent is allowed to fully expand applying maximal retention force, at which point the prosthetic valve is immediately functional. Rapid ventricular pacing is not required during implantation. Valve retrieval and/or repositioning remain possible until final release of the prosthesis. With the device in place, the native leaflets are entrapped between the feelers and the body of the stent providing sufficient anchoring and thus preventing downward movement into the left ventricle. The flared shape of the base and high radial force of the JenaClip stent are designed to prevent distal migration.

Successful implantations have been reported in an experimental setting [13], but clinical experience is still limited to 15 patients, with no published reports.

43.6.9 Engager™ Valve

The Engager™ Aortic Valve Bioprosthesis (Medtronic, Inc., Minneapolis, MN previously Embracer (Ventor)) is a bovine pericardial three leaflet valve, sewn to a polyester sleeve, and mounted on a compressible and self-expanding nitinol frame (Fig. 43.16). The stent assembly consists of a mainframe and a support frame which are coupled together so as to form the commissural posts for the valve. For the first-in-man clinical trial, the valve was only available one size (23 mm), to fit an aortic annulus size of 19–24 mm [14]. The introducer sheath (overtube) containing the dilator is introduced over the guidewire and positioned across the aortic valve using fluoroscopic guidance. The Engager™

delivery system is inserted into the overtube via the cone-shaped entrance. Commissural alignment is performed under fluoroscopic guidance with the valve still in the overtube. Once the delivery system leaves the overtube, the Engager support arms are exposed in the aortic root, expand laterally. With gentle pull, the support arms engage against the floor of the aortic sinuses (Fig. 43.17). Exact positioning is verified by aortic root angiography in LAO and RAO position and echocardiography. If necessary, repositioning can be performed by rotating the valve and realigning the commissural posts with the commissures. Under a period of rapid ventricular pacing and under constant pull to ensure stable position, the valve is gradually released. Postoperative device-specific medical therapy consists of aspirin 100 mg daily indefinitely and clopidogrel 75 mg daily for 3 months except in patients older than 85 years. In the initial series including 30 patients, valve placement was achieved in 29/30 cases (97%). Mean fluoroscopy time was 7.5 ± 2.6 min; 129 ± 58 ml of contrast dye was used per procedure. Time for surgery was 100 ± 81 min (excluding conversions to sternotomy 74 ± 26 min). The invasively measured peak-to-peak gradient after valve implantation was 13.3 ± 9.3 mmHg; corresponding to a Doppler mean pressure gradient of 12.6 ± 5.9 mmHg, aortic regurgitation due to paravalvular leak grade 1 or less was present in 80%, grades I–II in 13%, and grade II in 3% of the patients. Aortic insufficiency greater than grade II was not observed. Ten percent of the patients required permanent pacemaker implantation for

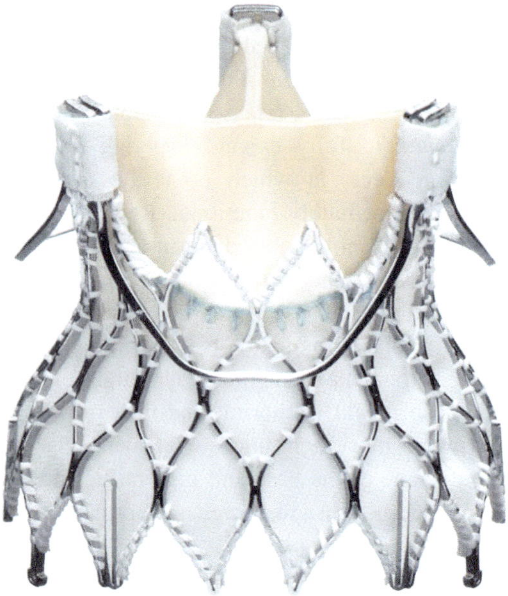

Fig. 43.16 Engager Valve

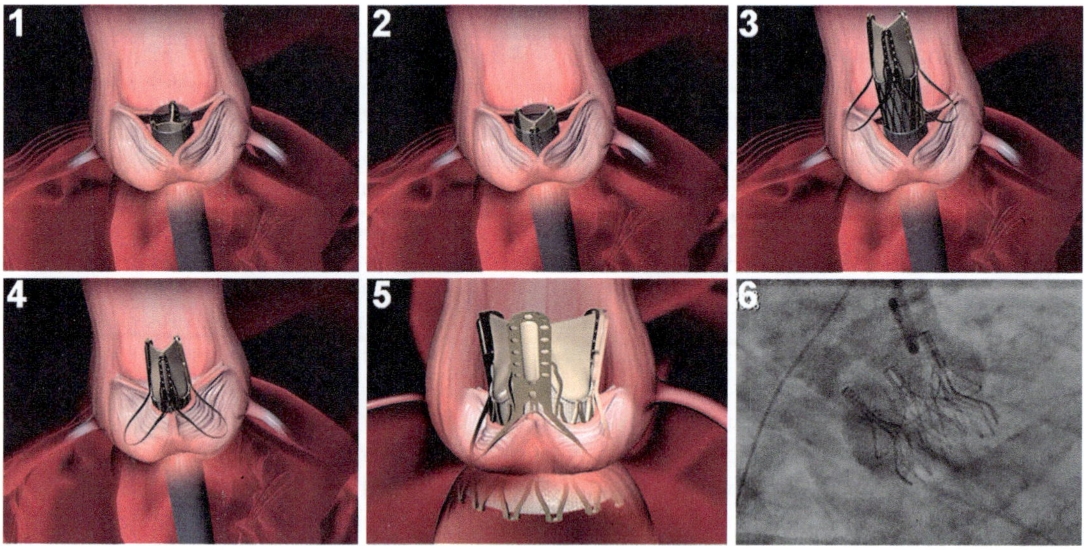

Fig. 43.17 Stepwise implantation of the Engager Valve

AV-block. Four patients (12.5%) experienced aortic dissection that was treated surgically in three cases. Retrospective review of the intraoperative angiograms revealed local dissection above the noncoronary sinus during device positioning as the most likely cause. Thirty-day mortality was 20% (in-hospital mortality 23%). Survival at 6 months was 56.7%. Meanwhile, the system has been redesigned as to avoid the risk of aortic dissection. The straight and rigid delivery system was abandoned in favor of a delivery system with a flexible shaft for over-the-wire tracking, thus conforming to the ventriculo-aortic angle and allowing coaxial alignment with the ascending aorta. A protective cover over the prosthetic commissural posts secures the posts until the valve's final position prior to the deployment of the mainframe is confirmed. In addition, several design modifications have been implemented in the valve prosthesis itself, including an increase in the space between support arms and mainframe to accommodate bulkier calcified leaflets and commissures, an increase in radial strength at the waist (native annulus) level to avoid the potential need for post-dilatation, and a reduction of the length of the support arms to improve prosthesis conformance to the native root anatomy.

43.7 Results

Information on early and midterm results is mainly available for the CoreValve and the Edwards Sapien. Data come from large registries, single and multicenter reports, and few matched pair comparisons. No randomized controlled trials have as yet been reported.

Procedural success for the CoreValve™ has substantially increased over time and with refinements in technology. For TF implantations of the SAPIEN prosthesis, Webb reported a procedural success rate of 76% in the first 25 patients and 96% success rate for the subsequent 25. Thirty-day mortality decreased from 16% to 8%, respectively [15, 16]. In a recent multicenter study on 646 patients receiving the third-generation CoreValve™, the overall procedural success rate was 97%, procedural mortality was 1.5%, and the 30-day all-cause mortality was 8% [2].

In the initial US feasibility trial for the Sapien valve, a 17.5% 30-day and 22.5% in-hospital mortality was reported [17]. In the Partner EU trial, a multicentre trial that included 69 patients receiving an Edwards Sapien valve, a similar mortality of 18.8% was reported. Large single center studies and registry data show more recently mortality rates in the range of 8–15% [18]. The Canadian multicenter experience including 345 procedures using the Sapien valve (TF: 168, TA: 177) was published in 2009. The predicted surgical mortality using the STS score was 9.8 ± 6.4%. The procedural success rate was 93.3%. Procedural, post-procedural, and cumulative 30-day mortality were 1.7%, 8.7%, and 10.4% (TF: 9.5%, TA: 11.3%), respectively. In this context, it is to mention that results of most trials match predicted risk (according to STS score) but rarely exceed the results of conventional AVR for similar risk groups. The reasons leading to procedural death in the Canadian Multicenter Registry were major vascular complications (0.6%), severe left ventricular dysfunction after valve implantation (0.6%), cardiac perforation (0.3%), and acute severe MR after balloon valvuloplasty (0.3%). After a median follow-up of 8 months, the mortality rate was 22.1%. In this cohort, the predictors of cumulative late mortality were periprocedural sepsis (HR: 3.49, 95% CI: 1.48–8.28) or need for hemodynamic support (HR: 2.58, 95% CI: 1.11–6), pulmonary hypertension (PH) (HR: 1.88, 95% CI: 1.17–3), chronic renal failure (CRF) (HR: 2.30, 95% CI: 1.38–3.84), and COPD (HR: 1.75, 95% CI: 1.09–2.83). Interestingly, frail patients (25%) had the same acute outcomes as the rest of the study population [19].

The SOURCE-registry data including 1,038 patients (TA = 575 TF = 463) enrolled at 32 centers showed a procedural success rate of 93.8% for implantation of the Sapien valve. Thirty-day mortality was 6.3% in transfemoral patients and 10.3% in transapical patients but not comparable due to significant differences in perioperative risk profile (logistic ES TA 29.1% vs. TF 25.7%; $p < 0.001$).

The hemodynamic performance of transcatheter valves is excellent. All major studies report low transvalvular gradients both for the Sapien (10±4 mmHg) as well as for the CoreValve™ (4–7 mmHg) and an improvement of LVEF as well as NYHA functional class. Few studies report echocardiographic findings at 12 months or later with no evidence of structural valve failure and persistent low gradients [20–22]. Quality of life is improved after TAVI similar to the experience after conventional AVR [23].

Perioperative access- and device-related complications can create life-threatening situations and are sometimes challenging to treat.

Access-related complications include perforation of the iliac or femoral vessels for the TF approach. Depending on the site of injury and the severity of bleeding, intermittent balloon occlusion of the abdominal aorta and stenting (using a covered stent) or open surgical repair may become necessary. It is advisable to maintain contralateral arterial access until sufficient femoral closure and hemostasis have been achieved. The reported incidence of major vascular injury using the Sapien valve is reported in the range of 10.6% for the transfemoral and 2.4% for the transapical cohort. Major vascular complications that doubled the perioperative mortality in earlier registries still impact mortality in the TAVI group [24].

Apical ventricular injury is rare but can result from apical manipulation and cause major hemorrhage. If the ventricular defect cannot be readily repaired by additional felt-pledgeted sutures, decompression of the heart using CPB is advisable, and repair should be carried out using large patches and tension-free suturing.

The stiff wire used for placing the implant can cause perforation or rupture of the left ventricle leading to tamponade and ventricular rupture. The reported incidence ranges from 0.3% to 1% [19, 21]. This may happen during valve insertion and balloon valvuloplasty or valve placement as these maneuvers can be associated with forces that push the wire against the free ventricular wall. Distal wire tip control throughout the implantation procedure and manual wire shaping forming a less traumatic pigtail-like wire tip is therefore recommended. Ventricular rupture can only be treated by emergency surgery but even under the best circumstances has a dismal prognosis.

Overinflation or excess oversizing can cause annular rupture demanding for immediate implementation of CPB and surgical repair which in this case usually involves complete root replacement and ventricular repair.

Aortic dissection is rare but incidence may vary depending on the type of implant and the deployment mode. In the SOURCE registry, aortic dissection occurred in 1.9% of patients undergoing transfemoral and 0.7% of the patients undergoing transapical aortic valve implantation [23]. In the Engager series, aortic dissection occurred in 4/30 patients and has triggered reengineering of both the valve and the delivery system. Aortic dissection is best treated with immediate subclavian arterial cannulation, antegrade cerebral perfusion, and replacement of the aortic root and the ascending aorta. Hemiarch or full arch replacement may become necessary.

Paravalvular leak resulting in aortic insufficiency of grade II or more is reported at an incidence of 10–30% [20, 25] and may lead to LV dysfunction and hemolysis and may even be a cause for endocarditis [26]. However, valve endocarditis is seen rather infrequently with transcatheter AVI.

The incidence of permanent pacemaker implantation is reported in the range from 7% for the Sapien Valve [23] to up to 33% for the self-expanding CoreValve [27]. Acute onset of AV-Block or new onset of LBBB is best treated by temporary pacing using the pacing wires that are placed for rapid ventricular pacing. Careful perioperative monitoring is required, and persistent block should trigger an early decision for permanent pacemaker implantation. AV-block can occur anytime during the first few days after transcatheter valve implantation, and therefore these patients should remain on telemetry for at least 4–5 days.

Coronary occlusion, partial or total, has infrequently been reported. In the SOURCE registry, the incidence of coronary occlusion was 0.6% [23]. In case of a very low insertion of the left coronary ostium and heavy calcification of the left coronary cusp, it can be useful to place a guidewire into the left coronary artery prior to balloon inflation to secure access for emergent PCI should coronary obstruction result from valvuloplasty or valve implantation. PCI is the method of choice to treat acute coronary occlusion [28]. If not feasible, the patient should be placed on CPB, and coronary artery bypass grafting should be performed immediately to minimize the time to reperfusion.

Acute LV dysfunction can result from acute aortic insufficiency after balloon dilatation, coronary obstruction, or ventricular pacing. In the Canadian multicenter study, extracorporeal circulation for acute LV failure was required in 2.9% [19]. If aortic insufficiency is the cause for acute LV dysfunction, prompt placement of the valve is required.

Device embolization is reported at an incidence of 0.3–2.0% [19, 23, 29]. The management of device misplacement (into the LV or into the aorta) depends on the type of implant. In some cases, distal embolization is treated best by pulling the device back from the aortic arch into the descending aorta where it should not cause potential damage. Nevertheless, full retrievability remains a top priority for future developments.

Device malfunctioning due to incomplete closure, leaflet damage, or incomplete expansion may be treated with balloon inflation or require a second implant (valve in valve). The decision to implant a second valve, however, demands for some expertise.

The stroke rate is reported in the range from 0% to 10% but averages around 2.5% in the larger registries [20, 23]. Retrograde passage of the aortic arch in the presence of severe atherosclerosis causing embolism is thought to be one of the leading mechanisms. Dislodgement of debris from the native valve during balloon inflation or implantation is another potential cause. Sequential MRI has revealed small defects also in asymptomatic patients. Despite the fact that no CPB is used and the aorta is not clamped, the stroke rate remains high in TAVI and is currently not less than reported for standard open AVR.

43.8 Discussion

Transcatheter aortic valve implantation may provide benefit to higher risk patients by avoiding the need for cardiopulmonary bypass, cardiac ischemia, and sternotomy. The hemodynamic performance of transcatheter valves is favorable, and up to now no reports have indicated early structural valve failure. Functional improvement has been documented, and in patients with no complications early ambulation can be expected.

Besides major cardiac and noncardiac complications, the frequent occurrence of paravalvular leakage and atrioventricular block are of concern in transcatheter valve implantations. The presence of asymmetric calcification patterns, variations in aortic root geometry and mechanical properties of the aorta, the valve and the aortic annulus all may impact the final position of the valve and determine potential collateral damage such as leaks and AV-block. Improved valve designs and a better valve selection process based on individual anatomic criteria may improve results in the future. Enhanced imaging and modeling as well as augmented reality techniques will most likely help to improve the implant procedure.

With the expectation that technology is likely to improve within the next few years, the indication for TAVI is likely to shift to a younger population. However, controlled randomized clinical trials will be required beforehand. Another interesting indication are patients with degenerated xenografts. While this problem is less frequent with the current generation of biological valves, the trend for implantation in younger patient groups will generate an increasing patient cohort requiring a second operation. Redo AVR can be performed with excellent results, but alternative techniques may further decrease the risks associated with redo aortic valve surgery. Especially after root replacement, redo AVR can be challenging. A few studies demonstrated that for both mitral and aortic valve xenografts, TAVI can be performed successfully. The so-called valve-in-valve concept makes use of the stent of the implanted xenograft that serves as a marker during implantation of the transcatheter valve [30, 31]. This concept has also already been

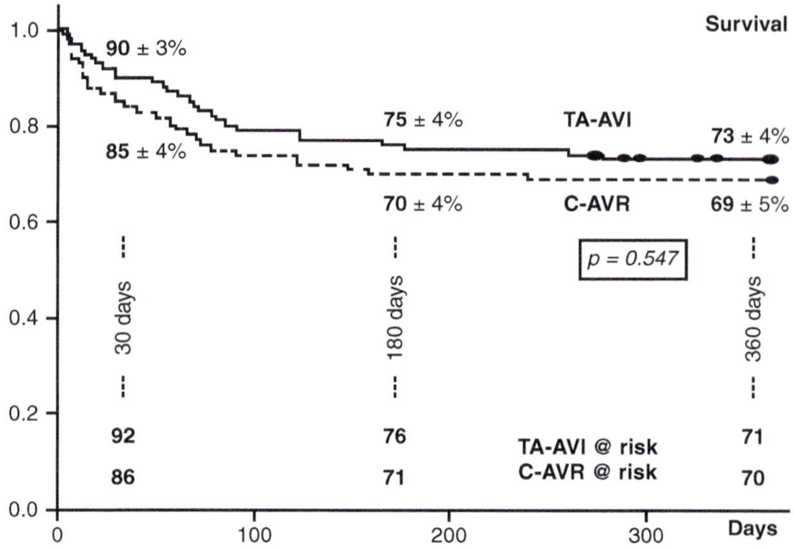

Fig. 43.18 Results of matched pair comparison for TAVI and conventional AVR (Taken from Walther et al. [3])

applied in an experimental setting as valve-in-a-ring for late mitral valve replacement after late failure of mitral valve repair [32].

Another promising approach is the transcatheter placement of autologous tissue engineered valve stents. A proof of concept has recently been shown. This approach may have important implications for the correction of congenital cardiac malformations [33].

In the absence of randomized trials and the few data on matched comparisons showing similar results for TAVI as for patients undergoing conventional surgery (Fig. 43.18) [3], TAVI can currently be considered an alternative approach for selected high-risk patients with severe aortic stenosis.

References

1. Cribier A, Eltchaninoff H, Bash A, Borenstein N, Tron C, Bauer F, Derumeaux G, Anselme F, Laborde F, Leon MB (2002) Percutaneous transcatheter implantation of an aortic valve prosthesis for calcific aortic stenosis: first human case description. Circulation 106:3006–3008
2. Piazza N, Grube E, Gerckens U, den Heijer P, Linke A, Luha O, Ramondo A, Ussia G, Wenaweser P, Windecker S, Laborde JC, de Jaegere P, Serruys PW (2008) Procedural and 30-day outcomes following transcatheter aortic valve implantation using the third generation (18 Fr) corevalve revalving system: results from the multicentre, expanded evaluation registry 1-year following CE mark approval. EuroIntervention 4(2): 242–249
3. Walther T, Schuler G, Borger MA, Kempfert J, Seeburger J, Rückert Y, Ender J, Linke A, Scholz M, Falk V, Mohr FW (2010) Transapical aortic valve implantation in 100 consecutive patients: comparison to propensity-matched conventional aortic valve replacement. Eur Heart J 31:1398–1403
4. Vahanian A, Alfieri OR, Al-Attar N, Antunes MJ, Bax J, Cormier B, Cribier A, De Jaegere P, Fournial G, Kappetein AP, Kovac J, Ludgate S, Maisano F, Moat N, Mohr FW, Nataf P, Pierard L, Pomar JL, Schofer J, Tornos P, Tuzcu M, van Hout B, von Segesser LK, Walther T (2008) Transcatheter valve implantation for patients with aortic stenosis: a position statement from the European Association of Cardio-Thoracic Surgery (EACTS) and the European Society of Cardiology (ESC), in collaboration with the European Association of Percutaneous Cardiovascular Interventions (EAPCI). Eur J Cardiothorac Surg 34:1–8
5. Vahanian A, Baumgartner H, Bax J, Butchart E, Dion R, Filippatos G, Flachskampf F, Hall R, Iung B, Kasprzak J, Nataf P, Tornos P, Torracca L, Wenink A (2007) Task Force on the Management of Valvular Heart Disease of the European Society of Cardiology; ESC Committee for Practice Guidelines. Guidelines on the management of valvular heart disease: the Task Force on the Management of Valvular Heart Disease of the European Society of Cardiology. Eur Heart J 28:230–268
6. Walther T, Dewey T, Borger MA, Kempfert J, Linke A, Becht R, Falk V, Schuler G, Mohr FW, Mack M (2009) Transapical aortic valve implantation: step by step. Ann Thorac Surg 87:276–283
7. Schultz CJ, Moelker A, Piazza N, Tzikas A, Otten A, Nuis RJ, Neefjes LA, von Geuns RJ, de Feyter P, Krestin G, Serruys PW, de Jaegere PT (2010) Three dimensional evaluation of the aortic annulus using multislice computer tomography: are manufacturer's guidelines for sizing for percutaneous aortic valve replacement helpful? Eur Heart J 31:849–856

8. Kempfert J, Falk V, Schuler G, Linke A, Merk D, Mohr FW, Walther T (2009) Dyna-CT during minimally invasive off-pump transapical aortic valve implantation. Ann Thorac Surg 88:2041
9. Gessat M, Karar ME, Walther T, Falk V, Burgert O (2009) Computer assisted transapical aortic valve implantation. Proc World Congr Med Phys Biomed Eng 25/VI:303–306
10. Grube E, Schuler G, Buellesfeld L, Gerckens U, Linke A, Wenaweser P, Sauren B, Mohr FW, Walther T, Zickmann B, Iversen S, Felderhoff T, Cartier R, Bonan R (2007) Percutaneous aortic valve replacement for severe aortic stenosis in high-risk patients using the second- and current third-generation self-expanding CoreValve prosthesis: device success and 30-day clinical outcome. J Am Coll Cardiol 50:69–76
11. Petronio AS, De Carlo M, Bedogni F, Marzocchi A, Klugmann S, Maisano F, Ramondo A, Ussia GP, Ettori F, Poli A, Brambilla N, Saia F, De Marco F, Colombo A (2010) Safety and efficacy of the subclavian approach for transcatheter aortic valve implantation with the CoreValve revalving system. Circ Cardiovasc Interv 3(4):359–366
12. Treede H, Tübler T, Reichenspurner H, Grube E, Pascotto A, Franzen O, Mueller R, Low R, Bolling SF, Meinertz T, Schofer J (2010) Six-month results of a repositionable and retrievable pericardial valve for transcatheter aortic valve replacement: the direct flow medical aortic valve. J Thorac Cardiovasc Surg 140(4):897–903
13. Lauten A, Ferrari M, Petri A, Ensminger SM, Gummert JF, Boudjemline Y, Schubert H, Schumm J, Hekmat K, Schlosser M, Figulla HR (2009) Experimental evaluation of the JenaClip transcatheter aortic valve. Catheter Cardiovasc Interv 74:514–519
14. Falk V, Schwammenthal EE, Kempfert J, Linke A, Schuler G, Mohr FW, Walther T (2009) New anatomically oriented transapical aortic valve implantation. Ann Thorac Surg 87:925–926
15. Webb JG, Chandavimol M, Thompson C, Ricci DR, Carere R, Munt B, Buller CE, Pasupati S, Lichtenstein S (2006) Percutaneous aortic valve implantation retrograde from the femoral artery. Circulation 113:842–850
16. Webb JG, Altwegg L, Boone RH, Cheung A, Ye J, Lichtenstein S, Lee M, Masson JB, Thompson C, Moss R, Carere R, Munt B, Nietlispach F, Humphries K (2009) Transcatheter aortic valve implantation: impact on clinical and valve-related outcomes. Circulation 16(119):3009–3016
17. Svensson LG, Dewey T, Kapadia S, Roselli EE, Stewart A, Williams M, Anderson WN, Brown D, Leon M, Lytle B, Moses J, Mack M, Tuzcu M, Smith C (2008) United States feasibility study of transcatheter insertion of a stented aortic valve by the left ventricular apex. Ann Thorac Surg 86:46–54
18. Wendler O, Walther T, Nataf P, Rubino P, Schroefel H, Thielmann M, Treede H, Thomas M (2010) Transapical aortic valve implantation: univariate and multivariate analyses of the early results from the SOURCE registry. Eur J Cardiothorac Surg 38(2):119–127
19. Rodés-Cabau J, Webb JG, Cheung A, Ye J, Dumont E, Feindel CM, Osten M, Natarajan MK, Velianou JL, Martucci G, DeVarennes B, Chisholm R, Peterson MD, Lichtenstein SV, Nietlispach F, Doyle D, DeLarochellière R, Teoh K, Chu V, Dancea A, Lachapelle K, Cheema A, Latter D, Horlick E (2010) Transcatheter aortic valve implantation for the treatment of severe symptomatic aortic stenosis in patients at very high or prohibitive surgical risk: acute and late outcomes of the multicenter Canadian experience. J Am Coll Cardiol 55:1080–1090
20. Clavel MA, Dumont E, Pibarot P, Doyle D, De Larochellière R, Villeneuve J, Bergeron S, Couture C, Rodés-Cabau J (2009) Severe valvular regurgitation and late prosthesis embolization after percutaneous aortic valve implantation. Ann Thorac Surg 87:618–621
21. Yan TD, Cao C, Martens-Nielsen J, Padang R, Ng M, Vallely MP, Bannon PG (2010) Transcatheter aortic valve implantation for high-risk patients with severe aortic stenosis: a systematic review. J Thorac Cardiovasc Surg 139(6):1519–1528
22. Ye J, Cheung A, Lichtenstein SV, Nietlispach F, Albugami S, Masson JB, Thompson CR, Munt B, Moss R, Carere RG, Jamieson WR, Webb JG (2010) Transapical transcatheter aortic valve implantation: follow-up to 3 years. J Thorac Cardiovasc Surg 139:1107–1113
23. Thomas M, Schymik G, Walther T, Himbert D, Lefèvre T, Cartier J, Treede H, Eggebrecht H, Rubino P, Michev L, Lange R, Wendler O (2010) 30 day results of the SOURCE registry: a European registry of transcatheter aortic valve implantation using the Edwards SAPIEN™ valve. Circulation 122:62–69
24. Gotzmann M, Hehen T, Germing A, Lindstaedt M, Yazar A, Laczkovics A, Mumme A, Mügge A, Bojara W (2010) Short-term effects of transcatheter aortic valve implantation on neurohormonal activation, quality of life and 6-minute walk test in severe and symptomatic aortic stenosis. Heart 96:1102–1106
25. Clavel MA, Webb JG, Pibarot P, Altwegg L, Dumont E, Thompson C, De Larochellière R, Doyle D, Masson JB, Bergeron S, Bertrand OF, Rodés-Cabau J (2009) Comparison of the hemodynamic performance of percutaneous and surgical bioprostheses for the treatment of severe aortic stenosis. J Am Coll Cardiol 53:1883–1891
26. Walther T, Falk V (2009) Hemodynamic evaluation of heart valve prostheses paradigm shift for transcatheter valves? J Am Coll Cardiol 53:1892–1893
27. Jilaihawi H, Chin D, Vasa-Nicotera M, Jeilan M, Spyt T, Ng GA, Bence J, Logtens E, Kovac J (2009) Predictors for permanent pacemaker requirement after transcatheter aortic valve implantation with the CoreValve bioprosthesis. Am Heart J 157:860–866
28. Kapadia SR, Svensson L, Tuzcu EM (2009) Successful percutaneous management of left main trunk occlusion during percutaneous aortic valve replacement. Catheter Cardiovasc Interv 73:966–972
29. Al Ali AM, Altwegg L, Horlick EM, Feindel C, Thompson CR, Cheung A, Carere RG, Humphries K, Ye J, Masson JB, Webb JG (2008) Prevention and

management of transcatheter balloon-expandable aortic valve malposition. Catheter Cardiovasc Interv 72:573–578
30. Seiffert M, Franzen O, Conradi L, Baldus S, Schirmer J, Meinertz T, Reichenspurner H, Treede H (2010) Series of transcatheter valve-in-valve implantations in high-risk patients with degenerated bioprostheses in aortic and mitral position. Catheter Cardiovasc Interv 76(4):608–615
31. Webb JG, Wood DA, Ye J, Gurvitch R, Masson JB, Rodés-Cabau J, Osten M, Horlick E, Wendler O, Dumont E, Carere RG, Wijesinghe N, Nietlispach F, Johnson M, Thompson CR, Moss R, Leipsic J, Munt B, Lichtenstein SV, Cheung A (2010) Transcatheter valve-in-valve implantation for failed bioprosthetic heart valves. Circulation 121:1848–1857
32. Kempfert J, Blumenstein J, Chu MW, Pritzwald-Stegmann P, Kobilke T, Falk V, Mohr FW, Walther T (2009) Minimally invasive off-pump valve-in-a-ring implantation: the atrial transcatheter approach for re-operative mitral valve replacement after failed repair. Eur J Cardiothorac Surg 35:965–969
33. Schmidt D, Dijkman PE, Driessen-Mol A, Stenger R, Mariani C, Puolakka A, Rissanen M, Deichmann T, Odermatt B, Weber B, Emmert MY, Zund G, Baaijens FTP, Hoerstrup SP (2010) Minimally invasive implantation of living tissue engineered heart valves. J Am Coll Cardiol 56(6):510–520

Robotic Coronary Revascularisation 44

Roberto Pasquale Casula and Thanos Athanasiou

Contents

R.P. Casula, M.D., FETCS, FRCS (✉)
Department of Cardiothoracic Surgery, St. Mary's Hospital, Imperial College Healthcare NHS Trust, Praed Street, London W2 1NY, UK

Hammersmith Hospital, Imperial Healthcare College NHS Trust, Imperial College of Science, Technology and Medicine, London, UK
e-mail: roberto.casula@imperial.nhs.uk

T. Athanasiou, M.D., Ph.D, FRCS FETCS
Cardiothoracic Department, Hammersmith Hospital, Imperial Healthcare Trust, Due Cane Rd, London W12 0HS, UK
e-mail: t.athanasiou@imperial.ac.uk

44.1 Clinical Background

In less than a decade, robotic surgical techniques have been established in coronary surgery. The first coronary artery bypass procedure in a closed-chest was performed in 1998 by Loulmet and Carpentier [1].

We performed the first eight consecutive beating heart totally endoscopic coronary artery bypass (BH TECAB) procedures in a beating heart with the da Vinci system in the UK between 2003 and 2004 at St. Mary's Hospital [2–4].

Robotic coronary revascularisation has been applied in selected elective patients without significant enlargement of the left ventricle, without either left ventricular dysfunction or intra-myocardial coronary vessels. Relative contraindications remain the presence of anatomically chest deformities or morbid obesity.

In recent years, the indications for TECAB have been expanded by offering this surgical procedure in the contest of a 'hybrid revascularisation' strategy in combination with a planned percutaneous coronary intervention (PCI) in patients with multi-vessel disease involving the LAD [5, 6]. The robotic procedure can be performed before, after or on the same setting of the percutaneous intervention to the non-LAD target vessel depending on anatomical, clinical urgency status, logistics and drug-related consideration which should be discussed in the setting of a multidisciplinary (MDT) meeting with cardiologists, interventional cardiologists and cardiac surgeons and offered on an individual patient basis [7].

R.G.C. Inderbitzi et al. (eds.), *Minimally Invasive Thoracic and Cardiac Surgery*, DOI 10.1007/978-3-642-11861-6_44, © Springer-Verlag Berlin Heidelberg 2012

The hybrid approach has several potential benefits for the cardiac patient including the avoidance of a full median sternotomy and mostly an advantage in the longer-term survival and freedom from target coronary re-intervention of the patients who receive a left internal thoracic artery (LITA) to the LAD surgical revascularisation. Furthermore, the need for both surgical and interventional cardiologist interventions will require that all potential hybrid cases are surely discussed at an MDT-type clinical case conference as recommended by the 2010 published guidelines on coronary revascularisation [8].

The long-term benefits of coronary artery bypass grafting (CABG) in treating coronary artery disease are related mainly to the use of the left internal thoracic artery bypass to the left anterior descending artery (LAD). The LITA graft patency rate has been shown to constantly be over 90% after 15 years of follow-up offering a significantly better freedom from major cardiovascular event and coronary re-intervention compared to the use of intra-coronary stents via percutaneous coronary interventions.

Furthermore, the use of bilateral internal thoracic arteries (BITA) as bypass conduits may offer superior patient survival and freedom from re-operation when compared to patients operated with the use of a single LITA and saphenous veins. Since its approval by FDA for thoracoscopic use in 2001, The da Vinci system (Intuitive Surgical, Mountain View, CA) has been increasingly used to harvest the left and/or right internal thoracic arteries as bypass conduits for coronary revascularisation in three continents over the last decade. The totally endoscopic harvesting and preparation of the LITA for revascularisation purposes is an established, fast, accurate and reproducible surgical procedure.

Despite minimal access, techniques of coronary revascularisation are widely adopted by a small community of cardiac surgeons world wise; at present, there is no consensus of what is the exact definition of minimally invasive cardiac surgery (MICS) for coronary revascularisation [9, 10].

As far as coronary surgery is concerned, it is acceptable to consider 'minimal invasive' all techniques that do avoid the use of cardiopulmonary bypass (CPB). Furthermore, techniques that use a minimal surgical access into the chest such as a mini-thoracotomy either with direct vision or video assistance or a partial sternotomy are commonly considered as less invasive. Robotically assisted technique such as totally endoscopic coronary artery bypass (TECAB) on a 'beating heart' combines the concept of all the above-mentioned categories and can be considered as the latest advance in MICS by combining a closed chest surgical strategy and the avoidance of cardiopulmonary bypass.

A beating heart TECAB procedure seems to achieve the ultimate goal of a minimal access revascularisation approach by combining a truly totally endoscopic access operating via four 1-cm skin incisions with the avoidance of cardiopulmonary bypass [9–11].

In the contest of robotic coronary artery bypass surgery, the endoscopic, robotic-enhanced harvesting of the left internal thoracic artery represents the first stage of three different coronary revascularisation surgical procedures as follows:

1. Totally endoscopic coronary artery bypass (TECAB) for single-vessel disease on the beating heart (BH-TECAB) (left internal thoracic artery to left anterior descending coronary artery) or with the use of cardiopulmonary bypass (arrested heart or AH-TECAB)
2. A minimally invasive direct coronary artery bypass procedure (MIDCAB) through small anterior thoracotomy without spreading the ribs known as 'atraumatic coronary artery bypass' (ACAB) or robotic single-vessel small thoracotomy (SVST)
3. Totally endoscopic coronary artery bypass (TECAB) for multi-vessel coronary artery disease with the assistance of cardiopulmonary bypass (CPB)

44.2 Patient Selection and Assessment

44.2.1 General Considerations

There are some anatomical and technical considerations that need to be taken into account in order to successfully achieve a totally endoscopic coronary artery bypass procedure on the beating heart:

1. The anatomical features and target vessel quality of the LAD vessel should be evaluated pre-operatively with a routine coronary angiography with or without the adjunct of a CT chest scan which can potentially offer further details as in the case of a deep intra-myocardial LAD.
2. Correct positioning of the patient, the robotic arms, camera, trocars, endoscopic stabiliser are mandatory in order to reduce the risk of conversion to an open thoracotomy or a traditional median sternotomy approach.
3. Intra-operative monitoring with trans-oesophageal echo (TOE) which is used also as a dynamic diagnostic tool to assess in real time both global and segmental myocardial wall function changes and valvular function during each stage of the performance of a totally endoscopic off-pump procedure.

A robotic cardiac operation requires a high level of teamwork in the operating room, and the following staff members are ideally required: a console surgeon, a patient-side surgeon, two nurses (the scrub nurse and the circulating nurse), anaesthesiologists and a cardio-pulmonary bypass perfusions technician on standby as routinely adopted in the case of an 'off-pump' coronary revascularisation procedure.

In our view, when performing a TECAB, the most recent da Vinci system Si HD got several advantages compared to the standard version which we have used in our initial first 7 years of robotic cardiac experience. It is less bulky with less voluminous robotic arms that allow a faster and easily reproducible set-up in the operating room with a reduced chance of external arm collision even while performing the wide range of internal chest surgical navigation required during the harvesting of the entire length of one or both internal thoracic arteries.

44.2.2 Anaesthetic Considerations

1. In patients with a mild to moderately reduced left ventricular systolic function, a Swan-Ganz catheter can be positioned in order to monitor pulmonary artery and left atrial venous pressures and cardiac output continuously.
2. In our 8-year clinical practice in robotic coronary revascularisation, it has been our preference not to use Swan-Ganz catheters, but instead to regularly use only non-invasive intra-operative TOE monitoring which offers the advantage to be a routinely used tool in most cardiac theatres and allows instantaneous myocardial left and right functional assessment, segmental wall motion abnormalities analysis and preload assessment in the setting of intra-thoracic pressure changes caused by the routine and systematic use of CO_2 continuous pleural space insufflation.
3. Arterial blood gas monitoring is intermittently and regularly performed as in routine cardiac operations.
4. The patient is intubated with a double-lumen endotracheal tube for single right lung ventilation. As an alternative, a bronchial blocker can be used to temporarily collapse the left lung instead of a double-lumen tube.
5. A central venous line, a right radial arterial line and a Foley urinary catheter are routinely used.
6. The correct functioning and positioning of external defibrillation pads is of paramount importance as in all minimal access cardiac operation. In this case it becomes necessary to defibrillate the patients from an episode of ventricular or atrial fibrillation, the robotic instruments and ports have to be temporarily and rapidly taken out of the chest; both lungs must be re-inflated to ensure successful defibrillation as the electrical current will not easily pass through a gas-filled chest cavity.

44.3 Patient Positioning

The patient is placed supine on the operating table. In the most common scenario in which a LITA takedown and its anastomosis to the LAD is planned, an inflatable bag is placed under the patient's left side to allow elevation the left chest by 20–30°.

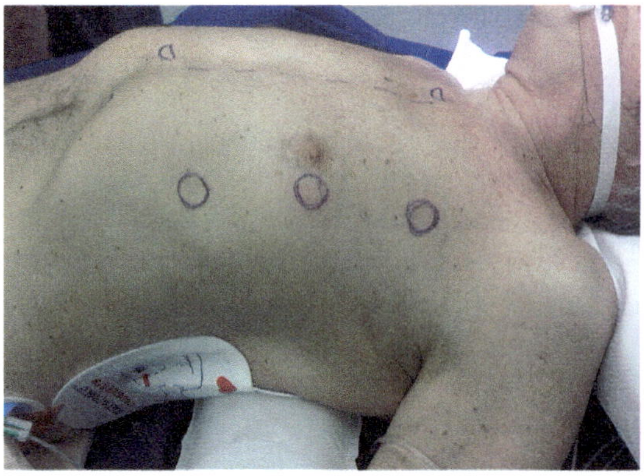

Fig. 44.1 Position of a patient for robotic LITA takedown followed by TECAB. Ink landmarks show the planned port location. The upper and lower edges of the sternal bone are shown as external reference points

The patient's left arm is slightly flexed at the elbow and supported on the side of the table below the left posterior axillary line. Such a position opens up the left chest and mainly aims to drop the left shoulder providing enough space for the right robotic arm to function without external collision.

The defibrillator pads are placed, one on the right anterolateral chest and the other pad on the left posterolateral chest.

A lower-body warming blanket system is applied, as in any off-pump procedure, attempts are made to prevent patients' rapid cooling which also increases the risk of cardiac rhythm disturbances.

Both groins are exposed for establishment of cardiopulmonary bypass if on-pump TECAB is performed or emergency cardiopulmonary bypass support is required in case of haemodynamic instability. The positioning of the patient as we described herein is presented in Fig. 44.1.

44.4 Surgical Techniques

44.4.1 Thoracic Port Placement

Precise port placement is a critical step in ensuring smooth manipulation of the robotic instruments in the chest without either external or internal instrument collision in view of the fact that the rigid bony thoraces and ribs limit instrument mobility. The third, fifth and seventh intercostal spaces are identified, and an approximate line along the left anterior axillary line is drawn.

Three trocar-size skin incisions are made most commonly along a straight line about 1 cm medial and parallel to the anterior axillary line (Fig. 44.1). Before the first trocar is introduced into the chest, single-lung ventilation is initiated by interrupting ventilation to the left lung which will deflate. The camera port is inserted always in the fifth space on the anterior axillary line followed by immediate but gradual intra-pleural space insufflation with CO_2.

A 12-mm disposable trocar is placed at the fifth intercostal space. In a man, this trocar is usually placed slightly inferior and lateral to the left nipple. In a woman, the skin incisions for the fifth and seventh intercostal trocars are made more laterally and inferiorly, respectively, to avoid the breast. The breast is then retracted medially and upward so that the trocar chest entry points are similarly positioned as described previously.

Through the fifth intercostal trocar, a 30° scope with 'looking-up' vision is inserted into the left pleural cavity. Inspection of the lung, chest wall, any visible portion of the LITA and pericardial sac is initially carried out.

Under direct scope vision, two 8-mm re-usable robotic trocars are placed separately in the seventh and third intercostal spaces, respectively, for the insertion of the two robotic instruments operated by the left and right robotic arms. The left-arm trocar location on an anteroposterior line in the chest is normally at the same level of the camera arm or marginally more posteriorly and inserted via the sixth or seventh intercostal space.

The left robotic instrument, either a microbipolar grasper or a Debakey tissue grasper, is inserted via the left-sided trocar. The right trocar is inserted in the third intercostal space usually halfway in a line between the left nipple and the shoulder in a man. The right instrument, a monopolar cautery, is inserted via the third intercostal trocar.

The three thoraco-ports more commonly lie on the same straight line on an anteroposterior plane.

An insufflation device is connected via the camera trocar to supply continuous CO_2 into the left pleural space. The CO_2 insufflation pressure is usually kept at 5 mmHg to start with and can occasionally be increased to 10–15 mmHg depending on the need to create a larger intra-thoracic working space between the chest wall and the pericardium. In case that both left and right internal thoracic arteries need to be harvested, the right thoracic artery is harvested first using the 0° endoscope and then changing to a 30° angled endoscope so that the left internal thoracic artery can be harvested too. Another port is required for the insertion of the epicardial stabiliser in order to stabilise epicardially the coronary targets and to perform the coronary anastomosis with or without cardiopulmonary bypass. The endostabiliser is operated by the fourth robotic arm.

44.4.2 Harvesting the Left and Right Internal Thoracic Arteries

It is important to identify the relevant anatomical landmarks:

- The LITA in any portion visible via the pleural fat
- The left phrenic nerve
- The first rib

This will allow full-length mobilisation of LITA, while avoiding injury to the left phrenic nerve.

The author's preference is to start the dissection of the LITA in any of his visible portion. The pleural fat is initially taken down to facilitate visualisation of the target. The LITA dissection of the chest wall can be started proximally at the level of the first rib and extending distally down to bifurcation, at the level of the sixth intercostal space.

The LITA can be dissected either using a totally skeletonised technique or as a pedicle surrounded by its satellite veins. In either case, the visualisation of the conduit can be achieved by dissecting the pleural reflection and the pleural fat pad from the anterior chest wall. This surgical step can significantly reduce the harvesting time especially if the skeletonisation technique has been chosen. A micro-bipolar vascular grasper and a monopolar cautery spatula can be used for this (Fig. 44.2).

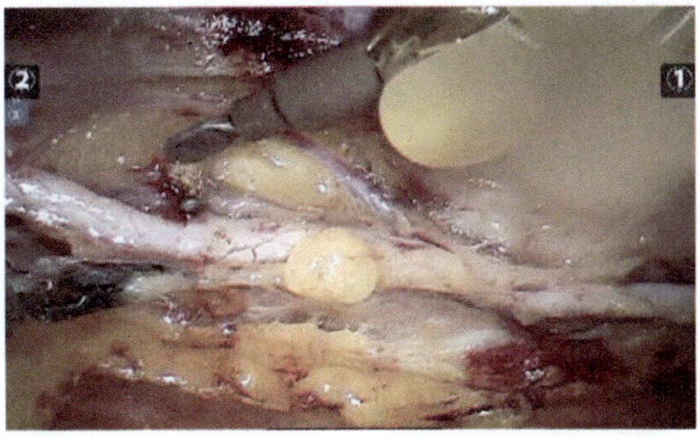

Fig. 44.2 A monopolar cautery spatula (on the right arm) can be used to skeletonise the LITA in all its length

The author has successfully harvested the first 100 LITA in a non-skeletonised fashion while preserving a tiny pedicle consisting of the two satellite veins and the small amount of fascia covering them. We would advise surgeons in their initial phase of their robotic experience to perform the LITA dissection as a pedicle so that they are less likely to accidently traumatise the LITA wall while still familiarising with the da Vinci Si instruments' capability and functions. The muscle pedicle and veins along the LITA are harvested together, and all the LITA and vein branches can be either clipped or cauterised. The diathermy energy used in the case of a LITA pedicle dissection is usually quite low at the level of 20 W, and coagulation of the branches at this setting is usually successfully carried out by dissecting around the branches and then coagulating them by touching the side branch with the flat part of the monopolar spatula. The skeletonised technique requires less traction during the manipulation of the LITA and should be used after the surgeon has acquired the relevant experience of dissecting the LITA as a pedicle. The cautery energy is kept low at 15 W in order to open the fascia just above the LITA for its entire length, then to gently separate the artery from the accompanying veins and surrounding fat. The skeletonised technique provides longer graft length and greater blood flow compared with the pedicle technique [11] (Fig. 44.3).

During BITA harvesting, the RITA is harvested first and usually left connected distally until the LITA is entirely dissected as well in order to allow

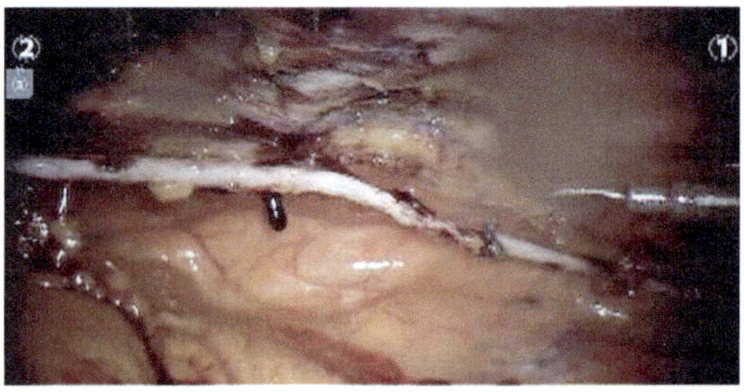

Fig. 44.3 Panoramic view of skeletonised LITA

blood nourishment of its vessel wall during the time required to dissect the LITA.

The harvesting of both internal thoracic arteries can be undertaken from the left side and requires the CO_2 insufflation pressure to be increased to 10–15 mmHg in order to improve the right pleural cavity visualisation if the patient's haemodynamic status allows. Both mediastinal pleural reflections are detached from the sternum, starting from the first rib to the sixth intercostal space. It is preferable for the RITA to be harvested in a skeletonised fashion, and the proximal part of the internal thoracic vein can be divided allowing extra length to be gained. Heparin is given i.v. to maintain an ACT between 300 and 400 s. The distal parts of the LITA or RITA are clipped while a *Scanlan* padded mini-green bulldog vessel clamp is applied to the LITA and/or RITA distal third; the LITA is then divided with robotic Potts scissors. In this stage, the LITA distal part is prepared for the anastomosis, and after transection of the vessel the distal end is opened longitudinally by a few millimetres. This step is facilitated by the fact that the LITA is held in close proximity to the chest wall having left a small fat or fascial bridge as a support during its dissection. Also the robotic Potts are marked on the side to conveniently show 1–4-mm scale.

44.4.3 Pericardiectomy and Identification of Coronary Artery

The site of the pericardial opening can be decided depending on the target coronary arteries to be grafted. If the LAD is the target vessel, the pericardial incision is started more medially and near the apex of the heart. If the target vessel involves any of the coronary arteries of the lateral wall such as diagonal and/or obtuse marginal arteries in addition to the LAD, the pericardium can be conveniently opened more laterally, about 3–4 cm anterior to the left phrenic nerve. The pericardium incision is carried out from about the level of the apex of the heart and then cranially up to the level of right pulmonary outflow tract. Once the targeted LAD segment and other target vessels are identified, the CO_2 insufflation is temporarily reduced to minimise the shifting of the heart. An important aspect during the pericardial incision is that diathermy setting should be kept to a low power and with caution as the possibility of a sudden ventricular arrhythmia can occur. It is advisable to check both the serum potassium level and the correct positioning of the defibrillator pads before starting the pericardial opening. Other authors suggest to start a lignocaine infusion during pericardial opening.

44.4.3.1 Atraumatic Coronary Artery Bypass (ACAB): Surgical Steps

Following the dissection of the LITA by using thoraco-ports and preparation of the distal end of the LITA, opening of the pericardium and identification of the target coronary artery, the following surgical steps are carried out in order to perform an atraumatic coronary artery bypass also called single-vessel small thoracotomy (SVST):

- Our preference is to remove the left and right robotic instruments and while leaving the thoraco-ports briefly in situ to maintain positive pressure with CO_2 insufflation. We swap the camera for a 0° vision, and we point the camera at the target vessel roughly in the area where the arteriotomy will be carried out. The orientation and angle of the camera as observed from outside the chest will orient us in choosing the correct intercostal space, usually the fifth IC and the medial extent of the skin incision. With increasing team experience, it is common to limit the skin incision to 5–6 cm most commonly via the same IC space of the

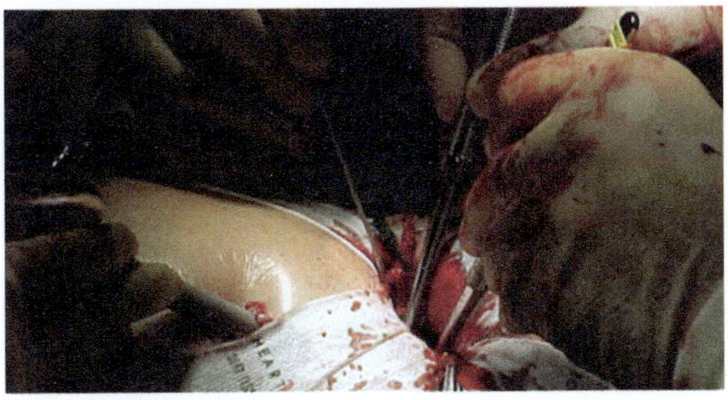

Fig. 44.4 View of an ACAB during the completion of the LITA to LAD anastomosis

camera incision but more medial and not in continuation with the camera port incision to contain the total length of the skin incision to a maximum of 5–6 cm.

- A more medial incision is also likely to preserve intact the more bulky part of the pectoralis major which is instead incised in its more medial part and in a parallel direction to its muscle fibres in order to maintain muscle integrity.
- The left pleural cavity is entered. The intercostal muscle incision can be extended to a larger size compared to the skin incision.
- A soft tissue retractor can be used (Fig. 44.4) or even a small-size thoracotomy retractor since the limited skin incision does prevent anything apart from a minimal rib spreading which we feel represent one of the major advantages compared to a MIDCAB approach in which a larger amount of ribs spreading is necessarily needed in order to harvest most of the length of the LITA. This invariably causes intercostal space trauma, cartilages dislocation or even rib fractures in older osteoporotic patients.
- As soon as the IC is entered, the pericardial opening should be easily identified, and firstly attention is drawn to the LITA which is visualised and taken in control by exteriorising it towards the level of the entered IC space.
- A few pericardial stitches can be used to bring the LAD target closer and in perfect proximity to the limited surgical incision.
- We advise to achieve the LAD epicardial stabilisation by positioning an endoscopic stabiliser such as the 'rod-mounted' Estech coronary stabiliser that can be entered into the chest via one of the previously created ports for robotic arm access. In our experience, the most common and suitable one is the third space right arm port which allows the stabiliser foot to lie nearly parallel to the LAD. In our experience, there is no need or advantage for using a suction device for stabilisation. The stabiliser arm is supported by a table-mounted arm.
- Proximal and distal silastic slings are passed around the LAD and gently retracted in order to temporarily stop the LAD blood flow during the arteriotomy and to maintain a dry operative field with the help of CO_2 blower. An intra-coronary shunt can be used in case of a non-total occlusion of the LAD on angiography or to better control LAD blood losses in case a time-consuming anastomosis is likely to be needed. The use of an intra-luminal shunt also reduces LAD territory ischaemia and is our preferred method of maintaining a dry arteriotomy site.
- The LITA to coronary anastomosis is routinely performed with either 7/0 or 8/0 Prolene. A *Scanlan* padded mini-green bulldog vessel clamp is released from the LITA, and blood flow is re-established into the LAD after releasing the two silastic slings. The anastomosis is checked with the help of the CO_2 blower. The endostabiliser is carefully removed.
- One- or two-size 24-Fr Blake drains through the existing left and right arm robotic ports, one apical and one basal in the left pleural space.
- A flow metre can be easily applied to the skeletonised LITA for flow characteristic assessment, and heparin action is then reversed with protamine sulphate.
- An important point before closure is to assess the position of the LITA which should lie just parallel and above the phrenic nerved and be covered by the left lung once carefully re-expanded.
- The mini-thoracotomy is closed without use of pericostal stitches that are not required since no or minimal rib spreading was required.

44.4.3.2 Total Endoscopic Coronary Artery Bypass (TECAB)

The TECAB operation can be safely performed without the use of cardiopulmonary bypass, on the beating heart. The use of cardiopulmonary bypass and cardioplegic arrest can be used for a single-vessel LITA to LAD procedure but is more likely to be reserved particularly for cases in which more than one anastomosis or sequential LITA grafting, in which the beating heart technique even if potentially technically feasible can be very time consuming and more technically demanding with significantly higher risk of conversion.

In the case of an on-pump totally endoscopic revascularisation case, the left femoral artery and vein are exposed. A 25-Fr multi-stage venous cannula and a 21–23-Fr arterial femoral cannula with 'endoclamp' balloon are correctly positioned under trans-oesophageal echocardiography guidance. The pericardium is opened, and the LAD is identified. Cardiopulmonary bypass is initiated; the ascending aortic balloon is inflated, and cardioplegia is given to arrest the heart.

44.4.4 'Beating Heart' (BH) TECAB Surgical Technique

Following the preparation of the distal end of the harvested LIMA and the identification of the LAD target as described in the case of the ACAB, the endoscopic coronary *EndoWrist stabiliser* is inserted into the chest via a sub-xiphoid 12-mm re-usable thoraco-port which is most commonly introduced sub-costally about 3–5 cm laterally on the left side of the xiphoid process. It is advisable that the table surgeon introduces a long thru-cut needle in order to identify the correct pathway into the chest while the console surgeon can help the introduction of the thoracoport by haemostatically dissecting some subcostal fat pad off the diaphragm. Once the port is in position, the coronary *EndoWrist stabiliser* is introduced into the chest via the da Vinci fourth arm. The console surgeon can take control of the navigation of the *EndoWrist stabiliser* which is

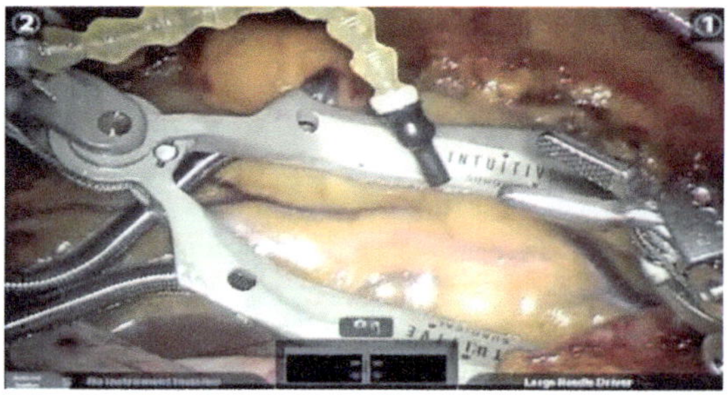

Fig. 44.5 Insertion of the *EndoWrist stabiliser* with irrigator to stabilise the coronary target

gently position in proximity of the LAD portion chosen for the arteriotomy. The *EndoWrist stabiliser* is a suction device, and vacuum is applied and kept up to 400 mmHg to the two stabiliser branches. Careful opening of the stabiliser jaw allows flattening of the epicardial fat surrounding the LAD and consequently better exposure and stabilisation. A coronary irrigator is used to flash warm normal saline and is introduced via a separate channel of the same *EndoWrist stabiliser* (Fig. 44.5). The flexible end of the coronary irrigator can be easily handled by the console surgeon and carefully positioned in a suitable position to continuously or intermittently irrigate the coronary target during the arteriotomy and the anastomosis if and when needed.

Once LAD stabilisation has been achieved to robotic silastic coronary occluders (Quest Medical *SaddleLoop*), their blunt tip needle is passed around the LAD just proximally and distally to the arteriotomy chosen site and then tightened to temporarily stop the coronary flow. The arteriotomy is started by perforating the front wall of the coronary by using a *Snap-fit* Blue Blade and then by continuing the arteriotomy with Potts scissors which with increasing experience can be easily and efficiently used from the same left or right robotic arm in both forward and reverse directions (Figs. 44.6a, b and 44.7).

It has been our preference in the most recent part of our experience to use an intra-coronary shunt. The insertion of the shunt into the LAD arteriotomy is usually straightforward due to the

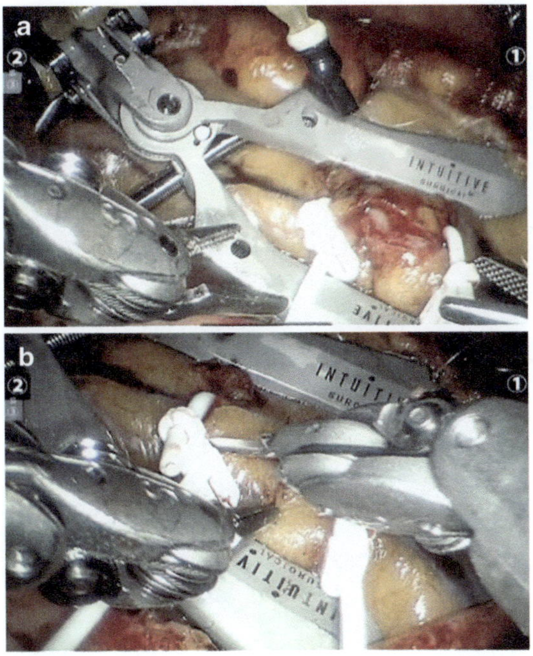

Fig. 44.6 (**a**) Positioning of proximal and distal silastic *SaddleLoops* to maintain a bloodless anastomotic site. (**b**) Coronary arteriotomy: a *Snap-fit* paddle 'beaver blade' is used to dissect the epicardial fat over the LAD chosen anastomotic site before the LAD is incised with a *Snap-fit* Blue Blade

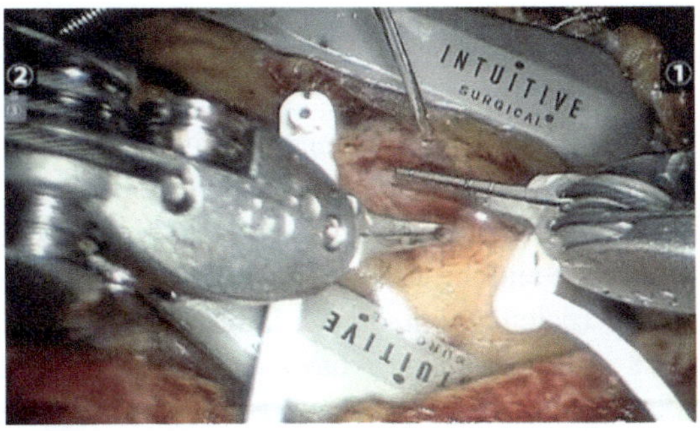

Fig. 44.7 Extension of arteriotomy with robotic Potts scissors

excellent vision and dexterity provided by the robotic arms and instruments. The advantages of the presence of an intra-coronary shunt have been shown and reported in the off-pump revascularisation literature, and also in a robotic TECAB set-up, a bloodless field and a gentle retraction of the shunt can help expose the intima in order to secure

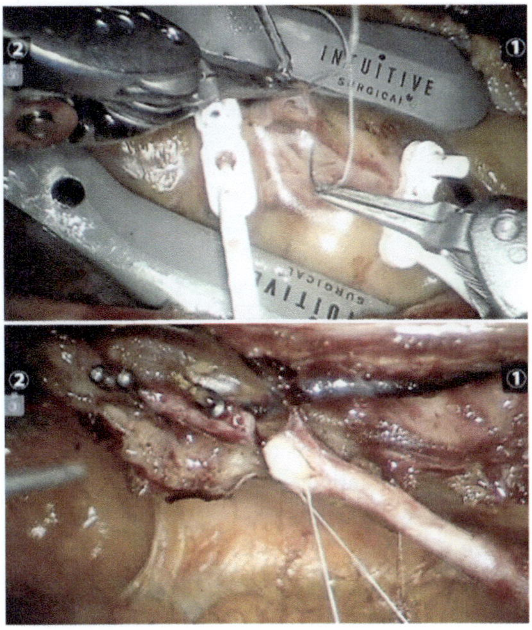

Fig. 44.8 Anastomosis with use of GORE-TEX CV-8 7-cm-length suture

each bite during the anastomosis. The coronary anastomosis is accomplished with GORE-TEX CV-8 suture or Ethicon 7/0 Prolene; both stitches are made in 7 cm length for robotic endoscopic use (Fig. 44.8).

In order to facilitate the execution of the very first part of the anastomosis with the 'parachuting technique', we suggest that the LITA is left attached to the chest wall by a tiny bridge of fascia or fat (Fig. 44.8). As an alternative, the table surgeon could insert an endo-grasper via a tiny stab incision in the anterior chest. With the aid of the endo-grasper, the distal LITA can be held and presented to the console surgeon effectively offering support when passing the first few stitches via the LITA and also improving the LAD exposure when stitching through the LAD anastomotic 'heel'.

Once the anastomosis has been accomplished, the distal LAD silastic *SaddleLoop* and the LITA mini-green bulldog are released and LAD flow re-established and the anastomosis is checked. Once haemostasis has been confirmed, also the proximal LAD silastic *SaddleLoop* is released and taken out (Fig. 44.9).

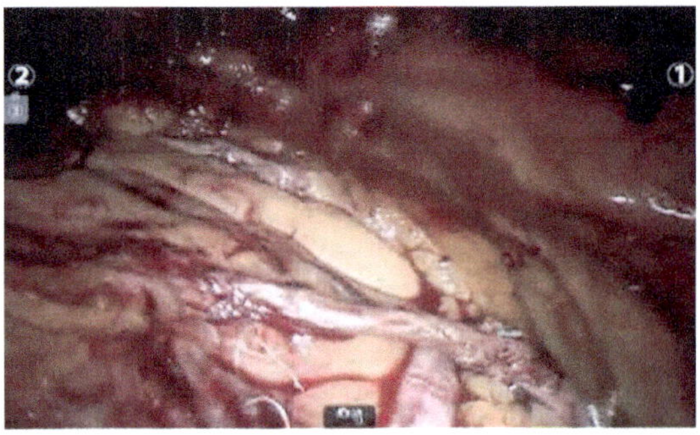

Fig. 44.9 View of a completed LITA to LAD anastomosis

The irrigator tube is retrieved outside the chest and the endostabiliser carefully released after interrupting the suction on both channels.

We routinely introduce into the pleural space one or two Blake 24-Fr chest drains via the left arm and stabiliser arm entry ports. Just before removing the camera, gentle re-expansion of the left lung should be achieved under endoscopic video guidance in order to confirm that the LITA lies over and parallel to the left phrenic nerve and is covered by the expanded left lung. Finally, the camera port is removed and secured.

The BH TECAB is performed via four skin incisions of 1–1.5 cm in length (Fig. 44.10).

44.5 Discussion

Robotic surgical systems seem to have important advantages when used in minimal access coronary revascularisation, but understandably, their clinical efficacy and precision, complication rate and reliability have all been questioned compared to conventional surgical or percutaneous alternatives. All these aspects have been evaluated favourably in various clinical trials although more evidence is required to demonstrate the superiority of patient reported and functional outcomes of robotic revascularisation procedures to justify the additional cost required.

Robotic coronary surgery on the beating heart has been extensively applied to perform the LITA-LAD anastomosis with the use of intraluminal shunt to achieve a bloodless operative field and reduce myocardial ischaemia.

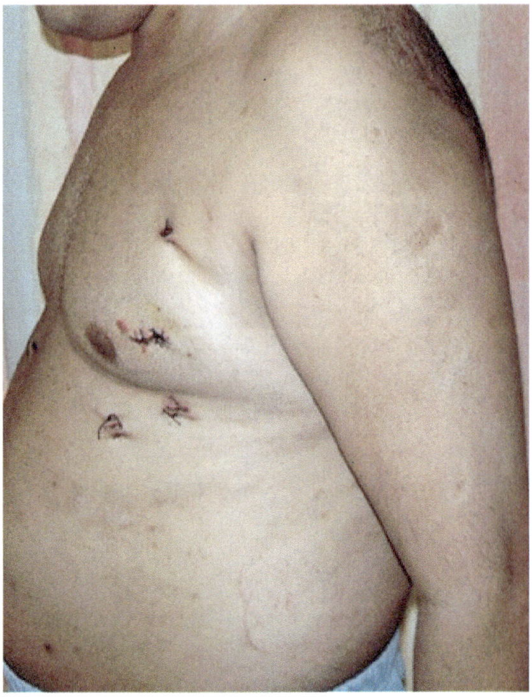

Fig. 44.10 A patient following TECAB

The da Vinci system has been used for harvesting bilateral internal mammary arteries with or without left anterior thoracotomy and CPB for multi-vessel coronary artery bypass grafting. This surgical strategy is attractive for diabetic patients where harvesting of bilateral internal thoracic arteries is associated with significant risk of sternotomy wound-related complications.

Studies on the arrested heart evaluating procedural time and the quality of the coronary anastomosis (patency, intactness, alignment, intimal tears and dehiscence) have demonstrated that robotic endoscopic anastomoses using telemanipulation systems are comparable to conventionally performed anastomoses [12].

The safety, feasibility and efficacy of beating heart total endoscopic coronary artery bypass grafting (BH-TECAB) were demonstrated in a multi-centre European study reported by de Canniere et al. in 2007 [13]. Of 74 patients who underwent off-pump TECAB, 93.6% achieved both angiographic patency and absence of ischaemic signs on stress electrocardiography at 6-month follow-up. In this study, the conversion rate for off-pump TECAB to a non-robotic procedure was 33.3%; however, a recent series by Gao et al. demonstrated that this technique may be refined to limit the conversion rate to as few as 3.4% (2/58) of patients [14]. Surgical cardiac centres that adopt BH-TECAB must be aware that a significant learning curve in robotic cardiac surgery is required also for experienced cardiac surgeons. Conversion strategies and emergency protocols must therefore be available in order to ensure that patient safety is always maintained also in challenging cases. Adoptions of standardised techniques and pre-operative patient selection have dramatically reduced conversion rates in more recent experiences who benefited the use of the da Vinci Si.

TECAB on the arrested heart may be performed as an alternative approach to beating heart robotic coronary revascularisation. Cardiopulmonary bypass is usually established through peripheral cannulation. The ascending aorta is clamped with an endovascular balloon, and anterograde cardioplegic solutions are delivered to achieve the cardiac arrest and consequently to facilitate robotic anastomosis. The arrested heart technique increases further the intra-operative costs of the TECAB procedure. Due to our long-term and established off-pump surgery experience, we believe that the use of cardiopulmonary bypass should be used only in case of multi-vessel coronary surgery with the use of multiple arterial grafting.

In 2006, Argenziano et al. published results from the only major prospective multi-centre trial to evaluate robotic TECAB with the use of cardiopulmonary bypass [15]. Eighty-five patients underwent robotic TECAB. There were no deaths or strokes, one early re-intervention and one myocardial infarction. The conversion rate to open surgery was 6%. Mean hospital stay was 5.1 ± 3.4 days. The safety and efficacy of on-pump TECAB has been confirmed in large case series from different centres around the world [16–18]. Interestingly this technique was also successfully applied to morbidly obese individuals with clinical outcomes comparable to non-obese individuals [18]. The avoidance of a full median sternotomy incision may be particularly beneficial in this cohort of individuals because of a potential association of obesity with impaired wound healing [19].

There is a growing body of evidence to suggest that TECAB with CPB (on-pump) and without CPB (off-pump) are safe, feasible and effective for single-vessel coronary revascularisation. However, there is a paucity of evidence to describe experience with robotic TECAB for treatment of multi-vessel coronary disease. Bonatti et al. report preliminary results in ten patients who underwent endoscopic placement of the right internal mammary artery (RIMA) to the left anterior descending artery in combination with left internal mammary artery (LIMA) grafting to an obtuse marginal (OM) branch [20, 21]. Seven procedures were completed endoscopically with no major adverse cardiac or cerebrovascular events. Mean total TECAB time was 477 min. This short series suggests that robotic TECAB may be reproducible for treatment of coronary artery disease in two distinct vessels. Given the success of single-vessel robotic procedures, multi-vessel TECAB is a desirable goal. Further research is required to assess the safety and feasibility of such techniques.

Hybrid coronary revascularisation describes the use of percutaneous coronary intervention plus robotic totally endoscopic coronary artery bypass to treat patients with multi-vessel coronary artery disease. These two procedures may be performed during the same anaesthetic setting [22] or in a staged approach where surgery and percutaneous intervention are two separate even in time [6]. Kiaii et al. have demonstrated the safety and feasibility of a one-stage technique involving simultaneous integrated coronary artery revascularisation following robotic harvesting of the internal thoracic artery. One patient suffered a stroke and three required re-operation for bleeding. There were no deaths or wound infections. All 58 patients were alive and symptom free at a median follow-up of 20.2 months [23]. Katz et al. report findings from a cohort of 27 patients with multi-vessel disease who underwent robotic TECAB of the LAD using the LITA as a pedicle conduit. In addition, percutaneous coronary intervention (PCI) was performed before, during or after surgery [24]. Angiographic LITA anastomotic patency rate was 96.3% at 3-month follow-up. There was no mortality and low perioperative morbidity. However, the re-intervention rate in these patients was as high as 23.5%. The authors concluded that this could have been influenced by the suitability of vessels, stent type and the timing of treatment.

It is important for the surgeon to explain to each patient exactly what the robotic procedure entails. Many patients could be under the impression that a surgical robot actually performs their operation. The understanding of the master–slave systems must be conveyed to the patient. As with any minimally invasive technique, the possibility of the procedure being converted either to an on-pump procedure or to a larger thoracotomy or even a sternotomy approach should be discussed with the patient when taking the patient's informed consent. Currently, robot-assisted procedures are performed in selected cases also in the larger volume robotic cardiac centres, and potential robotic patients should always be discussed at joint cardiology and cardiac surgery multidisciplinary meeting according to recently published European coronary revascularisation guidelines [8].

The issues of patient selection, hybrid revascularization, risk of conversion and important anatomical characteristics have an important role in deciding which conduit configuration and type of robotic procedure can be offered to each individual patient [25, 26].

The combination of teamwork and closed collaboration and communication between console and table surgeons and anaesthesiologists are of paramount importance in achieving a successful procedure while minimising the risk of conversion.

The authors firmly believe that mastering off-pump techniques and limited access techniques before approaching the use of robotic technology will allow a safe intra-operative shift from BH-TECAB to ACAB when clinically indicated and therefore retaining the clinical benefits and potential advantages of a minimal invasive off-pump surgical revascularisation even in the case of timely planned 'conversion'.

Since Falk et al. described robotic coronary revascularization at the turn of the millennium [27], computer technology has been used to enhance the basic TECAB protocol. One such technology is the endoscopic dynamic stabiliser, which facilitates vessel anastomosis on the beating heart [28]. 'Tissue deformation tracking' is an exciting technology that combines tracking of reference points based on stereo-thoracoscopic images and a constrained geometrical surface model that deforms with heart motion [29]. Reference points may be natural (prominent local features on the tissue surface) or fiducial (external markers with distinctive shape or colour placed in vivo). The use of natural landmarks, such as vessel junctions and surface textures, is preferred as external markers may interfere with the operative field of view. However, natural reference points may be distorted intra-operatively. The ideal reference points for accurate construction of a stable geometrical heart model are yet to be defined.

The safe adoption of robotic cardiac techniques such as the TECAB or ACAB requires a significant training commitment as cardiac surgeons have to undergo a demanding learning curve to achieve clinical proficiency in this robotic surgical modality. The robotic cardiac revascularisation procedures described herein are based on an established surgical platform and the use of presently available technologies; these robotic procedures are reproducible and should be safely performed following adequate theoretical and practical technical training under adequate mentoring guidance. The clinical results should be comparable to current results reported with more conventional techniques and standard surgical practice.

References

1. Loulmet D, Carpentier A, d'Attellis N, Berrebi A, Cardon C, Ponzio O, Aupècle B, Relland JY (1999) Endoscopic coronary artery bypass grafting with the aid of robotic assisted instruments. J Thorac Cardiovasc Surg 118(1):4–10
2. Casula RP, Athanasiou T, Cherian A, Bacon R, Foale R, Darzi A (2003) Totally endoscopic robotically enhanced coronary artery bypass on the beating heart. J R Soc Med 96(8):400–401

3. Casula R, Athanasiou T (2004) Totally endoscopic coronary artery bypass on the beating heart in Jehovah's Witness and HIV patients: case report. Heart Surg Forum 7(2):E174–E176
4. Deeba S, Aggarwal R, Sains P, Martin S, Athanasiou T, Casula R, Darzi A (2006) Cardiac robotics: a review and St Mary's experience. Int J Med Robot 2(1):16–20, Review
5. Bonatti J, Lehr E, Vesely MR, Friedrich G, Bonaros N, Zimrin D (2010) Hybrid coronary revascularization: which patients? When? How? Curr Opin Cardiol 25(6):568–574
6. Gao C, Yang M, Wu Y, Wang G, Xiao C, Liu H, Lu C (2009) Hybrid coronary revascularization by endoscopic robotic coronary artery bypass grafting on beating heart and stent placement. Ann Thorac Surg 87(3):737–741
7. Kiaii B, McClure RS, Stewart P, Rayman R, Swinamer SA, Suematsu Y, Fox S, Higgins J, Albion C, Kostuk WJ, Almond D, Sridhar K, Teefy P, Jablonsky G, Diamantouros P, Dobkowski WB, Jones P, Bainbridge D, Iglesias I, Murkin J, Cheng D, Novick RJ (2008) Simultaneous integrated coronary artery revascularization with long-term angiographic follow-up. J Thorac Cardiovasc Surg 136(3):702–708
8. The European task force on myocardial revascularisation of the European Society of Cardiology (ESC) and the European Association for Cardiothoracic Surgery (EACTS) (2010) Guidelines on myocardial revascularisation. Eur Heart J 31:2105–2555
9. Casula R, Athanasiou T, Darzi A (2004) Minimal access coronary revascularisation without cardiopulmonary bypass–the impact of robotic technology in the current clinical practice. Int J Med Robot 1(1):98–106, Review
10. Casula R, Athanasiou T, Foale R (2004) Recent advances in minimal-access cardiac surgery using robotic-enhanced surgical systems. Expert Rev Cardiovasc Ther 2(4):589–600, Review
11. Athanasiou T, Crossman MC, Asimakopoulos G, Cherian A, Weeresinghe A, Glenville B, Casula R (2004) Should the internal thoracic arteries be skeletonised? Ann Thorac Surg 77(6):2238–2243, Review
12. Falk V, Gummert JF, Walther T, Hayase M, Berry GJ, Mohr FW (1999) Quality of computer enhanced totally endoscopic coronary bypass graft anastomosis–comparison to conventional technique. Eur J Cardiothorac Surg 15(3):260–264; discussion 264–265
13. de Canniere D, Wimmer-Greinecker G, Cichon R et al (2007) Feasibility, safety, and efficacy of totally endoscopic coronary artery bypass grafting: multicenter European experience. J Thorac Cardiovasc Surg 134(3):710–716
14. Gao C, Yang M (2011) Wu Y *et al.* Early and midterm results of totally endoscopic coronary artery bypass grafting on the beating heart, J Thorac Cardiovasc Surg
15. Argenziano M, Katz M, Bonatti J et al (2006) Results of the prospective multicenter trial of robotically assisted totally endoscopic coronary artery bypass grafting. Ann Thorac Surg 81(5):1666–1674; discussion 1674–1665
16. Bonatti J, Schachner T, Bonaros N et al (2009) Effectiveness and safety of total endoscopic left internal mammary artery bypass graft to the left anterior descending artery. Am J Cardiol 104(12):1684–1688
17. Oehlinger A, Bonaros N, Schachner T et al (2007) Robotic endoscopic left internal mammary artery harvesting: what have we learned after 100 cases? Ann Thorac Surg 83(3):1030–1034
18. Wiedemann D, Schachner T, Bonaros N et al (2009) Does obesity affect operative times and perioperative outcome of patients undergoing totally endoscopic coronary artery bypass surgery? Interact Cardiovasc Thorac Surg 9(2):214–217
19. Assmann A, Boeken U, Feindt P, Schurr P, Akhyari P, Lichtenberg A (2011) Vacuum-assisted wound closure is superior to primary rewiring in patients with deep sternal wound infection. Thorac Cardiovasc Surg 59(1):25–29
20. Bonatti J, Schachner T, Bonaros N et al (2007) Robotic totally endoscopic double-vessel bypass grafting: a further step toward closed-chest surgical treatment of multivessel coronary artery disease. Heart Surg Forum 10(3):E239–E242
21. Bonatti J, Rehman A, Schwartz K et al (2010) Robotic totally endoscopic triple coronary artery bypass grafting on the arrested heart: report of the first successful clinical case. Heart Surg Forum 13(6):E394–E396
22. Bonatti J, Schachner T, Bonaros N et al (2005) Treatment of double vessel coronary artery disease by totally endoscopic bypass surgery and drug-eluting stent placement in one simultaneous hybrid session. Heart Surg Forum 8(4):E284–E286
23. Kiaii B, McClure RS, Stewart P et al (2008) Simultaneous integrated coronary artery revascularization with long-term angiographic follow-up. J Thorac Cardiovasc Surg 136(3):702–708
24. Katz MR, Van Praet F, de Canniere D et al (2006) Integrated coronary revascularization: percutaneous coronary intervention plus robotic totally endoscopic coronary artery bypass. Circulation 114(1 Suppl): I473–I476
25. Schachner T, Bonaros N, Wiedemann D et al (2011) Predictors, causes, and consequences of conversions in robotically enhanced totally endoscopic coronary artery bypass graft surgery. Ann Thorac Surg 91(3): 647–653
26. Jegaden O, Wautot F, Sassard T, Szymanik I, Shafy A, Lapeze J, Farhat F (2011) Is there an optimal minimally invasive technique for left anterior descending coronary artery bypass? J Cardiothorac Surg 6(1):37
27. Falk V, Diegeler A, Walther T, Jacobs S, Raumans J, Mohr FW (2000) Total endoscopic off-pump coronary artery bypass grafting. Heart Surg Forum 3(1):29–31
28. Bachta W, Renaud P, Cuvillon L, Laroche E, Forgione A, Gangloff J (2009) Motion prediction for computer-assisted beating heart surgery. IEEE Trans Biomed Eng 56(11):2551–2563

Anastomotic Connectors in Robotically Assisted Coronary Surgery

45

Stefanos Demertzis and Husam H. Balkhy

Contents

S. Demertzis, M.D., Ph.D (✉)
Department of Cardiovascular Surgery, University Hospital Bern, Inselspital, CH-3010 Bern, Switzerland

Department of Cardiac Surgery, Cardiocentro Ticino, Via Tesserete 48, CH-6900 Lugano, Switzerland
e-mail: demertzis@cardiocentro.org

H.H. Balkhy, M.D.
Department of Surgery, Center for Robotic and Minimally Invasive Cardiac Surgery, The Wisconsin Heart Hospital, Milwaukee, WI 53227, USA
e-mail: skidoc@execpc.com

45.1 Introduction

The mission critical part of any coronary bypass surgery is the (micro) vascular anastomosis. While manual suturing of a coronary anastomosis is certainly feasible in the closed chest, the procedure is definitively time consuming and technically challenging. Anastomotic times are rather long (around 35 min in experienced hands) [2]. The use of U-clips® (Medtronic, Inc., Minneapolis, Minnesota, USA) facilitates distal anastomosis construction since it abolishes the need for tying knots; the anastomotic times are significantly shorter (around 13 min) [15]. Results with both techniques are favorable [2, 5, 9, 13, 15]. However, both techniques require careful logistics (suture transfer and parking) and a high level of technical dexterity with the robot. The use of an anastomotic connector offers a true alternative. Anastomotic connectors were developed with minimally invasive surgery in mind. Their purpose, i.e., enabling surgeons to perform easily and rapidly high quality and consistent anastomoses between a graft (venous or arterial) and a coronary artery, fits perfectly in a concept of coronary surgery in limited space such as robotically assisted closed-chest coronary surgery [6, 16].

Many attempts were made to perform the delicate and critical distal anastomosis in a facilitated mode [4, 7, 8, 10, 11]. Besides individual design flaws, one common characteristic of those devices was the increased blood-exposed

R.G.C. Inderbitzi et al. (eds.), *Minimally Invasive Thoracic and Cardiac Surgery*, DOI 10.1007/978-3-642-11861-6_45, © Springer-Verlag Berlin Heidelberg 2012

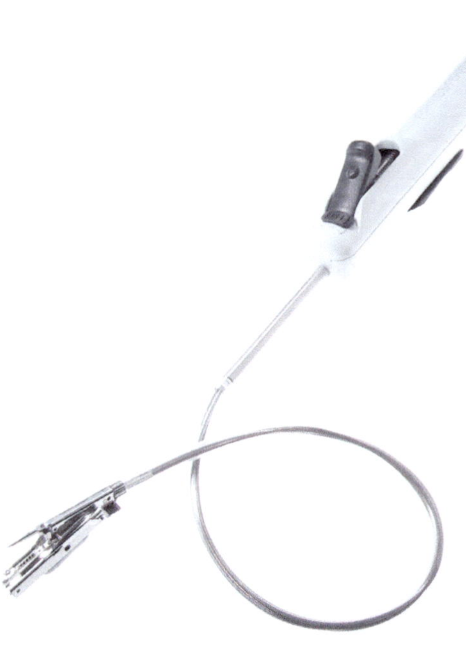

Fig. 45.1 Port Flex-A®

non-intimal surface (BENIS) which required aggressive antiplatelet treatment or anticoagulation immediately after surgery [16]. From all devices arrived at initial clinical applications, only one survived in the long term, Cardica's C-Port product line.

C-Port Flex-A (Fig. 45.1) is one iteration of the C-Port distal connector product family developed and marketed by Cardica, Inc. (www.cardica.com) specifically designed for minimally invasive CABG surgery. Its end effector or cartridge is identical to the C-Port xA designed for open-chest coronary surgery. Both devices are suitable for arterial and venous grafts, and both are CE-marked and FDA-cleared. There is already significant and growing clinical experience with the C-Port product line [1, 12] in both open-chest and closed-chest settings [3, 14]. The bottom line of these clinical studies is that short- and midterm results from facilitated distal anastomoses performed with C-Port devices are well comparable (and in subgroups of target vessels with diameter below 1.5 mm even superior) to traditionally handsewn anastomoses.

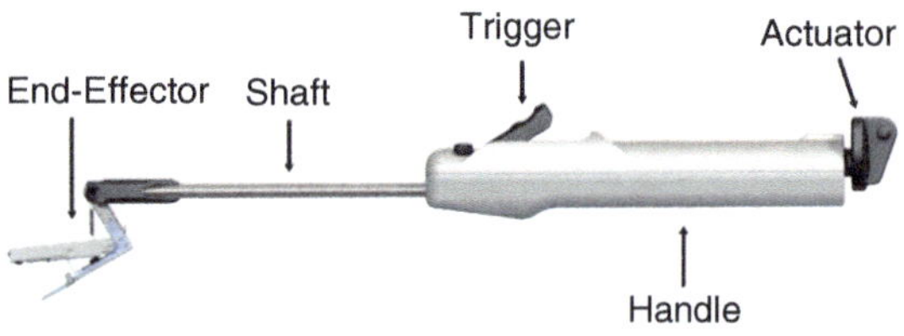

Fig. 45.2 Basic components of the C-Port product line

45.2 The Cardica C-Port Distal Anastomosis System

45.2.1 Background and Specific Indications

The C-Port product line delivers a series of staples that create an anastomosis between a small target vessel, such as the coronary artery, and a conduit, such as a venous or arterial graft. The stainless steel staples create an end-to-side anastomosis that is functionally equivalent to a hand-sutured interrupted stitch anastomosis. The C-Port allows the surgeon to create a distal anastomosis without interrupting blood flow through the target vessel. It produces a compliant anastomosis consisting of individual staples that are not connected to each other. The anastomosis can be completed rapidly with minimal user skills. The quality of the anastomosis is reflected by good medium-term patency rates, and therefore the indications for this product are in beating as well as arrested heart surgery. One product iteration, the C-Port Flex-A (Fig. 45.1), has been specifically developed to facilitate closed-chest revascularization.

All C-Port iterations have the same end effector and handle. They differ in the design of the shaft (rigid vs. flexible) and the reloadability. The basic components are depicted in Figs. 45.2, 45.3, and 45.4.

The handle consists of a manifold that utilizes CO_2 from a small canister to regulate the forces required to clamp and deploy this miniaturized stapler. The CO_2 canister holds sufficient gas to deploy four cartridges in the reloadable version. The CO_2 canister is pierced by rotating the actuator. Immediately in front of the trigger, which is the deployment button, is a safety

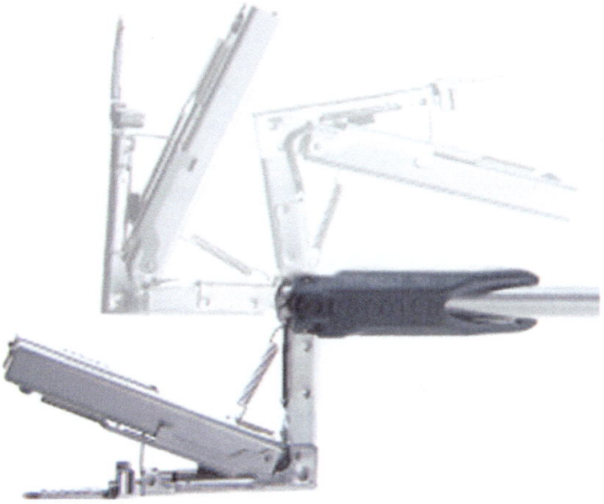

Fig. 45.3 Pivoting system of the end effector in the rigid shaft version (C-Port xA®)

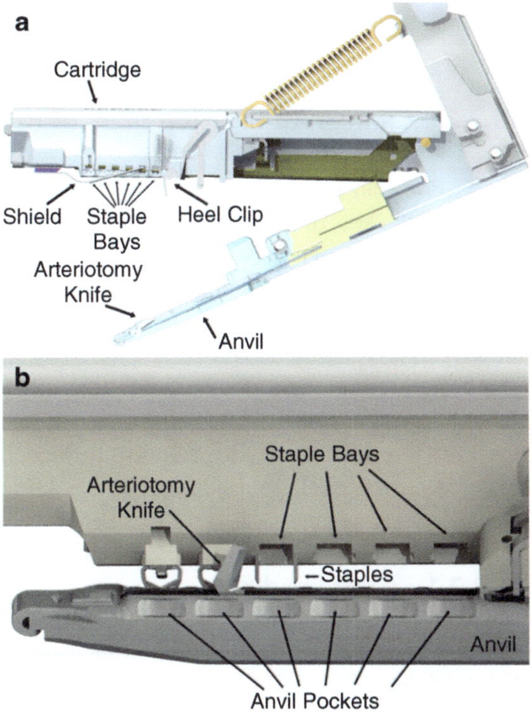

Fig. 45.4 Cut-through diagram of the C-Port end effector in open (**a**) and closed (**b**) position

switch that prevents inadvertent actuations of the device.

In the rigid shaft version, the end effector is connected to the shaft with a pivoting system that can be locked in various angles to aid in access and deployment.

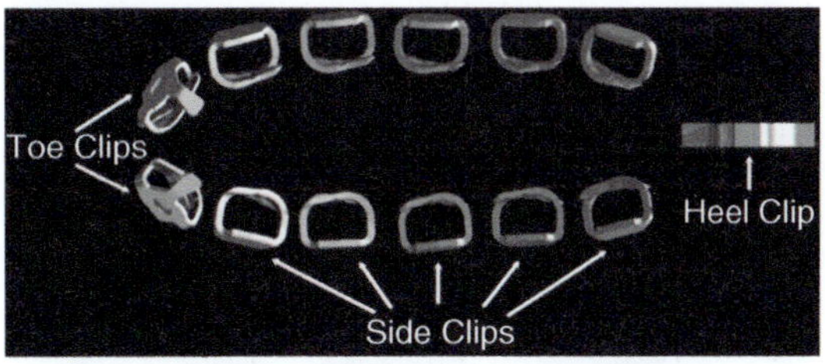

Fig. 45.5 The 13 formed staples of the C-Port device

The end effector is comprised of a cartridge with 13 staples and an anvil, which carries a hidden cutting blade. By depressing the trigger, the surgeon actuates the manifold, which through a cable mechanism, first clamps the cartridge against the anvil and then fires two rows of staples sequentially from the toe to the heel. The arteriotomy knife hidden in the anvil is activated shortly after the first staples are deployed to cut the coronary from the inside out.

All staples are made of medical grade 316 L stainless steel. While the typical staple in a conventional endostapler is bent out of wire, the C-Port staples are stamped out of sheet metal, which allows the staple to have a three-dimensional structure (Fig. 45.5).

The crown of the C-Port staple is widened to have a large contact surface and to prevent the staple from cutting through tissue. This allows a single row of staples to provide hemostasis that using a wired staple would require three rows of staples. In addition, the tines have been tapered to provide strength at the elbow but at the same time allow low forming forces.

Three different types of staples are used in the C-Port device: there are two sets of five side staples, which are two tine staples with a simple crown; there are two toe staples which are modified side staples with a single side-arm each to help seal at the toe of the anastomoses; and there is one heel staple that seals the heel and has been designed to allow the graft to be attached during the initial loading process.

The arteriotomy is performed with a double-edged knife that is initially hidden inside the anvil and that during deployment, is flipped up to perform the cut. At the end of its travel, it is flipped back down so it is hidden and cannot damage the

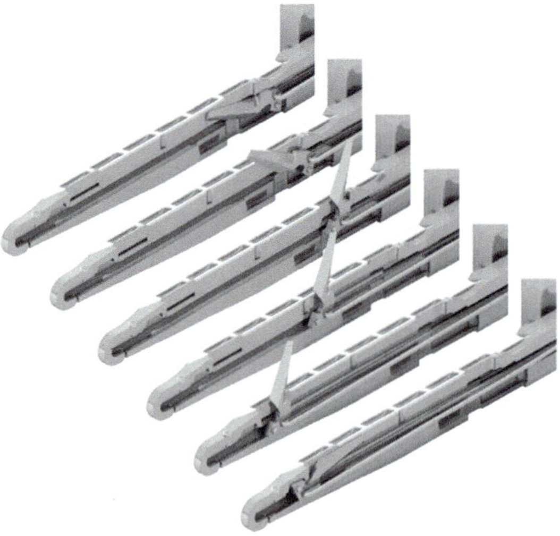

Fig. 45.6 Arteriotomy sequence of the C-Port (from the *top to the bottom*): the knife hidden in the anvil moves automatically from the heel to the toe during stapler application

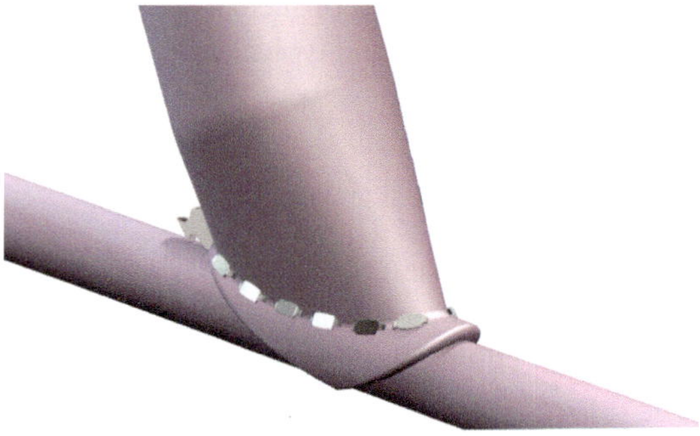

Fig. 45.7 Artist's impression of a distal coronary anastomosis performed with a C-Port device

coronary as the anvil is extracted from the coronary (Fig. 45.6).

Similar to hand-sewn anastomosis, only a simple cut is made in the coronary and with pressurization, turning the anastomotic orifice from a slit into an oval (Figs. 45.7 and 45.8).

The C-Port is approved for anastomosis of all types of grafts and for target vessel with at least an internal diameter of 1.3 mm and a single wall thickness of 0.75 mm.

Following deployment, the majority of the foreign material is located outside the bloodstream, and the graft is attached to the coronary in overlapping joint, where with the exception of one thickness of the coronary artery wall, there is a smooth intima-to-intima transition between graft and target vessel.

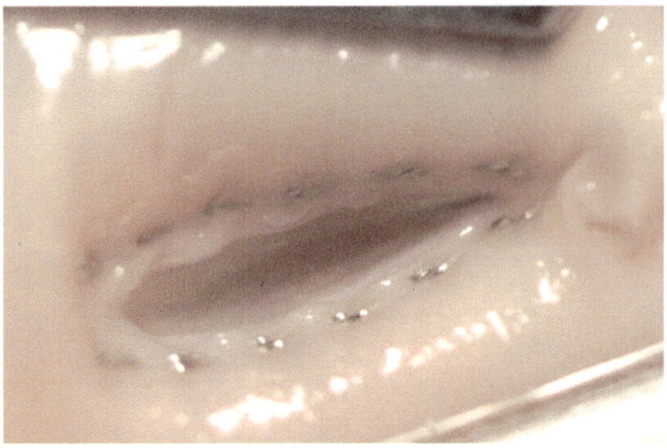

Fig. 45.8 Endoluminal view of an anastomosis performed with a C-Port device. The heel of the anastomosis is on the right picture side

45.2.2 Clinical Application

The C-Port can be used regardless whether the surgeon chooses to do the proximal or distal anastomoses first. There is a minimal free length of the graft required to be able to load the product, which, depending on the experience level of the surgeon, typically should be at least 3–4 cm. The system comes with loading aids that allow the C-Port to be loaded while being attached to a chest retractor, but the device can also be loaded inside the chest cavity with an assistant holding the device.

45.2.2.1 Graft Loading

The slot in between the two cartridge arms is 1.2 mm, which limits the maximum thickness of the graft that can be used with the C-Port. The same gauge used for the PAS-Port device can be used for the C-Port to determine that the double wall thickness of the graft is equal to or less than 1.4 mm. It is not recommended to use conduits that cannot be easily introduced in between the cartridge arms as following deployment, a graft that is too thick may be difficult to disengage from the cartridge, and in the process of doing so, one runs the risk of dislodging staples from the coronary and causing leaks. One should also ensure that there are no clips on side branches within 15 mm of the proposed distal end of the conduit, as these may interfere with the cartridge opening following deployment. The graft should be denuded and free of connective tissue, so it can

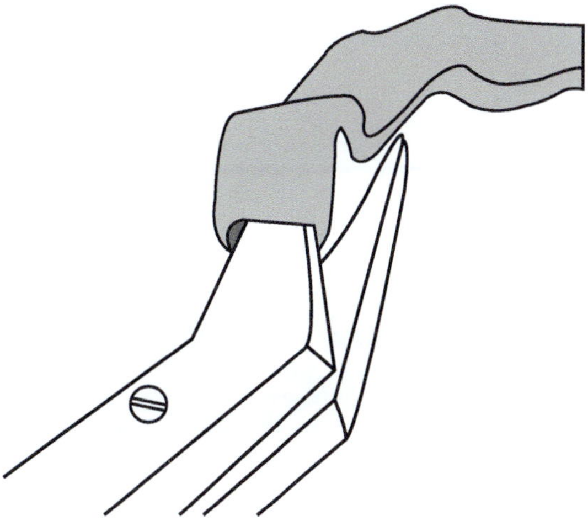

Fig. 45.9 The conduit is incised over a length of approximately 6–8 mm

easily be inserted into the cartridge. The conduit should then be cut at a 90° angle and incised on the surface that will be facing the coronary over a length of approximately 6–8 mm (Fig. 45.9).

The device is now removed from the packaging and either loaded onto the chest retractor mount or held by the first assistant. The CO_2 energy source is prepared by rotating the actuator knob in a clockwise direction until the indicator on the handle has been rotated past the indicator on the case halves (Fig. 45.10).

The cartridge is now rotated from the shipping position to the loading position, which resembles an S configuration relative to the shaft. The two graft clamps are rotated upward, and the graft shield is rotated out of the cartridge (Fig. 45.11).

The graft is now inserted with the incised edge first in between the cartridge arms, and the heel of the graft is everted over the heel clip. The assistant lowers the right graft clamp with the attached piercer and thereby pushes the graft onto the heel clip and secures it in this position (Fig. 45.12).

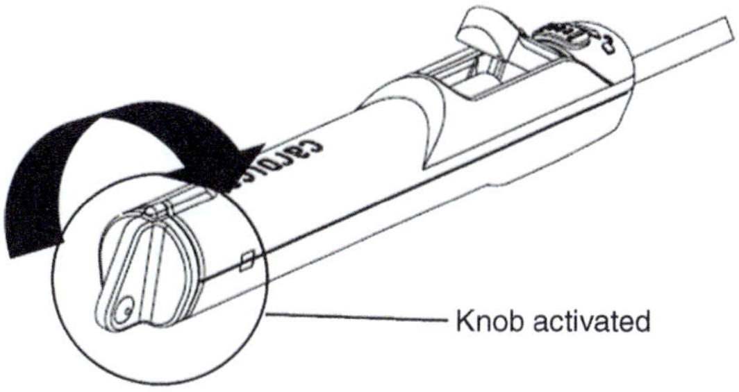

Fig. 45.10 Activation of the CO_2 energy source by turning the actuator knob in a clockwise direction

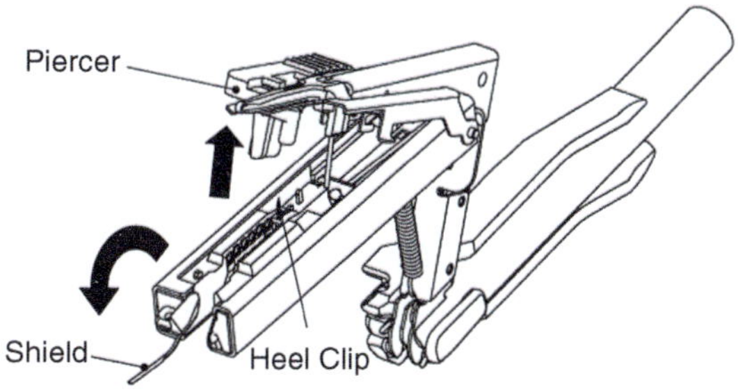

Fig. 45.11 Cartridge in position for loading

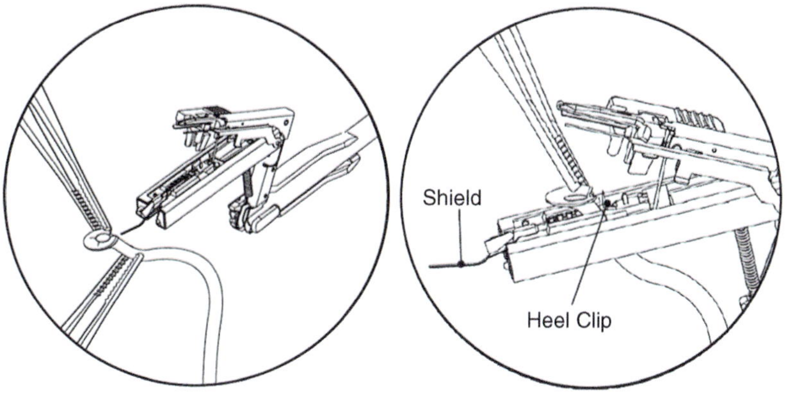

Fig. 45.12 Loading sequence. Graft insertion and eversion over the heel clip

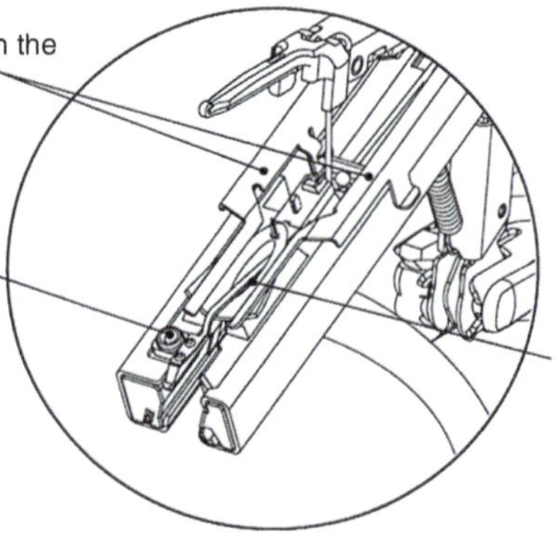

Fig. 45.13 Device loaded with the conduit

Slight traction on the graft from underneath the cartridge rotates the graft downward and brings the toe of the graft in line with the most forward facing staple bays. The side flaps of the graft are now spread over the cartridge and held in place first by the left graft clamp, and after removal of the piercer, later by the right graft clamp. The shield is now flipped into the lumen of the graft. Alternatively, the shield guard is flipped in first, and then the two wing guards are brought down. The shield basically serves two functions: first and foremost, it protects the hood of the graft from the arteriotomy knife; secondly, by tugging the shield into the graft lumen, it ensures that an adequate hood is formed in the anastomosis (Fig. 45.13).

45.2.2.2 C-Port Deployment

The C-Port can be deployed on any coronary with an internal diameter of at least 1.3 mm in a single wall thickness of not more than 0.75 mm. Heavily calcified sections and deep intramural coronary should be avoided.

The surgeon should expose the target vessel per standard surgical routine dissecting the top surface of the coronary over a length of approximately 15–18 mm. In order to deploy the C-Port device, a small arteriotomy has to be made at the very proximal end of the dissected area to insert the anvil. This arteriotomy is not part of the anastomosis and requires closure following removal of the anvil. The C-Port anastomosis can be performed without interrupting blood flow in the native coronary. By pre-placing a U-stitch at the location where the anvil insertion hole is intended to be made, the surgeon can facilitate later anvil insertion hole closure after removal of the anvil. The U-stitch should be placed very superficial and in immediate proximity to the anvil insertion hole. This will avoid any possibility of a stenosis following closure.

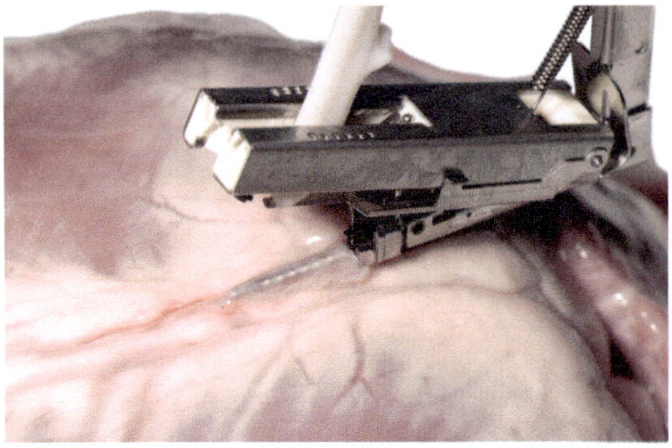

Fig. 45.14 Alignment of the cartridge within the stabilizer

In off-pump surgery, the surgeon should ensure that the stabilizer will not interfere with the deployment of the C-Port (Fig. 45.14).

The end effector is now rotated into an ideal configuration that will allow easy insertion and deployment of the device. For inferior coronary targets, the surgeon would typically use the L configuration; for lateral and posterior targets, most frequently U configurations are chosen. Occasionally the S configuration is best suited for anastomoses to the right coronary or the posterior descending artery.

The safety switch is now moved from the locked to the unlocked position and using a sharp

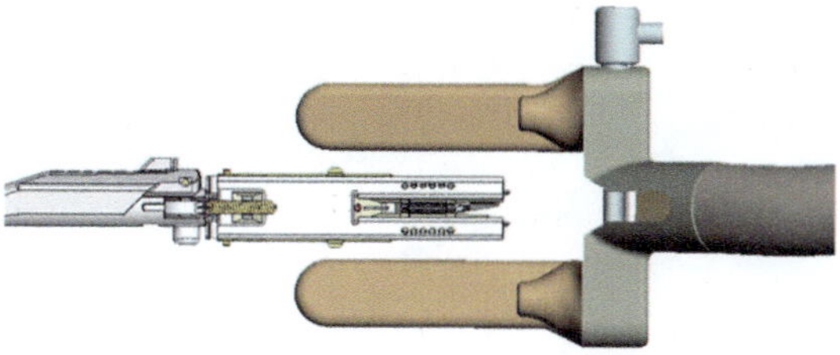

Fig. 45.15 Insertion of the anvil into the lumen of the target coronary artery through a 1.0–1.2 mm arteriotomy

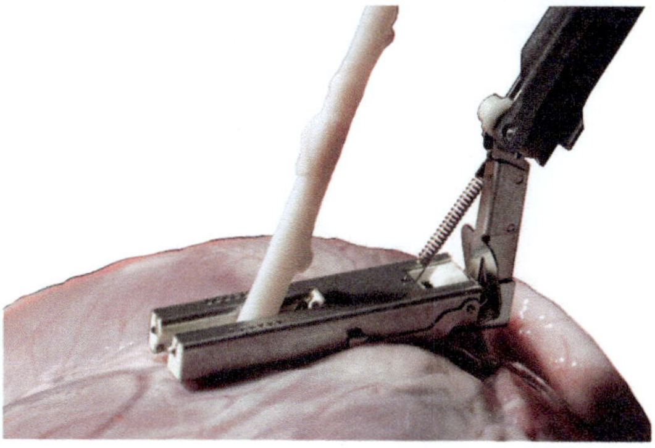

Fig. 45.16 Deployment. After double-trigger actuation (see text), the cartridge is closed on the anvil, the staples are fired, and the arteriotomy is created

Beaver blade, the surgeon creates a small arteriotomy inside the previously placed U-stitch. To verify that the arteriotomy is complete, one can elect to use a 1-mm probe to gain access into the coronary.

The anvil of the C-Port is now inserted gently into the arteriotomy and should be advanced freely until a hard stop is felt and the anvil is no longer visible (Fig. 45.15).

It is very important to ensure that the anvil is definitely free in the lumen of the coronary target at this time. If there is any doubt, the anvil should be removed and re-inserted.

After making sure that the anvil is truly intraluminal and that there is no interference of connective tissue, epicardium, or the stabilizer with the device, the trigger is actuated halfway until a small detent is felt and the cartridge has closed on the anvil. After waiting 3 s in the clamped position, the trigger is actuated its full stroke, which will result in the staples being fired and the arteriotomy being created (Fig. 45.16).

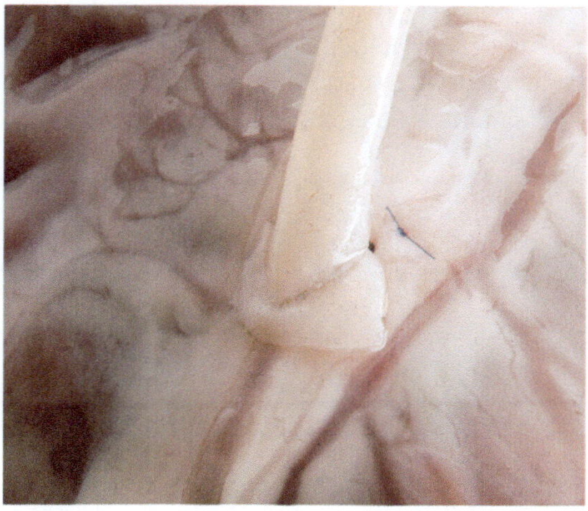

Fig. 45.17 Completed anastomosis with secured anvil insertion hole

The trigger can now be released which will open the cartridge. A forceps is used to first flip the shield out from under the graft and then grab the graft underneath the cartridge for counter traction as the cartridge and anvil are carefully withdrawn from the coronary and graft.

The previously placed U-stitch is then tied and the anastomosis inspected for hemostasis (Fig. 45.17).

If necessary, stitches can be placed to secure hemostasis, although in our experience, as this is an interrupted anastomoses, initial oozing and small leaks typically subside following gentle compression with gauze and later administration of protamine. It is strongly encouraged to determine adequate blood flow in the graft using appropriate equipment.

45.3 Technical Arrangements in the Robotic Set-Up

An additional 15-mm port access is required for the introduction of the C-Port Flex-A into the thorax. This port is placed in the second ICS (medioclavicular line) after the IMA is taken down. The C-Port Flex-A is introduced prior to its loading and is picked up by an EndoWrist® forceps and brought into the loading position by a turn towards the mediastinum. The C-Port Flex-A® is held firm

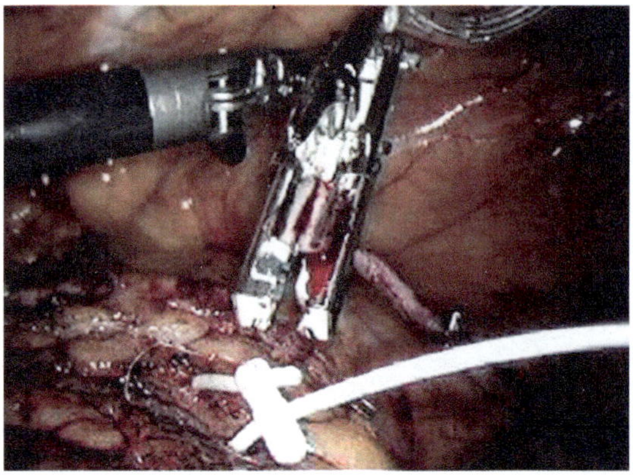

Fig. 45.18 The left internal mammary artery is loaded onto the C-Port Flex-A®. *Note* the loose SaddleLoop® placed around the LAD

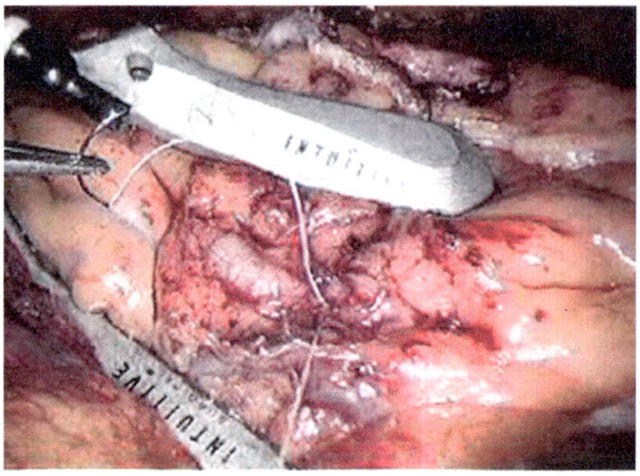

Fig. 45.19 Target artery stabilized and prepared. The suture for the control of the anvil insertion hole is in place

in its loading position by an EndoWrist® large-needle driver or long-tip forceps placed on the third da Vinci arm (12-mm subcostal da Vinci port). Loading is carried out as described above using two EndoWrist® microforceps (first and second da Vinci arms). The loaded C-Port Flex-A (Fig. 45.18) is then rotated back and parked safely on the posterior thoracic wall or in the mediastinum. It is important to have a standardized technique for rotating the Flex-A for loading and then rotating it back in preparation for firing. This will minimize the potential for creating a twist in the conduit between loading and firing.

45.3.1 Off-Pump Technique

The EndoWrist® stabilizer is introduced again (third da Vinci arm) for stabilization of the target coronary artery. The target artery is prepared either with the cautery blade or with a Beaver® knife. A SaddleLoop® silicone snare (Quest Medical, Inc., Allen, Texas, USA) can be placed proximally and/or distally around the artery for bleeding control. As next, there is the choice between placing in advance the suture to close the anvil insertion hole needed for the C-Port Flex-A deployment or closing the anvil insertion hole after the deployment. We would recommend the first approach: a U-stitch using a GORE-TEX CV-8 suture (7-cm thread length, W.L. Gore & Associates, Inc., Flagstaff, Arizona, USA) is placed at the most proximal site of the cleaned target coronary artery leaving safe space for the approximately 1 mm in diameter anvil insertion hole (Fig. 45.19). This suture will be tied after the removal of the C-Port Flex-A®. Alternatively Medtronic U-clips® (S18) can be used for the same purpose after deployment.

The target coronary artery is snared proximally by pulling tightly and secure the prior placed SaddleLoops®. The anvil insertion hole is created using the EndoWrist® 15° Blue Blade Scalpel. The anvil of the C-Port Flex-A® is introduced into the coronary artery. It is of paramount importance to ensure that the anvil is in the lumen and not in the wall of the artery. When the full length of the anvil is safely in the lumen of the target coronary artery, the table-side assistant actuates the trigger for deployment (Figs. 45.20 and 45.21).

Prior to releasing the trigger and initiate the ascent of the cartridge, it is strongly advisable to pick up the graft and elevate it. This protects the anastomosis from accidental tearing, which could occur when the friction between the cartridge arms and the graft is too high, usually due to connective tissue around the graft and/or bigger collateral branches. When the C-Port Flex-A® is retracted successfully, the anvil insertion hole is secured as described above. The anastomosis is inspected for residual bleeding (Fig. 45.22). Should bleeding be more than the

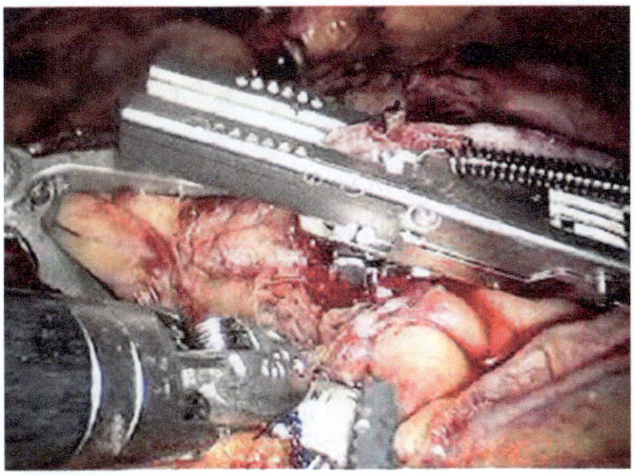

Fig. 45.20 The anvil of the C-Port Flex-A® is inserted into the lumen of the LAD (photograph courtesy Dr. H. Balkhy)

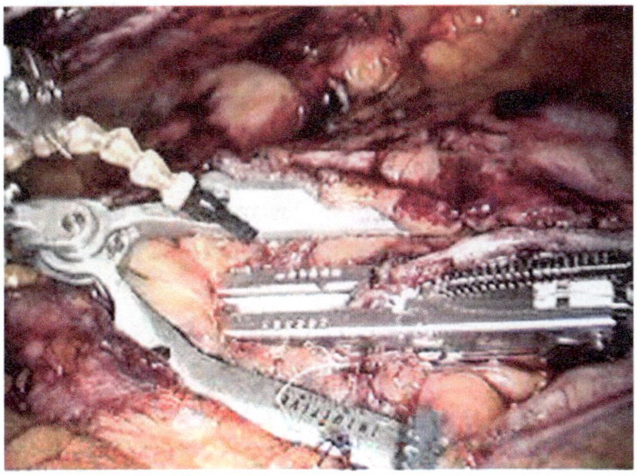

Fig. 45.21 After double actuation of the trigger, the cartridge is closed on the anvil, and deployment occurs (photograph courtesy Dr. H. Balkhy)

usual oozing between the clips, additional stitches with GORE-TEX® suture or U-clips® can be added to control it. In most cases, bleeding stops after a while and after reversal of the heparin effect with protamine. We recommend flow measurement for assuring the quality of the anastomosis (Fig. 45.23).

45.3.2 On-Pump Technique

Preparation of the internal mammary arteries (IMA) and loading of the C-Port xA® are performed as described above. The patient is placed on cardiopulmonary bypass (CPB) via

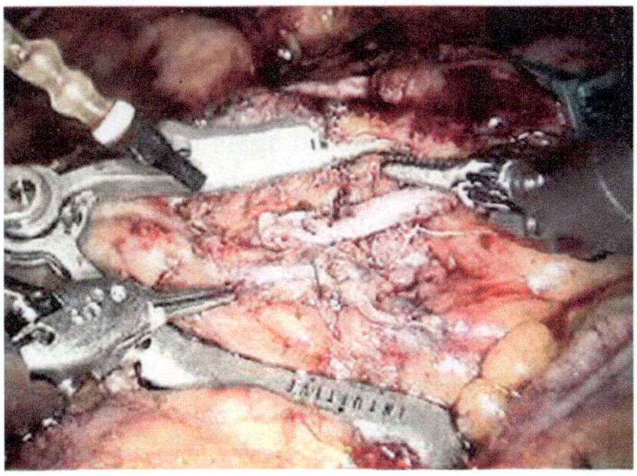

Fig. 45.22 Completed anastomosis (photograph courtesy Dr. H. Balkhy)

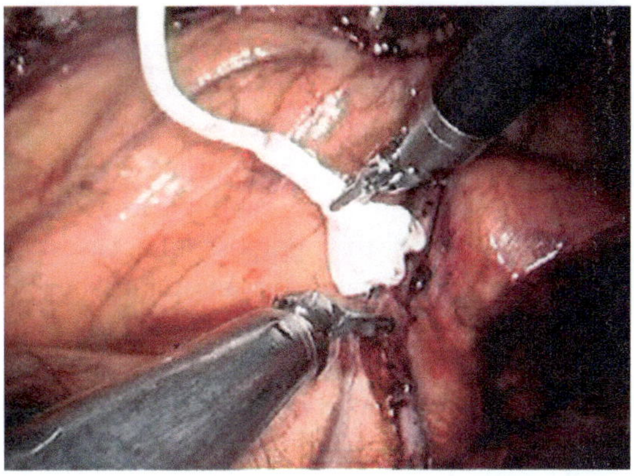

Fig. 45.23 Flow measurement using a Medistim® probe (Medtronic, Inc., Minneapolis, Minnesota, USA)

femoro-femoral cannulation. The right atrium is drained by a long multiperforated venous return cannula. Arterial return is provided by a 21F remote access perfusion cardiopulmonary bypass system (ESTECH, Danville, California, USA). The ascending aortic occlusion balloon is inflated, and antegrade cardioplegic solution is administered. The EndoWrist® stabilizer is introduced again (third da Vinci arm) for exposure of the target coronary artery. The coronary artery is prepared and incised for the anvil insertion (eventually under administration of cardioplegic solution for confirmation of the successful arteriotomy). Anastomosis creation with the C-Port Flex-A® is accomplished as described above. After deployment and successful retraction of the device, the anvil insertion hole is secured as described. The conduit is declamped and the anastomosis tested for significant bleeding. If significant bleeding has to be addressed surgically, the clamp is placed again on the conduit, and it might become necessary to readminister cardioplegic solution for cardiac arrest. The conduit is declamped, and the ascending aorta occlusion balloon is deflated.

45.4 Complications

The main specific complications of connector robotic revascularization include bleeding and nonsatisfactory flow through the anastomosis. Anastomotic oozing is frequent but as stated above in most cases stops spontaneously. More important bleeding has to be controlled by sutures. The graft flaps, which were held by the small graft clamps during loading and do not participate at the anastomosis, can serve as good tissue cushion for this purpose. In cases of inadequate flow through the anastomosis, graft spasm has to be ruled out first. Should flow characteristics such as a high pulsatility index point towards an anastomotic stenosis other possibilities have to be considered. Failure of inserting the anvil into the lumen and instead forcing it into the target vessel wall will result in a nonfunctional anastomosis. Tissue interference with cartridge movement or the extremely rare case of mechanical malfunction could also result in an incomplete arteriotomy presenting as anastomotic stenosis. In these cases, the anastomosis can be gently zipped open and inspected. A hand-sewn anastomosis (either robotically or after conversion to mini-thoracotomy or sternotomy) has to be created according to the local findings. Normally the same arteriotomy can be used.

45.5 Results

From January 2008 to June 2010, one of the authors (HHB) performed 123 robotic totally endoscopic beating heart CABG (BH TECAB) procedures with the aid of the C-Port Flex-A® anastomotic device (age range 43–86 years). In 63% of the patients, there was a single-vessel, and in 37%, a multivessel revascularization was performed (31% double vessel and 6% triple vessel). The majority of single-vessel cases were left IMA (LIMA) to the left anterior descending coronary artery (LAD). Three patients received isolated right IMA (RIMA) to the right coronary artery (RCA) grafts. The multivessel patients received either bilateral IMAs or sequential LIMA grafts. Bilateral IMAs were used in all triple-vessel revascularizations. No vein grafts were used. A total of 165 anastomoses were performed, 144 with the C-Port Flex-A® device, and 21 with U-clips®.

Mean graft flow was 76±44 ml/min (PI 1.4±0.5). Five out of 165 grafts required revision secondary to poor intraoperative flow.

All patients were completed off-pump except for one patient who required CPB support via femoro- femoral cannulation. There was one conversion to sternotomy. Two patients were re-explored for postoperative bleeding (via the same robotic ports).

There was one perioperative death within 30 days of surgery in an 86-year-old patient with peripheral vascular disease who underwent carotid endarterectomy prior to her uncomplicated single-vessel totally endoscopic CABG and suffered a large and eventually fatal ipsilateral cerebrovascular accident 5 days postoperatively. The average length of stay was 3.5 days (three outliers excluded). Patency evaluation was performed in 65 patients with 85 grafts by means of multidetector angio-CT or formal angiography at a mean of 4 months. Patency was 94.1%.

Conclusion

Robotically assisted coronary revascularization is gaining again the interest of cardiac surgeons. The use of the C-Port Flex-A® allows for easy facilitated end-to-side anastomosis with short anastomotic times and proven clinical results. This approach can become an integral part of totally endoscopic robotically assisted coronary surgery.

References

1. Balkhy HH, Wann LS, Arnsdorf S (2010) Early patency evaluation of new distal anastomotic device in internal mammary artery grafts using computed tomography angiography. Innovations (Phila) 5:109
2. Bonatti J, Schachner T, Bonaros N et al (2006) Technical challenges in totally endoscopic robotic coronary artery bypass grafting. J Thorac Cardiovasc Surg 131:146–153
3. Brunsting L III, Brunsting K, Rankin JS (2010) Beating heart TECAB: impact of an automated stapling device. Innovations (Phila) 5:195
4. Carrel T, Englberger L, Keller D et al (2004) Clinical and angiographic results after mechanical connection for distal anastomosis in coronary surgery. J Thorac Cardiovasc Surg 127:1632–1640
5. Caskey MP, Kirshner MS, Alderman EL et al (2002) Six-month angiographic evaluation of beating-heart coronary arterial graft interrupted anastomoses using the coalescent U-CLIP anastomotic device: a prospective clinical study. Heart Surg Forum 5:319–326; discussion 327
6. Falk V, Jacobs S, Gummert JF et al (2003) Computer-enhanced endoscopic coronary artery bypass grafting: the Da Vinci experience. Semin Thorac Cardiovasc Surg 15:104–111
7. Falk V, Walther T, Stein H et al (2003) Facilitated endoscopic beating heart coronary artery bypass grafting using a magnetic coupling device. J Thorac Cardiovasc Surg 126:1575–1579
8. Gill IS, Izutani H (2006) Internal thoracic artery to left anterior descending anastomosis performed on the beating heart by endoscopic robot assistance using a new distal connector. Can J Surg 49:37–40
9. Hill AC, Maroney TP, Virmani R (2001) Facilitated coronary anastomosis using a nitinol U-Clip device: bovine model. J Thorac Cardiovasc Surg 121:859–870
10. Kim KB, Cho KR, Choi JS et al (2004) Initial experience of an automated anastomotic distal device in off-pump CABG. Heart Surg Forum 7:E360–E363
11. Klima U, Falk V, Maringka M et al (2003) Magnetic vascular coupling for distal anastomosis in coronary artery bypass grafting: a multicenter trial. J Thorac Cardiovasc Surg 126:1568–1574
12. Matschke KE, Gummert JF, Demertzis S et al (2005) The cardica C-Port system: clinical and angiographic evaluation of a new device for automated, compliant distal anastomoses in coronary artery bypass grafting surgery – a multicenter prospective clinical trial. J Thorac Cardiovasc Surg 130:1645–1652
13. Smith JM, Stein H, Robinson JR et al (2006) Influence of anastomotic techniques in totally endoscopic coronary artery bypass. Int J Med Robot 2:197–201
14. Srivastava S, Barrera ZR, Quismundo S et al (2010) Beating heart totally endoscopic artery: comparison between first 350 and last 100 patients. What did we learn? Innovations(Phila) 5:194
15. Srivastava S, Gadasalli S, Agusala M et al (2008) Robotically assisted beating heart totally endoscopic coronary artery bypass (TECAB). Is there a future? Innovations (Phila) 3:52–58
16. Vassiliades T (2009) Enabling technology for minimally invasive coronary artery bypass grafting. Semin Thorac Cardiovasc Surg 21:237–244

Minimal Access Atrial Fibrillation Surgery

46

Thierry A. Folliguet, Borut Gersak, Andy C. Kiser, Gerhard Wimmer-Greinecker, Claudio Muneretto, Michael Zembala, and Marian Zembala

Contents

T.A. Folliguet, M.D., FACS (✉)
Départment de Pathologie Cardiaque,
Institut Mutualiste Montsouris, 42 Boulevard Jourdan,
Paris Cedex 14, 75674, France
e-mail: thierry.folliguet@imm.fr

B. Gersak, M.D., Ph.D
Department of Cardiovascular Surgery,
University Medical Center Ljubljana, Zaloska cesta 2,
1000 Ljubljana, Slovenia
e-mail: bgersak@maat.si

A.C. Kiser, M.D.
Division of Cardiothoracic Surgery,
University of North Carolina at Chapel Hill,
3040 Burnett-Womack Bldg., CB #7065, Chapel Hill,
NC 27599-7065, USA
e-mail: andy_kiser@med.unc.edu

G. Wimmer-Greinecker, M.D.
Klinik für Herz-Thorax-Chirurgie Herz,
Gefässzentrum Bad Bevensen, Roemstedter Str. 25,
29549 Bad Bevensen, Germany
e-mail: g.wimmer-greinecker@hgz-bb.de

C. Muneretto, M.D.
Department of Cardiac Surgery,
University of Brescia Medical School,
P.le Spedali Civili, 1, 25123 Brescia, Italy
e-mail: munerett@med.unibs.it

M. Zembala • M. Zembala, M.D., Ph.D
Department of Surgery, Silesian University Center
for Heart Disease, Szpitalna Street 2,
41800 Zabrze (Silesia), Poland
e-mail: m.zembala@sccs.pl

46.1 Introduction

Atrial fibrillation (AF) is a common supraventricular arrhythmia associated with symptoms of varying severity. AF is the most common sustained arrhythmia in the United States. Paroxysmal AF is defined as recurrent AF (·2 episodes) that terminates spontaneously within 7 days. Persistent AF is defined as AF which is sustained beyond 7 days or lasting less than 7 days but necessitating pharmacologic or electrical cardioversion. Long-standing persistent AF is defined as continuous AF of greater than 1 year duration. Permanent AF refers to long-standing AF and where the decision was made not too convert in sinus rhythm by any means. Mechanisms of AF are incompletely understood; however two major mechanisms predominate which are multiple random propagating wavelets and focal triggers. Paroxysmal AF represents 12% of the patients with AF and can be due to either focal AF or wavelet AF, while patients with persistent or permanent AF represent 88% and have multiple wavelets AF. This has important therapeutic implications since focal AF is often triggered by a focal source originating usually around the pulmonary veins, and the ablation of that focal trigger can

R.G.C. Inderbitzi et al. (eds.), *Minimally Invasive Thoracic and Cardiac Surgery*,
DOI 10.1007/978-3-642-11861-6_46,

eliminate AF. In the multiple wavelet hypotheses, AF results from the presence of multiple reentrant wavelets occurring simultaneously in the left and right atria, and treatment will require more ablation than the pulmonary veins which include the creation of an anatomical pattern of myocardial scar. The corridor procedure, the radial maze procedure, and the Cox maze I-III surgically create anatomical patterns designed to disrupt the reentry circuits of AF by dividing the atria into non-conductive segments [1, 2]. Despite its proven efficacy, the Cox maze procedure did not gain widespread application due to its complexity and technical difficulty [1]. Therefore many groups worldwide replaced the "cut and saw technique," with linear lines of ablation [3, 4]. These ablations lines are created using a variety of energy sources including radiofrequency energy, microwave, cryoablation, laser, and high-intensity focused ultrasound (HIFU). Surgical ablation is based on the principle that the predominant mechanism of development and persistent AF is reentry stimulated by ectopic triggers [5, 6]. Thus the techniques consist of creating an intricate pattern of lesions inducing scarring in predefined areas in the atrial wall which effectively blocks the propagation of reentrant circuits while preserving normal conduction from the sinus to the AV node.

The success of any surgical treatment for persistent or long-standing permanent AF is dependent upon the transmurality and contiguity of the ablation lines and the completeness of the lesion pattern [6–9].

Epidemiologic studies showed that atrial fibrillation is associated with an increased risk of cerebral thromboembolism, development of heart failure, and mortality.

Although a straightforward cause and effect relationship is often uncertain, AF is frequently a sign of the severity of the underlying cardiovascular disease. Many patients with either persistent or permanent AF will have structural heart disease, and atrial fibrillation may in fact be the first sign of underlying structural heart disease.

Goal of rhythm control drugs is to restore sinus rhythm; however multiple antiarrhythmic drugs (AADs) are effective in only 62% of patients at 5 years and are associated with a significant morbidity and mortality.

Multiple randomized clinical trials demonstrated that rate control drugs were not inferior to rhythm control drugs (PIAF, RACE AFFIRM). However a recent new analysis of the AFFIRM trial data showed that the presence of sinus rhythm dramatically lowered the risk of death; this effect was not seen in the original analysis as the concomitant use of AAD simultaneously resulted in increased mortality balancing the positive effects of SR on mortality. Although the AAD trials failed to show lower mortality despite restoring SR, it can be speculated that if SR can be achieved safely, mortality will be lowered. Restoring SR could restore atrial contractility and improve hemodynamics by restoring AV synchrony. Furthermore by restoring SR, atrial remodeling may be prevented (or even reversed), and in case AF does not recur, anticoagulant drugs may be stopped.

Ablation strategy has been employed with the intention of "curing" atrial fibrillation in several patient populations [10–13]. The majority of studies have concentrated on paroxysmal AF in patients without structural heart disease.

Prior to an ablation procedure, all patients should undergo a 12-lead ECG and/or Holter recording to demonstrate the nature of the arrhythmia and a transthoracic echocardiogram to identify or exclude an underlying structural heart disease. Additional imaging studies, e.g., magnetic resonance or computer tomography, demonstrate individual 3D geometry and some quantification of atrial fibrosis.

46.2 Indications

The endocardial, catheter-based AF ablations, not unlike the surgical procedures, remain long and technically difficult procedures performed by a relatively few electrophysiologists, and in persistent or permanent AF, successful ablation is more difficult. The high rate of repeat procedures and less-than-desirable long-term outcomes has been disappointing. Unfortunately, surgeons and electrophysiologists seldom collaborate in the development of new technologies and innovative approaches to overcome these individual procedural shortcomings.

A multidisciplinary team of electrophysiologists and cardiac surgeons has developed the Convergent procedure to address existing procedural and communication barriers. The Convergent procedure is the simultaneous creation of a surgeon's epicardial ablation pattern and electrophysiologist's endocardial ablation pattern. The surgeon's ability to effectively create robust and visible 2–5- cm epicardial ablation lines has greatly reduced the amount of endocardial tissue which must be ablated to complete pulmonary vein isolation, coronary sinus ablation, posterior left atrial ablation, and ablation of the cavotricuspid isthmus. The integration of a surgeon's anatomical approach to AF with the physiological approach of the electrophysiologists has led to the development of the Convergent procedure.

46.3 Description of the Convergent Procedure

During paracardioscopy, the patient is positioned supine under single lumen, general endotracheal anesthesia. Procedures are performed in either a "hybrid" operating theater or a "hybrid EP laboratory" with integrated fluoroscopy, endoscopy, general anesthesia, and CARTe™ (Biosense Webster, Inc. Diamond Bar, CA) mapping and imaging technologies (Fig. 46.1). A 2-cm incision is made 3 cm below the xiphoid and extended into the peritoneum under direct visualization and two 5-mm laparoscopic ports are placed in the left and right subcostal areas with the assistance

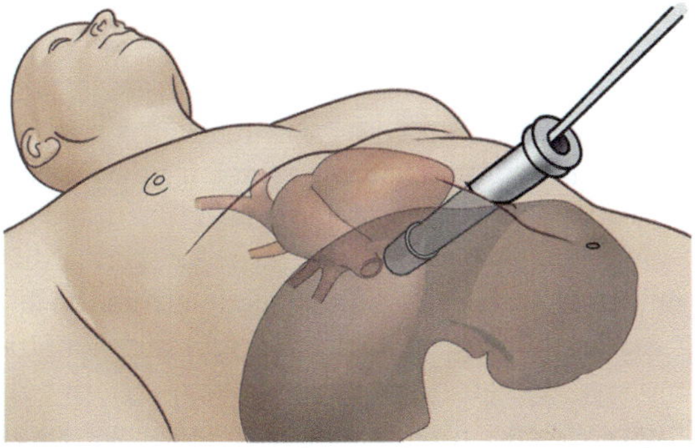

Fig. 46.1 Hybrid suite schematic for the Convergent procedure

of a finger inside the peritoneum. A 10-mm port is placed in the midline incision and the abdomen is insufflated with Ce_2 to 12 mmHg. Using a 10-mm endoscope, the central fibrous region of the diaphragm is identified anterior to the left lobe of the liver and left of the falciform ligament. Utilizing standard laparoscopic scissors and graspers in the 5-mm ports, the central diaphragmatic tendon is opened longitudinally 3 cm. The incision should be 1–2 cm anterior to the reflection of the hepatic ligament to allow later closure of the diaphragm, if desired. The incision in the pericardium should be made directly behind the diaphragmatic incision. The pericardium is opened longitudinally as well, providing access to the posterior region of the heart. Once opened, the pericardium will be filled with Ce_2 from the abdomen. The first direct view of the heart is at the acute margin of the right ventricle.

The paracardioscopic cannula provides direct access to the heart. The 10-mm port is removed and the cannula positioned through the midline incision. Once the abdomen is reinsufflated, the cannula is positioned through the defect in the diaphragm and into the pericardium under the direct visualization of a 5-mm laparoscope in the left subcostal port. The abdominal insufflation is discontinued and a rigid endoscope is inserted into the cannula providing direct visualization and access to the left atrium, coronary sinus, the superior (SVC) and inferior (IVC) vena cava, the aorta, the right main pulmonary artery, the right and left pulmonary veins, the transverse sinus, the ligament of Marshall, and the left and right atrial appendages. Since the tip of the cannula is soft and flexible, it can be manipulated within the pericardium without injury to the epicardial surface of the heart. There is minimal compromise of cardiac function during paracardioscopy.

A guide wire, incorporated at the tip of the cannula, provides a platform over which the Visitrax™ (nContact Surgical, Morrisville, NC, USA) ablation device can be positioned. Because these ablation lines are visible, a contiguous epicardial ablation pattern can be created (Figs. 46.2, 46.3, 46.4, 46.5, and 46.6).

Utilizing the cannula and associated guide wire, ablation lines are created from the atrial

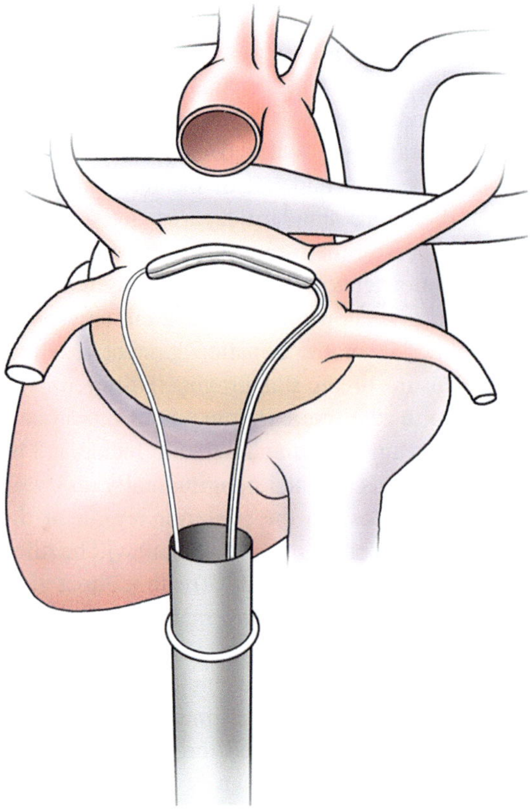

Fig. 46.2 The Convergent procedure epicardial and endocardial pattern. Posterior ablation lesions in blue

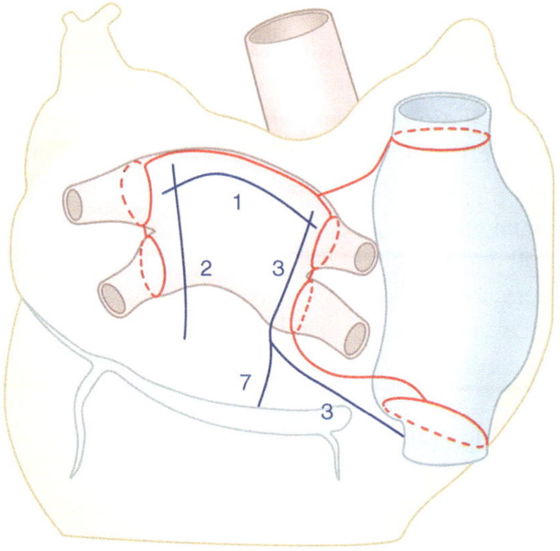

Fig. 46.3 The Convergent procedure epicardial and endocardial pattern. Right pulmonary vein ablation line in blue

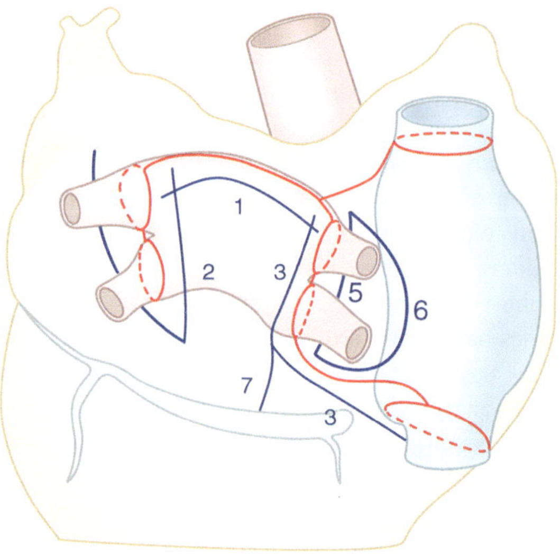

Fig. 46.4 The Convergent procedure epicardial and endocardial pattern. Anterior left pulmonary vein ablation line in blue

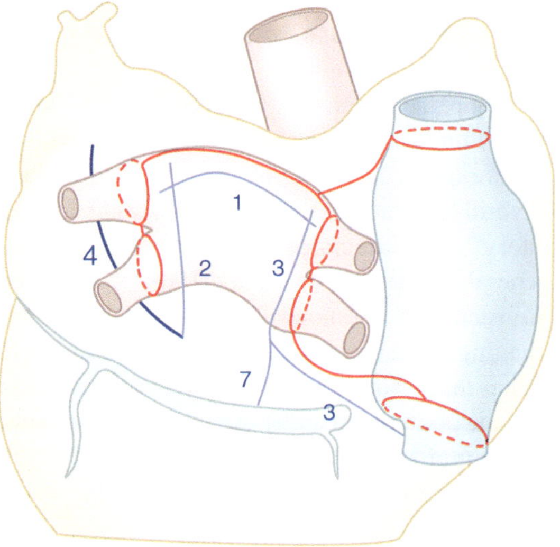

Fig. 46.5 The Convergent procedure epicardial and endocardial pattern

side of the coronary sinus to the left inferior pulmonary vein (2b)g, behind the left pulmonary veins cephalad toward the posterior pericardial reflection (2a)g, along the reflection from the left superior pulmonary vein to the right superior pulmonary vein (1a)g, along the posterior right pulmonary veins (3a)g, along the coronary sinus from the right to the left inferior pulmonary veins

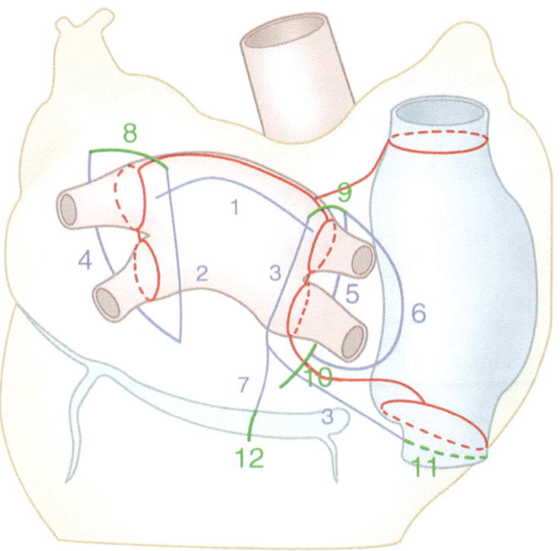

Fig. 46.6 The Convergent procedure epicardial and endocardial pattern. Endocardial lesions ablation lines in green. Epicardial ablation lines in blue. Pericardial reflections in red

(1b)g, from the right inferior pulmonary vein onto the inferior vena cava (3b), and to the inferior right atrium near the Thebesian valve (7).

The cannula is moved anteriorly over the IVC into the space between the right atrium and right pericardium. In this location, an ablation line is created along the anterior surface of the right pulmonary veins from the top of the superior pulmonary vein to the oblique sinus (5).

A second line of ablation is created upon the fat in Waterston's groove (6). The cannula is repositioned behind the left atrium where the left inferior pulmonary vein is again identified. From here, the cannula is directed along the anterior left pulmonary veins as far cephalad as possible to identify the base of the left atrial appendage and the ligament of Marshall. The ligament of Marshall is thoroughly ablated, and an ablation line is extended from the highest point on the left superior pulmonary vein along the antrum to the first ablation line on the inferior left pulmonary vein (4).

The cannula is then repositioned anterior to the IVC then along the anterior right atrium to the SVC. The cannula is then carefully positioned medial to the SVC and into the transverse sinus until the left atrial appendage is visualized. A flexible guide wire is positioned through the cannula and the transverse sinus and behind the left atrial appendage to be in position along the anterior left pulmonary veins. The cannula is repositioned behind the left atrium and the wire is identified and pulled into the cannula, thus providing a platform for positioning the ablation device. Ablation at the anterior left pulmonary veins along the ligament of Marshall and across the dome of the left atrium in the transverse sinus is completed, and all ablation lines are reexamined to verify contiguity. Upon the completion of the epicardial, surgical portion of the procedure, the electrophysiologist begins the endocardial portion of the Convergent procedure (Figs. 46.7 and 46.8).

Femoral venous access is obtained percutaneously at both the right and left groins. After the transvenous placement of mapping catheters into the right atrium and coronary sinus, the electrophysiologist gains transseptal access to position circular mapping and ablation catheters into the left atrium. The patient is anticoagulated with unfractionated heparin and the ACT is maintained h350 s. Because of the pericardial reflections, the epicardial ablations may not be

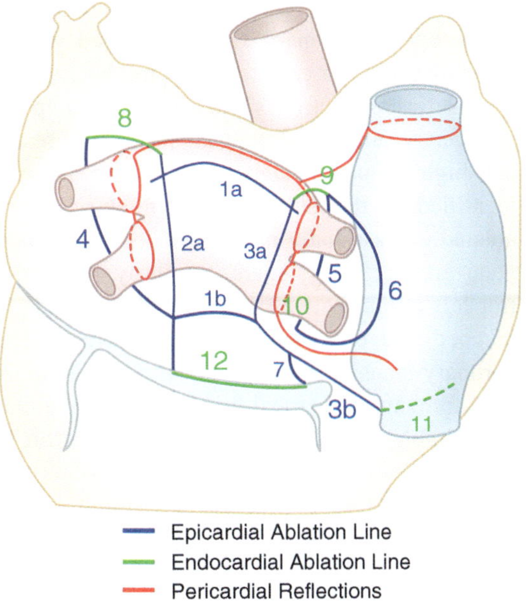

Fig. 46.7 Introduction of trocar in the abdominal and pericardium

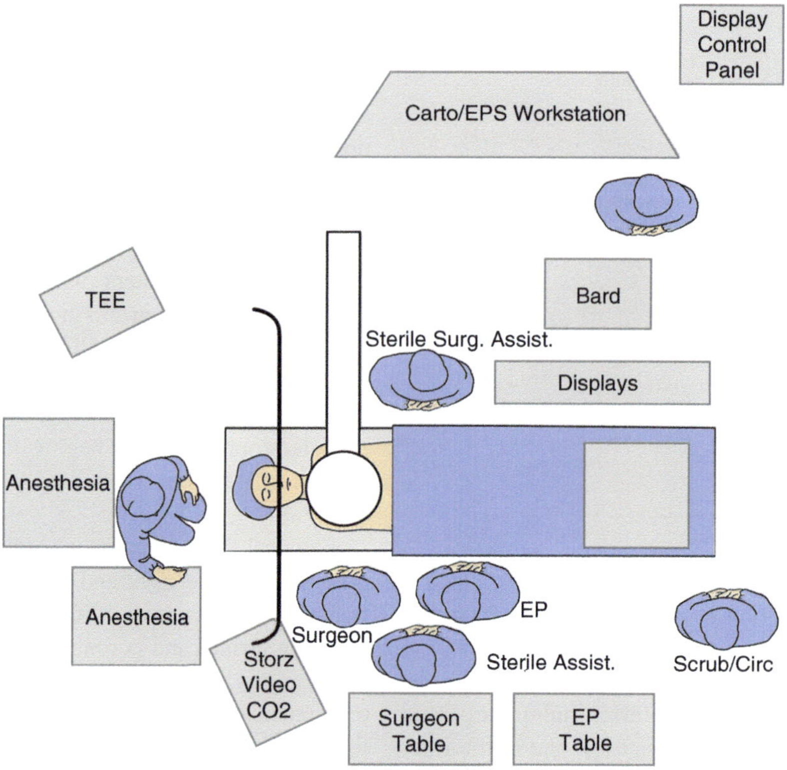

Fig. 46.8 Radiofrequency catheter for epicardial ablation

contiguous at the superior right and left pulmonary veins and at the right inferior pulmonary veins. Each pulmonary vein is mapped with a multipolar circular catheter. The circular catheter has a series of electrodes that are used to map the pulmonary veins and left atrial surface for residual high-frequency signals. Areas of activity identified in the pulmonary vein antrums are ablated endocardially until all of the pulmonary veins are electrically silent. Similarly, the posterior left atrium between the pulmonary veins is mapped and electrical silence confirmed. The coronary sinus is mapped and, if demonstrating high-frequency electrical firing, a series of endocardial ablation lesions is applied in an effort to isolate the structure. Finally, a line of ablation is created at the cavotricuspid isthmus with confirmation of a line of block. The metrics of procedural completion are electrical silence of the four pulmonary veins, electrical silence of the posterior left atrium, ablation of the coronary sinus with debulking or electrical isolation, and conduction block at the cavotricuspid isthmus.

If sinus rhythm is not attained, the patient is cardioverted and further electrophysiologic study with and without Isuprel (Sanofi-Aventis, Bridgewater, NJ, USA) is performed with targeting of arrhythmias as indicated. Various mapping and visualization systems are used during the electrophysiologist's portion. Fluoroscopy and ultrasound, either transesophageal or intracardiac, are utilized during transseptal puncture. Three-dimensional mapping systems are utilized with fluoroscopy during atrial mapping and endocardial ablation.

Upon completion of the endocardial portion of the Convergent procedure, anticoagulation is corrected and the venous sheaths are removed when the ACT is less than 200. The midline fascia is closed securely with nonabsorbable, interrupted suture and the skin closed routinely. The patient is generally extubated in the operating room and is usually ready for discharge in 3–5 days. Using an Enoxaparin (Sanofi-Aventis, Bridgewater, NJ, USA) bridge, Warfarin (Bristol-Myers Squib, New York, NY, USA) therapy is

Table 46.1 Postoperative results. Medium term results

Results	6-month Holter ECG	6 month or Holter reveal	12-month/Holter ECG	12-month reveal
Sinus rhythm	91% (48/53)	88%* (36/41)	90%* (35/39)	81%* (30/37)
Sinus rhythm and freedom from antiarrhythmic medications	79% (42/53)	73%* (30/41)	77%* (30/39)	76%* (28/37)

Table 46.2 Convergent patient outcomes

	1 month ECG	3 month Holter	6 month Holter/Tele
Freedom from AF (%)	94	100	100
# free from AF	17	9	3
Total # of patients	18	9	3
Sinus rhythm (%)	89	100	100
# in sinus rhythm	16	9	3
Total # of patients	18	9	3
%Freedom from AF & AADs (%)	46	67	100
# from AF & AADS	6	6	3
Total # of patients	13	9	3

initiated the night of the procedure and continued at least 3 months. Antiarrhythmic medications are initiated at the discretion of the electrophysiologist but are discontinued by 3 months. The patients are evaluated at 1, 3, 6, and 12 months with routine ECG evaluation and with a 24- h Holter before the end of the first 3-month postoperative period. Seven-day, or longer, monitoring is conducted at the 6- and 12-month visits and annually thereafter.

46.4 Results

Sixty five patients (92% persistent AF) have successfully undergone the Convergent procedure. The average duration of AF was 5.2 years and the average left atrial size was 5.3 cm. The average ablation time for the surgical portion was 102 min while the average endocardial ablation time was 85 min. The average total fluoroscopy time was 35.1 min. One patient underwent the Convergent procedure and, simultaneously, underwent minimally invasive mitral valve repair via a 7-cm right submammary incision and remains in sinus rhythm at 3 months. Two patients developed a pericardial effusion 2 weeks postprocedure requiring percutaneous drainage. Both recovered fully and remain in sinus rhythm at 3 months. No hemodynamically significant pericardial effusions have occurred since drainage of the pericardium postprocedure became standard. One patient has demonstrated right phrenic nerve paresis at 3 months.

Early clinical results are presented in Tables 46.1 and 46.2. Although less than 50% of patients are free from AF and antiarrhythmic medications (AADs) at 1 month, 89% are in sinus rhythm. Most patients at 3 and 6 months with 24-h continuous rhythm evaluation remain in sinus rhythm.

46.5 Discussion

This convergence of technologies and expertise (1) allows the creation of a complete, biatrial, endocardial, and epicardial ablation pattern without a chest incision or cardiopulmonary bypass, (2) provides intraoperative metrics to confirm procedural success, (3) encourages integrated patient care by cardiology and cardiac surgery, and (4) potentially decreases length of hospital stay and the number of repeat ablation procedures.

While the early results reported here are encouraging, the number of patients evaluated remains small. The development of symptomatic pericardial effusions, perhaps directly related to the degree of pericardial irritation combined with immediate anticoagulation, has been addressed successfully by draining the pericardium for 36 h. We must, however, continue to evaluate these patients for procedural-related complications, such as phrenic nerve injury or intraoperative cardiac injury. Paracardioscopy with epicardial ablation is early in development, thus requires appropriate initial training and guidance but can be quickly mastered by surgeons with little minimally invasive procedural experience. Careful evaluation of outcomes and procedural proficiency is crucial to the long-term success of this new hybrid approach to chronic AF.

References

1. Barnett SD, Ad F (2006) Surgical ablation as treatment for the elimination of atrial fibrillation a meta-analysis. J Thorac Cardiovasc Surg 31:1029–1035
2. Calkins H, Brugada J, Packer DL, et al., HRS/EHRA/ECAS Expert Consensus Statement on catheter and surgical ablation of Atrial fibrillation recommendations for personnel, policy, procedures and follow-up a report of the Heart Rhythm Society (HRS) Task Force on Catheter and Surgical Ablation of Atrial Fibrillation. Developed in partnership with the European Heart Rhythm Association (EHRA) and the European Cardiac Arrhythmia Society (ECAS); in collaboration with the American College of Cardiology (ACC), American Heart Association (AHA), and the Society of Thoracic Surgeons (STS) (2007) Endorsed and approved by the governing bodies of the American College of Cardiology, the American Heart Association, the European Cardiac Arrhythmia Society, the European Heart Rhythm Association, the Society of Thoracic Surgeons, and the Heart Rhythm Society. Heart Rhythm 4(6): 1547-5271. doi: 10.1016/j.hrthm.2007.04.005/$ – see front matter o 2007 by the Heart Rhythm Society and the European Heart Rhythm Association, registered branch of the European Society of Cardiology
3. Calo I, Lamberti F, Loricchio ML et al (2006) Left atrial ablation versus biatrial ablation for persistent and permanent atrial fibrillation a prospective and randomized study. J Am Coll Cardiol 47:2504–2512
4. Cappato R, Calkins H, Chen SA et al (2005) Worldwide survey on the methods, efficacy, and safety of catheter ablation for human atrial fibrillation. Circulation 111:1100–1105
5. Cox JL (2004) The role of surgical intervention in the management of atrial fibrillation. Tex Heart Inst J 31:257–265
6. Cox JL, Boineau JP, Schuessler RB et al (1995) Modification of the Maze procedure for atrial flutter and atrial fibrillation I. Rationale and surgical results. J Thorac Cardiovasc Surg 110:485–495
7. Cox JL, Schuessler RB, D'Agostino HJ Jr et al (1991) The surgical treatment of atrial fibrillation. III. Development of a definitive surgical procedure. J Thorac Cardiovasc Surg 101:569–583
8. Defauw JJ, Guiraudon GM, van Hemel FM et al (1992) Surgical therapy of paroxysmal atrial fibrillation with the corridor operation. Ann Thorac Surg 53:564–570
9. Edgerton JR, Edgerton ZJ, Weaver T et al (2008) Minimally invasive pulmonary vein isolation and partial autonomic denervation for surgical treatment of atrial fibrillation. Ann Thorac Surg 86:35–39
10. Kosakai J (2000) Treatment of atrial fibrillation using the maze procedure the Japanese experience. Semin Thorac Cardiovasc Surg 12:44–52
11. Fitta T, Lee R, Schuessler RB et al (1999) Radial approach a new concept in surgical treatment for atrial fibrillation I. Concept, anatomic and physiologic bases and development of a procedure. Ann Thorac Surg 67:27–35
12. Prasad SM, Maniar HS, Camillo CJ et al (2003) The Cox maze III procedure for atrial fibrillation long-term efficacy in patients undergoing lone versus concomitant procedures. J Thorac Cardiovasc Surg 126:1822–1828
13. Wolf RK, Schneeberger EW, Esterday R et al (2005) Video-assisted bilateral pulmonary vein isolation and left atrial appendage exclusion for atrial fibrillation. J Thorac Cardiovasc Surg 130:797–802

Robotically Cardiac Resynchronization Therapy for Heart Failure

47

Jean-Luc Jansens

Contents

J.-L. Jansens, M.D.
Department of Cardiac Surgery, Europe Hospitals, 206, Avenue de Fré, 1180 Brussels, Belgium
e-mail: jl.jansens@gmail.com

47.1 Clinical Background

Cardiac resynchronization therapy (CRT) is an emergent therapeutic option for a very selected population of heart failure patients. More and more studies are showing the beneficial impact of this treatment in terms of exercise tolerance, cardiac function improvement, symptom relief, and decrease in hospital stay.

Still many questions about CRT remain unsolved: the actual mechanism, the best technical way of achieving CRT, the high nonresponder rate, etc.

After a first positive experience of surgical epicardial lead implantation in the very first studies related to biventricular pacing [1], a decade ago, the percutaneous approach has been preferred, for its minimally invasive approach.

Unfortunately, the percutaneous approach has shown several drawbacks and complications, and the minimally invasive surgical procedure has become a serious option again.

Among these surgical techniques, robotically assisted thoracoscopy represents one of the most elegant ways of implanting the left ventricular lead, and recently some articles have shown its advantage, over the percutaneous approach, in terms of accuracy of targeting the optimal LV area and reproducibility of the procedure. It is currently considered to be a minimally invasive rescue in the setting of failed CS leads.

R.G.C. Inderbitzi et al. (eds.), *Minimally Invasive Thoracic and Cardiac Surgery*,
DOI 10.1007/978-3-642-11861-6_47, © Springer-Verlag Berlin Heidelberg 2012

What is heart failure?

Despite many encouraging advances in its understanding and treatment – pharmacologic and nonpharmacologic – prognosis of heart failure remains poor.

HF incidence approaches 10 per 1,000 in people over the age of 65 years [2].

In people diagnosed with HF, sudden death occurs at 6–9 times the rate of the general population.

Hospital discharge for HF rose from 377,000 in 1979 to 970,000 in 2002, an increase of 157%.

In 2005, the estimated direct and indirect cost of HF in the United States is 27.9 billion.

What is cardiac dyssynchrony?

About *10%* [3, 4] of these heart failure patients have segmental delayed myocardial activation and contraction, either because the dilation of the ventricles or because of the presence of ischemic myocardial areas. This cardiac dyssynchrony leads to impaired heart failure symptoms (fatigue, dyspnea, etc.) and ventricular function, decreased exercise tolerance, poor quality of life, and increased hospital stay.

What is cardiac resynchronization therapy?

Cardiac resynchronization therapy (CRT) aims at restoring a synchronous contraction of both ventricles. This treatment has been under investigation since the early 1990s, and recently many well-conducted studies have shown its clinical benefit for patients with New York Heart Association (NYHA) class III or IV. Such benefits have included improvement in symptomatology, reduced complications, reduced risk of mortality, and reduction in hospital stay [5–7].

Generally, according to major studies, patients are eligible for CRT in case of stable NYHA class III or IV despite standard pharmacologic therapy, with a left ventricular ejection fraction (LVEF) of less than 35%, and a QRS interval of more than 120 ms on the electrocardiogram. Recently, other echocardiographic criteria have been added in many studies: an interventricular mechanical delay of more than 40 ms, an aortic pre-ejection delay of more than 140 ms, a delayed activation of the lateral or posterolateral left ventricular wall, etc.

Technically, resynchronization is obtained by the placement of a specially designed pacemaker (or defibrillator). Two conventional endocardial leads are positioned just as the classical pacemaker (or defibrillator) indications: the right atrial lead, placed in the right atrial appendage, and the right ventricular (RV) lead, generally inserted in the RV apex.

A third lead is also placed on the epicardial side of the left ventricle (LV), either through the coronary sinus (CS) into a lateral coronary vein, under fluoroscopy guidance, or surgically fixed on the LV epicardial surface.

This lead configuration allows pacing of both ventricles in a synchronous way, beat to beat, in relation to the atrial sensing and thanks to the programming of a shorter AV delay than spontaneously obtained.

47.1.1 Studies Results and Questions Raised About CRT

Since the early 1990s, many studies have tried to evaluate and demonstrate the clinical benefit of cardiac resynchronization therapy. None of these were really suggestive enough to make this new treatment become a standard in such patients until the final results from studies such as the COMPANION trial [7]. This trial revealed that in patients with advanced heart failure and a prolonged QRS interval, CRT decreases the combined risk of death from any cause or first hospitalization and, when combined with an implantable defibrillator, significantly reduces mortality.

Also, according to the CARE-HF Study [5], CRT improves symptoms and quality of life and reduces complications and mortality, as compared to standard medical treatment.

Finally, CRT combined to ICD, as compared to ICD alone, was found to decrease HF events in relatively asymptomatic patients with a low ejection fraction and a QRS duration of 130 ms or more [8].

However, about 30% of patients do not respond to CRT, even when the CS lead has properly been placed with a percutaneous technique.

This fairly high nonresponder rate has probably multiple explanations, and among these, the selection criteria and the optimal placement of the LV lead may play an important role [9].

Currently, patients are selected mainly on electrocardiogram criteria (wide QRS complex, left bundle branch block configuration).

In order to decrease the 30% of nonresponders rate, additional selection criteria are needed.

Echocardiography (and, in particular, tissue Doppler imaging, known as TDI) may allow further identification of potential responders to CRT, based on an assessment of inter- and intraventricular dyssynchrony [10].

Also, echocardiography may allow optimal LV lead positioning and follow-up after CRT.

Moreover, accurate LV lead position may be an important point to have a more effective response to CRT. In that case, the surgical approach could be more suitable in terms of treatment efficacy.

47.2 Techniques

As written above, CRT can be achieved by two different approaches, with their advantages, disadvantages, and complications.

Initially, CRT was first tried through thoracotomies [1] but rapidly moved to percutaneous attempts mainly because of the importance of the surgical invasiveness.

During 1990s, major advances and efforts have been made by the different companies involved in CRT in making percutaneous tools enabling easier and more reproducible CS lead placement for cardiologists.

The venue of minimally invasive cardiac surgery in the field of CRT a few years later changed somewhat the perspective of obtaining a more accurate CRT in several types of patients.

47.2.1 Percutaneous Approach

47.2.1.1 Implantation Techniques

The right atrial and ventricular leads are placed using a standard method, through the (right or left) cephalic or subclavian vein.

The same subclavian approach is used to insert the LV lead, but as it has to be placed through the coronary sinus os, several other tools are needed to facilitate the implantation (see Fig. 47.1).

Different consecutive steps are needed to have an LV lead placed into the desired LV vein:

- Entering the coronary sinus
- To catheterize the CS os, either a long stylet delivery tool or preshaped guiding catheters may be used.
- Obtaining a CS venogram
- In order to have a good overview of the venous distribution, the CS is occluded with a special balloon catheter, and the CS is visualized with dye injection. The decision about the target tributary of the CS is determined at this time.
- Placement of the LV lead

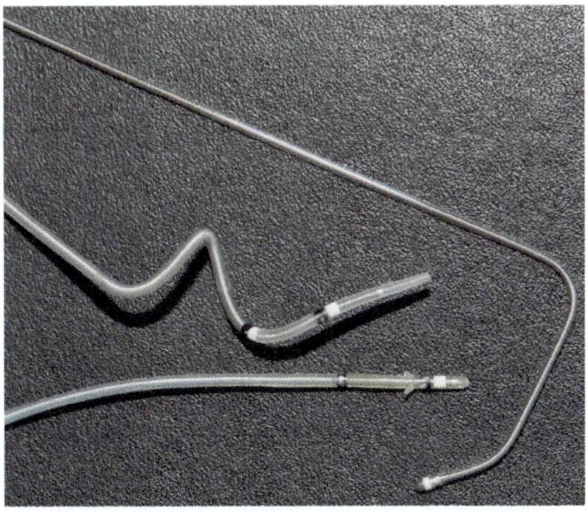

Fig. 47.1 Three different models of coronary sinus leads, with various stabilizing systems

Two different techniques are currently available: the "over-the-wire" *technique* allowing the lead implantation by pushing it over a guide wire to its final location, and the *stylet delivery system*, enabling the implantation of a specially shaped lead directly from a stylet placed into the CS os.

Usually the lead is placed as far as possible in the LV venous circulation, preferably in a lateral or posterolateral vein, in order to have the longest interventricular conduction time and the shortest QRS duration when pacing with both ventricular leads.

47.2.1.2 Technical Problems

Although there are advantages of placing the three leads through the same way (subclavian vein), and also of being really as minimally invasive as possible, this method carries drawbacks and complications (see Table 47.1). Among them, coronary venous anatomy is an important problem for such an approach, as the veins are unpredictable in their locations from one patient to another.

As a consequence, if, as mentioned above, accuracy of LV lead placement is mandatory to decrease the nonresponder rate of CRT, the percutaneous approach could probably not offer such precision as any other surgical placement strategy.

Table 47.1 Major reasons for percutaneous left ventricular lead implantation failure

Unability to cannulate the coronary sinus	49%
Anatomic cardiac venous anomaly	24%
Phrenic stimulation or ventricular dyssynchrony	17%
Perforation or dissection	5%
Dislodgement	5%

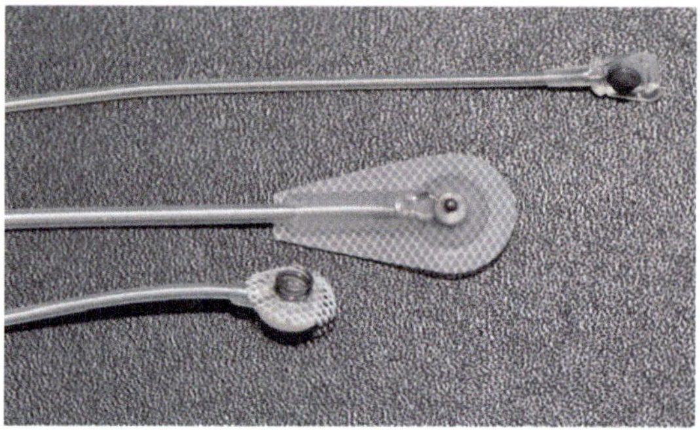

Fig. 47.2 Three different models of epicardial leads: a steroid-eluting tip (*upper*), a fractal coating device (*middle*), and a screw-in lead (*inferior*)

47.2.2 Surgical Approach

47.2.2.1 Epicardial Leads

Epicardial leads have been developed during the 1950s [11] and were routinely used for classical pacemaker implantations. After the new developments of the endocardial lead technology, the use of epicardial leads was more confined in the pediatric population.

Epicardial leads have been developed according to two different concepts:

1. *The type of fixation*

Basically two different types of fixation have been developed in order to have a constant and reliable contact with the epicardium (see Fig. 47.2):

(i) The *screw-in leads*
(ii) The leads that must be stitched onto the epicardial surface

The screw-in lead certainly has the advantage of being easily placed through a classical sternotomy, a mini-thoracotomy, or even through video-assisted thoracoscopy (VATS). Several handling tools have even been designed recently in order to facilitate a less invasive approach of surgical LV lead placement. Unfortunately, there is a risk of potential local damage of the pacing target area, thus scar tissue formation on the mid- and long term, leading to high electrical (sensing and pacing) thresholds.

Moreover, there are no recent data about the late outcome of such leads implanted on large and fragile ventricular cavities.

The non-screw-in lead would be more challenging to place with less invasive surgical tools, especially without any intrathoracic tools equipped with wrists.

2. *The presence of steroids at the distal end of the electrode*

Different distal electrode ends have been developed in order to improve the pacing and sensing thresholds; some are relying only on their fixation system (screw-in devices), some have increased the contact surface between the electrode and the heart (fractal coating), and finally some have added steroids to avoid a major inflammatory response at implant and several weeks after the procedure (see Fig. 47.2).

Several studies have shown the benefit in terms of threshold profile in favor of the epicardial leads having their distal end eluting steroids in a couple of weeks after the implant [12].

Based upon these findings, one can assume that the less aggressive for the myocardium the fixation system is, the better the thresholds will be, which will be a determinant factor of the best response to CRT. Moreover, it seems well accepted in the literature that steroids added at the distal end of the electrode also play an important role in preserving the best thresholds, in the acute and the more chronic phase [13].

47.2.2.2 Implantation Techniques

There are different surgical approaches for an epicardial lead fixation on the left ventricle. These will be depending on the surgical team, the surgical tools at their disposal, and the type of epicardial lead fixation chosen.

Thoracotomy

Thoracotomy was formerly the most common surgical approach used for CRT [1]: the procedure is easy, and every cardiac surgeon is able to perform it. Unfortunately, this procedure has some disadvantages, such as the postoperative pain with the risk of pulmonary complications and the limited visual field allowing only a restricted LV target zone. Nevertheless, this approach allows the use of screw-in and active fixation devices.

Conventional Thoracoscopy

Video-assisted thoracoscopy is certainly a step forward in a less invasive surgical setting but, because of its relatively cumbersome movements, does not allow an active fixation technique with stitches. For teams favoring screw-in methods, this technique is for sure valuable, easy, and fast, thanks to the industry that has developed specific tools allowing a simple way of screwing the lead.

Robotic Thoracoscopy

By its ease of intrathoracic motions, robotics allows every kind of fixation technique, thus certainly represents the most attractive way of performing minimally invasive surgical CRT.

Incidentally, this easy robotic procedure may represent a first step in the learning course of this surgical tool for teams who want to start a robotic program in the cardiosurgical field.

Two different approaches are possible: the anterior and the posterior.

The posterior approach [14] aims for more reproducibility in the placement: the purpose is to place the epicardial lead on the LV posterobasal side, the more refined resynchronization being made postoperatively by the cardiologist with the optimization of the V-V delay between both right and left ventricular leads.

The main purpose of the anterior approach [15] is to be as accurate as possible in the lead placement, basing the LV target zone on the perioperative assessment, with a preoperative TDI, or an intraoperative sensing tool (allowing to look at the longest activation zone) which seems to be an elegant surgical way of defining, intraoperatively, the best resynchronization point. The trocar incisions will be more anterior than the first approach because this target point could be more anterior than expected (Fig. 47.3).

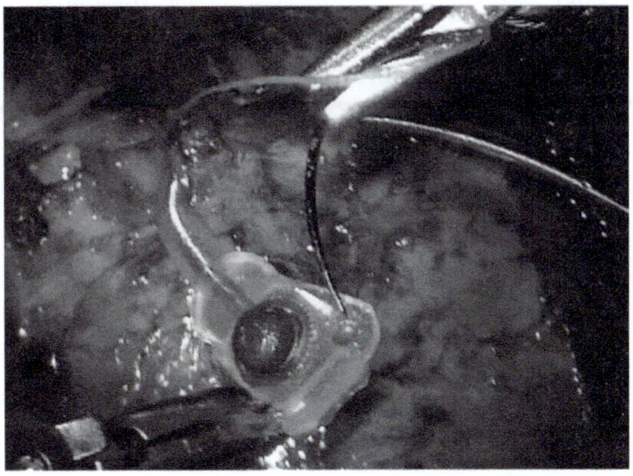

Fig. 47.3 Robotic fixation with a stitch of a steroid-eluting epicardial lead on the LV surface

47.2.2.3 Operative Technique

- After conventional, percutaneous, fluoroscopy-guided implantation of the right atrial and ventricular leads, three 1-cm incisions are made in the intercostal spaces, along the left mid- or posterior axillary line, allowing the introduction of two lateral robotic arms and one central 3-D camera into the chest.
- If the percutaneous step has been performed in the first operation, the left deltopectoral incision (for the pacemaker pocket) may be reopened in order to insert the distal end of the epicardial lead. Another option is to make a fourth intercostal incision for the lead and tunnelize it to the pacemaker at the end of the procedure.
- Gentle CO_2 insufflation and right lateral tilting of the patients are mandatory to provide a sufficient amount of working space between the dilated LV and the chest wall.
- The surgeon, placed at a distance from the patient at the operating console, performs the operation by remotely telemanipulating the endoscopic arms and camera as described elsewhere [16].
- A left posterior or lateral pericardiotomy is performed with an articulated cautery tool to expose the LV lateral wall, and the lead is positioned under direct vision after having been inserted into the thorax as abovementioned.
- The lead is either attached to the epicardium according to visual assessment of local viability (aspect and contractility) by means of a simple suture, which is secured in the myocardium (in the anterior approach), or by screwing it (in the posterior approach). A second lead may be screwed in the LV, as a backup.
- Threshold measurements are completed, and echocardiographic assessment of resynchronization efficiency may be performed.
- The proximal end of the lead is then brought through the intercostal space to be connected to the stimulator and placed in a conventional pectoral position.

47.2.2.4 Clinical Data

As this procedure is relatively new, only a few series of robotic CRT have been recently reported [14, 15]. Recently, short- and long-term thresholds were proven to be performed well in a 78-patient population [17].

In summary, these reports show that this procedure is not only feasible but represents a safe, easy, and reproducible method of obtaining an efficient CRT.

47.2.3 Possible Developments of Resynchronization

It has recently been reported that the fairly high number (30%) of nonresponders in CRT was due to several factors: the absence of electrical conduction delay or mechanical dyssynchrony despite wide QRS complexes, failure to optimize the CRT settings after device implantation, and the placement of the left ventricular pacing lead in an inappropriate location [9].

For this last cause, it seems obvious that any new development of the percutaneous approach would not adequately answer this problem simply because of the anatomic constraints.

On the contrary, the surgical approach, and more precisely robotic implantation, may offer an added value in terms of adequate positioning of the lead. It certainly gives the ability of choosing the best possible site in relation with the flexibility of robotic use and with the perioperative assessment.

Concerning this last part, many recent reports have been focusing on TDI as an excellent tool to determine the LV latest activation zone, which would a priori determine the best resynchronization point. Unfortunately this diagnostic tool is quite difficult to use, as it requires a long postprocessing time and is very operator-dependent. For these reasons, it is not quite established yet that TDI will remain the only diagnostic tool for CRT optimization. Robotics could therefore even play a role in an operative assessment, before final implantation.

Moreover, since 2008, an increasing number of studies [18, 19] are carried on about multiple site pacing in CRT: more than one (usually two) lead are placed on the left ventricle in order to expect a better response to resynchronization therapy. So far, only few results have been published, in particular, about increasing left ventricular reverse remodeling as compared to conventional CRT.

One possible drawback of this technique might be the technical difficulties of implanting several leads into specific coronary veins. Again, surgery and more particularly robotics could help develop this new encouraging way for CRT.

47.3 Discussion

Heart failure is a serious health-care problem. Many efforts are made to solve definitively this disease or to slow down its progression. Among them, cardiac resynchronization therapy certainly represents a new hope for many patients suffering from heart failure with intracardiac conduction disturbances. In order to obtain a biventricular resynchronization, the conventional percutaneous implantation of a left ventricular lead is the standard. Nevertheless, this procedure encounters many unsolvable technical difficulties, especially in terms of lead positioning and catheterization of the coronary sinus.

Thanks to its ease of manipulation, robotic implantation of the left ventricular epicardial lead can overcome these anatomic issues and may be a very competitive alternative not only as a backup therapy after percutaneous attempts, but also as the first-line treatment.

In addition, this simple procedure can be part of a learning process in robotic cardiac surgery, leading to the ability to use the device in broader applications of cardiac surgery, reported in other chapters of this book.

References

1. Auricchio A, Stellbrink C, Sack S, Block M, Vogt J, Bakker P, Mortensen P, Klein H et al (1999) The Pacing Therapies for Congestive Heart Failure (PATH-CHF) study: rationale, design, and endpoints of a prospective randomized multicenter study. Am J Cardiol 83(5B):130D–135D
2. American Heart Association (2005) Congestive heart failure. Heart Disease and Stroke Statistics — 2005 Update. Dallas, Texas: American Heart Association, pp 26–27
3. Bleeker GB, Schalij MJ, Nihoyannopoulos P et al (2005) Left ventricular dyssynchrony predicts right ventricular remodeling after cardiac resynchronization therapy. J Am Coll Cardiol 46(12):2264–2269
4. Vitarelli A, Franciosa P, Conde Y, Cimino E, Nguyen BL, Ciccaglione A, Morichetti MC, Chachques JC, Rosanio S et al (2005) Echocardiographic assessment of ventricular asynchrony in dilated cardiomyopathy and congenital heart disease: tools and hopes. J Am Soc Echocardiogr 18(12):1424–1439
5. Cleland JG, Daubert JC, Erdmann E, Cardiac Resynchronization-Heart Failure (CARE-HF) Study Investigators et al (2005) The effect of cardiac resynchronization on morbidity and mortality in heart failure. N Engl J Med 352(15):1539–1549
6. Ellenbogen KA, Wood MA, Klein HU (2005) Why should we care about CARE-HF? J Am Coll Cardiol 46(12):2199–2203
7. Carson P, Anand I, O'Connor C, Jaski B, Steinberg J, Lwin A, Lindenfeld J, Ghali J, Barnet JH, Feldman AM, Bristow MR (2005) Mode of death in advanced heart failure: the Comparison of Medical, Pacing, and Defibrillation Therapies in Heart Failure (COMPANION) trial. J Am Coll Cardiol 46(12):2329–2334
8. Moss AJ, Hall WJ, Cannom DS, Klein H, Brown MW, Daubert JP, Estes M III, Foster E, Greenberg H, Higgins SL, Pfeffer MA, Solomon SD, Wilber D, Zareba W (2009) Cardiac-resynchronization therapy for the prevention of heart-failure events. N Engl J Med 361(14):1329–1338
9. Yu CM, Wing-Hong Fung J et al (2005) Understanding nonresponders of cardiac resynchronization therapy–current and future perspectives. J Cardiovasc Electrophysiol 16(10):1117–1124
10. Bax JJ, Ansalone G, Breithardt OA et al (2004) Echocardiographic evaluation of cardiac resynchronization therapy: ready for routine clinical use? A critical appraisal. J Am Coll Cardiol 44(1):1–9
11. Jouve A, Corriol J, Velasque P et al (1957) Comparative study of epicardial and intramural leads in man and dog; synchronous epicardial recordings of the ventricles, anterior and posterior surface. Physiol (Paris) 49(1):223–226
12. Cohen MI et al (2001) Permanent epicardial pacing in pediatric patients: seventeen years of experience and 1200 outpatient visits. Circulation 103(21):2585–2590
13. Beaufort-Krol GC et al (1999) Comparison of longevity, pacing, and sensing characteristics of steroid-eluting epicardial versus conventional endocardial pacing leads in children. J Thorac Cardiovasc Surg 117(3): 523–528
14. Derose JJ Jr, Belsley S, Swistel DG et al (2004) Robotically assisted left ventricular epicardial lead implantation for biventricular pacing: the posterior approach. Ann Thorac Surg 77(4):1472–1474
15. Jansens JL, Jottrand M, Preumont N et al (2003) Robotic-enhanced biventricular resynchronization: an alternative to endovenous cardiac resynchronization therapy in chronic heart failure. Ann Thorac Surg 76(2):413–417
16. Falk V, Diegler A, Walther T et al (2000) Developments in robotic surgery. Curr Opin Cardiol 15(6):378–387

17. Kamath GS, Balaram S, Choi A, Kuteyeva O, Garikipati NV, Steinberg JS, Mittal S (2011) Long-term outcome of leads and patients following robotic epicardial left ventricular lead placement for cardiac resynchronization therapy. Pacing Clin Electrophysiol 34(2):235–240
18. Leclercq C, Gadler F, Kranig W, Ellery S, Gras D, Lazarus A, Clémenty J, Boulogne E, Daubert JC, TRIP-HF (Triple Resynchronization In Paced Heart Failure Patients) Study Group (2008) A randomized comparison of triple-site versus dual-site ventricular stimulation in patients with congestive heart failure. J Am Coll Cardiol 51(15):1455–1462
19. Sanaa I, Franceschi F, Prevot S, Bastard E, Deharo JC (2009) Is there a need for more than one left ventricular lead in some patients? Europace 11:29–31

Endovascular Hybrid Aortic Arch Repair

48

Martin Czerny, Michael Grimm, and Martin Funovics

Contents

M. Czerny, M.D. (✉)
Department of Cardiovascular Surgery,
University Hospital Berne, Freiburgstrasse,
Berne 3010, Switzerland
e-mail: martin.czerny@meduniwien.ac.at

M. Grimm, M.D.
Department of Cardiothoracic Surgery,
Medical University of Vienna, Währinger Gürtel 18-20,
1090 Vienna, Austria

Department of Cardiac Surgery,
Medical University of Vienna, Vienna, Austria
e-mail: michael.grimm@meduniwien.ac.at

M. Funovics, M.D.
Department of Interventional Radiology,
Medical University of Vienna, Währinger Gürtel 18-20,
1090 Vienna, Austria
e-mail: martin.funovics@meduniwien.ac.at

48.1 Background

Despite substantial advances in refining conventional surgical technique, there still remain elderly or physiologically frail patients who should probably not undergo standard arch replacement. This may be true in particular for patients with multisegmental thoracic aortic disease originating at the level of the aortic arch.

TEVAR has broadened treatment options in acute and chronic thoracic aortic disease and has proven durability [1–9]. As a prerequisite, the potential of the method, its limitations, as well as strict indications have to be known and followed. As such, a long landing zone, proximal and distal, has turned out to be a prerequisite for stable results [1]. If anatomy is unsuitable, suitability may be created by transposition of supraaortic branches [7–10]. By this clinical need, subclavian-to-carotid transposition regained popularity, and a new indication for this operation was present [11]. It was soon realized that there was clinical need for extending reroutings more proximal. As such, autologous double transposition entered the stage in 2002 and became the standard approach for distal arch disease [12]. However,

R.G.C. Inderbitzi et al. (eds.), *Minimally Invasive Thoracic and Cardiac Surgery*,
DOI 10.1007/978-3-642-11861-6_48, © Springer-Verlag Berlin Heidelberg 2012

some patients required an even more proximal extension of therapy. Finally, total arch rerouting was established soon afterward [13, 14].

48.2 Indications for Combined Approaches

48.2.1 Patient Selection

Primarily we should remain aware that we are treating a most often asymptomatic disease. As such, it is of utmost importance to preserve quality of life. This should be our major drive to recommend one treatment strategy or the other. The approach was primarily thought for patients not suitable for conventional surgery. Both has changed, more patients are now suitable for conventional surgery, and many patients are not suitable for any kind of therapy due to other limiting factors such as malignancy. The role for combined approaches is therefore – in our opinion – exactly in between. Furthermore, indication is closely associated with the underlying pathology. As such, it is mandatory to differentiate between dilatative and obliterative disease. Patients suffering from aneurysmal arch and descending aortic disease are not as likely to suffer from significant obliterative components of the disease in other vascular territories. Patients with acute dissections or patients with aneurysms on the basis of chronic type B dissections are – regarding atherosclerotic comorbidity – probably the most privileged ones as this fact is a rare exception. The situation is different in patients suffering from penetrating atherosclerotic ulcers (PAU). This disease is an expression of a fairly advanced aggressive form of obliterative arteriopathy. As such, these patients are the sickest ones and may have additional problems making treatment more complex such as significant carotid artery stenosis or iliac occlusive disease.

48.2.2 Preoperative Evaluation

Primarily patients are seen clinically, and an initial assessment of their willingness and ability of treatment is done. Afterward, an angio-CT scan from subcranially to the groin is being performed. By that, all essential questions regarding need and extent of rerouting, vascular abnormalities (lusorian artery, right-sided arch), anatomy of supraaortic branches, lesion per se, as well as access vessels are answered. A carotid artery duplex scan completes vascular diagnostics. Regarding cardiologic examinations, an echocardiogram is done routinely. Continuative diagnostics such as left heart catheterization are not performed routinely. Finally, lung function is not being assessed in order to prevent potential pressure exposition and rupture of the lesion (since this mechanism could once be observed).

48.2.3 Imaging

All CT examinations prior to treatment should be performed on a 64-row CT scanner. To allow pulsation free visualization of the thoracic aorta up to the aortic root, a retrospective ECG-gating technique should be used.

In our setting, all CT angiograms are performed in the arterial phase during the intravenous administration of nonionic iodinated contrast material. A bolus-triggering technique assesses the contrast medium transit time. A threshold of 150 HU (absolute) is used. 130 ml of contrast agent is administered in a biphasic fashion: the first 30 ml is injected at a flow rate of 6 ml/s followed by the second 100 ml administered at 5 ml/s. A saline flush of 40 ml is given in all the patients after the contrast medium injection to optimize contrast utilization. With a post-threshold delay of 8 s, ECG-gated CT angiography of the entire aorta is performed using the following imaging parameters: a slice collimation of 64×0.625 and a Pitch of 0.29 are used. The matrix size is 512×512. Images are reconstructed with a slice thickness of 1.4 and a slice increment of 1 mm, as well as with a slice thickness of 3 and a slice increment of 2 mm without using the ECG-triggering ("untagged images"). Additionally, image redistribution according to the heart action is performed after scanning (retrospective ECG-triggering). Usually, images are triggered in a mid-phase at 55% of an RR interval. If pulsation artifacts occur, other phases of the heart cycle are reconstructed. For every phase, two series are reconstructed (1.4/1 as well as 3/2 mm).

48.3 Surgical Approach

48.3.1 Subclavian-to-Carotid Transposition

If the extent of the lesion involves the origin of the left subclavian artery, routine subclavian-to-carotid transposition is performed usually using a lateral surgical approach with transection of the anterior scalene muscle. After transection of the proximal portion, the vessel is guided dorsally to the jugular vein and an end-to-side anastomosis between the common carotid and the subclavian artery is being performed. Care has to be taken not to lacerate the thoracic duct as this may result in tedious lymphatic fistulation. In rare cases with difficulties to expose the proximal portion of the left subclavian, it may be wise to perform a carotid-to-subclavian alloplastic graft. If this has to be done, it is imperative not to forget to insert a plug into the proximal left subclavian after TEVAR not in order to risk type II endoleakage by retrograde perfusion of the lesion.

48.3.2 Double Transposition

If the extent of the lesion involves the origin of the left common carotid artery, an autologous procedure to maintain cerebral perfusion may be performed. We developed this approach in 2002. In the initial two patients, a median sternotomy approach was used, and the pericardium was opened. Skin incision was extended parallel to the left clavicula to gain sufficient access to the left subclavian artery. From the third patient onward, an upper hemisternotomy instead of a complete sternotomy was chosen. The intraoperative situs is shown in Fig. 48.1. Afterward, the supraaortic branches are circumferentially dissected and encircled with silastic tapes (Fig. 48.2). After systemic heparinization with 80 IU/kg body weight, the left common carotid artery is dissected free and clamped. The vessel is transversely divided.

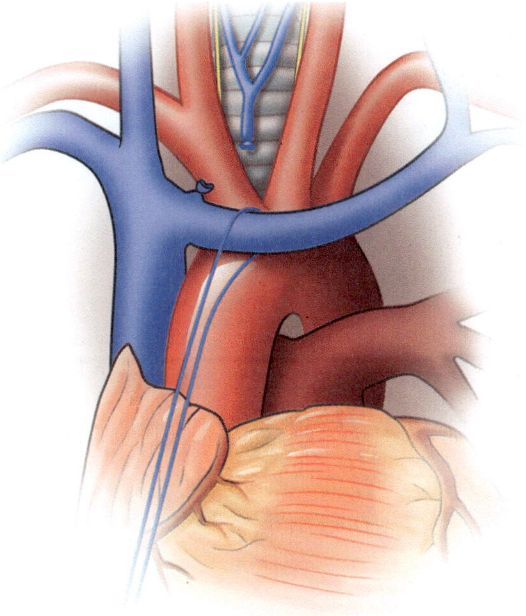

Fig. 48.1 Schematic view of the aortic arch and supraaortic branches and their relation to the anonymous vein, the trachea, as well as the recurring laryngeal nerves

The proximal portion is being closed with a 4-0 Prolene running suture (Ethicon, Inc, Somerville, NJ). Consecutively, the brachiocephalic trunk is partially clamped, longitudinally opened, and a

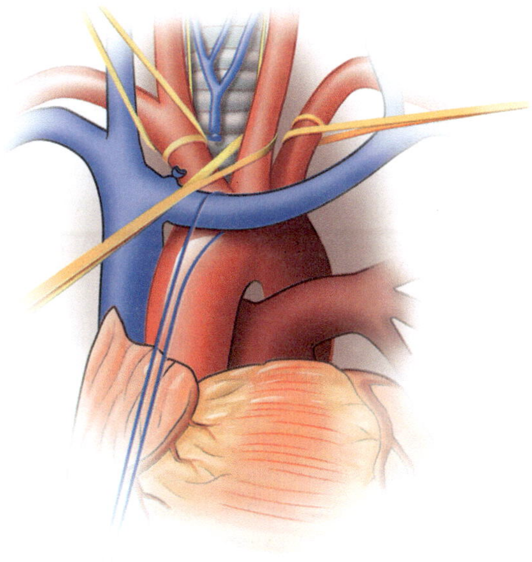

Fig. 48.2 Similar schematic view after surgical mobilization of the supraaortic branches and the anonymous vein having been encircled with silastic tapes

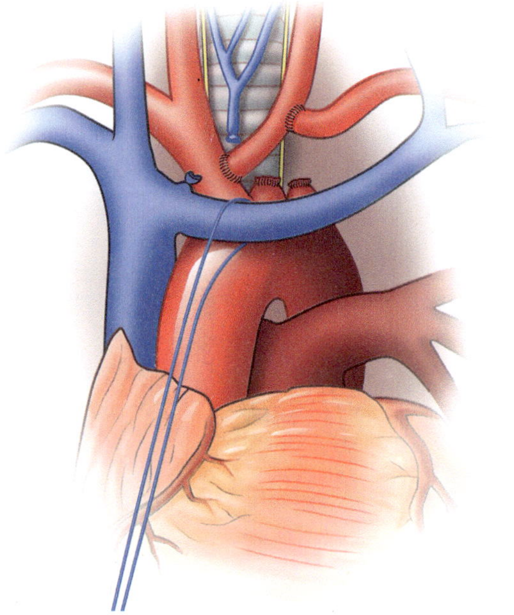

Fig. 48.3 Schematic view after autologous double transposition of the supraaortic branches with an end-to-side anastomosis between the left common carotid artery and the brachiocephalic trunk as well as an end-to-side anastomosis between the left subclavian artery and the already transposed left common carotid artery

side-to-end anastomosis is performed. After flushing and deairing, blood flow is reinstalled. An analogous procedure is carried out between the left subclavian artery and the already transposed left common carotid artery (Fig. 48.3). Due to differences in maximum diameter between the left common carotid and the subclavian artery, a side-to-side anastomosis between the two vessels may be chosen. In these cases, the left subclavian artery is ligated and additionally oversewn at its origin. After chest tube insertion, the wound is closed in layers.

The main advantage of this approach, besides the less invasiveness of the procedure, is the avoidance of alloplastic material to maintain perfusion of the arch vessels. As alloplastic replacement of native blood vessels always bears the risk of infection with deleterious consequences [15], this vascular surgical approach elegantly maintains supraaortic perfusion extending a standard arterial transposition between the left subclavian and left common carotid artery to the brachiocephalic trunk. Additionally, the potential risk of clot formation on the artificial surface of an alloplastic vascular prosthesis is avoided. Nevertheless, several authors have described excellent results with alloplastic reconstructions in this particular subgroup of patients [13, 16–19].

48.3.3 Involvement of the Brachiocephalic Trunk

If the extent of the lesion involves the origin of the brachiocephalic trunk, an autologous procedure is not deemed suitable for gaining sufficient proximal length. Therefore, alloplastic material has to be used in order to maintain cerebral perfusion. In these patients, we use a reversed aortobifemoral prosthesis. Patients undergo a complete sternotomy and opening of the pericardium. The ascending aorta is partially clamped, and the anastomosis between the proximal portion of the prosthesis and the ascending aorta is performed with a 4-0 Prolene running suture. Using a Teflon felt strip for accomplishment of the anastomosis remains optional. Afterward, the anastomosis between the first branch of the prosthesis and brachiocephalic trunk is being performed with a 5-0 Prolene running suture. It may be the best solution to transversely divide the trunk and to perform an end-to-end anastomosis. A secure closure of the proximal portion of the supraaortic vessels by a double-layer running suture with additional patch–counter patch sutures is highly recommended. Cerebral monitoring during this particular step of the operation is by intra-arterial blood pressure monitoring via the radial artery. The branch of the prosthesis is guided superior to the anonymous vein. After flushing and deairing, blood flow is reinstalled. Afterward, the second branch is guided inferior to the anonymous vein in order to avoid compression and consecutive inflow obstruction, the left common carotid artery is being clamped at its origin, transversely divided, and an end-to-end anastomosis is being performed with a 5-0 Prolene

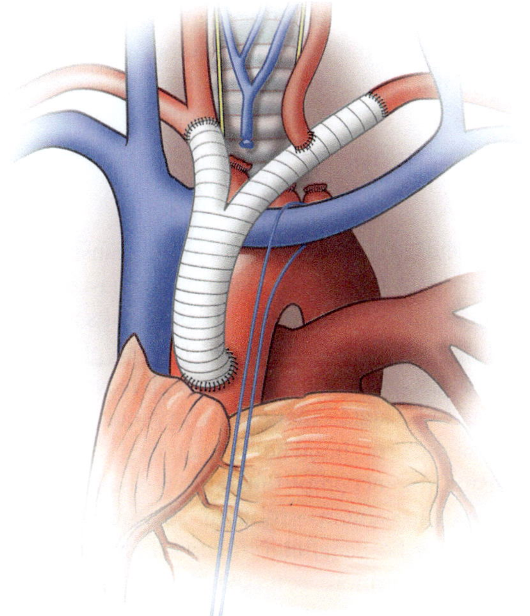

Fig. 48.4 Schematic view after total arch rerouting using an inversed bifurcated Dacron prosthesis end-to-side to the ascending aorta with an end-to-end anastomosis between the first branch of the prosthesis to the brachiocephalic trunk, an end-to-end anastomosis of the second branch to the left subclavian artery with reinsertion of the left common carotid artery into the branch to the left subclavian artery

running suture. The final intraoperative situs is shown in Fig. 48.4. In our experience, a 14/7-mm or a 16/8-mm bifurcated graft provides sufficient flow in this region, irrespective if Dacron or PTFE grafts are being used.

We highly recommend preservation of the left subclavian artery in each and every elective setting. Our rationale is not upper extremity perfusion, as this is hardly ever a problem, due to sufficient collateralization, but due to preservation of left posterior cerebellar circulation as well as maintaining an important spinal cord supplying vessel.

Arch rerouting and endovascular stent-graft placement are performed metachronously. A period of recovery for 7 days may be sufficient. Within this period, a completion CT scan is performed in order to reconfirm patency of the reconstructions performed.

48.3.4 Stent-Graft Systems

It is beyond the scope of this chapter to encourage or discourage the interested reader to use one product rather than another one. For us, the only important issue is that the more proximal the prosthesis has to be deployed, the more accurate the deployment mechanism has to be. As such, we do recommend to use a prosthesis with a "two-stage" deployment mode where – during deployment of the main body of the stent graft – the proximal portions are still controlled by a tip capture, thereby providing better stability and potentially allowing retraction of the device.

48.3.5 Details of Deployment

Stent grafts are placed under anesthesia. Access vessel exposure is being performed surgically. A 5-French pigtail catheter is advanced via the right brachial artery into the aortic arch to reconfirm characterization of the morphology and extent of the lesions. After systemic heparinization with 80 IU/kg, arteriotomy is performed, and the catheter is advanced under fluoroscopic guidance. Afterward, a change to an ultra-stiff guidewire (Backup Meier) is being performed. Stent grafts are deployed during systemic hypotension with a systolic pressure of 70 mmHg. The more proximal the stent graft is being deployed, the more liberal we do use rapid pacing via a temporary pacemaker electrode being inserted via the right subclavian vein into the right ventricle. Pacing is performed up to 180 beats per min. With this method, blood pressure control seems most effective.

48.4 Summary of Outcomes

48.4.1 Arch Rerouting

In general, morbidity after supraaortic reconstructions, both, autologous as well as alloplastic, is low [1–10, 16–19]. In our patient cohort, recovery was uneventful without any signs of permanent neurologic injury. One patient sustained a transient neurologic deficit due to partial clamping of a heavily calcified ascending aorta. No adverse events were observed after subclavian-to-carotid artery transposition as well as after double transposition.

However, total arch rerouting has to be regarded differently as despite avoiding CPB and hypothermic arrest, the procedure remains a big operation. In this series of 79 patients, we had to observe three retrograde type-A dissections, two of them with fatal outcome. Causes may be multifactorial including clamp injury by the side biting clamp, alterations of hemodynamics, as well as some sort of compliance mismatch between the stent graft and the very elastic ascending aorta. Current work will bring more insight into this issue. Nevertheless, we recommend that an ascending aorta with a diameter bigger than 40 mm should be replaced during total arch rerouting as this will definitely solve the issue, and it may be well presumed that a short period of normothermic CPB with a cross-clamp time of 20 min for ascending replacement will not dramatically increase risk [10].

48.4.2 Endoleak Formation and Treatment Options

Endoleak formation is directly related to the length of the landing zone – the longer the better at least 2 cm – as well as to the number of prostheses and may be reduced by longer devices [1]. Each type of arch rerouting, irrespective of extent, has turned out to be effective [7] to reach the aim of extending landing zone without subjecting these patients to cumulative increased risk.

The best way to approach endoleaks is to avoid them. This self-evident statement is the results of more than 10 years dealing with this specific issue and the knowledge that when endoleakage has occurred, options to treat them sufficiently are rare. As a consequence, exact planning of such procedures cannot be overemphasized. This includes reflection onto the anatomy such as steep angulation of aortic arches. Even if the prosthesis may be advanced into the correct position, the procedure may fail due to self-injury of the fabric by bending and by arroding of the fabric by the stents.

48.5 Comment

No death related to supraaortic transposition occurred in this series, thereby emphasizing the safety of these procedures. These results are well in line with the results after stent-graft placement without arch involvement [16–19]. Nevertheless, it has to be stated that extensive mobilization of the supraaortic branches is mandatory to enable tension-free accomplishment of vascular anastomoses [20]. Interposition of an 8-mm Dacron graft may be beneficial in certain clinical situations. Furthermore, reversed-T hemisternotomies may be more prone to dehiscence than full sternotomies, especially the osteosynthesis between the two upper parts of the sternum, and the caudal common part may be problematic. Therefore, in selected patients, we do use titanium sternal plates for stabilization. Recently, we have switched to a left-sided L-shaped upper hemisternotomy to avoid these challenges.

Notably, three patients died after total arch rerouting. We do think that despite avoiding cardiopulmonary bypass and hypothermic circulatory arrest, total arch rerouting is a more invasive procedure compared with double transposition and subclavian transposition owing to extended stress burden, resulting from surgical access as well as expenditure of time. Only one temporary neurologic injury was observed in this series. We do think that the risk of neurologic injury is in direct relation to the underlying disease. Dilatative arteriopathies are hardly ever related, with severe calcification affecting the ascending aorta as well as the supraaortic branches, whereas obliterative arteriopathies such as penetrating ulcers frequently are leading to potential embolization during clamping.

Conflicting evidence exists with regard to an ideal length of landing zones. Nevertheless, it is generally accepted that a landing zone of 1.5 cm is sufficient. We do proceed one step further and demand at least 2 cm, as data are available showing a direct correlation between the length of the landing zone and persisting or newly developing endoleaks [1]. Furthermore, we aim for an overlap between prostheses of at least 5 cm for the same reason. Interestingly, the length of landing zone after total arch rerouting was substantially longer than after the other types of transposition. This can be explained by the end-to-side anastomosis between the ascending aorta and the proximal portion of the Dacron prosthesis being routinely performed within the midportion of the ascending aorta because of technical reasons and because the majority of arch pathologies originate at the level of the brachiocephalic trunk and not within the cranial ascending aorta.

Our persistent primary endoleak rate is acceptably low and well in line with other published [16–19]. In two patients, after 45 and after 51 months, late surgical conversion had to be performed owing to progressive dilation of the aneurysmal sac. Both patients underwent stent-graft placement in 1997, thereby deriving from the very early series with regard to technical understanding and technology availability, as well as perception of the potential trade-offs of treatment.

Our mean follow-up is 54 months, to date, including some patients being observed for as long as 10 years. Survival is also in line with other recently published series. Interestingly, the more proximal extension of the landing zone was required, the higher EuroSCORE levels could be observed. Nevertheless, the type of arch rerouting had no adverse effect on survival, thereby reflecting the safety and efficacy of even these advanced procedures. Logistic regression analysis revealed a higher number of prostheses used as the only independent risk factor of early endoleak formation. With increased device length available up to 25 cm in the meantime, the number of prostheses used can be substantially reduced, thereby improving lateral stability and augmenting overlapping zones.

As a consequence, probability of endoleak formation may be substantially reduced. Interestingly, an earlier year of treatment did not predict early endoleak formation proving our principle of extensive landing zone requirement even in the early days. Likewise, a higher number of prostheses used were the only independent predictor of late endoleak formation. This becomes clear after reflection onto the anatomy of the arch and the tortuosities that may be observed in this region. Interestingly, an earlier year of implantation did not predict late endoleak formation. Furthermore, the length of the proximal landing zone did not predict either early or late endoleak formation, moreover underlining the accuracy of the concept.

Survival was independently predicted by higher logistic EuroSCORE levels and reached borderline significance with regard to earlier year of implantation. This becomes clear as the majority of patients in the early days have been at an advanced age already. Furthermore, the comorbidities associated with higher EuroSCORE levels may be limitating despite aggressive secondary medical preventive therapy. After comparison of supraaortic transpositions in various extents followed by endovascular stent-graft placement with the current literature of conventional repair of isolated arch and distal arch pathology, some striking differences become available [21–24]. Mean age of patients undergoing the new approach is substantially higher. Neurologic injury is neglectable low, and mortality is comparable and in the lower range of the spectrum. Furthermore, as there is a clear correlation between age and death, a substantially higher mortality could be expected if these patients would have undergone any kind of conventional treatment. Without doubt, conventional aortic arch and proximal descending aortic replacement will have their unaffected value in the future in younger patients as well as in patients with connective tissue diseases. However, recovery in patients at high risk for conventional repair is striking, especially as the majority of these patients represent a new cohort that would not have been treated by mere antihypertensive therapy even recently.

Summarizing, results after supraaortic transpositions in various extents followed by endovascular stent-graft placement for the treatment of pathology affecting the aortic arch are promising. Endoleak formation is directly related to the number of prostheses and may be reduced by longer devices. Each type of arch rerouting, irrespective of extent, has turned out to be effective. Therefore, extended applications of these combined treatment strategies substantially augment the therapeutic options especially in patients with multisegmental thoracic aortic disease originating at the level of the aortic arch.

References

1. Czerny M, Grimm M, Zimpfer D, Rodler S, Gottardi R, Hutschala D, Lammer J, Wolner E, Schoder M (2007) Results after endovascular stent graft placement in atherosclerotic aneurysms involving the descending aorta. Ann Thorac Surg 83:450–455
2. Schoder M, Czerny M, Cejna M, Rand T, Stadler A, Sodeck GH, Gottardi R, Loewe C, Lammer J (2007) Endovascular repair of acute type B aortic dissection: long-term follow-up of true and false lumen diameter changes. Ann Thorac Surg 83:1059–1066
3. Czerny M, Zimpfer D, Rodler S, Funovics M, Dorfmeister M, Schoder M, Marta G, Weigang E, Gottardi R, Lammer J, Wolner E, Grimm M (2007) Endovascular stent-graft placement of aneurysms involving the descending aorta originating from chronic type B dissections. Ann Thorac Surg 83:1635–1639
4. Gottardi R, Zimpfer D, Funovics M, Schoder M, Lammer J, Wolner E, Czerny M, Grimm M (2008) Mid-term results after endovascular stent-graft placement due to penetrating atherosclerotic ulcers of the thoracic aorta. Eur J Cardiothorac Surg 33:1019–1024
5. Holfeld J, Gottardi R, Zimpfer D, Dorfmeister M, Dumfarth J, Funovics M, Schoder M, Weigang E, Lammer J, Wolner E, Czerny M, Grimm M (2008) Treatment of symptomatic coral reef aorta by endovascular stent-graft placement. Ann Thorac Surg 85:1817–1819
6. Grimm M, Loewe C, Gottardi R, Funovics M, Zimpfer D, Rodler S, Dorfmeister M, Schoder M, Lammer J, Aharinejad S, Czerny M (2008) Novel insights into the mechanisms and treatment of intramural hematoma affecting the entire thoracic aorta. Ann Thorac Surg 86:453–456
7. Gottardi R, Funovics M, Eggers N, Hirner A, Dorfmeister M, Holfeld J, Zimpfer D, Schoder M, Donas K, Weigang E, Lammer J, Grimm M, Czerny M (2008) Supra-aortic transposition for combined vascular and endovascular repair of aortic arch pathology. Ann Thorac Surg 86:1524–1529
8. Weigang E, Parker J, Czerny M, Peivandi AA, Dorweiler B, Beyersdorf F, Siegenthaler MP (2009) Endovascular aortic arch repair after aortic arch debranching. Ann Thorac Surg 87:603–607
9. Schoder M, Lammer J, Czerny M (2009) Endovascular aortic arch repair: hopes and certainties. Eur J Vasc Endovasc Surg 38:255–261
10. Szeto WY, Bavaria JE (2009) Hybrid repair of aortic arch aneurysms: combined open arch reconstruction and endovascular repair. Semin Thorac Cardiovasc Surg 21(4):347–354
11. Czerny M, Cejna M, Hutschala D, Fleck T, Holzenbein T, Schoder M, Lammer J, Zimpfer D, Ehrlich M, Wolner E, Grabenwoger M (2004) Stent-graft placement in atherosclerotic descending thoracic aortic aneurysms: midterm results. J Endovasc Ther 11:26–32
12. Czerny M, Fleck T, Zimpfer D, Kilo J, Sandner D, Cejna M, Lammer J, Wolner E, Grabenwoger M (2003) Combined repair of an aortic arch aneurysm by sequential transposition of the supra-aortic branches and endovascular stent-graft placement. J Thorac Cardiovasc Surg 126(3):916–918
13. Dambrin C, Marcheix B, Hollington L, Rousseau H (2005) Surgical treatment of an aortic arch aneurysm without cardio-pulmonary bypass: endovascular stent-grafting after extra-anatomic bypass of supra-aortic vessels. Eur J Cardiothorac Surg 27:159–161
14. Gottardi R, Seitelberger R, Zimpfer D et al (2005) An alternative approach in treating an aortic arch aneurysm with an anatomic variant by supraaortic reconstruction and stent-graft placement. J Vasc Surg 42(2):357–360
15. Vogt PR, Brunner-La Rocca HP et al (1998) Cryopreserved vascular allograft in the treatment of major vascular infection: a comparison with conventional surgical techniques. J Thorac Cardiovasc Surg 116:965–972
16. Criado FJ, Barnatan MF, Rizk Y, Clark NS, Wang C (2002) Technical strategies to expand stent-graft applicability in the aortic arch and proximal descending thoracic aorta. J Endovasc Ther 9:II32–II38
17. Buth J, Penn O, Tielbeek A, Mersman M (1998) Combined approach to stent-graft treatment of an aortic arch aneurysm. J Endovasc Surg 5:329–332
18. Iguro Y, Arata K, Yamamoto H, Masuda H, Sakata R (2002) A new concept in distal arch aneurysm repair with a stent graft. J Thorac Cardiovasc Surg 123:378–380
19. Okada K, Sueda T, Orihashi K, Watari M, Ishii O (2001) An alternative procedure of endovascular stent-graft repair for distal arch aortic aneurysm involving arch vessels. J Thorac Cardiovasc Surg 121: 182–184
20. Czerny M, Zimpfer D, Fleck T et al (2004) Initial results after combined repair of aortic arch aneurysms by sequential transposition of the supra-aortic branches and consecutive endovascular stent-graft placement. Ann Thorac Surg 78:1256–1260
21. Kazui T, Washiyama N, Muhammad BA, Terada H, Yamashita K, Takinami M (2001) Improved results of atherosclerotic arch aneurysm operations with a refined technique. J Thorac Cardiovasc Surg 121: 491–499

22. Westaby S, Katsumata T (1998) Proximal aortic perfusion for complex arch and descending aortic disease. J Thorac Cardiovasc Surg 115:162–167
23. Czerny M, Fleck T, Zimpfer D et al (2003) Risk factors of mortality and permanent neurologic injury in patients undergoing ascending aortic and arch repair. J Thorac Cardiovasc Surg 126:1296–1301
24. Kouchoukos N, Mauney MC, Masetti P, Castner CF (2007) Optimization of aortic arch replacement with a one-stage approach. Ann Thorac Surg 83:S811–S814

Videothoracoscopic Closure of Patent Ductus Arteriosus

49

Thierry A. Folliguet and François Laborde

Contents

T.A. Folliguet, M.D., FACS (✉)
Pole Territorial Lorrain,
Chirurgie Cardiaque Vasculaire et Transplantations,
ILCV, CHU Brabois Nancy, France
e-mail: thierry.folligue@imm.fr

F. Laborde, M.D.
Department of Surgery, Institut Mutualiste Montsouris,
42 Boulevard Jourdan, Paris, 75014, France
e-mail: francois.laborde@imm.fr

Patent ductus arteriosus (PDA) was first surgically ligated in 1939 by Gross and Hubbard [1]. Since then, the surgical technique of choice was the left thoracotomy with simple ligation, multiple transfixed ligatures, titanium clipping occlusion, or suture and division. The advantages given are its low lack of mortality and reliable PDA closure, but the potential morbidity of thoracotomy is important especially in infants. The long-term postthoracotomy pain is common [2], and the risk of postoperative pulmonary complication represented by atelectasis and pneumonia is increased [3]. In addition, the incidence of thoracic scoliosis as a long-term complication in premature infants [4] is above 20–30%.

Percutaneous catheter closure of the PDA was first described in 1971 [5]. The advantages offered by this technique are avoidance of any incision, but the main disadvantage remains persistent shunting, on the order of 27% at 6-week follow-up, which decreases generally to 15% at 6 months. In addition, this technique is applicable only for patients weighting more than 10 kg because the size of these small vessels makes the use of the device difficult [6].

To circumvent these problems, we present here our technique [7] of PDA closure by videothoracoscopic surgery (VTS) in infants and children, which involves less discomfort and morbidity than the classic surgical thoracotomy and which provides an optimal rate of success.

R.G.C. Inderbitzi et al. (eds.), *Minimally Invasive Thoracic and Cardiac Surgery*,
DOI 10.1007/978-3-642-11861-6_49, © Springer-Verlag Berlin Heidelberg 2012

49.1 Technique

49.1.1 Anesthesia Preparation

General anesthesia is performed with Pentothal at a dose of 5–10 mg/kg, vecuronium (Norcuron) at a dose of 0.1 mg/kg, fentanyl (Fentanyl) at a dose of 0.5–1 mg/kg, and 1–2% enflurane (Ethrane). A central line is placed via the jugular vein without any arterial line. Electrocardiogram monitoring, oxymeter, and capnograph are routinely placed.

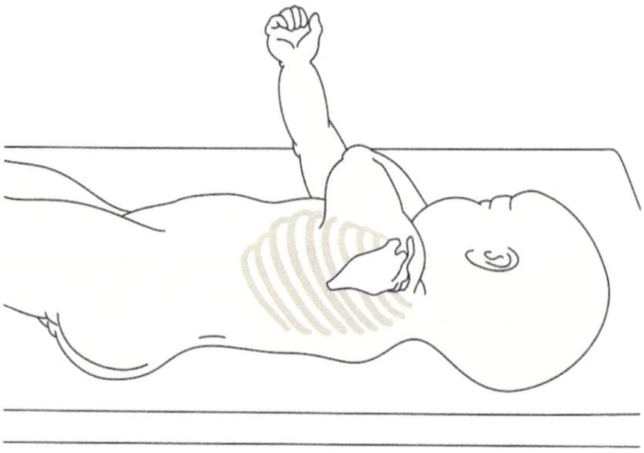

Fig. 49.1 Position of trocar sleeves in the 3rd intercostal space behind the scapula, the 5th intercostal space underneath the angle of scapula, and 3rd intercostal space along the midmammary line

49.1.2 Procedure

After induction of general anesthesia and standard intubation, the patient is positioned on his or her right side, as for a posterolateral thoracotomy. The skin is prepared with two Betadine scrubs, and a regular Vi-Drape is placed. The surgeon and the scrub nurse are on the left side of the patient, the assistant on the right.

At first, two 5-mm incisions are made in the left hemithorax (Fig. 49.1). The first incision is made just posterior to the scapula in the third intercostal space for the videothoracoscope (4 mm in diameter) introduced via a 5-mm trocar (Fig. 49.2). A second incision is performed in the fourth intercostal space underneath the angle of the scapula for the electrocautery hook introduced via a 5-mm trocar. Two or three 60° angled hooks, 1 mm in diameter, are introduced directly through the third intercostal space in its middle part, just in front of the scapula, for lung retraction.

The monitor is placed on the right side of the patient facing the surgeon; the cables come also from the right side and are clamped to the drape. Instruments used for VTS include scissors, dissectors, electrocautery hooks, a clip applier, a lung retractor, and a suction device. The operative field is viewed on the video screen by means of the video camera and can be stored on a video recorder.

The upper lobe of the left lung is retracted inferomedially with the angled hooks, the PDA is identified, and the mediastinal pleura is opened with the electrocautery hook. The PDA is dissected from the surrounding tissues, and the aorta is dissected at its junction with the PDA. The pericardium is dissected on the pulmonary side to protect the recurrent laryngeal nerve from any traumatic injury (Fig. 49.3). It is essential to dissect on both sides of the PDA to place the clip adequately. The clip applier is then introduced without any trocar through the access of the

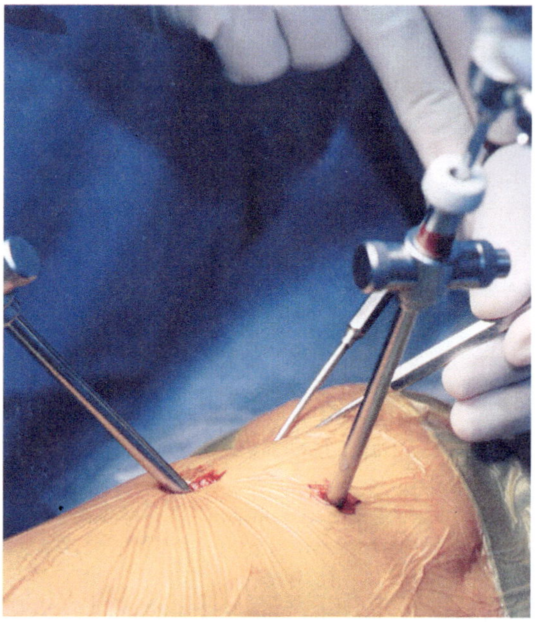

Fig. 49.2 Use of trocar sleeves. Thoracoscope in the 3rd intercostal space behind the scapula. Electrocautery hook in the 5th intercostal space. Two or three 60°hooks with 1-mm diameter in the 3rd intercostal space in its middle part

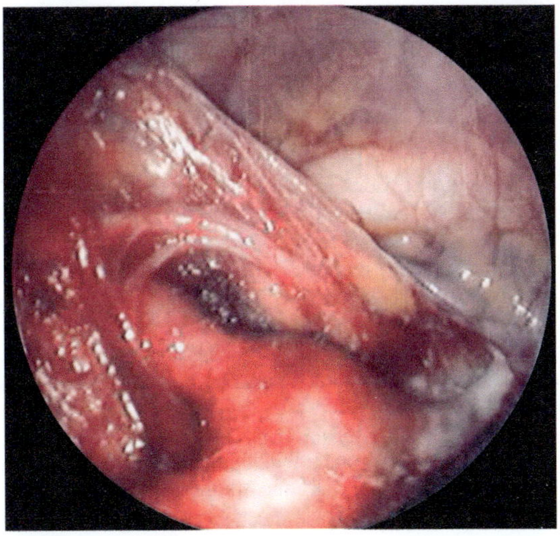

Fig. 49.3 The PDA is dissected from surrounding tissues and the recurrent laryngeal nerve is visualized and respected

fourth intercostal space. A first titanium clip (9 mm) is placed as distal as possible from the aortic junction on the pulmonary side of the PDA (Fig. 49.3) and a second clip is applied on the side close to the aorta. After visual confirmation that both clips are well in place, the lung is inflated and a 2-mm-diameter pleural suction catheter is placed before closure of the 5-mm skin incisions with sutures (Fig. 49.4).

49.1.3 Postoperative Care

Color-flow Doppler echocardiography is performed in the operating room or in the recovery room before extubation to assess the completeness of closure of the PDA. If there is a persistent shunt, the patient is taken back immediately to the operative room for reapplication of a new clip by VTS. Otherwise, if complete interruption is seen, extubation is performed and patients are placed either in the intensive care unit or in a regular pediatric room, according to age and previous symptoms of pulmonary hypertension. The pleural suction catheter is removed a few hours after extubation, a routine chest X ray is obtained, and a transthoracic echocardiogram is done before being discharged. All patients are then regularly followed up by their own pediatric cardiologist who performs a complete physical and transthoracic echocardiogram examination.

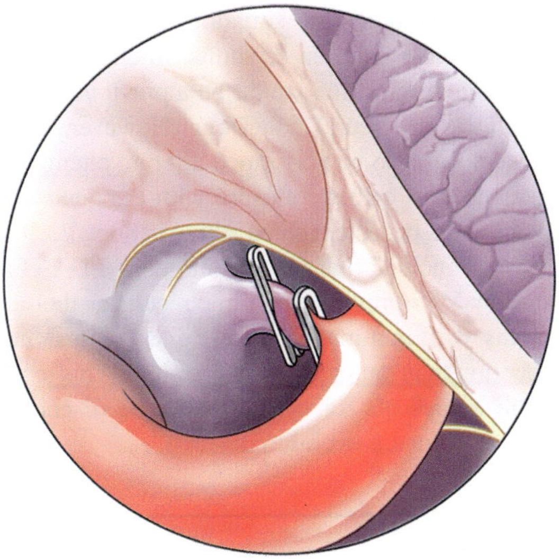

Fig. 49.4 Two titanium clips (9 mm) are placed: the first as distal as possible from the aortic junction, the second next to aorta

49.2 Comment

We have used this technique from 1991 for more than 340 patients. More than 30% were younger than 6 months, and the mean weight for the entire series was 12.6 kg with three patients weighting less than 1.9 kg. The mean operating time was 20 min. There were no deaths, hemorrhages, transfusions required, or episode of chylothorax. Six patients had a persistent PDA after VTS procedure, all early in our experience and related to insufficient dissection resulting in inadequate clip placement. This complication cannot be seen actually since we perform routine transthoracic echocardiography before extubation. Recurrent laryngeal nerve dysfunction was noted in six patients (five transient and one persistent). No complication or sequelae occurred in our last 300 patients. We believe that dissection must be sufficient in order to place the clip correctly, but not too extensive to avoid a transient left vocal cord paralysis. The only contraindication to this procedure is if the diameter of the ductus is greater than the size of the clip (9 mm) or if the ductus is calcified. Both of these situations can be encountered in older children or adults. In children, the only contraindication would be a previous thoracotomy with pleural adhesions. However, VTS closure can also be performed after an attempt at percutaneous catheter closure with the device in place and a persistent shunt (three patients).

We conclude that our technique of PDA closure by VTS provides the same results as thoracotomy with minimal morbidity and less residual shunting than endovascular procedure. This technique represents for us the technique of choice for PDA closure in children.

References

1. Gross RE, Hubbard JP (1939) Surgical ligation of a patent ductus arteriosus. Report of first successful case. JAMA 112:729–731
2. Dajczman E, Gordon A, Kreisman H, Wolkove N (1991) Long-term post-thoracotomy pain. Chest 99:270–274
3. Nomori H, Horio H, Fuyuno G, Kobayashi R, Yashima H (1996) Respiratory muscle strength after lung resection with special reference to age and procedures of thoracotomy. Eur J Cardiothorac Surg 10:352–358
4. Shelton JE, Walburg JR, Schneider E (1986) Functional scoliosis as a long term complication of surgical ligation for patent ductus arteriosus in premature infant. J Pediatr Surg 48A:855–857
5. Porstmann W, Wierny L, Warnake H et al (1971) Catheter closure of patent ductus arteriosus; 62 cases treated without thoracotomy. Radiol Clin North Am 9:203–218
6. Hosking MC, Benson LN, Musewe N, Dyck JD, Freedom RM (1991) Transcatheter occlusion of the persistently patent ductus arteriosus: forty month follow-up and prevalence of residual shunting. Circulation 84:2313–2317
7. Laborde F, Folliguet T, Batisse A et al (1995) Video-assisted thoracoscopic surgical interruption: the technique of choice for patent ductus arteriosus. J Thorac Cardiovasc Surg 110:1681–1685

Index

R.G.C. Inderbitzi et al. (eds.), *Minimally Invasive Thoracic and Cardiac Surgery*,
DOI 10.1007/978-3-642-11861-6, © Springer-Verlag Berlin Heidelberg 2012

N

O

P

Printed by Printforce, the Netherlands